Dental Materials In Vivo:
Aging and Related Phenomena

Edited by

George Eliades, DDS, Dr Dent
Associate Professor and Director
Biomaterials Laboratory
School of Dentistry
University of Athens
Athens, Greece

Theodore Eliades, DDS, MS, Dr Med, PhD
Honorary Research Fellow
Biomaterials Science Unit
Turner Dental School
University of Manchester
Manchester, United Kingdom

William A. Brantley, PhD
Professor
Section of Restorative and Prosthetic Dentistry
College of Dentistry
The Ohio State University
Columbus, Ohio

David C. Watts, PhD
Professor
Biomaterials Science Unit
Turner Dental School
University of Manchester
Manchester, United Kingdom

Quintessence Publishing Co, Inc
Chicago, Berlin, Tokyo, Copenhagen, London, Paris, Milan, Barcelona,
Istanbul, São Paulo, New Delhi, Moscow, Prague, and Warsaw

Library of Congress Cataloging-in-Publication Data

Dental materials in vivo : aging and related phenomena / edited by
George Eliades ... [et al.].
            p. ; cm.
Includes bibliographical references and index.
   ISBN 0-86715-399-7 (pbk.)
 1. Dental materials.
   [DNLM: 1. Dental Materials. 2. Research Design. WU 190 D4145 2003]
I. Eliades, George.
   RK652.5 .D4535 2003
   617.6'95—dc21

                                        2002152682

quintessence books

©2003 Quintessence Publishing Co, Inc

Quintessence Publishing Co, Inc
551 Kimberly Drive
Carol Stream, IL 60188
www.quintpub.com

Editor: Kathryn O'Malley
Internal Design and Production: Susan Robinson
Cover Design: Dawn Hartman

Printed in Hong Kong

Dental Materials in Vivo:

Aging and Related Phenomena

TABLE OF CONTENTS

DEDICATION

To Maria, Anna, and Konstantinos, who make it all so worthwhile.
—*GE*

To Zeev Davidovitch, paying back a long-due debt.
—*TE*

To Vivian, for her constant patience and support.
—*WAB*

To my dear wife, Wendy.
—*DCW*

FOREWORD

Dental materials science must be regarded as the conscience of restorative dentistry. Natural teeth, as well as all restorations, are composed of materials that are subject to deterioration. It is the aging of these materials that is the dominant mechanism for these structures' eventual failure. The lifetime of a construction depends on the nature of its materials and the acting fatigue process.

It is therefore clear that knowledge of the static properties of materials is inadequate for applying them in biologic systems. For such applications, one must also understand how these materials *live* and ultimately *die*. However, up to the time of this writing, the subject of in vivo aging of dental biomaterials has not received the attention it merits. This book, which explores new questions and offers many ground-breaking answers, provides a valuable contribution to our clinical and scientific knowledge about this highly important topic.

One of the most laudable attributes of this book is its integration of the various aspects of in vivo aging of dental biomaterials in numerous applications, including prosthodontics, implant and restorative dentistry, orthodontics, endodontics, oral and maxillofacial surgery, and periodontology. It is meritorious that the editors, all well known and highly respected in contemporary dental science, sought out expert assistance among their colleagues to uncover many specific material-scientific and clinical aspects of the unavoidable aging phenomenon and possible methods to control them.

In addition to presenting valuable scientific research, this text serves as a practical manual, providing stepwise instruction in the management of the aging of materials as it applies to the various fields of dentistry. Therefore, *Dental Materials In Vivo: Aging and Related Phenomena* is unmistakably a timely must-read for scientists as well as clinicians.

Carel L. Davidson, PhD
Professor
Department of Dental Materials Science
Academic Center for Dentistry at Amsterdam (ACTA)
Amsterdam, The Netherlands

PREFACE

Although several well-known and highly respected textbooks on dental biomaterials are available—some with multiple editions over several decades—none of these texts focuses to a significant extent upon the effect of the oral environment on these biomaterials over extended periods of time, ie, the effect of in vivo aging on their properties and clinical performance. Individuals teaching and performing research on the wide range of dental biomaterials have long been aware of this deficit, as well as its root cause: a general lack of research on the subject. However, within the past decade, more investigators have begun to carefully study the in vivo performance of dental biomaterials and have demonstrated that striking differences can exist with respect to the performance found in conventional in vitro laboratory tests, even when these tests are performed at normal oral temperature (37°C).

The oral environment represents a combination of complex conditions that cannot be duplicated in the research laboratory: *(1)* complex intraoral flora that lead to plaque accumulation and its by-products; *(2)* highly variable alterations in pH that can arise from the ingestion and decomposition of foods, particularly in crevices around restorations; and *(3)* the warm, moist nature of the oral environment, which, when subjected to fluctuating stresses during mastication, leads to irregular cyclic fatigue conditions that may be further exacerbated by stress corrosion processes. Such an aggressive environment can cause failure processes in metallic, ceramic, or polymeric materials that would not be observed under the in vitro laboratory testing conditions used over the past decades.

This text presents the results of recent in vivo research, which has uncovered many aspects of the role of oral flora and their by-products in the aging of dental biomaterials. For example, the action of microbiota colonization on metallic dental biomaterials has been found to be twofold: Certain species can metabolize individual component metallic elements from alloys, while microbial by-products and metabolic processes may alter the microenvironment, such as by decreasing the local pH and thereby contributing to the initiation of corrosion. The implication of bacterial metabolism has been reported for the surface alteration of dental alloys and endodontic silver points. It is also known that sulfate-reducing and nitrate-reducing bacteria are inflammatory to host tissues and can also affect the corrosion processes of various alloys. The effects of the biofilm found on all dental materials in vivo on the materials' surface structures and properties also have recently begun to be appreciated; however, considerable further work is needed to elucidate its role in the clinical behavior of these biomaterials.

Also presented is research on environmental factors in addition to dietary habits that recently have been found to have important consequences for dental biomaterials. For example, it has been estimated that an urban mouth-breather inhales in 2 hours approximately 1 m^3 of air, with a potential sulfur dioxide intake of up to 2.3 mg. Hence, differences in the ambient air quality potentially can have considerable effects on the long-term clinical performance of dental biomaterials.

The purpose of this book is to provide a comprehensive discussion, based upon current research findings, of the in vivo aging processes of dental biomaterials in the oral environment and to provide a scientifically plausible extrapolation to likely occurrences for situations where appropriate in vivo research has not yet been performed. Moreover, the chapters in this book are intended to stimulate new research investigations into the many facets of this exciting field and to inspire a much greater appreciation for the need to investigate the long-term performance of dental biomaterials, rather than to rely upon shorter-term in vitro investigations in which experimental results may bear little relationship to the clinical situation. In particular, research on the in vivo behavior of ceramic and polymeric dental biomaterials is strongly encouraged, since such investigations to date have frequently tended to focus on metallic materials.

Lastly, the editors wish to express their enormous gratitude to Quintessence Publishing Company for supporting this research-oriented book, which is somewhat out of the mainstream of the publisher's highly popular, more clinically oriented dental books, and for their patient assistance with the myriad details associated with bringing the chapter manuscripts to their final form.

CONTRIBUTORS

William A. Brantley, PhD
Professor
Section of Restorative and Prosthetic Dentistry
College of Dentistry
Graduate Faculty
Oral Biology and Integrated Biomedical
    Science Graduate Program
Participating Faculty
Department of Biomedical Engineering
Adjunct Faculty
Department of Materials Science and
    Engineering
The Ohio State University
Columbus, Ohio

James L. Drummond, DDS, PhD
Professor
Department of Restorative Dentistry
College of Dentistry
University of Illinois at Chicago
Chicago, Illinois

George Eliades, DDS, Dr Dent
Associate Professor and Director
Biomaterials Laboratory
Section of Basic Sciences and Oral Biology
School of Dentistry
University of Athens
Athens, Greece

Theodore Eliades, DDS, MS, Dr Med, PhD
Honorary Research Fellow
Biomaterials Science Unit
Turner Dental School
University of Manchester
Manchester, United Kingdom

Research Associate
Biomaterials Laboratory
Section of Basic Sciences and Oral Biology
School of Dentistry
University of Athens
Athens, Greece

Arne Hensten-Pettersen, DDS, MS, Dr Odont, Odont Dr HC (Lund)
Director
NIOM—Scandinavian Institute of Dental
    Materials
Haslum, Norway

Nils Jacobsen, DDS, MS, Dr Odont
Professor
Institute of Clinical Dentistry
Faculty of Dentistry
University of Oslo
Oslo, Norway

Aphrodite I. Kakaboura, DDS, Dr Dent
Associate Professor
Department of Operative Dentistry
School of Dentistry
University of Athens
Athens, Greece

Miroslav I. Marek, PhD
Professor
School of Materials Science and Engineering
College of Engineering
Georgia Institute of Technology
Atlanta, Georgia

John Margelos, DDS
Private Practice in Endodontics
Athens, Greece

Claude G. Matasa, D Chem Eng, D Tech Sci
Lecturer
Department of Orthodontics
College of Dentistry
University of Illinois at Chicago
Chicago, Illinois

Adjunct Assistant Professor
Department of Orthodontics
Nova Southeastern University College of
    Dental Medicine
Fort Lauderdale, Florida

Ian R. Matthew, PhD, M Dent Sc, BDS, FDS, RCS
   (England and Edinburgh)
Assistant Professor
Head of Oral and Maxillofacial Surgery
Faculty of Dentistry
The University of British Columbia
Vancouver, British Columbia
Canada

Edwin A. McGlumphy, DDS, MS
Associate Professor
Section of Restorative and Prosthetic Dentistry
College of Dentistry
The Ohio State University
Columbus, Ohio

John C. Mitchell, PhD
Assistant Professor
Department of Biomaterials and Biomechanics
School of Dentistry
Oregon Health & Science University
Portland, Oregon

Efstratios Papazoglou, DDS, MS, PhD
Assistant Professor
Department of Operative Dentistry
School of Dentistry
University of Athens
Athens, Greece

Karl-Johan Söderholm, DDS, MPhil, Odont Dr
Professor
Department of Dental Biomaterials
College of Dentistry
University of Florida
Gainesville, Florida

Elliott J. Sutow, PhD, MEd
Professor of Biomaterials Science
Department of Applied Oral Sciences
Faculty of Dentistry
Dalhousie University
Halifax, Nova Scotia
Canada

Manolis Vavuranakis, MD
Staff Cardiologist
Hippokrateion General Hospital
Athens, Greece

Clinical Assistant Professor
Division of Cardiology
College of Medicine
The Ohio State University
Columbus, Ohio

J. Anthony von Fraunhofer, PhD
Professor and Director
Biomaterials Science
College of Dental Surgery
University of Maryland
Baltimore, Maryland

David C. Watts, PhD
Professor
Biomaterials Science Unit
Turner Dental School
University of Manchester
Manchester, United Kingdom

Spiros Zinelis, PhD
Metallurgical Engineer
Research Associate
Biomaterials Laboratory
Section of Basic Sciences and Oral Biology
School of Dentistry
University of Athens
Athens, Greece

Section I

OVERVIEW

1

General Aspects of Biomaterial Surface Alterations Following Exposure to Biologic Fluids

George Eliades, DDS, Dr Dent

Theodore Eliades, DDS, MS, Dr Med, PhD

Manolis Vavuranakis, MD

When a biomaterial is exposed to a biologic system, a noncellular acquired biofilm is rapidly organized on the biomaterial surface by spontaneous adsorption of extracellular macromolecules composed of glycoproteins and proteoglycans.[1] These films induce a conditioning effect that modifies the biomaterial surface properties and alters both the response of the subsequently attached cells and the interactions occurring at the biomaterial-host interface.[2,3] This conditioning effect is based on the differing capacities of artificial surfaces to fractionate proteins from biologic fluids, such as saliva or blood, as well as on the ability to induce conformation and orientation changes of adsorbed proteins.[4,5]

The outcome of biofilm adsorption depends on the biologic fluid flow rate at the site of contact, the type of interfacial interactions involved, and the attachment strength with the substrate. The fundamental factor affecting the composition and organization of acquired biofilms under static conditions or low flow rates is the biomaterial surface chemistry, whereas substrate surface molecular motion and roughness are also important factors in environments with high flow rates. In addition, with long exposure periods, material properties such as porosity, sorption, corrosion,

and biodegradation may further modify the biomaterial-host interactions.[6] Finally, the attachment strength of biofilms formed on biomaterial surfaces is capable of regulating the vitality of the contact. When there is continuous adsorption/desorption of biomolecules from an artificial surface, conformational changes in the desorbed biomolecules may trigger a biochemical response from structures that are not in physical contact with the surface.[7]

The bioadhesive activity of biofilms in the biologic environment depends mainly on the composition and surface reactivity of the outer monolayers. It has been proposed that when strong bioadhesion is required, the biomaterial surface should demonstrate a critical surface tension in the range of 30 to 40 dynes/cm, with a high proportion of polar interactive sites. In contrast, when minimal bioadhesion is desirable, materials with a critical surface tension of 20 to 30 dynes/cm and reduced polar interactive sites should be chosen.[8] Biomaterials with high critical surface tension may still be within the bioadhesive range following biofilm formation, and the biofilms formed will be dense and more coherent; the conformationally changed macromolecules will promote cell attachment. In contrast, where critical surface tension is low, the biofilms developed are more loose and more easily detached under flowing conditions; the macromolecules formed have a more native conformation and retain fewer microorganisms.[9,10]

Biofilm maturation may induce differences in the film quality and self-organization states. However, in the absence of inhibitors, biofilm maturation may also result in calcification of the adsorbed species, either by contact activation and thrombosis on surfaces conducting blood[11] or by nonspecific ectopic calcification through nucleation of calcium phosphates on charged groups of macromolecules having a particular stereochemical geometry.[12,13]

Once adsorption equilibrium has been established between the surfaces involved, biofilms at biomaterial-host interfaces seem capable in the long term not only of influencing cell attachment and proliferation but also, in many cases, of modulating the phenotypic expression of attached cells and, consequently, the potential of interfacial tissue remodeling.[6]

This chapter will review the general aspects of development and maturation of biofilms formed on biomaterial surfaces in relation to the biologic environment. This approach will facilitate understanding of the complex mechanisms involved in the in vivo aging phenomena discussed in subsequent chapters—phenomena that eventually determine whether a biomaterial is clinically functional or nonfunctional.

Basic Principles of Biomaterial Surface Properties and Biologic Responses

The term *surface* commonly refers to a boundary defined by the outer atomic layer that separates a bulk solid from an adjacent phase. However, a more realistic approach is to consider the surface as a region of variable depth and having a degree of flexibility that depends on the nature of the material.[14]

Material surfaces should be considered special states of matter with unique chemistry, organization, dynamics, and electrical properties. The major differences between surface and bulk structures arise from (1) the direct accessibility of surface molecules for reaction with adjacent phases and (2) the tendency for surface energy minimization to reach equilibrium, as mediated by the rearrangement of chemical groups, additive migration, and spontaneous adsorption of low-energy layers from the environment.[15] The effective depth of the biologically important region of biomaterials involved in interactions with protein functional groups is usually considered to be the outermost layer extending 10 nm into the material. Nevertheless, the near-surface region of 0.1 to 10.0 μm plays a significant role as well, because it is involved in corrosion, biodegradation, controlled release, and cell contact guidance phenomena.[14] The biomaterial properties that influence the biologic response by selectively promoting interfacial interactions are listed in Fig 1-1 and discussed below.

Biomaterial Surface Properties: Substrate Definition

The molecular and elemental composition of biomaterial surfaces is considered the determinant factor of the early response of the biologic environment. The polar or nonpolar nature, the hydrogen-bonding capacity, and the electron donor or acceptor potential seem to control the hydrophilic or hydrophobic character and energetic state of the surfaces. Surface electrical properties, such as the zeta and streaming potentials and surface charges, also are involved in interfacial interactions with biologic fluids and living cells.[16]

Surface thermal mobility is found with materials having a very low elastic modulus, such as polymers in the colloidal state or soft-chain segments of hard polymers, where the majority of the material or specific regions may demonstrate active Brownian motion. These molecular regions are permeable to small molecules capable of modifying the conformation of biologic fluids by steric or fluctuation forces, and they demonstrate less adsorption energy. Surface mobility correlates with the degree of crystallinity, because rigid solid

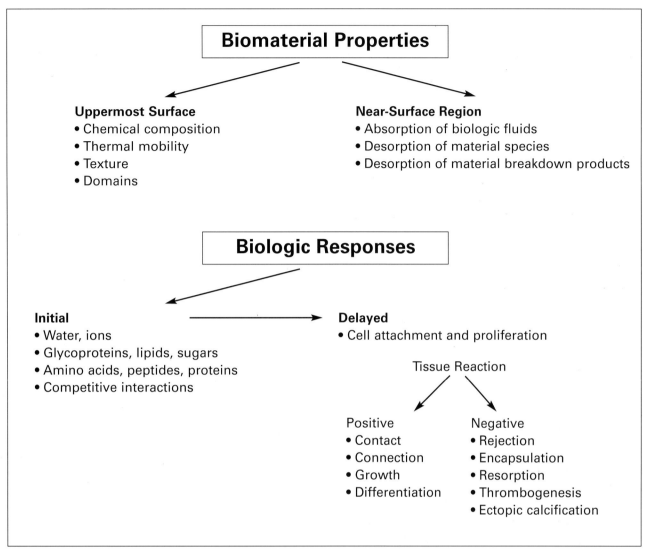

Fig 1-1 Important biomaterial surface properties and biologic responses.

crystalline phases demonstrate higher adsorption energy compared with amorphous phases, with some exceptions in materials exposed to high flow rates.[17]

Surface texture incorporates both ultrastructural and macroscopic features; vacancies, other structural imperfections, gas entrapment, and adsorbed layers alter the surface composition on an ultrastructural scale. Macroscopically, surface roughness and porosity interfere with the biologic fluid flow rate by producing local secondary fluid motions of enhanced or reduced shear, which at high flow rates may affect the shape, distribution, and aggregation of the attaching particles. At low flow rates or under static conditions, the grooves of rough surfaces may act as stagnation points, thereby promoting biofilm maturation.[18] Because most surfaces are heterogeneous at the microscopic level, the regional surface distribution of the foregoing properties may produce domains with different characteristics and thus induce a variable biologic response.

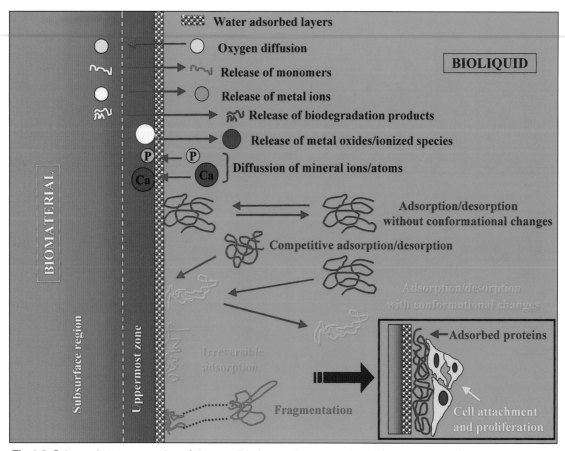

Fig 1-2 Schematic representation of the possible interactions occurring at biomaterial surfaces exposed to a biologic environment.

Initial Biologic Responses to Biomaterial Surfaces: Substrate Modification

The biologic responses to biomaterial surfaces involve a great variety of chemical species. A time sequence based on experimental data and logical hypotheses has been described for the phenomena occurring on biomaterial surfaces placed in a biologic environment (Fig 1-2).[19]

Initially, within nanoseconds, either oxygen or hydrogen bonding binds a water monolayer to a biomaterial surface. Some water molecules may dissociate to hydroxyl groups, which may form surface hydroxyls. Next, a second water layer binds to the first monolayer. The orientation and density of water molecules in the first adsorbed monolayer may regulate the overall hydration state of the surface, because the unique properties of water offer a wide spectrum of solvation forces in aqueous systems. For example, when two hydrophilic surfaces come in contact, repulsive hydration (long-range) and steric (short-range) forces are generated because of the energy required to dehydrate the surfaces; the presence of cations, or pH, controls these forces. On hydrophobic surfaces, in contrast, the orientation of water molecules toward the surface is entropically unfavorable. Thus, when two hydrophobic surfaces approach each other, water is ejected into the bulk solution, reducing the total free energy of the system and establishing attractive long-range hydrophobic forces between the two surfaces.[20] These phenomena are of paramount importance for biologic systems and control protein adsorption, which proceeds by nonspecific physicochemical interactions with the water- and ion-modified biomaterial surfaces.[7]

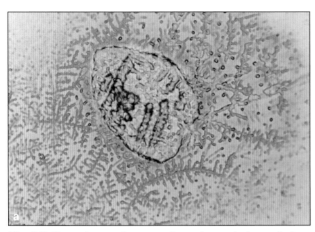 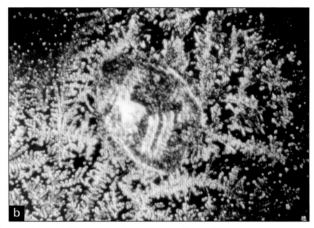

Fig 1-3 Crystal growth on surface-charged sites of dental plaque bacterial aggregations formed in vivo on germanium minicrystals: reflected light microscope images in bright-field *(a)* and dark-field *(b)* observation modes (original magnification × 400).

Protein adsorption is initiated within a few milliseconds of contact with biologic fluids. The protein layers adsorbed are complex and may vary depending on the nature of the surface. In an aqueous environment, the interaction between hydrophilic surfaces with strongly attached water molecules and hydrated protein cores is weak because of the development of hydrophilic repulsive forces. Thus, on hydrated surfaces, hydrophobic and electrostatic interactions are expected to govern protein adsorption. Heavily charged macromolecules are probably the first species to be adsorbed; however, the first protein adsorbed does not determine the potential for attachment or the overall response at later stages. Competitive adsorption usually occurs, with rapidly decreasing protein affinity accompanying increasing surface occupancy. The result is sequential adsorption/desorption and an exchange of proteins on surfaces, a phenomenon known as the *Vroman effect*.[21] The adsorption/desorption sequence of proteins is not distinct. All proteins are adsorbed simultaneously at different rates, and displacement occurs according to the proteins' binding affinity, which depends on the spreading capacity and the energy required to denature the proteins in the solution.[22]

Proteins with high carbohydrate content and relatively uniform carbohydrate distribution around the molecule show increased solubility, conformational stability, and minimal adsorption on hydrophobic and negatively charged surfaces, characteristics that can be attributed to the carbohydrate's shielding effect. However, when carbohydrate groups are localized, the protective effect diminishes. Lipoproteins make up another important group having preferential adsorption on hydrophobic surfaces, especially surfaces possessing thermal mobility. Lipid phase transition at body temperature and denaturing reactions seem to control the adsorption process.[22]

At protein adsorption equilibrium, biomaterial surfaces are dominated by high-molecular-weight proteins. These proteins demonstrate a great number of statistical contact points in a denaturable or conformational labile state and are readily capable of interacting with the interfacial microenvironment.[22]

Adsorbed proteins may induce crystalline formation on chemical groups of their structures that fulfill the stereochemical and surface charge requirements for crystal nucleation.[12] The crystals grow if these conditions occur within a range sufficient for crystal nucleus stabilization and growth at a defined spatial orientation.[13] Extracellular noncollagenous proteins are believed to be the principal components regulating crystal growth. Protein-induced mineralization in the oral environment proceeds by the initial formation of potassium chloride crystals[23] (Fig 1-3), whereas calcium phosphate precipitation may take place at later stages. This mode of extracellular mineralization participates in the formation of ectopic calcified deposits on tissues and materials, including teeth, dental materials, acetabular components of hip-joint arthroplasty, and bioprosthetic valves.[23]

Prolonged Biologic Responses to Biomaterial Surfaces: Cell Attachment and Organization

Because cell attachment onto biomaterial surfaces coordinates and integrates cellular differentiation, shape, movement, and biosynthetic activity, it is a fundamental biologic process underlying numerous homeostatic functions in living organisms.[24] A cell's approach to a biofilm-modified biomaterial surface requires considerably more time than does protein adsorption. This cell attachment may be classified into three groups, depending on the distance between the two elements. The first group incorporates the far-distance effects (> 100 nm); the second group, the intermediate-distance effects (20 to 100 nm); and the third group, the short-distance effects (< 20 nm).[25]

At far distances exceeding 100 nm, cell movement is controlled by fluid dynamics and chemotaxis, which compete with repulsion forces of electrostatic origin, as both acquired protein films and cells are mostly negatively charged. At intermediate distances, between 20 and 100 nm, the effect of fluid dynamics forces is reduced, and the competitive action of van der Waals attraction, electrical repulsion, and water solvation forces determines the overall response leading to the occurrence or absence of cell attachment. At short distances of less than 20 nm, cell attachment occurs through nonspecific and specific bonding mechanisms.[24] The latter involve signaling transactions to cell-surface binding proteins or activation of specific transmembrane receptors, such as integrins. Of particular importance is the role of heparin sulfate proteoglycans, which participate in many cellular events such as focal contacts and modification of the extracellular matrix, where they serve as reservoirs for growth factors and cytokines. Receptor mobility, cell deformability, biofluid ionic strength, and the osmotic tendency of water play important roles as well. The initial

cell-substrate and cell-cell contact is small. At equilibrium, maximization of the number of bonds and minimization of the surface area of contact lead to a balance between thermodynamics and intra-aggregating factors.[25]

Apparently, any change in the surface-adsorbed protein composition during the lifetime of a biomaterial may lead to the utilization of different cell adhesion receptors, thus altering cell behavior. This consequence is especially important for implantable devices, where an array of reactions related to tissue inflammatory response, activation of wound-healing mechanisms, and tissue remodeling take place. The presence of inflammatory cells at the interface initiates secondary reactions on a biomaterial surface and the surrounding cell population by secretion of proteins, enzymes, and oxidizing agents, as well as the production of oxygen radicals.[26] These agents may change the biomaterial surface reactivity by altering the types of proteins adsorbed onto the original surface or by affecting the structure of this surface.

The most common mechanisms of structural biomaterial modification by biologic fluids involve the near-surface regions. In general, these mechanisms may be subdivided into three groups: (1) the absorption of biologic species; (2) the desorption of ions, monomers, additives, and impurities; and (3) the release of breakdown products because of corrosion, wear, or enzymatic attack.

The production of wear debris at tissue-implant interfaces activates foreign-body granulomatous reactions and the release of active proinflammatory substances implicated in pathologic procedures and tissue remodeling. The composition, size, and shape of the biomaterial particles released modulate the cell and tissue responses. Moreover, uptake of metals from cells and charge-carrier species may affect cell differentiation and the regulation of gene expression.[24] With time, the intermediate bioliquid region diminishes, and the biomaterial comes in closer contact with the tissue. At this point, cell differentiation and regulation depend on tissue vascularity and implant stability, as in skeletal tissue repair, where the distortional and hydrostatic cell strains produced at a tissue-mobile implant interface may result in fibrous growth rather than the desired osseous tissue formation.[27] The same mechanism may be responsible for the synovium-like structures that develop around artificial joints.

Surface roughness also may contribute to the strength of cell and tissue attachment to the substrate. For certain types of cells, variations in substrate roughness may influence cell locomotion by contact guidance phenomena. These responses are subject to the mechanical restrictions imposed on the formation of cell microfilament bundles at cell focal points. Contact guidance may modify the secretory and proliferative activities of cells.[28] Thus, implant mobility and surface roughness are two of the complex biomechanical mechanisms governing tissue response to implants.

The basic principles of biomaterial-host interactions reviewed above have regional variations that depend on the dynamic activity of biologic fluids and the nature of tissue response. The following discussion focuses on the interactions of dental biomaterials with saliva, soft tissues, and bone.

Biomaterials in Contact with Saliva

The intraoral biofilm that forms naturally on teeth and restorative materials is dental plaque, a diverse community of bacteria embedded in an organic matrix that prevents colonization by exogenous microorganisms.[29] Plaque development involves the formation of a conditioning film (acquired pellicle), early microbial colonization, and maturation and late colonization leading to a dynamic equilibrium. Major shifts in equilibrium lead to disease of hard and soft dental tissue.[29,30]

The significance of surface properties in intraoral biofilm formation was discovered more than three decades ago by Glantz,[31] who first adopted the analytical methodology used for traditional surface chemistry to study the surface reactivity of teeth and restorative materials. From that time, researchers have systematically investigated the interactions of hard dental tissues and restorative materials with saliva in an attempt to

understand the interfacial phenomena involved and to regulate the complex saliva-substrate interactions. Most of these studies have investigated the effect of the substrate surface properties on pellicle composition, microorganism colonization, and plaque maturation.

Effect of Biomaterial Surface Properties on Pellicle Formation

Any natural or artificial surface exposed in the oral cavity will be covered within seconds by a noncellular salivary biofilm rich in acidic proteins and lipids, known as *acquired pellicle*.[32,33] Pellicle has a major role in intraoral physiologic functions because of the following characteristics:

1. It is a permeability barrier for ionic or macromolecular transport between surfaces and the intraoral environment.[34]
2. It may act as a lubricating agent to reduce mechanical friction.[35]
3. It reduces bacterial colonization by minimizing the bacteria's interfacial free energy of adhesion with the substrate.[36]
4. It may promote attachment of specific bacteria strains.[37]

Pellicle formation involves selective protein adsorption, employing nonspecific electrostatic and hydrophobic interactions and protein conformational changes, and it is affected by the saliva flow rate and pH.[38] It has been proposed that pellicle development proceeds through three phases.[39] Initially, low-molecular-weight phosphoproteins are adsorbed at a high rate, producing a tightly bound layer. Next, competitive interactions take place mainly between phosphoproteins and low-molecular-weight glycoproteins, creating a second, less tightly bound layer. Finally, high-molecular-weight glycoproteins are adsorbed, forming a third, loosely bound layer. On enamel, the rapid pellicle adsorption period ends within 30 minutes, whereas the time required for adsorption equilibrium has been estimated to be 90 minutes.[40]

Pellicle has a micellar structure composed of negatively charged globular clusters 20 to 300 nm

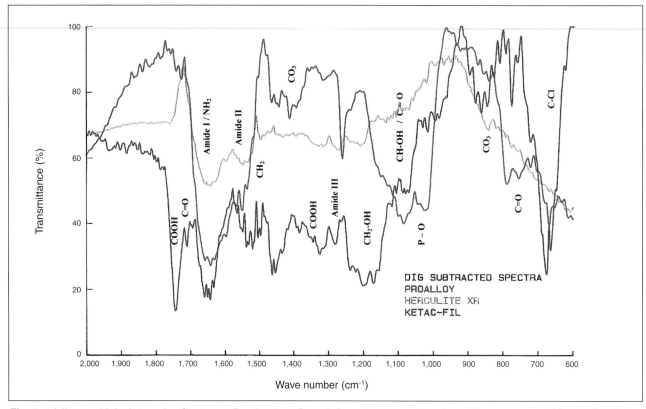

Fig 1-4 Micromultiple internal reflectance Fourier transform infrared spectra showing different compositions of pellicles formed on amalgam (ProAlloy [DMP, Athens, Greece]), resin composite (Herculite XR [Kerr, Orange, CA]), and glass-ionomer (Ketac-Fil [ESPE, Norristown, PA]) surfaces after a 60-minute simultaneous exposure of the restorative materials to the same intraoral conditions. Spectra were acquired from material surfaces and then subjected to digital subtraction interpretation to remove original material and water interferences. Note the complex profile of the adsorbed species on the hydrophilic surfaces of amalgam and glass ionomer in comparison with the hydrophobic resin composite surface.

in diameter, which are stabilized by calcium ions. Upon maturation, a homogeneous layer replaces the globular structure, possibly as a result of proteolytic activity.[41] The composition of pellicle varies on surfaces with different characteristics. Compared with cementum pellicle, enamel pellicle contains considerably higher amounts of the acidic proline–rich proteins, cystine, and lysozyme.[42] Extensive in vivo studies of pellicle formation on surfaces with well-defined characteristics, including composition, roughness, and critical surface tension, have documented that the amino acid composition[43] and packing distribution, as well as the pellicle configuration, may vary substantially.[44–46] These studies found that even though the same amount of protein was adsorbed on high- and low-energy surfaces during pellicle for-

mation, films on low-energy surfaces were thicker and more loosely bound. These differences in pellicle composition and organization may reflect an inherent biologic response that transforms all intraorally exposed solid surfaces to the same state of bioadhesiveness.[47]

Despite the extensive study of pellicle formation on reference materials, information on pellicle composition, interaction, and organization in relation to restorative materials is scarce. Experiments employing chemical characterization techniques, which were conducted on pellicles formed in vivo on various dental materials, revealed significant differences in composition[48–52] (Fig 1-4). A transmission electron microscopy investigation of in vivo pellicle formation on a variety of restorative materials revealed no ultrastructural

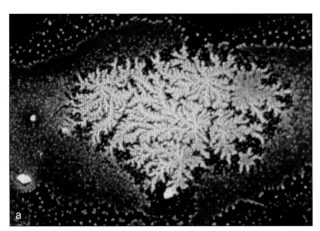
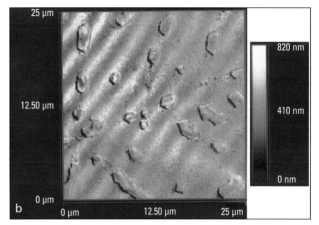

Fig 1-5 Early microbial colonization of pellicle formed on germanium minicrystals after a 90-minute intraoral exposure. *(a)* Dark-field reflected light microscope image. Note the dendritic bacterial aggregation onto the adsorbed amorphous fraction of salivary proteins (original magnification × 50). *(b)* Atomic force microscope image of dendritic bacterial aggregation under lateral-force (frictional) imaging mode. Note the differences in the morphology of adsorbed pellicle relative to the orientation of bacteria (scan size: 25 μm; z-range: 820 nm).

differences, implying that the initially adsorbed protein layer effectively masked the substrate surface properties.[53] Nonetheless, in a recent in vitro study of pellicle formation on flat and unpolished surfaces of glass-ionomer and resin composite restoratives, more bacteria-binding proteins (agglutinins, proline-rich proteins, and mucins) were recovered from the pellicle adjacent to the glass ionomer.[54] These findings suggest that pellicle demonstrates a "memory" effect of the substrate surface properties, as mediated by the surface-protein interactions.

Effect of Biomaterial Surface Properties on Plaque Formation

Early microbial colonization of acquired pellicle (Fig 1-5) involves nonspecific forces that transfer microorganisms close to the substrate to establish specific bonding.[55] During this phase, the main factors controlling microorganism retention rate include the detachment shear forces (originating from salivary flow, buccal and lingual tongue movements, and hard food) and the surface energetic state of the substrate, as modified by pellicle.[56] Interactions of different microbial species and strains in the bioliquid (coaggregation) or with surface-attached microorganisms (coadhesion), re-

lease of biosurfactants, production of extracellular matrix polymers, and various competitive reactions are considered important factors for the formation and rapid growth of plaque.[55] After 18 to 48 hours in vivo, an equilibrium is reached; plaque organized in cell microcolonies is entrapped in a dense polysaccharide-based matrix interspersed with water channels.[57,58]

The plaque-retention capacity of restorative materials has long been recognized as a major factor influencing oral health, and efforts have been undertaken to design materials with minimal plaque growth potential. The important role of substrate surface roughness and surface free energy for plaque formation in vivo has been demonstrated in a series of studies on surfaces with well-defined characteristics. These studies showed that in supragingival regions, roughness contributes more to plaque formation than does the surface energy state, whereas in subgingival regions, surface free energy is the determinant factor.[59] In plaque formation, roughness generates flow stagnation points on surface irregularities (eg, pores, grooves, cracks, and scratches), which promote cell attachment (Fig 1-6), although the response of individual bacteria biofilms on rough substrates varies.[60]

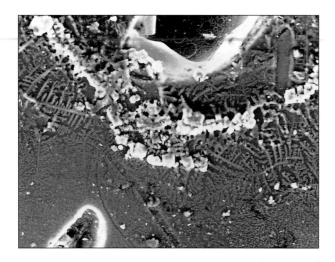

Fig 1-6 Secondary electron image of dental plaque formed in vivo at the protruding edges of a craterlike defect of a resin composite surface. Note the excessive plaque maturation and crystal development at the region (original magnification × 360).

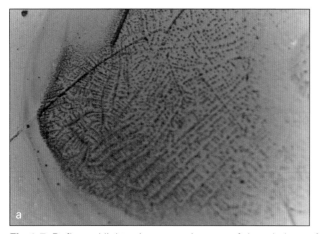
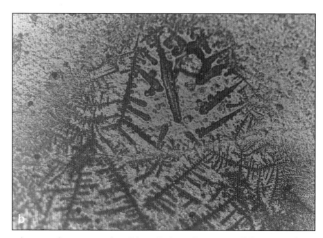

Fig 1-7 Reflected light microscope images of dental plaque formed on resin composite (a) and glass-ionomer (b) restoratives prepared against a flat surface covered with a polystyrene matrix strip, after a 90-minute intraoral exposure. Bacterial colonization is much more pronounced on the glass-ionomer surface (bright-field observation mode, original magnification × 50).

Moreover, the surface area of plaque accumulation is less on low-energy (hydrophobic) surfaces than on high-energy (hydrophilic) surfaces (Fig 1-7).[10] Four possible explanations may be given for this finding:

1. The microbial binding strength is lower on low-energy surfaces.
2. High-surface-energy microorganisms bind with high-energy surfaces, and vice versa. Because most of the bacteria found in human dental plaque have high surface energy,[61] colonization on low-surface-energy regions is limited.

3. The surface energy regulates the cohesive strength of pellicle films against the shear detachment forces; thus, on low-energy surfaces, films with low cohesive strength are formed.
4. The increased surface area and decreased protruding height of well-spread cells may produce a geometric configuration with decreased flow resistance.

A limited number of in vivo studies have documented such interactions between dental materials and developing plaque.[49,50,62] However, other in vivo studies find no major structural or bacteriologic differences in the early plaque formed on various dental materials.[63–65] These findings may suggest that plaque formation is influenced predominantly by the oral environment rather than the type of substrate.[65] In any case, such a mechanism fails to explain the low plaque retention clinically experienced with porcelain and other ceramics.[66] Many in vitro plaque formation experiments involving saliva incubation on dental material surfaces have been performed as well and have yielded contradictory conclusions. The results of these studies should be interpreted with caution, because shear force gradients are missing, and the pellicles formed contain more intact protein species than pellicles developed under in vivo conditions.[67] It seems that some material surface properties are transferred through pellicle to plaque, but the detailed mechanism is not fully understood.[68]

When intraoral exposure periods are long, the phenomena occurring at plaque-material interfaces become more complex through interactions at the near-surface region. These phenomena include the release of ions, monomers, and biodegradation and fretting corrosion products, which may reorganize interfacial protein adsorption and subsequently lead to the formation of new plaque. These interactions proceed at higher rates in regions where pellicle and plaque are continuously renewed, thus establishing a more aggressive environment.[69] Of particular importance is the role of pellicle and plaque on the selective release of material species with a therapeutic effect, such as fluoride. The rate of such ion-exchange interactions drops sharply in the presence of these natural intraoral integuments.[70]

Effect of Biomaterial Surface Properties on Calculus, Organic Deposits, and Stains

Mature plaque calcification and calculus formation involve calcium and phosphate uptake from the oral environment, supersaturation, and crystal nucleation and growth. It is believed that pellicle and plaque calcification proceed only after enzymatic deactivation of certain inhibitors, such as saliva phosphoproteins and pyrophosphate,

noncollagenous components (including proteoglycans), and plaque lipoteichoic acid.[55,71] Plaque calcification begins at extracellular regions with deposition of the soluble calcium phosphates (octacalcium phosphate and dicalcium phosphate dehydrate). Upon maturation, carbonated hydroxyapatite and magnesium-substituted beta-tricalcium phosphate form as well. This structure is organized in needlelike, rodlike, and platelike crystals that form layers separated by organic-rich material resembling pellicle.[71]

Information on the composition of the intraoral calculus on dental materials is limited. On denture resin polymers, the inorganic part of denture calculus is composed of carbonated hydroxyapatite and magnesium-substituted beta-tricalcium phosphate.[72,73] Studies on orthodontic wires and elastomers show that initial mineral deposition occurs by the formation of potassium chloride microcrystallites on adsorbed biofilms, followed by the precipitation of calcium phosphates.[74,75] On dental alloys, the cathodic protection offered by cationic saliva corrosion inhibitors determines calculus formation and may explain the common clinical observation that in patients with poor oral health, calculus forms more frequently on gold than on amalgam.[76] No information is available for resin composites and glass ionomers. However, an in vivo study has documented the contribution of surface roughness in creating salivary flow stagnation points and biofilm calcification on resin composites.[50]

After prolonged intraoral exposure, denture polymers have been found to accumulate amorphous dark and yellow deposits, in addition to calculus.[77] These deposits are strongly attached and removed only by sodium hypochlorite solutions. Chemical analysis revealed that the deposits' composition differed from calculus and contained much more organic material. The surface extent of these deposits did not correlate with the surface roughness of the substrate but was strongly influenced by the water absorption properties of these polymers, suggesting the role of diffusion-driven phenomena.

Extrinsic staining of dental alloys is common and has been associated[76] with the surface interactions of certain elements in the alloys with thiol groups of biologic origin, resulting in the formation of nonsoluble products. With the advent of esthetic restorative materials, surface resistance to extrinsic staining has become important. It is thought that surface texture and surface free energy control the complex mechanisms for staining of tooth-colored restorative materials in the oral environment.[77] Generally, although rough surfaces are more susceptible to staining, the surface energetic effect may overwhelm the effect of roughness. For example, resin composites containing acid-modified monomers (compomers), although having the same surface roughness characteristics as conventional resin composites, exhibited more staining, which extended to a greater depth. This finding was attributed to the presence of hydrophilic carboxyl groups on the compomers and their slow neutralization rate in the oral environment.[78] Commonly used antiseptics and mouthrinses contribute greatly to surface staining by interacting either with plaque and pellicle or with the restorative material surfaces.[79]

Dental Implants in Contact with Soft Tissues and Bone

The transmucosal placement of dental implants sets some unique healing requirements for the establishment and maintenance of an adequate biologic seal and an effective load-bearing capacity.[80] Biologic sealing at the gingival-implant interface is of paramount importance to prevent diffusion of microorganisms and toxins to the bone-implant interface. Several in vivo and in vitro studies have documented the development of a hemidesmosome–basal lamina attachment complex between the junctional epithelium and a variety of implant materials, which is similar to the complex bond between the epithelium and normal hard dental tissues. Ultramicroscopic investigations on hemidesmosome–basal lamina complex structures have demonstrated the presence of a basal lamina layer 15 to 25 nm thick and rich in glycosaminoglycans; this layer acts as a conditioning film between implant surfaces and hemidesmosomes. This biofilm seems to control the hemidesmosome response to local environmental conditions, such as the presence of plaque and inflammation, and thus establishes a dynamic equilibrium modulated by interfacial protein adsorption and desorption processes.[81]

The early formation of the hemidesmosomal complex and the high proliferation rate of epithelial cells compared with osseous cells may result in undesired apical epithelial migration and intrusion at the bone-implant interface. When there are no bone crestal defects, an implant design that uses cell contact guidance principles may optimize both biologic sealing and implant-bone integration in this region.[28]

An effective implant load-bearing mechanism requires structural and functional integration between the implant material and bone without the initiation of rejection mechanisms. This condition, called *osseointegration*, is usually fulfilled by titanium, titanium alloys, and ceramic implant materials. Based on the ultrastructure of the bone-biomaterial interface, implant materials may be classified as *biotolerant*, *bioinert*, and *bioactive* (Table 1-1).[82]

Metallic dental implants principally are manufactured from commercially pure (CP) titanium and Ti-6Al-4V, which rapidly form an amorphous, dense titanium dioxide passivating film that is stable in the biologic environment. After implantation, it is believed that selective adsorption of water, O_2^-, HPO_4^{2-}, and $H_2PO_4^-$ and the release of titanium as $Ti(OH)_4$ occur[83] at the outer oxide layer under the adsorbed protein film, whereas oxide growth takes place at the oxide-metal interface. These interactions result in titanium dioxide films with an outermost layer rich in titanium hydrogen phosphates, along with an increased thickness and a more crystalline and insoluble nature. Calcium phosphate precipitates subsequently form on this structure, changing the outer oxide layer to a complex of titanium phosphates and calcium phosphates, the latter being similar to hydroxyapatite. The calcium precipitation kinetics on titanium-rich surfaces are much slower than on bioactive ceramics. Because of the effective electronic shielding of the thin precipitated film by bulk titanium and the titanium dioxide film, the layer formed cannot exhibit the

Table 1-1 Classification of dental implants based on bone response

CATEGORY	COMPOSITION	BONE RESPONSE
Biotolerant	Co-Cr-Mo, Au, Pt, polymers	Distal osteogenesis; connective tissue interface
Bioinert	Ti, Ta, alumina, zirconia, ceramics	Close contact between bone and implant
Bioactive	Ca-P ceramics, bioglass, bioceramics	Bonding osteogenesis; chemical bonding between bone and implant

properties of calcium phosphates. Similar interactions have been documented on stainless steel, cobalt-chromium, and nickel-chromium alloys. However, calcium adsorption occurs later, and the stoichiometry of the calcium phosphates formed (Ca:P ratio) differs from that of hydroxyapatite, probably because of the presence of Cr_2O_3 passivating films.[84]

The adsorption process described above is strongly influenced by inflammatory reactions. The reduced pH of the early exudative phases; the activation of cells, including polymorphonuclear granulocytes and macrophages; and the release of proteins, enzymes, and oxidizing agents all modify implant surface reactivity. Of particular importance is the secretion of reactive oxygen intermediates from inflammatory cells. These species rapidly oxidize titanium through a specific mechanism, forming titanium-peroxy compounds that inhibit inflammation. However, in the presence of halides or secretory enzymes like myeloperoxidase and lactoperoxidase, the peroxide compounds may either decompose to titanium hydroxide and hydrogen peroxide or directly form halide compounds with microbicidal action. This mechanism may explain the low infection incidence reported after placement of titanium dental implants. Yet the same mechanism may form soluble titanium compounds that may be transferred through phagocytosis to sites far from the implant surface.[85]

For other bioinert materials such as alumina and zirconia, a narrow interfacial layer 20 to 40 nm thick and composed of a calcified noncollagenous interfacial zone rich in proteoglycans and glycosaminoglycans has been identified. For interfaces between CP titanium or Ti-6Al-4V implants and bone, an amorphous zone has been detected between the implant surface and cells labeled strongly for osteocalcin and weakly for osteopontin.[86]

For bioactive glasses, rapid exchange occurs between Na^+ and K^+ from the implant with H^+ and H_3O^+ from the tissue fluid, leading to the release of $Si(OH)_4$ in solution and the formation of silanols at the glass-solution interface. Silanol groups form an Si-O-Si–rich layer through a polycondensation reaction. During this stage, metastable hydrated silica species such as $Si(OH)_5^-$ may provide nucleation sites for biologic mineralization onto this layer by migration of calcium and phosphate ions, forming an amorphous $CaO-P_2O_5$ film, which crystallizes by incorporation of OH^-, CO_3^{2-}, and F^-. The optimum bioactivity of these glasses requires very specific ratios of oxides, especially of P_2O_5, and depends on the times required for calcium phosphate film formation, hydroxyapatite crystallization, and protein adsorption equilibrium.[87]

For calcium phosphate ceramic implants (beta-tricalcium phosphate, biphasic calcium phosphate, and hydroxyapatite), the proposed interfacial events occurring at the implantation site are quite different. The sequence of interaction steps includes the following:

1. A reduction in pH and partial dissolution of calcium phosphate macrocrystals
2. An increase in the concentration of calcium and phosphate ions in the vicinity
3. The formation of carbonated hydroxyapatite crystals
4. The association of the carbonated hydroxyapatite minicrystals with an organic matrix
5. The incorporation of these minicrystals and calcium phosphate macrocrystals into the collagen matrix during new bond formation, possibly by epitaxial growth onto these sites

The extent of calcium phosphate dissolution depends on composition, particle size, and crystallinity. Several mechanisms have been described for carbonated hydroxyapatite minicrystal formation, including precipitation, phase transformation, seeded growth, and ion incorporation from biologic fluids.[88,89]

As healing proceeds, the exudative phase diminishes, and the tissue adjacent to the implant becomes organized. At this point, the application of functional loading may produce micromovements that modify the surrounding cell response. Particle detachment from an implant due to wear may initiate inflammatory reactions and influence cell response as well. Implant surface topography strongly modifies cell adhesion, migration, and proliferation. The migration and orientation movements of fibroblasts and leukocytes are influenced by contact guidance phenomena. Inflammatory cells such as macrophages better adhere to irregular surfaces and release more bone-resorbing factors there. Moreover, an irregular surface topography promotes rigid implant fixation.[28]

The application of stress to a healing implant may induce adverse, clinically important, time-dependent phenomena. Distortional strains may influence tissue differentiation by altering cell gene expression and biosynthetic activity, whereas hydrostatic pressure may additionally inhibit capillary blood flow, thereby decreasing tissue oxygenation. It is believed that implants with rigid fixation experience minimal distortional strain and interference with hydrostatic stress, resulting in the regenerative response of bone formation; in contrast, poorly fixed implants are subject to the repair response of fibrous tissue formation.[27]

Implant micromotion is extremely important for bone regeneration and influences bone healing much more than do biomaterial properties per se. Without micromotion, an osseointegrated bone-biomaterial interface arises more from the inherent healing potential of bone than a unique phenomenon induced by an implant biomaterial.[90,91]

Osteoconductive glasses and calcium phosphate ceramics have been used as coatings on titanium implants to combine the benefits of a bioactive surface with the favorable properties of the titanium substrate (Fig 1-8). Coatings seem to modify the tissue response around the implant, accelerating bone attachment, increasing osteoblast precursor activity, and leading to more extracellular matrix mineralization.[92,93] Nevertheless, bone resorption, cohesive fracture, and debonding of the ceramic coatings have been reported in several cases.[94,95] Recently, these coatings have been used as carriers of biologically active molecules with osteoinductive potential, such as recombinant bone morphogenetic protein type 2 (BMP-2) and other growth factors[96,97]; however, the long-term biologic activity of these coatings has not been confirmed.

Resorbable and nonresorbable membranes for guided-tissue regeneration constitute another interesting group of dental implant materials. Nonresorbable membranes are prepared from expanded polytetrafluoroethylene, whereas resorbable membranes are either synthetic copolymers of lactide-polylactic acid, glycolide-polylactic acid, or collagen. Resorbable membranes, especially those composed of type I collagen, become actively engaged in the bone reconstruction process. The hydrophilic structure of resorbable membranes seems to accelerate protein adsorption and hence shorten the time required to reach adsorption equilibrium.[98] Nonresorbable membranes

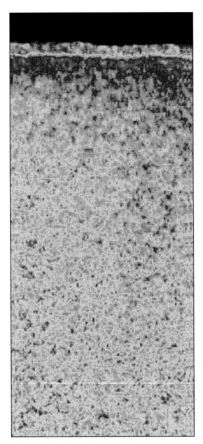

Fig 1-8 Two-dimensional reconstruction of x-ray microtomographic images of a hydroxyapatite-coated titanium dental implant. Note the morphology at the coating-metal transitional zone (80 kV/100 µA, original magnification × 60).

have the disadvantage of necessitating a second surgical procedure for their removal. However, the biologic activity of the biodegradation products released from resorbable copolymers and the compatibility of the collagen extractions used are also concerns. Currently, both types of membranes are used experimentally as carrier materials for bone growth–stimulation substances.

References

1. Baier RE. On the formation of biological films. Swed Dent J 1977;1:261–271.
2. Baier RE. Selected methods of investigation of blood-contact surfaces. Ann N Y Acad Sci 1987;516:68–77.
3. Schakenraad JM, Noordmans J, Wildevuur CRH, Arends J, Busscher JH. The effect of protein adsorption on substratum surface free energy, infrared adsorption and cell spreading. Biofuling 1986;1:193–201.
4. Schakenraad JM, Busscher HJ, Wildevuur CRH, Arends J. The influence of substrate surface free energy on growth and spreading of human fibroblasts in the presence and absence of serum proteins. J Biomed Mater Res 1989;20:773–784.
5. Chittur KR. Surface techniques to examine the biomaterial-host interface: An introduction to the papers. Biomaterials 1998;19:301–305.
6. Hoffman A. Modification of material surfaces to affect how they interact with blood. Ann N Y Acad Sci 1987;516:96–101.
7. Kasemo B, Lausmaa J. Biomaterials from a surface science perspective. In: Ratner BD (ed). Progress in Biomedical Engineering. Vol 6: Surface Characterization of Biomaterials. Amsterdam: Elsevier, 1988:1–12.
8. Baier RE, Meyer AE, Natiella JR, Natiella PR, Carter JM. Surface properties determine bioadhesive outcomes: Methods and results. J Biomed Mater Res 1984;18:337–355.
9. Baier RE. Surface chemical factors presaging bioadhesive events. Ann N Y Acad Sci 1983;416:34–57.
10. Quirynen M, Marecal M, Busscher HJ, et al. The influence of surface free-energy on planimetric plaque growth in man. J Dent Res 1989;68:796–799.
11. Colman RW, Scott CF, Schmaier AH, Wachtfogel YT, Pixley RA, Edmunds LH Jr. Initiation of blood coagulation at artificial surfaces. Ann N Y Acad Sci 1987;516:253–267.
12. Addadi L, Weiner S. Interactions between acidic proteins and crystals: Stereochemical requirements for mineralization. Proc Natl Acad Sci USA 1985;82:4110–4114.
13. Addadi L, Borman A, Moradian O, Idak J, Weiner S. Structural and stereochemical relations between acidic macromolecules of organic matrices and crystals. Connect Tissue Res 1989;21:127–135.
14. Klauber C, Smart RStC. Solid systems: Their structure and composition. In: O'Connor DI, Sexton BA, Smart RStC (eds). Springer Series in Surface Sciences. Vol 23: Surface Analysis Methods in Materials Science. Berlin: Springer-Verlag, 1992:3–65.
15. Ratner BD. The surface characterization of biomaterials: How finely can we resolve surface structure? In: Ratner BD (ed). Progress in Biomedical Engineering. Vol 6: Surface Characterization of Biomaterials. Amsterdam: Elsevier, 1988:13–36.

16. Davis JE. The importance and measurement of surface charge species in cell behaviour at the biomaterial interface. In: Ratner BD (ed). Progress in Biomedical Engineering. Vol 6: Surface Characterization of Biomaterials. Amsterdam: Elsevier, 1988:219–234.

17. Merrill EW. Distinctions and correspondences among surfaces containing blood. Ann N Y Acad Sci 1987;516:196–203.

18. Karino T, Goldsmith HL, Motomiya M, Mabuchi S, Sohara Y. Flow patterns in vessels of simple and complex geometries. Ann N Y Acad Sci 1987;516:422–441.

19. Kasemo B, Lausmaa J. The biomaterial-tissue interface and its analogues in surface science and technology. In: Davies JE (ed). The Bone-Biomaterial Interface. Toronto: University of Toronto Press, 1991:19–32.

20. Israelachvili J. Intermolecular and Surface Forces, ed 3. San Diego: Academic Press, 1991:275–286.

21. Brash JL. Studies on protein adsorption to blood compatible materials. In: Missirlis YF, Lemm W (eds). Modern Aspects of Protein Adsorption on Biomaterials. Dordrecht, The Netherlands: Kluwer Academic Press, 1991:39–47.

22. Andrade JD, Hlady V. Plasma protein adsorption: The big twelve. Ann N Y Acad Sci 1987;516:158–172.

23. Vasin M, Rosanova J, Sevastianov V. The role of proteins in the nucleation and formation of calcium-containing deposits on biomaterial surfaces. J Biomed Mater Res 1998;39: 491–497.

24. Leonard EF, Rahmin I, Angarska JK, Vassilief CS, Ivanov IB. The close approach of cells to surfaces. Ann N Y Acad Sci 1987;516:502–512.

25. Sauk JJ, Van Kampen CL, Somerman MJ. Role of adhesive proteins and integrins in bone and ligament cell behavior at the material surface. In: Davies JE (ed). The Bone-Biomaterial Interface. Toronto: University of Toronto Press, 1991:111–119.

26. Thomsen P, Ericson LE. Inflammatory cell response to bone implant surfaces. In: Davies JE (ed). The Bone-Biomaterial Interface. Toronto: University of Toronto Press, 1991:153–164.

27. Carter DR, Giori NJ. Effect of mechanical stress on tissue differentiation in the bony implant bed. In: Davies JE (ed). The Bone-Biomaterial Interface. Toronto: University of Toronto Press, 1991:367–376.

28. Brunette DM. The effect of surface topography on cell migration and adhesion. In: Ratner BD (ed). Progress in Biomedical Engineering. Vol 6: Surface Characterization of Biomaterials. Amsterdam: Elsevier, 1988:203–217.

29. Marsh PD. Host defenses and microbial homeostasis role of microbial interactions. J Dent Res 1989;68:1567–1575.

30. Gibbons RJ. Bacterial adhesion to oral tissues: A model for infectious diseases. J Dent Res 1989;68:750–760.

31. Glantz P-O. On wettability and adhesiveness. Odontol Revy 1969;20(suppl 17):1–132.

32. Eggen KH, Rölla G. Gel filtration, ion exchange chromatography and chemical analysis of macromolecules present in acquired enamel pellicle (2 hour-pellicle). Scand J Dent Res 1982;90:182–188.

33. Slomiany BL, Murty VLN, Zdebska E, Slomiany A, Gwozdzinski K, Mandel ID. Tooth surface pellicle lipids and their role in the protection of dental enamel against lactic acid diffusion in man. Arch Oral Biol 1986;3:187–191.

34. Tabak LA, Levine MJ, Mandel ID, Ellison SA. Role of salivary mucins in the protection of the oral cavity. J Oral Pathol 1982;11:1–17.

35. Hatton MN, Levine MJ, Margarone JE, Argurre A. Lubrication and viscosity features of human saliva and commercially available saliva substitutes. J Oral Maxillofac Surg 1987;45:496–499.

36. Pratt-Terpstra IH, Weerkamp AH, Busscher HJ. Microbial factors in a thermodynamic approach of oral streptococcal adhesion to solid substrata. J Coll Interfac Sci 1989;129: 568–574.

37. Pratt-Terpstra IH, Weerkamp AH, Busscher HJ. The effects of pellicle formation on streptococcal adhesion to enamel and artificial substrata with various surface free energies. J Dent Res 1989;68:463–467.

38. Vassilakos N. Some Biophysical Aspects of Salivary Film Formation [dissertation]. Malmo, Sweden: Graphic Systems AB, 1992.

39. Embery G, Hogg SD, Heaney TG, Stanbuty JB, Green RDJ. Some considerations on dental pellicle formation and early bacterial colonization: The role of high and low molecular weight proteins of the major and minor salivary glands. In: Leach SA, Arends J (eds). Bacterial Adhesion and Preventive Dentistry. Oxford, England: IRL Press, 1984:73–84.

40. Kuboki Y, Teraoka K, Okada S. X–ray photoelectron spectroscopic studies of the adsorption of salivary constituents on enamel. J Dent Res 1987;66:1016–1019.

41. Rölla G, Rykke M, Gaare D. The role of acquired enamel pellicle in calculus formation. Adv Dent Res 1995;9:403–409.

42. Ruan MS, Paola C, Mandel I. Quantitative immunochemistry of salivary proteins in vitro to enamel and cementum from caries resistant and caries susceptible human adults. Arch Oral Biol 1986;31:597–601.

43. Sönju T, Glantz P-O. Chemical composition of salivary integuments formed in vivo on solids with some established surface characteristics. Arch Oral Biol 1975;20:687–691.

44. Baier RE, Glantz P-O. Characterization of oral in vivo films formed on different types of solid samples. Acta Odontol Scand 1978;76:289–301.

45. Glantz P-O. Adhesion to the surfaces of teeth. In: Leach SA (ed). Dental Plaque and Surface Interactions in the Oral Cavity. London: IRL Press, 1980:49–64.

46. Glantz P-O, Baier RE, Christersson CE. Biochemical and physiological considerations for modeling biofilms in the oral cavity: A review. Dent Mater 1996;12:208–214.

47. Jendresen MD, Glantz P-O. Clinical adhesiveness of selected dental materials: An in vivo study. Acta Odontol Scand 1981;39:39–45.

48. Sönju T, Skjörland K. Pellicle composition and initial bacterial colonization on composite and amalgam in vivo. In: Stiles HM, Loesche WJ, O'Brien TC (eds). Microbial Aspects of Dental Caries. London: IRL Press, 1976:133–141.

49. Skjörland K. Auger analysis of the integuments formed on different dental materials in vivo. Acta Odontol Scand 1982;40:129–134.

50. Palaghias G, Eliades G. Characterization of oral films adsorbed on surfaces of dental materials in vivo [abstract 668]. J Dent Res 1992;71:599.

51. Eliades T, Eliades G, Brantley WA. Microbial attachment on orthodontic appliances, I. Wettability and early pellicle formation on bracket materials. Am J Orthod Dentofacial Orthop 1995;108:351–360.

52. Lee SJ, Kho HS, Lee SW, Yong WS. Experimental salivary pellicles on the surface of orthodontic materials. Am J Orthod Dentofacial Orthop 2001;119:59–66.

53. Hannig M. Transmission electron microscopic study of in vivo pellicle formation on dental restorative materials. Eur J Oral Sci 1997;105:422–433.

54. Carlen A, Nikdel K, Wennerberg A, Holmberg K, Olsson J. Surface characteristics and in vitro biofilm formation on glass ionomer and composite resin. Biomaterials 2001;22:481–487.

55. Busscher HJ, van der Mei HC. Physico-chemical interactions on initial microbial adhesion and relevance for biofilm formation. Adv Dent Res 1997;11:24–32.

56. Christersson CE, Dunford RG, Glantz P-O, Baier RE. Effect of critical surface tension on retention of oral microorganisms. Scand J Dent Res 1989;97:247–256.

57. Bowden GMW, Li YH. Nutritional influences on biofilm development. Adv Dent Res 1997;11:81–99.

58. Wood SR, Kirkham J, Marsh PD, Shore RC, Nattress B, Robinson C. Architecture of intact natural human plaque biofilms studied by confocal laser scanning microscopy. J Dent Res 2000;79:21–27.

59. Quirynen M, Marechal M, Busscher HJ, Weerkamp AH, Darius PL, Van Steenberghe D. The influence of surface free energy and surface roughness on early plaque formation. J Clin Periodontol 1990;17:138–144.

60. Yamauchi M, Yamamoto K, Wakabayashi M, Kawano J. In vitro adherence of microorganisms to denture base resin with different surface texture. Dent Mater J 1990;9:19–24.

61. Weerkamp AH, Quirynen M, Marechal M, van der Mei HC, Van Steenberghe D, Busscher HJ. The role of surface energy in the early in vivo formation of dental plaque on human enamel and polymeric substrata. Microb Ecol Health Disease 1989;2:11–18.

62. Skjörland KK, Sönju T. Effect of sucrose rinses on bacterial colonization on amalgam and composite. Acta Odontol Scand 1982;40:193–196.

63. Siegrist BE, Brecx MC, Gusberti FA, Joss A, Lang NP. In vivo early human dental plaque formation on different supporting substances: A scanning electron microscopic and bacteriological study. Clin Oral Implants Res 1991;2:38–46.

64. Leonhardt Å, Olsson J, Dahlén G. Bacterial colonization on titanium, hydroxyapatite and amalgam surfaces in vivo. J Dent Res 1995;74:321–326.

65. Hannig M. Transmission electron microscopy of early plaque formation on dental materials in vivo. Eur J Oral Sci 1999; 107:55–64.

66. Hahn R, Weiger R, Netuschil L, Bruch M. Microbial accumulation and vitality on different restorative materials. Dent Mater 1993;9:312–316.

67. Yao Y, Grogan J, Zehnder M, et al. Compositional analysis of human acquired enamel pellicle by mass spectrometry. Arch Oral Biol 2001;46:293–303.

68. Quirynen M, Bollen CML. The influence of surface roughness and surface-free energy on supra- and subgingival plaque formation in man. J Clin Periodontol 1995;22:1–14.

69. Jenkins GN. The Physiology and Biochemistry of the Mouth, ed 4. Oxford, England: Blackwell, 1978:486–487.

70. Eliades G. Chemical and biological properties of glass-ionomer cements. In: Davidson CL, Mjör IA (eds). Advances in Glass-Ionomer Cements. Chicago: Quintessence, 1999:85–101.

71. White DJ. Dental calculus: Recent insights on occurrence, formation, prevention, removal and oral health effects of supragingival and subgingival deposits. Eur J Oral Sci 1997;105:508–522.

72. Hayashi Y. High resolution electron microscopy of the interface between dental calculus and denture resin. Scanning Microsc 1995;9:419–427.

73. Gaffar A, LeGeros RJ, Gambogi RJ, Afflitto J. Inhibition of formation of calcium phosphate deposits on teeth and dental materials: Recent advances. Adv Dent Res 1995;9:419–426.

74. Eliades T, Eliades G, Watts DC. Structural conformation of in vitro and in vivo aged orthodontic elastomeric modules. Eur J Orthod 1999;21:649–658.

75. Eliades T, Eliades G, Athanasiou AE, Bradley TG. Surface characterization of retrieved NiTi orthodontic archwires. Eur J Orthod 2000;22:317–326.

76. Palaghias G. Oral corrosion and corrosion inhibition processes—An in vitro study. Swed Dent J 1985;30(suppl):1–72.

77. Zanghellini G, Dykman AG, Reinberger V, Arends J. Deposit formation on prosthetic materials in vivo after one year: A quantitative study of twelve materials. Adv Dent Res 1995;9:443–449.

78. Gladys S, Van Meerbeek B, Lambrechts P, Vanherle G. Marginal adaptation and retention of a glass-ionomer, resin-modified glass-ionomer and polyacid-modified resin composite in cervical Class-V lesions. Dent Mater 1998;14:294–306.

79. Addy M, Moran J. Mechanisms of stain formation on teeth, in particular associated with metal ions and antiseptics. Adv Dent Res 1995;9:450–456.

80. Steflik DE, McKinney RV Jr. Epithelial attachment to ceramic dental implants. Ann N Y Acad Sci 1988;523:4–18.

81. Steflik DE, McKinney RV Jr, Koth DL. Histological and ultrastructural observations of the tissue responses to endosteal dental implants. In: Kawahara H (ed). Progress in Biomedical Engineering. Vol. 7: Oral Implantology and Biomaterials. Amsterdam: Elsevier, 1988:203–217.

82. Letic-Gavrilovic A, Scandurra R, Abe K. Genetic potential of interfacial guided osteogenesis in implant devices. Dent Mater J 2000;19:99–132.

83. Eliades T. Passive film growth on titanium alloys: Physico-chemical and biologic considerations. Int J Oral Maxillofac Implants 1997;12:621–627.
84. Hanawa T. Titanium and its oxide film: A substrate for formation of apatite. In: Davies JE (ed). The Bone-Biomaterial Interface. Toronto: University of Toronto Press, 1991:49–60.
85. Bjursten LM, Tengvall P. Modulation of cell activity by titanium peroxy compounds. In: Davies JE (ed). The Bone-Biomaterial Interface. Toronto: University of Toronto Press, 1991:165–168.
86. Ayukawa Y, Takeshita F, Inoue T, et al. An immunoelectron microscopic localization of noncollagenous bone proteins (osteocalcin and osteopontin) at the bone-titanium interface of rat tibiae. J Biomed Mater Res 1998;41:111–119.
87. Hench L. Surface reaction kinetics and adsorption of biological moieties: A mechanistic approach to tissue attachment. In: Davies JE (ed). The Bone-Biomaterial Interface. Toronto: University of Toronto Press, 1991:33–44.
88. Daculsi G, LeGeros R, Heughebaert M, Barbieux N. Formation of carbonate-apatite crystals after implantation of calcium phosphate ceramics. Calcif Tissue Int 1990;24:471–488.
89. LeGeros R, Orly I, Gregoire M, Daculsi G. Substrate surface dissolution and interfacial biological mineralization. In: Davies JE (ed). The Bone-Biomaterial Interface. Toronto: University of Toronto Press, 1991:76–87.
90. Brunski JB, Hipp JA, Cochran GVB. The influence of biomechanical factors at the tissue-biomaterial interface. In: Hanker JS, Giammara BL (eds). Materials Research Society Symposium. Vol 110: Biomedical Materials and Devices. Pittsburgh: Materials Research Society, 1989:505–515.

91. Brunski JB. Influence of biomechanical factors at the bone-biomaterial interface. In: Davies JE (ed). The Bone-Biomaterial Interface. Toronto: University of Toronto Press, 1991:391–404.
92. Yan WQ, Nakamura T, Kobayashi M, Kim HM, Miyaji F, Kokubo T. Bonding of chemically treated titanium implants to bone. J Biomed Mater Res 1997;37:267–275.
93. Ong JL, Hoppe CA, Cardenas HL, et al. Osteoblast precursor cell activity on HA surfaces of different treatments. J Biomed Mater Res 1998;39:176–183.
94. Ichikawa T, Hirota K, Kanitani H, et al. Rapid bone resorption adjacent to hydroxyapatite-coated implants. J Oral Implantol 1996;22:279–285.
95. Biesbrock AR, Edgerton M. Evaluation of the clinical predictability of hydroxyapatite-coated endosseous dental implants: A review of the literature. Int J Oral Maxillofac Implants 1995;10:712–720.
96. Ono I, Ohura T, Murata M, Yamaguchi H, Ohmura Y, Kuboki Y. A study of bone induction in hydroxyapatite combined with bone morphogenetic protein. Plast Reconstr Surg 1992;90:870–879.
97. Asahina I, Watanabe M, Sakurai N, Mori M, Enomoto S. Repair of bone defect in primate mandible using a bone morphogenetic protein (BMP)-hydroxyapatite-collagen composite. J Med Dent Sci 1997;44:63–70.
98. Zambelis G, Eliades G, Palaghias G. Characterization of blood films formed on GTR materials in vivo [abstract 49]. Presented at the Europerio Conference, Paris, 1994.

Section II

PROSTHODONTICS AND IMPLANT DENTISTRY

2

AGING OF CASTING ALLOYS USED IN PROSTHODONTICS AND RESTORATIVE DENTISTRY

William A. Brantley, PhD

Dental restorations and prostheses use many different types of noble metal and base metal casting alloys. The compositions and properties of these alloys are described in detail in textbooks on dental materials.[1–3] The mechanical and physical properties needed for various clinical applications can be inferred from the information sheets provided by major manufacturers, which have extensive experience with alloy development and performance in the oral environment. The American National Standards Institute/American Dental Association (ANSI/ADA) specifications and the International Organization for Standardization (ISO) standards stipulate minimum values of clinically relevant alloy properties.

The principal element by weight in noble metal casting alloys is gold, palladium, or silver; the excellent in vivo corrosion resistance of these alloys arises from the inherent noble character of the major component elements. Although both all-metal and metal-ceramic restorations employ noble metal alloys, their alloy compositions differ. For example, alloys for metal-ceramic restorations must have melting temperatures higher than the firing temperatures for the dental porcelain, as well as thermal contraction coefficients closely matched to those of the porcelain. These alloys also contain small amounts of certain oxidizable elements that form strong chemical bonds with

the porcelain during the initial oxidation step and subsequent firing steps. In addition to obvious requirements for in vivo corrosion resistance and biocompatibility, alloys for both all-metal and metal-ceramic restorations must have sufficient strength to withstand mastication forces.

The principal element in the traditional (ie, non-titanium) base metal casting alloys is nickel, cobalt, or iron; these alloys also contain chromium, which provides corrosion resistance from a thin, passivating surface oxide film that blocks the diffusion of oxygen and the penetration of other corrosive species to the underlying bulk alloy. These base metal alloys are the usual choice for removable partial denture frameworks, where their high elastic modulus, high strength, and low cost make them particularly attractive compared with traditional type IV high-gold alloys. Other base metal casting alloys may be preferred over noble metal casting alloys for metal-ceramic applications because of their much lower cost. However, this economic advantage can be offset by the greater difficulty of manipulating these alloys in the dental laboratory.

Casting titanium for dental restorations is limited by the need for special casting machines, investments, laboratory procedures, and the presence of a very hard near-surface region (the α-case that arises from reaction with the investment) on the castings, as well as by difficulties with porcelain adherence.[4-8] The interest in casting titanium arises from its excellent strength-to-weight ratio[9] and biocompatibility,[10] which is associated with a thin, passivating titanium oxide film. Dental applications of the popular Ti-6Al-4V alloy,[9] which is much stronger than pure titanium, also have been investigated.[11,12]

Many published articles have described the microstructures and properties of the noble metal and base metal alloys in the as-cast and heat-treated conditions, the latter often involving simulation of the clinically relevant porcelain-firing cycles. However, only a few published studies have directly examined the aging of dental casting alloys (noble metal alloys only) at intraoral or room temperatures. Studies of low-temperature aging of gold- and palladium-based alloys are discussed in detail in the next section of this chapter. The final section summarizes the relevant principles of materials science for the aging processes. It also applies these principles to extrapolate the results from previous studies of noble metal and base metal alloys aged at elevated temperatures in order to obtain predictions about long-term alloy aging processes in the oral environment and their potential effects on clinically relevant properties.

Intraoral and Room Temperature Aging of Noble Metal Casting Alloys

Gold-Based Alloys

The traditional Type I to Type IV high-gold dental casting alloys for all-metal restorations are strengthened in the quenched as-cast condition by the incorporation of other elements (silver, copper, platinum, palladium, and zinc) in the face-centered-cubic (fcc) gold solid solution.[1] Type III and Type IV high-gold alloys contain sufficient copper to gain additional increases in hardness and strength from heat treatment at elevated temperatures by the formation of ordered regions of AuCu, which has been shown by x-ray diffraction[13] and high-resolution transmission electron

microscopy (TEM).[14] There are two ordered AuCu superlattices: AuCu II at higher temperatures and AuCu I at lower temperatures.[15] The ordered $AuCu_3$ structure is relevant for age hardening of popular casting alloys with lower gold content (eg, Midas [Jelenko, Armonk, NY]),[16] and its role in age hardening also has been studied by TEM.[17]

High-resolution TEM has established that the hardening and strengthening of aged high-gold alloys arise from interactions of dislocations with elastic strain fields at the interfaces between ordered AuCu I platelets, which have a face-centered-tetragonal (fct) structure, and the disordered fcc gold solid solution matrix.[14] Analogous dislocation interactions with elastic strain fields at interfaces with the ordered $AuCu_3$ regions[17] are assumed to be responsible for age hardening of alloys of reduced gold content, such as Midas and products of similar composition.

However, although dental manufacturers provide information about appropriate heat treatments to harden and strengthen specific gold alloy products, these procedures are time-consuming and generally not performed on cast restorations. The dimensional changes in restorations that such heat treatments would produce are another concern.[18]

During typical dental laboratory procedures,[1] the cast gold alloy restoration is quenched when the sprue button loses its "red heat" appearance, which leaves the casting in the softened condition. This is the customary alloy condition after final adjustments of the cast restoration when it is cemented to the prepared tooth. To obtain the highest hardness and strength possible with the Type III or Type IV gold alloy, the cast restoration is subjected to heat treatment, typically at a temperature between 200°C and 450°C for 15 to 30 minutes, depending on the product and manufacturer. It is recommended that the alloy be in the fully softened condition before the hardening heat treatment is performed. A solution heat treatment is performed, typically of 10 minutes duration at 700°C, followed by quenching to room temperature to prevent the ordering that would occur with slow cooling. The solution heat treatment converts the gold alloy to a single-phase, disordered fcc gold solid solution.

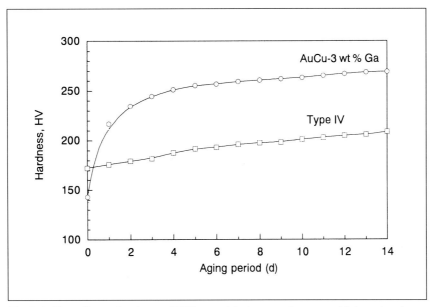

Fig 2-1 The effect of aging at 37°C over 14 days on the mean Vickers hardness (HV) (300-gm load) of AuCu-3 wt % Ga alloy and commercial Type IV high-gold alloy. (Adapted from Watanabe et al[18] with permission.)

Watanabe et al[18] compared increases in surface hardness, dimensional changes in the mesiodistal direction, and increases in surface roughness during aging at 37°C for two-unit fixed partial denture specimens of an Au-22Cu-3Ga-0.5Ir (wt %) alloy designed to undergo age hardening at intraoral temperatures and a commercial Type IV Au-15Cu-7Ag-5Pt-2Pd alloy. The decrease in linear dimensions during aging at 37°C was also reported for fixed partial denture–type and rod-shaped specimens of each alloy.

Figure 2-1 shows that rapid hardening of the AuCu-3 wt % Ga alloy occurred during the first 4 days of aging at 37°C, with the Vickers hardness increasing from 140 to 270.[18] The lower subsequent rate of age hardening for this alloy was similar to the gradual rate for the commercial Type IV gold alloy, for which the Vickers hardness increased from approximately 170 to 210 during the 2-week aging period. The decrease in linear dimensions over a 5-day aging period was much greater for the AuCu-3 wt % Ga alloy than

the commercial Type IV gold alloy, as shown in Fig 2-2, and the dimensional changes were similar for the fixed partial denture–type and rod-shaped specimens of each alloy.

The observed changes (generally < 20 µm) in several relevant dimensions in the mesiodistal direction (distortions) of the two-unit fixed partial denture specimens over the 2-week aging period at 37°C would have no clinical significance for the commercial Type IV gold alloy, but much larger distortions (often > 50 µm at the longer aging times) occurred for the AuCu-3 wt % Ga alloy.[18] Very small increases (mean values < 0.10 µm) in average surface roughness were measured for the AuCu-3 wt % Ga alloy during the 2-week aging period at 37°C, and the mean increases were less than 0.03 µm for the commercial Type IV gold alloy during the same aging period. For the AuCu-3 wt % Ga alloy, a rapid increase in average surface roughness occurred at about 3 days of aging, resulting in nearly two times the initial value. Much smaller increases in

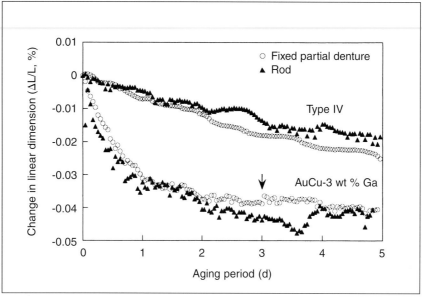

Fig 2-2 Percentage linear contraction (L/L) for fixed partial denture and rod specimens of AuCu-3 wt % Ga alloy and a commercial Type IV high-gold alloy during 5 days of aging at 37°C. These changes no longer appeared to occur for the AuCu-3 wt % Ga alloy after 3 days *(arrow)*. (Adapted from Watanabe et al[18] with permission.)

average surface roughness for the commercial Type IV gold alloy occurred during the same aging period.

The rate of hardening (see Fig 2-1) and the change in linear dimensions (see Fig 2-2) during aging at 37°C for both gold alloys corresponded well to the time periods for occurrence of the distortions and the increase in average surface roughness for the two-unit fixed partial denture–type castings.[18] Both AuCu I and AuCu II (which has a long-period orthorhombic structure[15]) ordered regions were observed by TEM in the AuCu-3 wt% Ga alloy after aging for 30 days at 37°C. For both alloys, the changes in average surface roughness were attributed to the relief of elastic coherency stresses that arise between the ordered regions and the disordered solid solution matrix.[18] The authors concluded that the mode of distortion for the AuCu-3 wt % Ga alloy would be more advantageous for crown-type restorations than inlay-type restorations and that the amount of contraction during intraoral aging of this alloy may not cause clinical problems. Future research to investigate in vivo aging and its clinical signif-

icance for other commercial Type III and Type IV gold casting alloys over longer times would be worthwhile.

Palladium-Based Alloys

Since their introduction in the early 1980s, high-palladium alloys containing more than approximately 75 wt % palladium have been popular alternatives to gold-based or gold-palladium alloys[1–3] for metal-ceramic restorations,[19] and they have been recommended for implant-supported prostheses[20] because of their excellent mechanical properties[21,22] and good porcelain adherence.[23,24] The attractive unit metal cost of these alloys compared with the gold-based alloys was a pivotal factor in their earlier widespread adoption,[19] but the recent price volatility of palladium has led to decreased clinical use.

Commercial high-palladium dental alloys are based on the Pd-Cu-Ga and Pd-Ga systems,[19,25] for which the starting point is the Pd-Ga phase diagram.[26,27] The presence of copper in the Pd-Cu-Ga alloy compositions,[26] along with the rapid solidification conditions because of the large temperature difference between the molten alloy and the investment mold,[1-3] typically results in the formation of a substantial near-surface lamellar eutectic constituent in small dental castings prepared from alloys that have an equiaxed fine-grained structure.[19,25,28] This eutectic constituent was not observed in larger Pd-Cu-Ga alloy specimens used with the tension test for measurement of mechanical properties,[22] where the cooling rate for the castings was much lower. Other Pd-Cu-Ga alloys that do not contain a grain-refining element solidify with a dendritic as-cast microstructure that contains the lamellar eutectic constituent in the interdendritic regions.[25,29] The observation of "hot tears" (microscopic fractures along the interdendritic regions at elevated temperatures) in bench-cooled small castings of a Pd-Cu-Ga alloy with a dendritic microstructure suggests that it is important that these alloys have sufficient bulk to resist stresses imposed by the investment as the casting cools to room temperature.[30] The near-surface eutectic structure in small castings, consisting of the palladium solid solution matrix and the Pd_2Ga phase[19,25] in both equiaxed fine-grained and dendritic as-cast Pd-Cu-Ga alloys, is largely eliminated when these high-palladium alloys are subjected to heat treatment simulating the porcelain-firing cycles.[25,30]

Because small Pd-Ga alloy castings (or those with thin cross sections) do not contain substantial amounts of near-surface eutectic constituent in the as-cast condition,[19,25,31] in the oral environment they may have biocompatibility superior to that of the as-cast Pd-Cu-Ga alloys,[32] although this hypothesis remains to be proven. The Pd-Ga alloys generally have lower hardness than the Pd-Cu-Ga alloys, a characteristic that facilitates finishing and final adjustments to the castings in the dental laboratory[19]; however, composition control can yield a Pd-Cu-Ga alloy with hardness very similar to that of Pd-Ga alloys.[27]

Scanning electron microscope (SEM) examination of as-cast simulated coping specimens for maxillary central incisor restorations prepared[19] from three Pd-Cu-Ga alloys (Athenium, 74Pd-14.5Cu-1.5Ga-5In-5Sn [Williams/Ivoclar, now Ivoclar Vivadent, Amherst, NY]; Spartan, 79Pd-10Cu-9Ga-2Au [Ivoclar Vivadent]; and Liberty, 76Pd-10Cu-5.5Ga-6Sn-2Au [Jelenko]) and stored at room temperature for 5 years revealed remarkable evidence of aging.[33] In the as-cast condition, the Athenium and Liberty alloys have equiaxed fine-grained microstructures due to the presence of approximately 0.5 wt % ruthenium as a grain-refining element. The Spartan alloy, which does not contain a grain-refining element, has a dendritic as-cast microstructure.[19,25]

Figure 2-3 shows the microstructure near the surface of an Athenium alloy casting that was aged for 5 years at room temperature. A subsurface oxidation region about 5 µm thick is followed by a denuded region that does not contain the eutectic constituent, which is a dominant microstructural feature in the bulk alloy.[33] Figure 2-4 shows the microstructure near the surface of a Liberty alloy casting that was aged for 5 years at room temperature. Again, there is a denuded region adjacent to the surface that does not contain the eutectic constituent in the bulk microstructure.[33] Figure 2-5 shows the near-surface microstructure of a Spartan alloy casting that was aged for 5 years at room temperature; some eutectic interdendritic constituent is still present. Partial transformation of this constituent appears to have occurred, although there may have been some loss of the lamellar phases during the etching procedure.[33] No near-surface oxidation regions were observed for the Liberty or Spartan alloy castings that were aged for 5 years at room temperature, although this relatively fragile feature may have been lost during metallographic preparation.[33]

Table 2-1 shows a comparison, using x-ray energy-dispersive spectroscopic analysis, of elemental compositions for bulk and near-surface regions of the Athenium alloy aged for 5 years at room temperature. Note that the near-surface region is enriched in copper, gallium, tin, and possibly ruthenium.[33] X-ray diffraction analysis of oxidized Liberty and Spartan Plus Pd-Cu-Ga alloys in another study[34] suggests that the near-surface region of the aged Athenium alloy in Fig 2-3 might contain particles of $CuGa_2O_4$, β-Ga_2O_3, and SnO_2. (The Spartan Plus alloy has a composition identical to that of the Spartan alloy

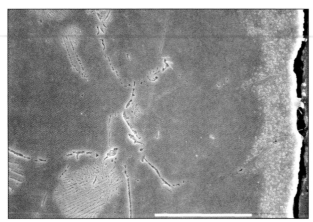

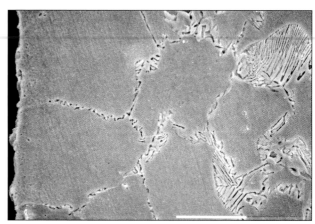

Fig 2-3 Scanning electron microscope secondary electron image of the near-surface microstructure of as-cast Athenium Pd-Cu-Ga alloy after aging 5 years at room temperature. A subsurface oxidation region at the right side of the specimen and a denuded region to its left that does not contain the lamellar eutectic constituent are evident. The gap near the right edge of the image was caused by shrinkage of the metallographic mounting resin (bar = 10 μm). The microstructures in Figs 2-3, 2-4, and 2-5 were revealed by etching in aqua regia solutions. (Adapted from Brantley et al[33] with permission.)

Fig 2-4 Scanning electron microscope secondary electron image of the near-surface region of as-cast Liberty Pd-Cu-Ga alloy after aging at room temperature for 5 years. As in Fig 2-3, a denuded region can be seen (now on the left side of the image) that does not contain the lamellar eutectic constituent. The gap between the specimen surface and the metallographic mounting resin is at the left edge of the image (bar = 10 μm). (Adapted from Brantley et al[33] with permission.)

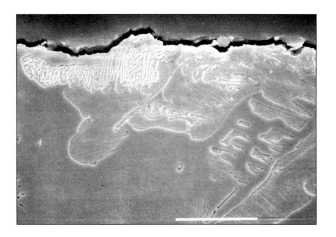

Fig 2-5 Scanning electron microscope secondary electron image of the near-surface microstructure of as-cast Spartan Pd-Cu-Ga alloy after aging at room temperature for 5 years, showing the presence of the remaining lamellar eutectic interdendritic constituent. This constituent may have been lost at the right side of this image during metallographic preparation, but some aging transformation appears to have occurred. The gap between the specimen surface and the metallographic mounting resin is at the top of the image (bar = 10 μm). (Adapted from Brantley et al[33] with permission.)

except for the absence of a very small amount of boron.[29]) Because in the same study,[34] x-ray diffraction analysis of two Pd-Ga alloys that contained indium showed that In_2O_3 formed readily when the alloys were subjected to the elevated-temperature oxidation procedure, perhaps this oxide was also present in the near-surface region of the Athenium alloy after aging at room temperature, despite the lack of indium enrichment (see Table 2-1). The apparent near-surface enrich-

ment of ruthenium in the aged Athenium alloy may arise from energy-dispersive spectroscopic spot analysis of some ruthenium-rich particles, which are a common microstructural constituent in high-palladium alloys.[25,27] This conjecture is supported by the large standard deviation for the mean ruthenium concentration in Table 2-1.

No differences in Vickers hardness were found[33] for the three Pd-Cu-Ga alloys after 5 years of aging at room temperature, compared with val-

Table 2-1 Comparison of compositions for bulk and near-surface regions of aged Athenium determined by x-ray energy-dispersive spectroscopic analysis*†

REGION	PALLADIUM	COPPER	GALLIUM	INDIUM	TIN	RUTHENIUM
Bulk	76.7 (0.6)	11.4 (0.6)	1.4 (0.2)	5.5 (0.2)	4.8 (0.8)	1.0 (0.1)
Near-surface	70.0 (2.4)	11.4 (0.6)	2.3 (0.6)	5.8 (0.9)	6.3 (0.9)	3.7 (2.0)

*Reproduced from Brantley et al[33] with permission.
†Entries are mean value (standard deviation) for a total of six analyses in the bulk region and five analyses in the near-surface region for two different specimens.

Table 2-2 Summary of Vickers hardness measurements (1-kg load) for aged Pd-Cu-Ga alloys*†

ALLOY	HARDNESS
Athenium	252 ± 6
Liberty	326 ± 9
Spartan	403 ± 20

*Reproduced from Brantley et al[33] with permission.
†Each entry is mean ± standard deviation for measurements on two specimens (N = 20). For the original as-cast specimens, the mean values of pooled Vickers hardness were Athenium (260), Liberty (330), and Spartan (409).[19]

ues for the initial[19] as-cast condition (Table 2-2). This result is not surprising, because only small differences were previously found[30] in the Vickers hardness of these three alloys for the as-cast condition and the heat-treated condition that simulated the firing cycles for dental porcelain. After this heat-treatment procedure, the Vickers hardness experienced small decreases of approximately 10% and 7% for the Athenium and Spartan alloys, respectively. The earlier study found a larger decrease in Vickers hardness—approximately 13%—for the Liberty alloy after the simulated porcelain-firing cycles,[30] but this finding would have little practical significance for dental laboratories adjusting cast restorations prepared from this alloy.

Hence, room temperature aging of these three Pd-Cu-Ga high-palladium alloys has minimal effect on the Vickers hardness (and, presumably, on the yield strength[35]), in contrast to the low-temperature age hardening previously described for high-gold alloys. The lack of effect for low-temperature aging on the hardness of the Pd-Cu-Ga alloys can be explained by the hardening mechanisms of these alloys.

Examination by TEM revealed that commercial high-palladium alloys are dominated by a tweed structure, which is found in both as-cast and heat-treated conditions of Pd-Cu-Ga and Pd-Ga alloys that differ substantially in hardness.[36,37] Consequently, this tweed structure is not the principal mechanism for providing increased hardness and strength beyond that achieved by solid solution incorporation of other elements in the palladium solid solution matrix. The mechanism for increased hardening and strengthening of high-palladium alloys was discovered by Wu et al[27] from experiments in which overall Vickers hardness (1-kg load) was obtained as a function of temperature for several high-palladium alloys, and a light indenting load (10 gm) permitted the determination of hardness measurements for the individual microstructural phases. The increased hardness of the as-cast Liberty alloy over that of the palladium solid solution arises from a hard grain-boundary phase (Vickers hardness > 400), whose composition approximately matches Pd_5Ga_2; this phase is surrounded by another grain-boundary phase that is assumed to be Pd_2Ga.[27] The hard phase was not observed in two Pd-Ga alloys or in one Pd-Cu-Ga alloy with substantially lower Vickers hardness (approximately 250 to 270) than the Liberty alloy; the hardness of these as-cast alloys is determined by the composition of the palladium solid solution.[27] Discontinuous precipitates formed from the supersaturated palladium solid solution in the four high-palladium alloys investigated during heat treatment at 1,200°F and 1,400°F, but these precipitates had the same Vickers hardness as the palladium solid solution. Likewise, there was no difference in the hardness of the eutectic structure in as-cast Liberty alloy compared with the palladium solid solution matrix for this alloy. The high hardness of the Spartan Pd-Cu-Ga alloy is attributed to a similar Pd_5Ga_2 phase in the interdendritic regions.[29]

The absence of a significant effect of room temperature aging on the Vickers hardness of the three Pd-Cu-Ga alloys is plausible, because such aging should have no effect on the hard Pd_5Ga_2 microstructural phase. Although room temperature aging over long periods might alter the tweed microstructure, this hypothesis would need to be verified by TEM experiments. Moreover, transformation of the tweed structure might affect the biocompatibility of the high-palladium alloys, because this relatively stable structure may contribute to the excellent in vitro corrosion resistance of these alloys.[37–39] Future research on these aspects of the high-palladium alloys is important.

Examination of Figs 2-3 and 2-4 reveals that the alloy surface has a central role in room temperature aging over a 5-year period for the Athenium and Liberty alloys. Observations with the scanning electron microscope revealed that a substantial eutectic constituent remained in both aged alloys at depths greater than approximately

20 µm.[33] The most likely modes of rapid diffusion would be first along the grain boundaries (which intersect the specimen surface), then along the interlamellar boundaries of the eutectic constituent, and finally perpendicular to the lamellae, the latter facilitated by the very small interlamellar distances of approximately 0.25 µm. During the 5-year period, the failure of room temperature aging to completely eliminate the eutectic constituent in the interdendritic regions of the Spartan alloy (see Fig 2-5) is attributed to the absence of a comparably efficient mode for rapid diffusion similar to the mode provided by the network of grain boundaries in the fine-grained Athenium and Liberty alloys.[33] Nonetheless, the eutectic interdendritic constituent appears to be somewhat transformed by rapid diffusion processes between the fine-scale lamellae during the room temperature aging of this alloy.

Because diffusion processes are thermally activated and there is little difference between room temperature and intraoral temperature on the absolute scale (°K), the foregoing results would also be expected for the in vivo aging of as-cast Athenium, Liberty, and Spartan alloys over 5 years. It must be emphasized that the major use of the high-palladium alloys in the United States has been in metal-ceramic restorations, where the alloys are subjected to a series of rapid elevated-temperature heat treatments during the initial oxidation step and the subsequent porcelain-firing cycles.[23] High-palladium alloys used for implant-supported prostheses may also be subjected to the same heat treatments for porcelain firing or to other heating regimens for soldering. In the past 2 decades, high-palladium alloys have been used only minimally in the United States for all-metal restorations and removable partial denture frameworks, where the alloys would most likely be in the as-cast condition.

Because the bulk microstructures of the high-palladium alloys retain some multiphase character after simulated porcelain firing,[19,25] further aging in the oral environment may occur as these alloys attempt to return to their equilibrium microstructures; this process is discussed in the next section. Scanning and transmission electron microscopy studies of high-palladium alloys in metal-ceramic restorations that have been subjected to clinical aging for several years are needed. Although short-term in vitro experiments have not revealed any effect of storage in a saliva-substitute medium on the porcelain adherence to high-palladium alloys,[24] the degradation of the metal-ceramic bond for these alloys over extended periods of in vivo use requires further investigation.

Application of Materials Science Principles to In Vivo Aging of Casting Alloys

Relevance of Phase Diagrams and Elevated-Temperature Heat-Treatment Studies

All conventional noble metal and base metal dental casting alloys contain multiple component elements.[1-3] (This section will not discuss the single-phase commercially pure titanium alloys that contain several important interstitial elements.[9]) According to the Gibbs phase rule,[9] these alloys will contain multiple phases at intraoral or room temperatures under equilibrium conditions. Even if complex multiple-component phase diagrams were available for dental casting alloys (which they are not), they would not provide completely relevant information. Because there is insufficient time for elemental diffusion to maintain equilibrium phase compositions under the rapid solidification conditions in the dental laboratory, the microstructures of cast dental alloys necessarily have elemental microsegregation and contain non-equilibrium phases. These phenomena are evident when microstructures of gold-based[40] and high-palladium[25] alloys are compared in the as-cast condition and after heat treatment simulating the porcelain-firing cycles, where substantial microstructural homogenization is typically observed.

Conventional base metal alloys for metal-ceramic applications[41] and removable partial denture frameworks[42,43] generally have as-cast dendritic microstructures. One study found that elevated-temperature heat treatment of several base metal casting alloys for removable partial den-

ture frameworks caused microstructural alterations, with reductions in strength and varying changes in elongation.[42] However, the results of that study suggest that clinically significant mechanical property changes in as-cast base metal alloys after extended service in the oral environment are unlikely. Significant in vivo aging of cast titanium and Ti-6Al-4V also seems unlikely because of their very high melting temperatures.

Residual Stresses in Cast Alloys and Their Role in Aging

Residual stresses exist in all cast dental alloys because of the rapid rates of solidification and the constraint of the solidifying alloy by the investment mold.[1-3] As previously noted, the development of stresses in solidifying Pd-Cu-Ga alloys with a dendritic microstructure can lead to hot tears when there is insufficient metal bulk to withstand these stresses,[30] and this problem is also expected for other high-palladium dental alloys with as-cast dendritic microstructures. Processing steps in the dental laboratory (such as air abrasion, polishing, and adjustments of cast restorations) that cause permanent surface deformation of the alloy impart residual stresses in the near-surface region. Although some residual stresses may be relieved during the porcelain-firing cycles for an alloy in a metal-ceramic restoration, other residual stresses will be created in the alloy during cooling of the metal-ceramic restoration because of the small mismatch between its thermal contraction coefficient and that of the porcelain. These stresses provide an additional driving force for phase transformations during elevated-temperature heat treatment, and also during in vivo aging, as the alloys attempt to form equilibrium phases.

Phase Transformation Principles and Relevance to In Vivo Aging of Casting Alloys

At intraoral temperatures, age hardening of dental gold casting alloys is facilitated by the relatively small atomic distances[15] the gold and copper atoms must move for regions in the disordered solid solution to transform to the AuCu I, AuCu II, and AuCu$_3$ superlattices. This suggests that intraoral aging would be found in dental gold alloys,[14,17,44,45] where complex phase transformations occur during age hardening at elevated temperatures.

Essential requirements for room temperature (or in vivo) aging of Pd-Cu-Ga high-palladium alloys are small diffusion lengths in the lamellar eutectic constituent and the existence of high-diffusivity paths at the surface and grain boundaries.[33] Although low-temperature aging studies have not been reported for the Pd-Ga high-palladium alloys, changes in the fine-scale microstructural constituents observed[19,25,27,31] at the grain boundaries might be expected, as the alloys seek equilibrium phase relationships. For Pd-Ga alloys, the effects on hardness and strength from in vivo aging should be minimal, based on studies comparing these alloys in the as-cast condition and after simulated porcelain-firing heat treatments.[22,25,27,29,30]

Recent TEM research[46–48] on two Pd-Ag alloys (Super Star [Jelenko] and Rx 91 [Jeneric/Pentron, Wallingford, CT]) revealed complex as-cast microstructures containing other phases in addition to the palladium solid solution matrix. Microstructural changes occurred after annealing at various elevated temperatures, with corresponding changes in Vickers hardness. The Pd-Ag binary alloys form solid solution systems with complete mutual solid solubility[1]; consequently, the microstructural phases and heat-treatment response may vary for each Pd-Ag alloy, depending on the proportions of the secondary alloying elements. The very small secondary phases observed by TEM suggest that Pd-Ag alloy castings might undergo in vivo aging, because elemental diffusion over relatively short distances could cause significant microstructural changes. Research in this area is recommended. However, in another study,[49] heat treatment of the Super Star alloy that simulated the porcelain-firing cycles caused a small decrease of only about 13% in Vickers hardness (1-kg load) compared with that for the as-cast alloy, and in vivo aging might not induce clinically significant changes in mechanical properties.

In Vivo Aging and Clinical Corrosion Resistance of Casting Alloys

Evidence to date suggests that in vivo aging will not significantly alter the corrosion resistance of dental casting alloys. Holland et al[50] found that the in vitro corrosion resistance of a low-gold alloy in artificial saliva was inferior when the alloy was prepared with a single-phase microstructure compared with the alloy prepared with a multiphase microstructure; this finding contrasts with what would be expected from the principles of corrosion science. These authors attributed this result to the formation of a protective surface tarnish layer that limited the corrosion of the multiphase alloy.

In vitro studies of high-palladium alloys in saline solutions and an artificial saliva have shown essentially no difference[38,39] in the corrosion behavior for the alloys in the as-cast condition and after simulated porcelain-firing heat treatment. The corrosion of these alloys is determined principally by the noble character of the major component elements, although some dissolution of less-noble secondary phases is expected.

Recent cyclic polarization studies by Sarkar and his associates[51,52] have shown that dealloying occurs during in vitro corrosion of high-palladium alloys in phosphate-buffered saline solution, leading to palladium enrichment at the surface; this finding has important implications for the biocompatibility of these alloys for patients with palladium allergy. In contrast, these investigators found that in vitro corrosion of Pd-Ag or Au-Pd alloys resulted in a silver- or gold-enriched surface, respectively, which is considered more biocompatible. Future research is needed to confirm that these mechanisms are applicable to intraoral corrosion as the alloy ages so that only biologically safe casting alloys are placed in the oral environment.

Acknowledgments

Support of Grant DE 10147 from the National Institute of Dental and Craniofacial Research (NIDCR) for investigation of the high-palladium alloys is acknowledged. The author wishes to thank Zhuo Cai, Alan Carr, William Clark, Wenhua Guo, Susan Kerber, John Mitchell, Suryanarayana Nitta, Efstratios Papazoglou, Desheng Sun, Stanley Vermilyea, and Qiang Wu for their extensive contributions to the research on palladium alloys discussed in this chapter.

References

1. Anusavice KJ. Phillips' Science of Dental Materials, ed 10. Philadelphia: Saunders, 1996:chap 15, 20, 23.

2. Craig RG, Powers JM (eds). Restorative Dental Materials, ed 11. St Louis: Mosby, 2002:chap 15–17.

3. O'Brien WJ (ed). Dental Materials and Their Selection, ed 3. Chicago: Quintessence, 2002:chap 13, 14, 16, 17.

4. Takahashi J, Kimura H, Lautenschlager EP, Chern Lin JH, Moser JB, Greener EH. Casting pure titanium into commercial phosphate-bonded SiO_2 investment molds. J Dent Res 1990;69:1800–1805.

5. Nakajima H, Okabe T. Titanium in dentistry: Development and research in the U.S.A. Dent Mater 1996;15:77–90.

6. Low D, Mori T. Titanium full crown casting: Thermal expansion of investments and crown accuracy. Dent Mater 1999;15:185–190.

7. Wang RR, Welsch GE, Monteiro O. Silicon nitride coating on titanium to enable titanium-ceramic bonding. J Biomed Mater Res 1999;46:262–270.

8. Brantley WA, Laub LW. Metal selection. In: Rosenstiel SF, Land MF, Fujimoto J (eds). Contemporary Fixed Prosthodontics, ed 3. St Louis: Mosby, 2001:497–509.

9. Brick RM, Pense AW, Gordon RB. Structure and Properties of Engineering Materials, ed 4. New York: McGraw-Hill, 1977:chap 2, 10.

10. Eliades T. Passive film growth on titanium alloys: Physicochemical and biologic considerations. Int J Oral Maxillofac Implants 1997;12:621–627.

11. Syverud M, Okabe T, Herø H. Casting of Ti-6Al-4V alloy compared with pure Ti in an Ar-arc casting machine. Eur J Oral Sci 1995;103:327–330.

12. Shimizu H, Habu T, Takada Y, Watanabe K, Okuno O, Okabe T. Mold filling of titanium alloys in two different wedge-shaped molds. Biomaterials 2002;23:2275–2281.

13. Leinfelder KF, O'Brien WJ, Taylor DF. Hardening of dental gold-copper alloys. J Dent Res 1972;51:900–905.

14. Yasuda K, van Tendeloo G, van Landuyt J, Amelinckx S. High-resolution electron microscopic study of age-hardening in a commercial dental gold alloy. J Dent Res 1986;65:1179–1185.

15. Cullity BD. Elements of X-Ray Diffraction, ed 2. Reading, MA: Addison-Wesley, 1978:chap 13.

16. Reisbick MH, Brantley WA. Mechanical property and microstructural variations for recast low-gold alloy. Int J Prosthodont 1995;8:346–350.

17. Winn H, Udoh K, Tanaka Y, Hernandez RI, Takuma Y, Hisatsune K. Phase transformations and age-hardening behaviors related to Au_3Cu in Au-Cu-Pd alloys. Dent Mater J 1999;18:218–234.

18. Watanabe I, Atsuta M, Yasuda K, Hisatsune K. Dimensional changes related to ordering in an AuCu-3 wt% Ga alloy at intraoral temperature. Dent Mater 1994;10:369–374.

19. Carr AB, Brantley WA. New high-palladium casting alloys: Part I. Overview and initial studies. Int J Prosthodont 1991;4:265–275.

20. Stewart RB, Gretz K, Brantley WA. A new high-palladium alloy for implant-supported prostheses [abstract 423]. J Dent Res 1992;71:158.

21. Papazoglou E, Wu Q, Brantley WA, Mitchell JC, Meyrick G. Mechanical properties of dendritic Pd-Cu-Ga dental alloys. Cells Mater 1999;9:43–54.

22. Papazoglou E, Wu Q, Brantley WA, Mitchell JC, Meyrick G. Comparison of mechanical properties for equiaxed fine-grained and dendritic high-palladium alloys. J Mater Sci Mater Med 2000;11:601–608.

23. Papazoglou E, Brantley WA, Carr AB, Johnston WM. Porcelain adherence to high-palladium alloys. J Prosthet Dent 1993;70:386–394.

24. Papazoglou E, Brantley WA, Johnston WM, Carr AB. Effects of dental laboratory processing variables and in vitro testing medium on the porcelain adherence of high-palladium casting alloys. J Prosthet Dent 1998;79:514–519.

25. Brantley WA, Cai Z, Carr AB, Mitchell JC. Metallurgical structures of as-cast and heat-treated high-palladium dental alloys. Cells Mater 1993;3:103–114.

26. Cascone PJ. Phase relations of the palladium-base, copper, gallium, indium alloy system [abstract 563]. J Dent Res 1984;63:233.

27. Wu Q, Brantley WA, Mitchell JC, Vermilyea SG, Xiao J, Guo W. Heat-treatment behavior of high-palladium dental alloys. Cells Mater 1997;7:161–174.

28. Brantley WA, Cai Z, Mitchell JC, Vermilyea SG. Mechanism for formation of lamellar constituents in grain-refined Pd-Cu-Ga dental alloys. Cells Mater 1997;7:63–67.

29. Brantley WA, Wu Q, Cai Z, Vermilyea SG, Mitchell JC, Comerford MC. Effects of casting conditions and annealing on microstructures and Vickers hardness of dendritic Pd-Cu-Ga dental alloys. Cells Mater 1999;9:83–92.

30. Carr AB, Cai Z, Brantley WA, Mitchell JC. New high-palladium casting alloys: Part II. Effects of heat treatment and burnout temperature. Int J Prosthodont 1993;6:233–241.

31. Brantley WA, Cai Z, Foreman DW, Mitchell JC, Papazoglou E, Carr AB. X-ray diffraction studies of as-cast high-palladium alloys. Dent Mater 1995;11:154–160.

32. Cai Z, Chu X, Bradway SD, Papazoglou E, Brantley WA. On the biocompatibility of high-palladium dental alloys. Cells Mater 1995;5:357–368.

33. Brantley WA, Cai Z, Wu Q, Carr AB, Mitchell JC. Room temperature aging of Pd-Cu-Ga dental alloys. Cells Mater 1995; 5:261–270.

34. Brantley WA, Cai Z, Papazoglou E, et al. X-ray diffraction studies of oxidized high-palladium alloys. Dent Mater 1996; 12:333–341.

35. Dieter GE. Mechanical Metallurgy, ed 3. New York: McGraw-Hill, 1986:329–331.

36. Cai Z, Brantley WA, Clark WAT, Colijn HO. Transmission electron microscopic investigation of high-palladium dental casting alloys. Dent Mater 1997;13:365–371.

37. Nitta SV, Clark WAT, Brantley WA, Grylls RJ, Cai Z. TEM analysis of tweed structure in high-palladium dental alloys. J Mater Sci Mater Med 1999;10:513–517.

38. Cai Z, Vermilyea SG, Brantley WA. In vitro corrosion resistance of high-palladium dental casting alloys. Dent Mater 1999;15:202–210.

39. Sun D, Monaghan P, Brantley WA, Johnston WM. Potentiodynamic polarization study of the in vitro corrosion behavior of 3 high-palladium alloys and a gold-palladium alloy in 5 media. J Prosthet Dent 2002;87:86–93.

40. Vermilyea SG, Huget EF, Vilca JM. Observations on gold-palladium-silver and gold-palladium alloys. J Prosthet Dent 1980;44:294–299.

41. Baran GR. Metallurgy of Ni-Cr alloys for fixed prosthodontics. J Prosthet Dent 1983;50:639–650.

42. Morris HF, Asgar K, Rowe AP, Nasjleti CE. The influence of heat treatments on several types of base-metal removable partial denture alloys. J Prosthet Dent 1979;41:388–395.

43. Bridgeport DA, Brantley WA, Herman PF. Cobalt-chromium and nickel-chromium alloys for removable prosthodontics. Part I. Mechanical properties of as-cast alloys. J Prosthodont 1993; 2:144–150.

44. Yasuda K, Ohta M. Difference in age-hardening mechanism in dental gold alloys. J Dent Res 1982;61:473–479.

45. Tani T, Udoh K, Yasuda K, Van Tendeloo G, Van Landuyt J. Age-hardening mechanisms in a commercial dental gold alloy containing platinum and palladium. J Dent Res 1991; 70:1350–1357.

46. Guo WH, Brantley WA, Clark WAT, Monaghan P, Mills MJ. Transmission electron microscopic investigation of a Pd-Ag-In-Sn dental alloy. Biomaterials (in press).

47. Guo WH, Brantley WA, Clark WAT, Sun D. TEM investigation of the hardening mechanisms for a Pd-Ag-Sn alloy [abstract 1229]. J Dent Res 2002;81:A-171.

48. Guo WH, Brantley WA, Clark WAT. TEM investigation of precipitation behavior of an annealed Pd-Ag alloy [abstract 2453]. J Dent Res 2002;81:A-309.

49. Vermilyea SG, Cai Z, Brantley WA, Mitchell JC. Metallurgical structure and microhardness of four new palladium-based alloys. J Prosthodont 1996;5:288–294.

50. Holland RI, Jørgensen RB, Herø H. Corrosion and structure of a low-gold dental alloy. Dent Mater 1986;2:143–146.

51. Berzins DW, Kawashima I, Graves R, Sarkar NK. Electrochemical characteristics of high-Pd alloys in relation to Pd-allergy. Dent Mater 2000;16:266–273.

52. Sarkar NK, Berzins DW, Prasad A. Dealloying and electroformation in high-Pd dental alloys. Dent Mater 2000;16: 374–379.

3

CERAMIC BEHAVIOR UNDER DIFFERENT ENVIRONMENTAL AND LOADING CONDITIONS

James L. Drummond, DDS, PhD

The degradation of ceramics in dental and orthopedic biomaterial applications can be evaluated based on different testing environments or loading conditions. This chapter focuses on the ceramics mainly used in dentistry—ie, feldspathic porcelain, alumina, and zirconia. Other sources cover the use of ceramics not only in dentistry but also in orthopedics, as well as the difficulties in developing clinically relevant in vitro testing.[1-3]

Ceramic materials fail when their ability to support an applied load is compromised by the presence of defects. Flaws in dental ceramics may be introduced by thermal processing during fabrication or by grinding during occlusal adjustments, or the flaws may be intrinsic and related to microstructural features. Upon loading, failure begins at the microscopic level through damage that results from the interaction of preexisting defects and the applied load. Ceramics also are subject to delayed failure due to subcritical crack growth,[4,5] and crack propagation is enhanced when ceramics are exposed to aqueous environments.[6,7] Dental ceramics used as restorative materials in the oral cavity are subject to average cyclic loads of approximately 60 to 250 N in a moist environment, and these loads can reach as high as 500 to 800 N for short periods.[8,9] The number of chewing cycles per day is estimated to be 800 to 1,400.[8,9]

Feldspathic Porcelains

Feldspathic porcelains, which are aluminosilicate glasses derived from feldspathic minerals, have been the subject of numerous studies concerning degradation with age or stress. The materials investigated have been the traditional porcelain or the newer pressable porcelains (eg, OPC [Jeneric/Pentron, Wallingford, CT], Empress [Ivoclar, Vivadent, Amherst, NY], and Finesse Pressable [Dentsply Ceramco, Burlington, NJ]). Using bar specimens and three-point bending in air, Campbell[10] determined the flexural strength (mean ± standard deviation) of feldspathic porcelain to be 88.6 ± 12.7 MPa. In another study of feldspathic porcelain in water, Morena et al[11] reported a fracture strength of 72.7 ± 8.2 MPa and a characteristic dynamic fatigue strength (at a constant stressing rate) of 44.0 MPa. Myers et al[12] used biaxial flexure to investigate Empress in water and determined a mean fracture strength of 96.6 ± 12.5 MPa and a mean fatigue strength of 83.3 ± 1.4 MPa. A conventional feldspathic porcelain in water had values of 70.8 ± 5.0 MPa for mean fracture strength and 49.1 ± 0.3 MPa for mean fatigue strength, indicating that the leucite-containing porcelain, Empress, had significantly improved mechanical properties over the conventional porcelain.

Ohyama et al[13] evaluated the effect of cyclic loading at 60% of the mean breaking load on a glass-infiltrated alumina core ceramic (In-Ceram [Vita Zahnfabrik, Bad Sackingen, Germany]) and a leucite-reinforced feldspathic porcelain (Empress). After 100,000 cycles in 37°C water, the alumina core ceramic exhibited more sensitivity to the cyclic loading, with 20% to 30% of the samples failing during cycling, whereas the cyclic loading had little effect on the leucite-reinforced porcelain. Other studies[14,15] examining dynamic and cyclic fatigue of conventional feldspathic dental porcelain found a corresponding decrease in mechanical properties.

Drummond et al[16] investigated the flexural strength under static and cyclic loading and the fracture toughness under static loading for six restorative ceramic materials. Four leucite ($K_2O \cdot Al_2O_3 \cdot 4SiO_2$)–strengthened feldspathic (pressable) porcelains, a low-fusing feldspathic porcelain, and an experimental lithium disilicate–containing ceramic were tested as controls in air and distilled water (without aging), as well as after 3 months of aging in air or distilled water, to determine flexural strength and fracture toughness. The investigators used a staircase approach to determine the cyclic flexural strength. The mean flexural strength for the controls in air and water (without aging or cyclic loading) ranged from 67 to 99 MPa for all the ceramics except for the lithium disilicate–containing ceramic, which was twice as strong, with a mean flexural strength of 191 to 205 MPa. For the mean fracture toughness, the range for the ceramics was generally 1.1 to 1.9 $MPa \cdot m^{0.5}$. The one exception was the lithium disilicate–containing ceramic, which had a mean value of 2.7 $MPa \cdot m^{0.5}$. Testing in water and aging for 3 months caused a moderate reduction in the mean flexural strength (6% to 17%) and a moderate to severe reduction in the mean fracture toughness (5% to 39%). The largest decrease (15% to 60%) in mean flexural strength was observed when the samples were subjected to cyclic loading. The lithium disilicate–containing ceramic had a significantly higher flexural strength and fracture toughness when compared with the four pressable leucite-strengthened ceramics and the low-fusing conventional porce-

lain. All the leucite-containing pressable ceramics provided an increase in mean flexural strength (17% to 19%) and mean fracture toughness (3% to 64%) compared with the conventional feldspathic porcelain.

To limit the susceptibility of ceramics to fracture, the number of surface defects are minimized through coatings (glazing), platinum foil–covered dies, reinforced ceramics, or ion exchange. A study[17] evaluated whether an ion exchange treatment of porcelain bars tested in static and cyclic fatigue in air and water affected the flexural strength. The porcelain bars were divided into two groups; the first group received the ion exchange coating, and the second group was uncoated. The specimens were aged for 12 months in air or distilled water at 37°C and tested in air or distilled water in three-point bending at a displacement rate of 0.5 mm/s. The specimens were cycled until fracture or 1,000 cycles, using a staircase approach. The results indicated that porcelain was weaker in water and cyclic fatigue, and that the ion exchange procedure did significantly increase the flexural strength (static and cyclic). No change in flexural strength was observed for the aging in water. The ion exchange treatment resulted in a 37% to 75% increase in flexural strength, with the greatest increase observed for the treated, aged specimens. Cyclic fatigue–tested specimens were found to have a flexural strength approximately 60% of the static strength.

Scherrer and de Rijk[18] evaluated the fracture resistance of all-ceramic crowns as a function of the elastic modulus of the supporting die. All-ceramic crowns were made for dies with three different elastic moduli and two different crown lengths. The occlusal surface was loaded in compression with a steel ball 12.7 mm in diameter. The fracture load increased markedly with increases in the elastic modulus of the supporting die. The investigators found the largest increase when only the occlusal surface of the crown was covered. The characteristic fracture load of the complete-crown restorations was more than double that of the occlusal-cover restorations in the dies with the lowest elastic modulus; in contrast, for the dies with the highest elastic modulus, the difference in the characteristic fracture load for the two configurations was not significant. Sobrinho et al[19] compared the strengths of crown shapes of different restorative ceramics (Empress, OPC, and In-Ceram) and found a significant decrease after fatiguing in both wet and dry environments.

Azer et al[20] investigated the effects of the use of dental amalgam, resin composite, and dentin as core buildup materials with OPC crowns to restore natural human teeth. The crowns supported by a dentin core showed a mean compressive strength of 22.7 ± 4.5 MPa when tested dry and 19.7 ± 4.7 MPa when tested wet. The dental amalgam core group showed a mean compressive strength of 25.2 ± 5.2 MPa when tested dry and 21.6 ± 6.3 MPa when tested wet. The resin composite core group showed a mean compressive strength of 20.9 ± 4.1 MPa when tested dry and 18.7 ± 4.9 MPa when tested wet. The investigators found no statistically significant difference in the effect of the three core materials on the compressive strength of the OPC crowns, whether tested in air or in water. These findings suggest that the elastic modulus of the core materials (dental amalgam, 52 to 60 GPa; dentin, 14 to 18 GPa; and resin composite, 6 to 16 GPa) may not influence the strength of all-ceramic crowns. In the same study, the mean fracture stress of OPC solid cylinders was $1{,}474 \pm 527$ MPa when tested in air and 794 ± 280 MPa when tested in water. One-way analysis of variance showed a statistically significant difference between the compressive failure load for wet versus dry testing conditions. The diametral tensile stress of the OPC cylinders in water was 42.2 ± 11.1 MPa.

In the same study, for cyclic loading in water, dentin core specimens showed a mean fatigue strength of 9.5 ± 1.5 MPa.[20] Amalgam core specimens showed a mean fatigue strength of 10.3 ± 1.6 MPa, whereas resin composite core specimens showed a mean fatigue strength of 13.3 ± 3.2 MPa. The statistical analysis again showed no significant difference between the cyclic fatigue strength of the three core materials, but it did find a significant difference between the static and cyclic strengths for each material. When the OPC crowns were cycled in water, their mean com-

pressive strength decreased significantly (approximately 44%).

Processing has also been shown to affect the flexural strength of dental ceramics. Giordano et al[21] investigated a feldspathic porcelain, an aluminous porcelain, and a computer-assisted design/computer-assisted manufacture (CAD/CAM) porcelain with as-fired, self-glazed, overglazed, ground, ground/annealed, and polished/annealed surface treatments. Overglazing, grinding, and polishing significantly increased (15% to 30%) the flexural strength (four-point bending) of the tested materials. Another study[22] found a significant correlation between the biaxial flexural strength and surface roughness of dental porcelain: the smoother the surface, the stronger the specimen. The CAD/CAM ceramic disk demonstrated[23] an increase in static biaxial flexural strength and biaxial flexural strength in cyclic fatigue when surface roughness decreased after polishing with pads of smaller diamond grain size (#200 to #1,000).

Alumina Ceramics

Because of the limited mechanical properties of feldspathic porcelain, dental and orthopedic applications have used other ceramics, such as alumina and zirconia. Drummond and Lenke[24] used dense alumina rods (99.9% α-alumina) in studies of steam-autoclaved specimens aged in distilled water and saline solution, as well as in Sprague-Dawley rats. One set of alumina specimens was not autoclaved. Specimens were aged in saline solution (400 mg/L sodium chloride and 190 mg/L potassium chloride) and in distilled water for 175, 367, 549, and 733 days, using 500 mL of the solution in sealed polyethylene containers at 37°C. The four-point bending strength or modulus of rupture (MOR) for autoclaved and nonautoclaved bars showed no significant difference when the test specimens were autoclaved before aging. Aging of the dense alumina for up to 2 years in distilled water or saline solution resulted in a significant decrease (20% to 25%) in the MOR compared with that for the autoclaved controls. The decrease was greatest in the first year, becoming more gradual as the aging time increased. No statistically significant change in the MOR was observed for aging in the Sprague-Dawley rats, which the investigators attributed to the buffering and encapsulating effect of the surrounding tissues, which prevented degradation from water.

More than two decades ago, Avigdor and Brown[25] conducted isothermal static fatigue experiments on porous alumina at three stress levels in distilled water. The rate-controlling reaction was an activated process sensitive to both temperature and applied stress, with the grain boundaries being the most likely sites of reaction. The activation energy (26.6 kcal/mol) for this reaction was found to be stress dependent, as was the activation entropy. Water analysis after the fatigue tests indicated a 25-fold increase in Ca^{2+} ion content and an increase in Si^{4+} ion content from below the detection limit in the original distilled water to a level of 15 ppm. No Al^{3+} ions were detected in the water. Scanning electron microscopic examination of the fracture surfaces of as-fired and fatigued alumina specimens revealed no notable differences.

At about the same time, Rockar and Pletka[26] investigated the fracture mechanics of dense alumina in simulated biologic environments. Although their results indicated more than one failure mechanism or flaw-size distribution, median strength values for dense alumina tested in water, Krebs-Ringer's solution, and bovine serum were not significantly different.

Subsequent research on dense alumina rods showed[27-29] a considerable decrease in MOR when the rods were exposed to steam, 50% steam and 50% carbon monoxide, and other gases at high temperatures and pressures. Examination of the external and fracture surfaces by Auger electron spectroscopy indicated that calcium segregation at or near these surfaces accounted for the decrease in strength, which was more pronounced with an increase in steam pressure.

Dalgleish and Rawlings[30] noted a 9% to 10% reduction in the MOR for three polycrystalline α-aluminas (97.5% to 99.9% purity) when tested in

liquids, compared with testing in air. Osterholm and Day[31] tested a 99.8% α-alumina aged 6, 12, and 23 weeks in vivo in the dorsa of rats and found significant strength reduction only for the bars aged 23 weeks. The MOR of dense alumina aged in deionized water and Ringer's solution at 40°C and 80°C showed an initial rapid decrease for the first 28 days, followed by a leveling or slight increase at longer periods (up to 420 days).[32] Fahr et al[33] aged two commercial orthopedic aluminas up to 52 weeks in simulated body fluids and by subcutaneous implantation in Sprague-Dawley rats, and they found that aging had no significant effect on the flexural strength of either alumina. Ferber and Brown[34] studied subcritical crack growth in dense alumina exposed to physiologic media and found greater stress corrosion in distilled water than in a complex buffered system.

A magnesia-alumina spinel was investigated[35] with respect to aging in air and water. After aging for 12 months, the MOR for testing in air (108.5 ± 16.1 MPa) versus water (96.9 ± 15.0 MPa) differed significantly. Weibull analysis of the data showed no difference between the Weibull constants (7.66 for air and 7.64 for water), but a significant difference between the characteristic strengths (115.2 MPa for air versus 103.0 MPa for water). An investigation[36] of two high-alumina core dental ceramics (Cerestore [Johnson and Johnson Dental Products, East Windsor, NJ] and Vitadur N [Vita Zahnfabrik, Bad Sackingen, Germany]) found a significant decrease in the fracture toughness when these ceramics were tested in water versus air. The investigators observed no significant decrease for testing in an artificial saliva, where values of fracture toughness were similar to those in air.

Single-crystal alumina was evaluated for subcritical crack growth by stress corrosion (static fatigue) and by cyclic fatigue in humid air and Ringer's solution.[37] The crack growth rates were significantly faster at a given stress intensity in Ringer's solution compared with the humid air environment.

Zirconia Ceramics

Compared with alumina, stabilized zirconia has the potential advantages of a lower elastic modulus, higher strength, better wear properties, and higher fracture toughness. At 1,000°C, zirconia undergoes a phase change on cooling from tetragonal to monoclinic, which necessitates stabilization in either the tetragonal or cubic form (the crystal structure at highest temperatures) with the aid of magnesia, yttria, or other additives. The strength degradation associated with this transformation from the tetragonal to the monoclinic phase (the crystal structure at lowest temperatures) has limited the use of high-strength zirconia for low-temperature (25°C to 100°C) applications. The aging of yttria-doped zirconia at 230°C for 400 hours in a water vapor environment resulted in a decrease in flexural strength from 819 ± 21 to 556 ± 67 MPa.[38] When some of these aged specimens were reheated to 1,000°C for 24 hours, the fracture strength in four-point loading increased to 717 ± 61 MPa. Several other studies of annealing zirconia at low temperatures,[39,40] in water,[41,42] in controlled humidity,[43] in hot water,[44] and in air[45] have attributed the decrease in fracture strength and fracture toughness to the formation of cracks on the surface, resulting from the transformation from the tetragonal phase to the monoclinic phase.

Garvie et al[46] aged a calcia-stabilized zirconia of 72% theoretical density in vitro in Ringer's solution for 1, 2, and 4 weeks and in vivo in rabbits for 12 weeks. The bars aged in vitro lost 16, 17, and 19% in fracture strength after 1, 2, and 4 weeks, respectively, and the bars aged in vivo decreased 25% in fracture strength. The investigators observed a 6% loss in strength for partially stabilized magnesia-zirconia after boiling in a 0.9 wt % saline solution for 1,000 hours, and there was no change in strength after aging in rabbits for 1 week and for 1, 3, and 6 months.

Yttria-stabilized zirconia was aged at 37°C in distilled water, saline solution (100 mg of potassium chloride and 4,500 mg of sodium chloride per liter), and Ringer's solution (100 mg of potassium chloride, 4,500 mg of sodium chloride, and 45 mg of calcium chloride per liter) for 140, 304, and 453 days; another set of specimens was aged in air for 730 days.[47] The control samples (not aged) and the samples aged 140 days showed no statistically significant difference. None of the samples aged longer than 140 days (304, 453, and 730 days) was significantly different from the others, but all were significantly different from the controls and from the samples aged 140 days. The aging solution had no significant effect on the MOR tested in four-point loading. The greatest decrease in the MOR occurred between 140 and 304 days. The decrease in strength (13% to 22%) for the yttria-stabilized zirconia was attributed to the tetragonal-to-monoclinic phase change, as reported in other studies for low-temperature annealing. The only difference was that at 37°C, the phase transformation occurred at some time between 140 and 304 days. This finding was supported by the results of the bars aged 730 days in air, which showed the same decrease in strength.

Thompson and Rawlings[48] compared the aging of zirconia-toughened alumina and three tetragonal zirconia polycrystalline ceramics in air and water. For periods up to 19 months, Ringer's solution promoted a surface layer of monoclinic zirconia, and the authors concluded that this strength decrease made the yttria-stabilized toughened alumina and tetragonal zirconia polycrystalline ceramics unsuitable as implant materials. Shimizu et al[49] aged yttria-stabilized zirconia for up to 3 years in 50°C and 95°C saline solutions and found no significant change in flexural strength. They did find that when the flexural strength declined, there was an increase in the amount of monoclinic zirconia on the surface.

Partially stabilized magnesia-zirconia was aged in distilled water for 6, 12, and 18 months.[50] The aging conditions were specimens autoclaved in air or distilled water and nonautoclaved specimens in distilled water, and the displacement rates during testing were 10.0, 1.0, or 0.1 mm/min (a two-decade range in the rate of stress application). The statistical analysis showed no significant difference in strength for the three aging times. The aging time data were then pooled, and a statistical analysis was run between the different aging conditions and rates of loading. The specimens tested in air (417.2 ± 43.6 MPa) were significantly stronger than the autoclaved specimens tested in water (382.6 ± 36.3 MPa) or the nonautoclaved specimens (382.0 ± 42.7 MPa). For the pooled data, all rates of stress application yielded statistically significant differences in strength. Analysis of the data using Weibull statistics demonstrated a higher characteristic strength for the specimens tested in air (437 MPa) versus water (autoclaved, 399 MPa; nonautoclaved, 401 MPa). The Weibull coefficient was essentially the same for each respective group: 10.3, 11.1, or 12.5.

Contact Loading

Contact loading, a new approach in the testing of dental ceramics, has been proposed by Lawn and associates.[51–56] This group used contact loading to investigate porcelain, micaceous glass-ceramic, glass-infiltrated alumina, and yttria-stabilized tetragonal polycrystalline zirconia. The authors showed that cone-crack and quasi-plastic damage modes operate in single-cycle loading, but more deleterious crack systems develop at large numbers of cycles, leading to accelerated failure. These additional crack systems include "radial" cracks associated with advanced quasi-plasticity, analogous to the radial cracks produced in "sharp" contacts. The authors did not observe the radial cracks in comparative static loading, which indicates a strong mechanical (in addition to chemical) component in the cyclic damage. Radial cracks that occur under severe cyclic loading conditions may not be easy to detect by conventional observational techniques. The authors hypothesized that cyclic damage accumulation limits the potentially long-lifetime performance of dental ceramics, because strength after multi-cycle contact damage is significantly lower than after single-cycle damage. They concluded that Hertzian contact tests more closely simulate oral function than do more traditional tests, such as dynamic fatigue, and thereby may provide deeper insights into relevant modes of failure in dental ceramics.

A summary of the contact loading research studies has indicated the following:

1. Contact damage mode analysis for fine-grain, low-toughness dental porcelain found that the fracture mode was conventional Hertzian cone fracture. Fractures in high-crystalline, higher-toughness, coarse-grain ceramics were caused by quasi-plastic deformation.
2. Stress-indentation curves of Hertzian contact damage confirmed the ranking from flexural strength data (ie, micaceous glass-ceramic < porcelain < alumina < zirconia).
3. For cyclic contact tests in dry versus wet environments, and for any given contact load, the strength of a ceramic degraded with an increase in the number of loading cycles. Most ceramic materials degraded significantly between 10,000 to 100,000 cycles. The presence of water enhanced damage accumulation in cyclic indentation.
4. Machining effects were shown to cause surface damage and reduce surface strength but to have only a secondary effect on the initiation and evolution of cone cracking and quasi-plasticity.

Multilayered Ceramics

Jung et al[55] examined the hypothesis that coating thickness and coating-substrate mismatch are key factors in the determination of contact-induced damage in clinically relevant bilayer composites. They designed crack patterns in two model coating-substrate bilayer systems to simulate crown and tooth structures at opposite extremes of elastic/plastic mismatch: porcelain on glass-infiltrated alumina (soft/hard) and glass-ceramic on resin composite (hard/soft). They used Hertzian contacts to investigate the evolution of fracture damage in the coating layers as functions of contact load and coating thickness. The crack patterns differed radically in the two bilayer systems: (1) in the porcelain coatings, cone cracks were initiated at the coating top surface, and (2) in the glass-ceramic coatings, cone cracks again were initiated at the top surface, but additional, upward-extending transverse cracks were initiated at the internal coating-substrate interface, with the latter dominant. The researchers thereby showed that the substrate has a profound influence on the damage evolution, which leads to ultimate failure in the bilayer systems. However, both systems had highly stabilized cracks and wide ranges between the loads required to initiate first cracking and cause final failure, implying damage-tolerant structures.

Thompson[57] examined the influence of testing methods (uniaxial and biaxial) and relative layer heights on the origin and mode of failure in bilayered ceramic composite beams and disks with relative layer heights of 1:2, 1:1, and 2:1, respectively, for In-Ceram and Vitadur Alpha (Vita Zahnfabrik) porcelain. Surface and interfacial failure origins were observed in three-point and biaxial disk test specimens, but not in four-point-bending specimens, where only surface failures occurred. None of the "clinically similar" specimens (1:2) failed at the interface. All testing methods resulted in delamination of Vitadur Alpha from In-Ceram, whereas only the three-point and biaxial disk testing methods resulted in crack propagation through the ceramic composite interface, without delamination. The bilayered material was still no stronger than the core material; the less core component there was, the weaker the material. Observation of different failure modes and failure origins with ceramic testing was dependent on testing methodology, relative layer heights, and very likely, the ceramic system being investigated.

White et al[58] determined the moduli of rupture of layered beams made of strong core materials veneered with weaker conventional feldspathic porcelain. They investigated two systems: (1) Vitadur N, a conventional feldspathic porcelain, and Dicor MGC (Caulk/Dentsply [Milford, DE]), a machinable glass-ceramic, and (2) Vitadur N and In-Ceram, a strong reinforced aluminous porcelain. The results indicated that the modulus of rupture was significantly affected by whether the materials forming the surface were subjected to tensile or compressive force, as well as by the interaction of these materials. The effect on the modulus of rupture of the material forming the surface subjected to tensile force was much greater than that of the material forming the surface subjected to compressive force. Theoretical curves describing the effects of the elastic moduli of the layers and their thickness on the force-bearing capacity of model beams indicated that for a wide range of thickness ratios and a wide variety of elastic modulus ratios, the material subjected to tensile force dominates the load-bearing capacity of layered beams, except when a material of much lower elastic modulus forms the layer subjected to compressive force. The authors concluded that layered prostheses made of strong cores veneered with weaker feldspathic porcelain may be prone to failure when the feldspathic porcelain surfaces are subjected to tensile force.

Wakabayashi and Anusavice[59] hypothesized that the fracture resistance of alumina core–porcelain veneer disks increased and that crack initiation shifted from veneer to core as the core-to-veneer thickness ratio increased from 0.5:1.0 to 1.3:0.2, or as the elastic modulus of the supporting substrate to which it was resin bonded increased from 5.1 to 226 GPa. When supported by a substrate of low elastic modulus, disks with low core-to-veneer thickness ratios exhibited cracks in the veneer and within the core, whereas disks with high core-to-veneer thickness ratios demonstrated core cracks but not veneer cracks. The investigators found that as the elastic modulus of the metal substrate increased, there was an increase in the load to cause failure, but no change in fracture origin. As the thickness ratio of ceramic core to veneer increased, the site of crack initiation shifted from the veneer porcelain to the core porcelain. The mean fracture strength increased as the core-to-veneer thickness ratio increased, but it did not exceed that of the core material.

Tsai et al[60] evaluated the influence of ceramic thickness on fracture mechanisms and found that as the thickness of the ceramic increased, the failure stress increased up to a thickness of 1.6 mm or greater, as well as that disks supported by a simulated dentin substrate had fractures initiated within the inner surface. Also, the failure loads required to produce Hertzian fracture were 50% to 200% greater than those required to produce fractures within the inner surface. The ceramic thicknesses evaluated ranged from 0.4 to 2.4 mm.

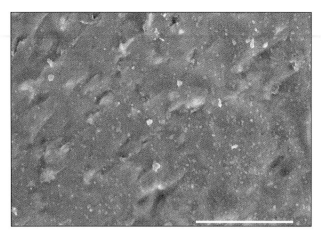

Fig 3-1 Fracture surface of a conventional porcelain (Finesse) (bar = 20 μm).

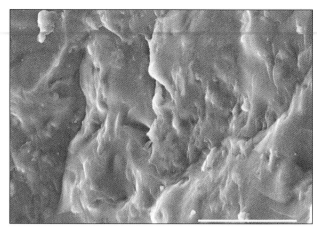

Fig 3-2 Fracture surface of a pressable porcelain (OPC) (bar = 20 μm).

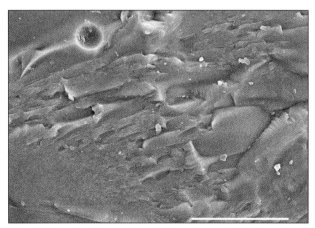

Fig 3-3 Fracture surface of a pressable porcelain (Empress) (bar = 20 μm).

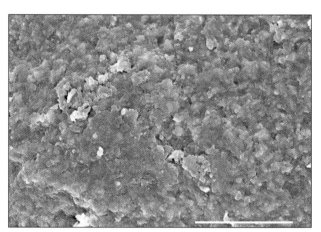

Fig 3-4 Fracture surface of lithium disilicate dental ceramic (bar = 20 μm).

Fracture Surfaces

The fracture surfaces of the ceramic materials discussed above differ considerably. Representative fracture surfaces are presented in Figs 3-1 to 3-9. Figure 3-1 shows a conventional porcelain (Finesse), characterized by a glassy, relatively smooth fracture surface. The pressable porcelains, OPC and Empress (see Figs 3-2 and 3-3), have slightly rougher fracture surfaces than the conventional porcelain, but the increase in fracture strength (17% to 19%) is minimal compared with the conventional porcelain. This increased strength is attributed to slightly more crystals of leucite and more uniform distribution of these crystals.

The experimental ceramic containing lithium disilicate has almost twice the strength of conventional porcelain (see Fig 3-4), partially because of a different composition and a more uniform and smaller grain size. Figure 3-5 shows the microstructure of In-Ceram, currently the strongest dental ceramic. The fracture surface is a mixture of large and small grains of alumina within the infiltrated glassy matrix. Cerestore (see Fig 3-6) is a magnesia-alumina spinel that had a short market life because its fracture strength was just slightly higher than conventional porcelain. As seen in the micrograph, this multicomponent material had a relatively large amount of porosity.

Figure 3-7 shows a dense alumina with very distinct grains and a rough fracture surface. This

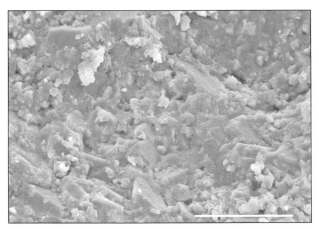

Fig 3-5 Fracture surface of In-Ceram (bar = 20 μm).

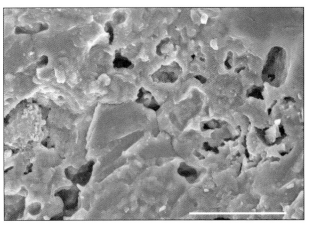

Fig 3-6 Fracture surface of Cerestore (bar = 20 μm).

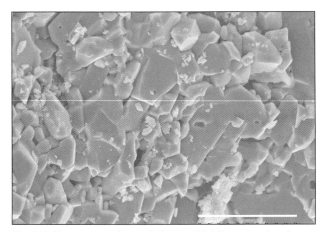

Fig 3-7 Fracture surface of dense, 99.9% α-alumina (bar = 20 μm).

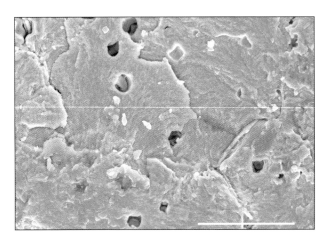

Fig 3-8 Fracture surface of magnesia-stabilized zirconia (bar = 20 μm).

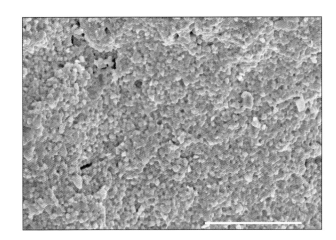

Fig 3-9 Fracture surface of yttria-stabilized zirconia (bar = 20 μm).

99.9% α-alumina, manufactured in the early 1980s, has a larger grain size than alumina dental ceramics manufactured today. Figure 3-8 (magnesia-stabilized zirconia [Zircon, Solon, OH]) and Fig 3-9 (yttria-stabilized zirconia [TZ-120, Batch 16089-57-1, AC Spark Plug, Flint, MI]) represent the ceramics with the highest fracture toughness and flexural strength. Their fracture patterns are completely different, even though both materials are composed of more than 90% zirconia. The magnesia-stabilized zirconia has a smoother fracture surface and is more porous than the yttria-stabilized zirconia, which has a rougher fracture surface and a smaller grain size.

Conclusions

Dental ceramic materials provide excellent esthetic results and have seen increasingly widespread clinical use. Their use is limited, however, by their susceptibility to subcritical crack growth and loss of strength when placed in a moist environment. Current research is investigating newer ceramic materials to take advantage of their strengths and minimize their weaknesses. The ultimate goal is to allow the use of dental ceramics throughout the entire oral cavity.

References

1. Kelly JR. Ceramics in restorative and prosthetic dentistry. Annu Rev Mater Sci 1997;27:443–468.
2. Kelly JR. Clinically relevant approach to failure testing of all-ceramic restorations. J Prosthet Dent 1999;81:652–661.
3. Drummond JL. Degradation of ceramic materials in physiological media. In: Rubin LR (ed). Biomaterials in Reconstructive Surgery. St. Louis: Mosby, 1983:273–280.
4. Evans AG. Slow crack growth in brittle materials under dynamic loading conditions. Int J Fract Mech 1974;10:251–259.
5. Evans AG, Johnson H. The fracture stress and its dependence on slow crack growth. J Mater Sci 1975;10:214–222.
6. Wiederhorn SM. Moisture assisted crack growth in ceramics. Int J Fracture Mech 1968;4:171–177.
7. Wiederhorn SM. Subcritical crack growth in ceramics. In: Bradt R, Hasselman DP, Lange FF (eds). Fracture Mechanics of Ceramics, vol 2. New York: Plenum Press, 1974:613–646.
8. Craig RG (ed). Restorative Dental Materials, ed 9. St. Louis: Mosby, 1993:54–55.
9. Anusavice KJ. Phillips' Science of Dental Materials, ed 10. Philadelphia: Saunders, 1996:65–66.
10. Campbell SD. A comparative strength study of metal ceramic and all-ceramic esthetic materials: Modulus of rupture. J Prosthet Dent 1989;62:476–479.
11. Morena R, Beaudreau GM, Lockwood PE, Evans AL, Fairhurst CW. Fatigue of dental ceramics in a simulated oral environment. J Dent Res 1986;65:993–997.
12. Myers ML, Ergle JW, Fairhurst CW, Ringle RD. Fatigue failure parameters of IPS-Empress porcelain. Int J Prosthodont 1994;7:549–553.
13. Ohyama T, Yoshinari M, Oda Y. Effects of cyclic loading on the strength of all-ceramic materials. Int J Prosthodont 1999;12:28–37.
14. Fairhurst CW, Lockwood PE, Ringle RD, Twiggs SW. Dynamic fatigue of feldspathic porcelain. Dent Mater 1993;9:269–273.
15. White SN, Li ZC, Yu Z, Kipnis V. Relationship between static chemical and cyclic mechanical fatigue in a feldspathic porcelain. Dent Mater 1997;13:103–110.
16. Drummond JL, King TJ, Bapna MS, Koperski RD. Mechanical property evaluation of pressable restorative ceramics. Dent Mater 2000;16:226–233.
17. Drummond JL, Van Scoyoc JP, Racean DC. Aging of ion exchanged porcelain. In: Fischman G, Clare A, Hench L (eds). Bioceramics: Materials and Applications, vol 48, Ceramic Transactions Series. [Proceedings of the Biomedical and Biological Applications of Ceramics and Glass Symposium, 1994, Indianapolis, IN]. Westerville, OH: American Ceramic Society, 1995:191–200.
18. Scherrer SS, de Rijk WG. The fracture resistance of all-ceramic crowns on supporting structures with different elastic moduli. Int J Prosthodont 1993;6:462–467.
19. Sobrinho LC, Cattell MJ, Glover RH, Knowles JC. Investigation of the dry and wet fatigue properties of three all-ceramic crown systems. Int J Prosthodont 1998;11:255–262.
20. Azer SS, Drummond JL, Campbell SD, El Moneim Zaki AM. Influence of core buildup material on the fatigue strength of an all-ceramic crown. J Prosthet Dent 2001;86:624–631.
21. Giordano R, Cima M, Pober R. Effect of surface finish on the flexural strength of feldspathic and aluminous dental ceramics. Int J Prosthodont 1995;8:311–319.
22. de Jager N, Feilzer AJ, Davidson CL. The influence of surface roughness on porcelain strength. Dent Mater 2000;16:381–388.
23. Nakazato T, Takahashi H, Yamamoto M, Nishimura F, Kurosaki N. Effect of polishing on cyclic fatigue strength of CAD/CAM ceramics. Dent Mater 1999;18:395–402.
24. Drummond JL, Lenke JW. Aging of dense alumina. Adv Ceram Mater 1988;3:159–161.
25. Avigdor D, Brown SD. Delayed failure of a porous alumina. J Am Ceram Soc 1978;61:97–99.

26. Rockar EM, Pletka BJ. Fracture mechanics of alumina in a simulated biological environment. Presented at the 2nd International Symposium on Fracture Mechanics of Ceramics, Pennsylvania State University, July 1977.

27. Sinharoy S, Levenson LL, Ballard VV, Day DE. Surface segregation of calcium in dense alumina exposed to steam and steam-CO. Ceram Bull 1978;57:231–233.

28. Wistrom KW, Day DE. Chemical reactivity of calcium aluminate cement bond phases in a steam-CO atmosphere at 199°C. Ceram Bull 1978;57:680–684.

29. Ballard VV, Day DE. Stability of the refractory-bond phases in high alumina refractories in steam-CO atmospheres. Ceram Bull 1978;57:660–666.

30. Dalgleish J, Rawlings RD. A comparison of the mechanical behavior of the aluminas in air and simulated body environments. J Biomed Mater Res 1981;15:527–542.

31. Osterholm HH, Day DE. Dense alumina aged in vivo. Am Ceram Soc Bull 1981;15:279–288.

32. Sinharoy S, Levenson LL, Day DE. Influence of calcium migration on the strength reduction of dense alumina exposed to steam. Am Ceram Soc Bull 1979;58:64–66.

33. Fahr A, Brown RF, Day DE. In vivo and in vitro aging of orthopedic aluminas. J Biomed Mater Res 1983;17:395–410.

34. Ferber MK, Brown SD. Subcritical crack growth in dense alumina exposed to physiological media. J Am Ceram Soc 1980;63:424–429.

35. Drummond JL, Novickas D, Lenke JW. Physiological aging of an all-ceramic restorative material. Dent Mater 1991;7: 133–137.

36. Mante FK, Brantley WA, Dhuru VB, Ziebert GJ. Fracture toughness of high alumina core dental ceramics: The effect of water and artificial saliva. Int J Prosthodont 1993; 6:546–552.

37. Asoo B, McNaney JM, Mitamura Y, Ritchie RO. Cyclic fatigue-crack propagation in sapphire in air and simulated physiological environments. J Biomed Mater Res 2000;52: 488–491.

38. Matsumoto RLK. Strength recovery in degraded yttria-doped tetragonal zirconia polycrystals. J Am Ceram Soc 1985;68:C213.

39. Sato T, Shimada M. Crystalline phase change in yttria-partially-stabilized zirconia by low-temperature annealing. J Am Ceram Soc 1984;67:C212–C313.

40. Sato T, Ohtaki S, Shimada M. Transformation of yttria partially stabilized zirconia by low temperature annealing in air. J Mater Sci 1985;20:1466–1470.

41. Sato T, Shimada M. Transformation of ceria-doped tetragonal zirconia polycrystals by annealing in water. Am Ceram Soc Bull 1985;64:1382–1384.

42. Sato T, Shimada M. Transformation of yttria-doped tetragonal ZrO_2 polycrystals by annealing in water. J Am Ceram Soc 1985;68:356–359.

43. Sato T, Ohtaki S, Endo T, Shimada M. Transformation of yttria-doped tetragonal ZrO_2 polycrystals by annealing under controlled humidity conditions. J Am Ceram Soc 1985;68: C320–C322.

44. Sato T, Shimada M. Control of the tetragonal-to-monoclinic phase transformation of yttria partially stabilized zirconia in hot water. J Mater Sci 1985;20:3988–3992.

45. Kenner GH, Pasco WD, Frakes JT, Brown SD. Mechanical properties of calcia stabilized zirconia following in vivo and in vitro aging. J Biomed Mater Res 1975;6:63–66.

46. Garvie RC, Urbani C, Kennedy DR, McNeuer JC. Biocompatibility of magnesia-partially stabilized zirconia (Mg-PSZ) ceramics. J Mater Sci 1984;19:3224–3228.

47. Drummond JL. In vitro aging of yttria stabilized zirconia. J Am Ceram Soc 1989;72:675–676.

48. Thompson I, Rawlings RD. Mechanical behaviour of zirconia and zirconia-toughened alumina in a simulated body environment. Biomaterials 1990;11:505–508.

49. Shimizu K, Oka M, Kumar P, et al. Time-dependent changes in the mechanical properties of zirconia ceramic. J Biomed Mater Res 1993;27:729–734.

50. Drummond JL. In vitro aging of magnesia stabilized zirconia. J Am Ceram Soc 1992;75:1278–1280.

51. Peterson IM, Pajares A, Lawn BR, Thompson VP, Rekow ED. Mechanical characterization of dental ceramics by Hertzian contacts. J Dent Res 1998;77:589–602.

52. Peterson IM, Wuttiphan S, Lawn BR, Chyung K. Role of microstructure on contact damage and strength degradation of micaceous glass-ceramics. Dent Mater 1998;14:80–89.

53. Jung YG, Peterson IM, Pajares A, Lawn BR. Contact damage resistance and strength degradation of glass-infiltrated alumina and spinel ceramics. J Dent Res 1999;78:804–814.

54. Kim DK, Jung YJ, Peterson IM, Lawn BR. Cyclic fatigue of intrinsically brittle ceramics in contact with spheres. Acta Mater 1999;99:1–15.

55. Jung YG, Wuttiphan S, Peterson IM, Lawn BR. Damage modes in dental layer structures. J Dent Res 1999;78: 887–897.

56. Jung YG, Peterson IM, Kim DK, Lawn BR. Lifetime-limiting strength degradation from contact fatigue in dental ceramics. J Dent Res 2000;79:722–731.

57. Thompson GA. Influence of relative layer height and testing method on the failure mode and origin in a bilayered dental ceramic composite. Dent Mater 2000;16:235–243.

58. White SN, Caputo AA, Vidjak FMA, Seghi RR. Moduli of rupture of layered dental ceramics. Dent Mater 1994;10:52–58.

59. Wakabayashi N, Anusavice KJ. Crack initiation modes in bilayered alumina/porcelain disks as a function of core/veneer thickness ratio and supporting substrate stiffness. J Dent Res 2000;79:1398–1404.

60. Tsai YL, Petsche PE, Anusavice KJ, Yang MC. Influence of glass-ceramic thickness on Hertzian and bulk fracture mechanisms. Int J Prosthodont 1998;11:27–32.

4

CHARACTERIZATION OF RETRIEVED IMPLANTS: TITANIUM, TITANIUM ALLOYS, AND HYDROXYAPATITE COATINGS

Efstratios Papazoglou, DDS, MS, PhD

William A. Brantley, PhD

Edwin A. McGlumphy, DDS, MS

The successful osseointegration of dental implants involves intimate adaptation and attachment of the surrounding bone to the implant. The success of this implant-bone connection dates from the pioneering studies of Brånemark and his associates[1-3] and has resulted in the widespread clinical use of implants. Because of the successful fabrication and osseointegration of the attached prostheses, dental implants are expected to be largely permanent restorations, as implied by current publications that report their long-term performance.[4,5] Dental implants can successfully replace a single tooth (Fig 4-1), multiple teeth (Fig 4-2), or an entire arch of missing teeth (Fig 4-3). However, implants and implant-supported superstructures are not immune to environmental abuse, design defects, treatment-planning defects, and materials limitations. The complications associated with long-term use of implant-supported restorations usually are of biologic origin or arise from biomechanical overload. Sometimes it is not clear whether biologic or mechanical factors initiated the problem. Other problems, such as wear and fatigue, are associated with the materials used for the construction of the dental implants and restorations.

This chapter characterizes retrieved dental implants, with an emphasis on the effects of the oral environment on the implant materials. To provide background for readers unfamiliar with this field, the following sections present the criteria for dental implant success, describe the possible biologic and mechanical complications of implants, and summarize the composition and properties of the implant materials commonly used today. Many textbooks describe the different types of dental implants, their clinical placement, and factors contributing to their success or failure.[6-9]

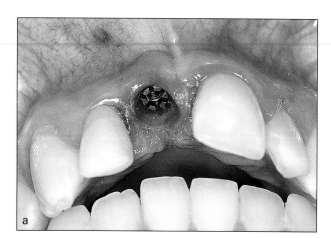
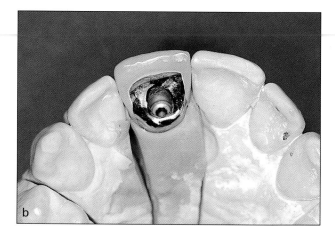

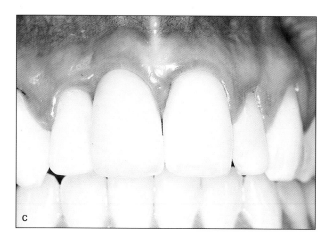

Fig 4-1 Implant replacing a single tooth. *(a)* Maxillary central incisor area for single-tooth implant. *(b)* Crown prepared in the dental laboratory to screw onto the single-tooth implant in *(a)*. *(c)* Single-implant crown screwed into place.

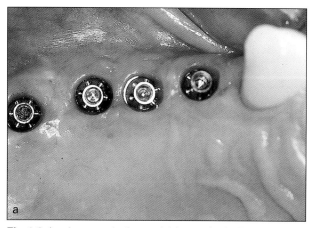
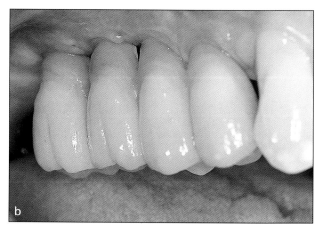

Fig 4-2 Implants replacing multiple teeth. *(a)* Four implants positioned in the posterior maxilla to accept a multiple-unit fixed partial denture. *(b)* Posterior fixed partial denture screwed into place.

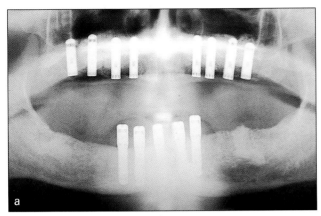
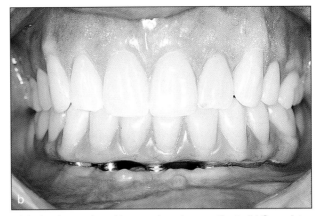

Fig 4-3 Implants replacing an entire arch of missing teeth. *(a)* Multiple implants placed in an edentulous patient. *(b)* Complete-arch implant restoration.

Dental Implants: Background Information

Criteria for Success of Dental Implants

Success criteria for dental implants were defined initially at the 1978 National Institutes of Health Consensus Conference[10] and later by Albrektsson et al[11] and by Smith and Zarb.[12] Current success criteria[13] include the following: clinical stability for an unsplinted implant; radiographic evidence of minimal bone loss; absence of pain, gingival inflammation, damage to surrounding tissues, and nerve damage; and satisfactory prosthetic rehabilitation. Conventional periodontal parameters (plaque index, gingival index, probing depth, and bleeding index) are not considered as important in implant success. Although analogous criteria for implant-supported restorations have not been published, such restorations obviously can be considered successful if they are intact and functioning properly.

Biologic Complications of Implants

Some bone loss occurs during the first year after implant placement, but in subsequent years a steady state exists, with minimal bone loss.[14] Well-controlled clinical studies are needed to determine the relative importance of various con-

tributions to early bone loss.[15] The etiologic factors associated with progressive bone loss around dental implants, or peri-implantitis, are bacterial infections and biomechanical overload. Plaque control is considered very important for individuals with implants, who are usually placed on a 3- to 6-month recall schedule. Clinical studies have shown that plaque accumulates around implants, and inflammation then can occur.[16,17] However, this condition may not be as destructive as it would be for teeth, and it may not increase periodontal probing depths or induce bone resorption. The microbial flora around teeth and implants differ between totally edentulous and partially edentulous individuals, and it is not clear if patients with a history of periodontal disease are predisposed to peri-implant pathologic conditions.

Mechanical Complications of Implants: Bone Resorption and Mechanical Failure

Biomechanical overloading—premature loading or repeated overloading—has been implicated in bone loss around endosseous implants.[18–20] Frost[21] described the compact bone adaptation to strain and distinguished four microstrain zones: the pathologic overload zone, the mild overload zone, the adapted window, and the acute disuse window. Pathologic overload causes microfractures and results in bone loss. Insufficient bone strain in the disuse zone decreases bone mass as well.

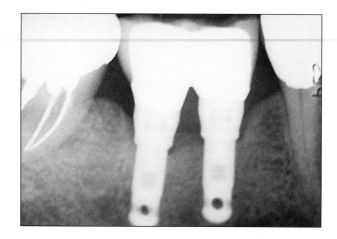

Fig 4-4 An unfavorable crown-to-root ratio can cause excessive leverage. Note beginning bone loss around short implants with long crowns.

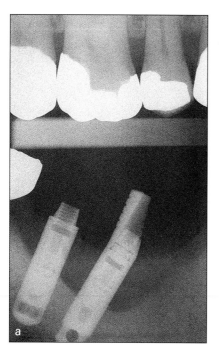

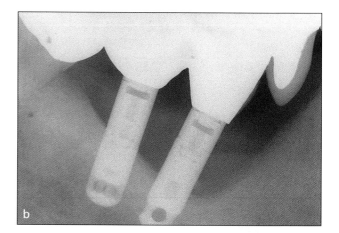

Fig 4-5 *(a)* Short implants placed at unfavorable angles in relation to the occlusal plane. *(b)* Without a third implant in this clinical situation, excessive cantilever forces can be generated, which may cause bone loss.

Bone surrounding an osseointegrated implant responds to strain by remodeling. This process of bone resorption and formation at the same site replaces existing bone. During remodeling, bone is less mineralized and thus weaker. The geometric design[22] and the bioactivity of the implant surface[23] affect the bone-remodeling rate. If the remodeling rate is high, as in Frost's mild overload zone,[21] the bone in proximity to the implant is immature; it is less organized and mineralized (woven bone). Lower remodeling rates, as in Frost's adapted window zone,[21] are more advan-

tageous biomechanically, because they create bone that is more mineralized and stronger, and thus has better load-bearing potential (lamellar bone).

A retrospective study[24] reported the fracture of 3.75-mm-diameter threaded implants fabricated from commercially pure (CP) titanium and noted that fracture was preceded by screw loosening. (The compositions and properties of CP titanium will be discussed in the next section on dental implant materials.) The study noted that although implant fracture is a major cause of clinical failure after long periods of time in vivo, threaded titanium screw–type implants rarely lose osseointegration after the first year.

Implant screw loosening, implant fracture, or bone loss may have many causes. Factors may include misfit of the screw-retained prosthetic framework, excessive occlusal forces, poor design of the prosthesis causing excessive leverage (Fig 4-4), an unfavorable number or angle of implants (Fig 4-5), and parafunctional activities. Interested readers may consult a review article[25] that describes practical methods for preventing screw loosening in dental implants. If screw loosening does occur, the practitioner should address the underlying etiology rather than merely retightening the screw.

A recent in vitro study[26] of hexed gold alloy implant prosthetic screws obtained from two major manufacturers found significant differences in fracture load, microhardness, microstructure, and alloy composition. The authors of this study suggest that variability in the properties of similar hexed screws from different manufacturers, or even from different lots from the same manufacturer, may affect the clinical success of implants.

Observations of clinically retrieved implants[27–29] reveal characteristic fracture patterns[30] that are representative of the functional loading in the oral environment. These observations will be discussed in the section on characterization of retrieved implants. The possibility that bending overload (cantilever load magnification) leads to failure of certain implant prosthesis configurations subjected to heavy occlusal forces or bruxism has been discussed.[31]

Dental Implant Materials

Titanium dental implants

Dental implants can be fabricated from many types of materials, some of which are illustrated in Fig 4-6. This section focuses on properties and compositions of CP titanium and the titanium-aluminium-vanadium (Ti-6Al-4V) alloy used for endosseous dental implants. Prosthesis frameworks have been fabricated from cobalt-chromium, high-palladium, and gold alloys, and articles describing these materials and their properties can be found using the PubMed search engine for the

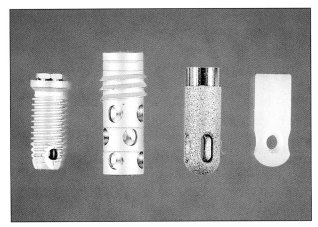

Fig 4-6 Examples of implant types and materials. *Left to right:* CP titanium screw, titanium alloy basket implant, titanium plasma–sprayed cylinder implant, and hydroxyapatite-coated implant.

National Library of Medicine of the National Institutes of Health (www.ncbi.nlm.nih.gov/PubMed). There are reports on the elongation and preload stress for gold and titanium abutment screws[32] and on the dynamic fatigue of the fastened implant–abutment interface,[33,34] but detailed mechanical property information for the screws is not available. Rambhia et al[26] described compositions for gold screws from two manufacturers, Implant Innovations and Nobel Biocare.

The original successful use of CP titanium for dental implants by Brånemark and associates[1–3] was a consequence of the excellent biocompatibility of this alloy, which is associated with its passivating titanium oxide surface film.[35] Albrektsson et al[36] originally described the electron microscopic appearance of the interface between titanium and bone as consisting of a proteoglycan layer 20 to 40 nm thick adjacent to the titanium oxide, followed by a region of collagen filaments and collagen bundles extending to approximately 100 nm from the interface, and then a fibrous tissue–free boundary zone. Klinger et al[37] described an alternative model in which titanium surfaces cause rapid degradation of a hyaluronan meshwork formed during the wound-healing response; they proposed that the adhesive strength of the collagen-free zone is provided by a bilayer of decorin proteoglycans that are tightly held by their overlapping glycosaminoglycan chains. The thickness, micropore configurations, surface roughness, crystal structure, and chemical composition of oxides on milled and electrochemically oxidized CP titanium implants recently have been reported.[38]

Researchers are exploring ingenious strategies to modify the surface titanium oxide to improve osseointegration. For example, one investigation[39] has employed surface treatment with a mixture of sulfuric acid and hydrogen peroxide to create a consistent oxide, followed by covalently bonding an intermediary aminoalkylsilane spacer molecule and then covalently bonding biologic molecules (alkaline phosphatase or albumin) to the free terminal NH_2 groups, using glutaraldehyde as a coupling agent.

There are four grades of CP titanium, classified under ASTM International (formerly American Society for Testing and Materials) Standard F67. From grade 1 to grade 4, the allowed amount of nitrogen in the alloy increases from 0.03% to 0.05%; the amount of oxygen, from 0.18% to 0.40%; and the amount of iron, from 0.20% to 0.50%. The allowed limits of carbon and hydrogen for all four grades are 0.10% and 0.015%, respectively (all values in wt %). The nitrogen, oxygen, carbon, and hydrogen atoms are located at interstitial sites within the hexagonal close-packed α-phase crystal structure of CP titanium, increasing yield strength and decreasing ductility.[40] From ASTM Standard F136, minimum allowed values for 0.2% yield strength increase from 240 MPa for grade 1 to 485 MPa for grade 4 CP titanium, whereas minimum allowed values for percentage elongation decrease from 24% for grade 1 to 15% for grade 4.[41]

Ti-6Al-4V has a duplex α-β microstructure at room temperature, because vanadium is a stabilizing element for the elevated-temperature body-centered cubic β-phase of titanium, which transforms to the α-phase at approximately 882°C for the pure metal; aluminum is a stabilizing element for the α-phase.[40] This alloy is substantially stronger and less ductile than CP titanium, with minimum values of 795 MPa for 0.2% yield strength and 10% for percentage elongation (ASTM Standard F136). This standard allows

maximum impurity contents (wt %) of 0.05% for nitrogen, 0.08% for carbon, 0.0125% for hydrogen, 0.25% for iron, and 0.25% for oxygen, with a tolerance of ±0.5% in the percentages of aluminum and vanadium.

Manufacturers can substantially modify the duplex microstructure of Ti-6Al-4V, depending on whether the alloy is cast or wrought and the processing regimen. As a consequence, the mechanical properties of Ti-6Al-4V alloys, including the fatigue life under cyclic loading conditions, can change significantly.[42] No studies of fatigue strength for dental implants fabricated entirely from wrought Ti-6Al-4V alloys have been reported in published articles, and no significant fatigue failure problems are observed clinically with the use of these dental implants.

Because of concerns and controversies about the relationship between aluminum and Alzheimer's disease,[43–46] the biocompatibility of Ti-6Al-4V dental implants has been questioned. No differences were reported[47,48] for CP titanium and Ti-6Al-4V surfaces with regard to the adaptation, growth, or morphology of fibroblasts, osteoblasts, or epithelial cells, although some studies[49,50] suggested that the differentiation of bone marrow cells harvested from rats was affected by exposure to solutions of ions representing Ti-6Al-4V. Particles of Ti-6Al-4V (simulating wear of joint-replacement prostheses) stimulated a significantly higher level of Prostaglandin E_2 release compared with CP titanium, as well as more release of IL-1, IL-6, and tumor necrosis factor.[51] Although neither Ti-6Al-4V nor CP titanium exhibited significant toxicity, the authors noted that the levels of inflammatory mediators released by phagocytic cells might influence the amount of bone loss.

Another study[52] that tested aqueous extracts of titanium, aluminum, and vanadium in phosphate-buffered saline solutions on polymorphonuclear leukocytes (PMNs) found that aluminum and vanadium increased the generation of reactive oxygen species by the PMNs, whereas signals not significantly different from unstimulated PMNs were found for titanium. Other investigators[53] measured blood levels of titanium, aluminum, and vanadium by atomic absorption spectrophotometry over 3 years in patients with endosseous implants. Although they found no change from preoperative levels, the investigators noted that their methodology could not detect local or remote accumulation of released ions.

Studies have found that surface roughness and texture can affect cell attachment to CP titanium and Ti-6Al-4V[54,55] and that surface treatment of Ti-6Al-4V can influence osteoblast proliferation and alkaline phosphatase activity[56]; the latter investigation suggested that the release of aluminum and vanadium ions may have an important effect. Another concern is the possibility of increased ion release from galvanically coupled superstructures on titanium dental implants. However, a recent in vitro study[57] found that the corrosion rates were very low for several superstructures with CP titanium and Ti-6Al-4V.

Hydroxyapatite coatings on titanium dental implants

The pure synthetic form of calcium hydroxylapatite (generally termed *hydroxyapatite*, or *HA*) has the chemical formula $Ca_{10}(PO_4)_6(OH)_2$. Biologic HA is the principal inorganic constituent of hard tissues in humans (tooth enamel and cortical bone) and, as such, would be the most biocompatible implant material. However, biologic HA is calcium deficient and nonstoichiometric, and it may contain trace inorganic elements.[58]

For more than 15 years, manufacturers have marketed endosseous dental implants in which HA is plasma-sprayed onto a titanium substrate.[59,60] Plasma-sprayed calcium phosphate coatings were found to significantly reduce in vitro ion release from the underlying Ti-6Al-4V substrate.[61] Coating thicknesses for two representative commercial products are approximately 70 μm,[62] which appears to be a compromise to prevent both the development of excessive interfacial stresses in thicker coatings and the premature resorption in thinner coatings. Current plasma-spraying technology appears to yield coatings that closely match the lattice parameters of HA[63] without the presence of the other crystalline calcium phosphates previously observed.[64] An amorphous calcium phosphate phase present in the coatings is more rapidly resorbed than crystalline HA.[63]

The HA coating–titanium substrate bond is considered to be primarily mechanical,[65] although interfacial interdiffusion during plasma spraying has been reported.[62,65,66] Differences in the limited interdiffusion in these studies can be attributed to the use of commercial implants[62,66] instead of laboratory specimens,[65] as well as to differing conditions during the coating process. The surface of the HA coatings is highly textured,[62,66] but examination of cross-sectioned specimens show[66] that surface porosity resulting from the incomplete coalesce of splat deposition regions during plasma-spraying did not extend through the bulk coating.

Recent studies[67,68] have investigated the fatigue behavior of Ti-6Al-4V with plasma-sprayed HA coatings. Coating thicknesses ranging from 25 to 100 μm were found to have no effect on the fatigue life of HA-coated Ti-6Al-4V, although a thickness of 150 μm reduced the fatigue life.[67] A 90-hour postdeposition annealing treatment at 400°C in air resulted in significant recovery of the crystalline HA structure in the plasma-deposited coating, but it significantly reduced the fatigue life of HA-coated Ti-6Al-4V.[68]

Substantial controversy has surrounded the use of plasma-sprayed HA coatings on titanium dental implants[62] because of concerns that the surface texture might harbor microorganisms that could cause periodontal disease or that resorption of the coating might cause implant failure. However, a recent investigation[69] that examined the results of 11 published clinical studies that met criteria for inclusion in a meta-analysis of the outcomes for HA-coated implants did not find decreasing yearly-interval survival rates with increasing numbers of years of follow-up. Thus, this detailed analysis of clinical trials did not show that the use of HA-coated titanium implants compromises long-term clinical survival. Nonetheless, because of these anecdotal concerns about plasma-sprayed HA-coated dental implants, many manufacturers offer titanium dental implants with titanium plasma–sprayed (TPS) coatings or acid-etched surfaces. Holloway and colleagues[70,71] employed an ingenious marker block technique to show that the mean number of cycles for fatigue failure was significantly higher for TPS-coated CP titanium compared with HA-coated CP titanium and uncoated CP titanium controls, which were not significantly different from each other.

Characterization of Retrieved Dental Implants

Numerous studies have investigated retrieved implants, but the major focus has been on histologic observation rather than on materials science characterization of the in vivo failures and the effects of the oral environment on the implant materials. The first part of this section describes some failure analysis observations for metallic implants, and the second part summarizes the reported changes in implant materials after in vivo use. The majority of recent articles have focused on plasma-sprayed HA-coated implants.

Examination of a fractured titanium prosthetic screw showed that crack initiation occurred at the root of the thread under shear loading and that subsequent propagation into the inner section of the screw caused implant failure.[27] In a comparison of the hydrogen content of as-received screws and the fractured screw, gas chromatography established that the titanium prosthetic screw had absorbed hydrogen from the oral environment. The authors suggest that this hydrogen absorption might have contributed to the implant failure, although corroborating studies of clinically fractured titanium abutment screws are necessary to support this hypothesis.

Our clinical observations suggest that dental implant fracture occurs near the end of the abutment stabilization screw (Fig 4-7), where stresses from cantilever bending are highest, and that a specific bone loss pattern occurs in these cases. We have observed striations on the screw fracture surface (Fig 4-8) that are characteristic of fatigue fracture in metals.[30] Each striation represents the movement of the advancing crack front during a single loading-unloading cycle. Other investigators[28,29] have reported similar fatigue striations on the fracture surfaces of clinically failed dental implants. The occurrence of fatigue failure in

dental implants is plausible because of the cyclic loading conditions in vivo and the long-term failure process, and the role of the implant design (holes) in the failure has been noted.[72,73] At present, it is not clear whether bone loss occurs because of biomechanical overload and then the implant fractures because of fatigue failure, or whether an initial infective process causes the observed pattern of bone loss, which worsens the crown-to-implant support ratio and causes a fatigue fracture. This area is important for future fundamental studies of failure in dental implants.

Aparicio and Olive[74] examined 11 Brånemark (CP titanium) implants retrieved after as long as 20 months in patients' mouths; the implants had been retrieved either because they initially failed to integrate or subsequently lost osseointegration. For these retrieved implants, the investigators found no significant differences in surface topography using scanning electron microscopy, and x-ray microanalysis yielded very similar compositions for the outermost layers compared with two control specimens that had not been implanted. Auger electron spectroscopy indicated considerable increases in the carbon and silicon content of the outermost atomic layers of the retrieved implants. The authors noted that this increase could have resulted from handling or surface cleaning, and they commented that in any case, there was some doubt with the long-term prognosis for retrieved implants that were reused clinically.

In a subsequent study, Esposito et al[75] examined failed Brånemark implants that exhibited a lack of osseointegration after longer periods because of clinical mobility. Ten implants were retrieved before loading (early failure), and 12 additional implants were retrieved after functioning for up to 8 years in patients' mouths. On radiographs, all these late failures exhibited peri-implant radiolucency, and the investigators considered no implant failure to result from peri-implantitis. They considered possible reasons for the implant failures to be impaired healing, asymptomatic infection, and biomechanical overload rather than any factors related to materials. Depth profiling using Auger electron spectroscopy indicated that the oxide thickness on the failed implants was in the same range (5 to 8 nm) expected for normal

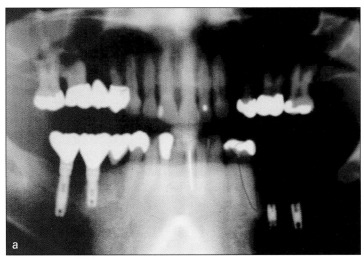
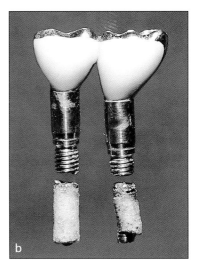

Fig 4-7 Dental implant fractures. *(a)* Panoramic radiograph showing remaining portion of fractured implants in bone. *(b)* Fractured implant prostheses corresponding to *(a)*. The bottom portions of the fractured implants have been retrieved.

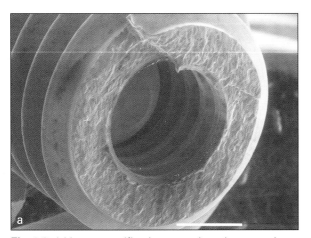
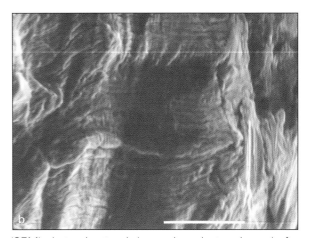

Fig 4-8 *(a)* Low-magnification scanning electron microscope (SEM) photomicrograph (secondary electron image) of a titanium implant abutment screw that fractured during the clinical function of one of the implants in Fig 4-7 (bar = 1 mm; original magnification × 25). *(b)* High-magnification SEM photomicrograph (secondary electron image) of the titanium implant abutment screw in *(a)*, showing characteristic striations associated with fatigue crack propagation (bar = 10 μm; original magnification × 3,000).

implants. No significant change in the composition of the oxide layer was observed, as determined by comparisons with control implants that had not been placed and that had been subjected to the same preparation procedures.

Denissen et al,[76] Proussaefs and associates,[77,78] and MacDonald et al[79,80] found much more complex changes in the HA coatings of retrieved implants, which have generally been reported to

display the expected integration with bone; however, some retrieved implants had partial or total loss of the HA coatings. MacDonald et al[79,80] found a loss of nonapatitic phases from the retrieved coatings with implantation time, resulting in a change in the ratio of calcium to phosphorus, along with an accumulation of bone as evidenced by the presence of proteins and carbonate apatite in the coatings. Leize et al[81] observed titanium grains 5 to 50 nm wide adjacent to the surface of bulk HA particles in the coatings and found that the crystal planes of these two constituents were continuous across the interface. Needlelike calcium phosphate grains within the porous layer of titanium grains suggested bone binding to the outer surface of the coated implant. Gaining a complete understanding of the structural changes in these retrieved implants remains a formidable task because of the potential multiphase complexity of the calcium phosphate coatings, which are in a nonequilibrium state and vary in phase relationships depending on the plasma-spraying procedure.

Acknowledgments

The authors are pleased to acknowledge the expert technical assistance of Dr John Mitchell in obtaining the SEMs of the fractured implant.

References

1. Brånemark PI, Hansson BO, Adell R, et al. Osseointegrated implants in the treatment of the edentulous jaw: Experience from a 10-year period. Scand J Plast Reconstr Surg 1977; 16(suppl):1–132.

2. Adell R, Lekholm U, Rockler B, Brånemark PI. A 15-year study of osseointegrated implants in the treatment of the edentulous jaw. Int J Oral Surg 1981;10:387–416.

3. Linder L, Albrektsson T, Brånemark PI, et al. Electron microscopic analysis of the bone-titanium interface. Acta Orthop Scand 1983;54:45–52.

4. Sullivan DY, Sherwood RL, Porter SS. Long-term performance of Osseotite implants: A 6-year clinical follow-up. Compend Contin Educ Dent 2000;22:326–328, 330, 332–334.

5. Norton MR. Biologic and mechanical stability of single-tooth implants: 4- to 7-year follow-up. Clin Implant Dent Relat Res 2001;3:214–220.

6. Albrektsson T, Zarb GA. The Brånemark Osseointegrated Implant. Chicago: Quintessence, 1989.

7. Spiekerman H. Implantology. Stuttgart: Thieme, 1995.

8. Watzek GW (ed). Endosseous Implants: Scientific and Clinical Aspects. Chicago: Quintessence, 1996.

9. Misch CE. Contemporary Implant Dentistry, ed 2. St. Louis: Mosby, 1999.

10. Dental implants: Benefit and risk. NIH Consensus Statement [online]. June 13–14, 1978;1(3):13–19.

11. Albrektsson T, Zarb G, Worthington P, Eriksson AR. The long-term efficacy of currently used dental implants: A review and proposed criteria of success. Int J Oral Maxillofac Implants 1986;1:11–25.

12. Smith DE, Zarb GA. Criteria for success for osseointegrated endosseous implants. J Prosthet Dent 1989;62:567–572.

13. McGlumphy EA, Larsen P, Peterson L. Etiology of implant complications: Anecdotal reports vs prospective clinical trials. Compend Contin Educ Dent 1993;15(suppl):S544–S548.

14. Lindquist LW, Rockler B, Carlsson GE. Bone resorption around fixtures in edentulous patients treated with mandibular fixed tissue-integrated prostheses. J Prosthet Dent 1988;59:59–63.

15. Oh TJ, Yoon J, Misch CE, Wang HL. The causes of early implant bone loss: Myth or science? J Periodontol 2002;73: 322–333.

16. Lekholm U, Adell R, Lindhe J, et al. Marginal tissue reactions at osseointegrated titanium fixtures, II. A cross-sectional retrospective study. Int J Oral Maxillofac Surg 1986;15:53–61.

17. Schou S, Holmstrup P, Hjorting-Hansen E, Lang NP. Plaque-induced marginal tissue reactions of osseointegrated oral implants: A review of the literature. Clin Oral Implants Res 1992;3:149–161.

18. Quirynen M, Naert I, van Steenberghe D. Fixture design and overload influence marginal bone loss and fixture success in the Brånemark system. Clin Oral Implants Res 1992;3: 104–111.

19. Hoshaw SJ, Brunski JB, Cochran GVB. Mechanical loading of Brånemark fixtures affects interfacial bone modeling and remodeling. Int J Oral Maxillofac Implants 1994;9:345–360.

20. Misch CE. Influence of biomechanics on implant complications. In: Proceedings of Conference on Dental Implant Treatments: Issues beyond ten years in vivo. Trans Acad Dent Mater 2000;14:49–62.

21. Frost HM. Mechanical adaptation: Frost's mechanostat theory. In: Martin RB, Burr DB (eds). Structure, Function and Adaptation of Compact Bone. New York: Raven Press, 1989:179–181.

22. Mihalko WM, May TC, Kay JF, Krause WR. Finite element analysis of interface geometry effects on the crestal bone surrounding a dental implant. Implant Dent 1992;1:212–217.

23. Kohn DH. Overview of factors important in implant design. J Oral Implantol 1992;18:204–219.

24. Eckert SE, Meraw SJ, Cal E, Ow RK. Analysis of incidence and associated factors with fractured implants: A retrospective study. Int J Oral Maxillofac Implants 2000;15:662–667.

25. McGlumphy EA, Mendel DA, Holloway JA. Implant screw mechanics. Dent Clin North Am 1998;42:71–89.

26. Rambhia SK, Nagy WW, Fournelle RA, Dhuru VB. Defects in hexed gold prosthetic screws: A metallographic and tensile analysis. J Prosthet Dent 2002;87:30–39.

27. Yokoyama K, Ichikawa T, Murakami H, Miyamoto Y, Asaoka K. Fracture mechanisms of retrieved titanium screw thread in dental implant. Biomaterials 2002;23:2459–2465.

28. Morgan MJ, James DF, Pilliar RM. Fractures of the fixture component of an osseointegrated implant. Int J Oral Maxillofac Implants 1993;8:409–414.

29. Piattelli A, Piattelli M, Scarano A, Montesani L. Light and scanning electron microscopic report of four fractured implants. Int J Oral Maxillofac Implants 1998;13:561–564.

30. Dieter GE. Mechanical Metallurgy, ed 3. New York: McGraw-Hill, 1986:394–398.

31. Rangert B, Krogh PH, Langer B, Van Roekel N. Bending overload and implant fracture: A retrospective clinical analysis. Int J Oral Maxillofac Implants 1995;10:326–334 [erratum 1996;11:575].

32. Haack JE, Sakaguchi RL, Sun T, Coffey JP. Elongation and preload stress in dental implant abutment screws. Int J Oral Maxillofac Implants 1995;10:529–536.

33. Gratton DG, Aquilino SA, Stanford CM. Micromotion and dynamic fatigue properties of the dental implant-abutment interface. J Prosthet Dent 2001;85:47–52.

34. Hoyer SA, Stanford CM, Buranadham S, Fridrich T, Wagner J, Gratton D. Dynamic fatigue properties of the dental implant-abutment interface: Joint opening in wide-diameter versus standard-diameter hex-type implants. J Prosthet Dent 2001;85:599–607.

35. Eliades T. Passive film growth on titanium alloys: Physicochemical and biologic considerations. Int J Oral Maxillofac Implants 1997;12:621–627.

36. Albrektsson T, Hansson HA, Ivarsson B. Interface analysis of titanium and zirconium bone implants. Biomaterials 1985;6:97–101.

37. Klinger MM, Rahemtulla F, Prince CW, Lucas LC, Lemons JE. Proteoglycans at the bone-implant interface. Crit Rev Oral Biol Med 1998;9:449–463.

38. Sul YT, Johansson CB, Petronis S, et al. Characteristics of the surface oxides on turned and electrochemically oxidized pure titanium implants up to dielectric breakdown: The oxide thickness, micropore configurations, surface roughness, crystal structure and chemical composition. Biomaterials 2002;23:491–501.

39. Nanci A, Wuest JD, Peru L, et al. Chemical modification of titanium surfaces for covalent attachment of biological molecules. J Biomed Mater Res 1998;40:324–335.

40. Brick RM, Pense AW, Gordon RB. Structure and Properties of Engineering Materials, ed 4. New York: McGraw-Hill, 1977:234–243.

41. Park JB, Lakes RS. Biomaterials: An Introduction, ed. 2. New York: Plenum Press, 1992:89–93.

42. Donachie MJ Jr. Titanium: A Technical Guide. Metals Park, OH: ASM International, 1988:chap 3, 4, 8, 11.

43. Munoz DG, Feldman H. Causes of Alzheimer's disease. Can Med Assoc J 2000;162:65–72.

44. Canales JJ, Corbalan R, Montoliu C, et al. Aluminium impairs the glutamate-nitric oxide-cGMP pathway in cultured neurons and in rat brain in vivo: Molecular mechanisms and implications for neuropathology. J Inorg Biochem 2001;87:63–69.

45. Flaten TP. Aluminium as a risk factor in Alzheimer's disease, with emphasis on drinking water. Brain Res Bull 2001;55: 187–196.

46. Carpenter DO. Effects of metals on the nervous system of humans and animals. Int J Occup Med Environ Health 2001; 14:209–218.

47. Hehner B, Heidemann D. Comparison of the biological tolerance of titanium and titanium alloys in human gingiva cell cultures [in German]. Dtsch Z Mund Kiefer Gesichtschir 1989;13:394–400.

48. Keller JC, Stanford CM, Wightman JP, Draughn RA, Zaharias R. Characterizations of titanium implant surfaces, III. J Biomed Mater Res 1994;28:939–946.

49. Thompson GJ, Puleo DA. Ti-6Al-4V ion solution inhibition of osteogenic cell phenotype as a function of differentiation timecourse in vitro. Biomaterials 1996;17:1949–1954.

50. Thompson GJ, Puleo DA. Effects of sublethal metal ion concentrations on osteogenic cells derived from bone marrow stromal cells. J Appl Biomater 1995;6:249–258.

51. Rogers SD, Howie DW, Graves SE, Pearcy MJ, Haynes DR. In vitro human monocyte response to wear particles of titanium alloy containing vanadium or niobium. J Bone Joint Surg Br 1997;79:311–315.

52. Ciapetti G, Granchi D, Verri E, et al. Fluorescent microplate assay for respiratory burst of PMNs challenged in vitro with orthopedic metals. J Biomed Mater Res 1998;41:455–460.

53. Smith DC, Lugowski S, McHugh A, Deporter D, Watson PA, Chipman M. Systemic metal ion levels in dental implant patients. Int J Oral Maxillofac Implants 1997;12:828–834.

54. Kononen M, Hormia M, Kivilahti J, Hautaniemi J, Thesleff I. Effect of surface processing on the attachment, orientation, and proliferation of human gingival fibroblasts on titanium. J Biomed Mater Res 1992;26:1325–1341.

55. Deligianni DD, Katsala N, Ladas S, Sotiropoulou D, Amedee J, Missirlis YF. Effect of surface roughness of the titanium alloy Ti-6Al-4V on human bone marrow cell response and on protein adsorption. Biomaterials 2001;22:1241–1251.

56. Ku CH, Pioletti DP, Browne M, Gregson PJ. Effect of different Ti-6Al-4V surface treatments on osteoblasts behaviour. Biomaterials 2002;23:1447–1454.

57. Grosgogeat B, Reclaru L, Lissac M, Dalard F. Measurement and evaluation of galvanic corrosion between titanium/Ti6Al4V implants and dental alloys by electrochemical techniques and auger spectrometry. Biomaterials 1999;20: 933–941.

58. LeGeros RZ. Calcium Phosphates in Oral Biology and Medicine, Monographs in Oral Science. Basel, Switzerland: Karger Press, 1991:1–3, 26–27.

59. Cook SD, Kay JF, Thomas KA, Jarcho M. Interface mechanics and histology of titanium and hydroxylapatite coated titanium for dental implant applications. Int J Oral Maxillofac Implants 1987;2:15–22.

60. de Groot K, Geesink R, Klein CPAT, Serekian P. Plasma sprayed coatings of hydroxylapatite. J Biomed Mater Res 1987;21:1375–1381.

61. Ducheyne P, Healy KE. The effect of plasma-sprayed calcium phosphate ceramic coatings on the metal ion release from porous titanium and cobalt-chromium alloys. J Biomed Mater Res 1988;22:1137–1163.

62. Tufekci E, Brantley WA, Mitchell JC, McGlumphy EA. Microstructures of plasma-sprayed hydroxyapatite-coated Ti–6Al–4V dental implants. Int J Oral Maxillofac Implants 1997;12:25–31.

63. Tufekci E, Brantley WA, Mitchell JC, Foreman DW, Georgette FS. Crystallographic characteristics of plasma-sprayed calcium phosphate coatings on Ti-6Al-4V. Int J Oral Maxillofac Implants 1999;14:661–672.

64. Koch B, Wolke JGC, de Groot K. X-ray diffraction studies on plasma-sprayed calcium phosphate-coated implants. J Biomed Mater Res 1990;24:655–667.

65. Filiaggi MJ, Coombs NA, Pilliar RM. Characterization of the interface in the plasma-sprayed HA coating/Ti-6Al-4V implant system. J Biomed Mater Res 1991;25:1211–1229.

66. Brantley WA, Tufekci E, Mitchell JC, Foreman DW, McGlumphy EA. Scanning electron microscopy studies of ceramic layers and interfacial regions for calcium phosphate-coated titanium dental implants. Cells Mater 1995;5:73–82.

67. Lynn AK, DuQuesnay DL. Hydroxyapatite-coated Ti-6Al-4V, Part I. The effect of coating thickness on mechanical fatigue behaviour. Biomaterials 2002;23:1937–1946.

68. Lynn AK, DuQuesnay DL. Hydroxyapatite-coated Ti-6Al-4V, Part II. The effects of post-deposition heat treatment at low temperatures. Biomaterials 2002;23:1947–1953.

69. Lee JJ, Rouhfar L, Beirne OR. Survival of hydroxyapatite-coated implants: A meta-analytic review. J Oral Maxillofac Surg 2000;58:1372–1379 [discussion 1379–1380].

70. Holloway JA, Litsky AS, Sosa MA, Brantley WA, Denry IL, McGlumphy EA. Effect of plasma-sprayed coatings on fatigue behavior of pure titanium for dental implants [extended abstract]. Trans Soc Biomater 1998;21:228.

71. Holloway JA, Litsky AS, Denry IL, Brantley WA, McGlumphy EA. Effect of plasma-sprayed coatings on fatigue behavior of titanium. In: Garetto LP, Turner CH, Duncan RL, Burr DB (eds). Bridging the Gap Between Dental and Orthopaedic Implants [Proceedings of the Third Annual Indiana Conference, May 1998, Indianapolis, IN]. Indianapolis: Indiana University School of Dentistry, 2002:232–234.

72. Piattelli A, Scarano A, Piattelli M, Vaia E, Matarasso S. Hollow implants retrieved for fracture: A light and scanning electron microscope analysis of 4 cases. J Periodontol 1998;69:185–189.

73. Brunel G, Armand S, Miller N, Rue J. Histologic analysis of a fractured implant: A case report. Int J Periodontics Restor Dent 2000;20:520–526.

74. Aparicio C, Olive J. Comparative surface microanalysis of failed Brånemark implants. Int J Oral Maxillofac Implants 1992;7:94–103.

75. Esposito M, Lausmaa J, Hirsch JM, Thomsen P. Surface analysis of failed oral titanium implants. J Biomed Mater Res 1999;48:559–568.

76. Denissen HW, Klein CP, Visch LL, van den Hooff A. Behavior of calcium phosphate coatings with different chemistries in bone. Int J Prosthodont 1996;9:142–148.

77. Proussaefs PT, Tatakis DN, Lozada J, Caplanis N, Rohrer MD. Histologic evaluation of hydroxyapatite-coated root-form implant retrieved after 7 years in function: A case report. Int J Oral Maxillofac Implants 2000;15:438–443.

78. Proussaefs P, Lozada J. Histologic evaluation of a 9-year-old hydroxyapatite-coated cylindric implant placed in conjunction with a subantral augmentation procedure: A case report. Int J Oral Maxillofac Implants 2001;16:737–741.

79. MacDonald DE, Betts F, Doty SB, Boskey AL. A methodological study for the analysis of apatite-coated dental implants retrieved from humans. Ann Periodontol 2000;5:175–184.

80. MacDonald DE, Betts F, Stranick M, Doty S, Boskey AL. Physicochemical study of plasma-sprayed hydroxyapatite-coated implants in humans. J Biomed Mater Res 2001;54:480–490.

81. Leize EM, Hemmerle J, Leize M. Characterization, at the bone crystal level, of the titanium-coating/bone interfacial zone. Clin Oral Implants Res 2000;11:279–288.

Section III

RESTORATIVE DENTISTRY

5

ALTERATIONS OF DENTAL AMALGAM

Miroslav I. Marek, PhD

On a worldwide scale, dental amalgam is the most common direct-filling restorative material, especially for premolar and molar teeth. Although the widespread use of dental amalgam is evidence of its substantial advantages, it also exhibits several undesirable properties, the most apparent of which is poor esthetic appearance. Like most metallic materials, dental amalgam does not match the teeth in appearance, an esthetic problem that becomes even more severe when the amalgam darkens due to tarnishing. Dental amalgam is also about the least resistant of all the common dental alloys to environmental degradation. The most serious recent challenge to dental amalgam is concern about the release of mercury into the human organism. Because dental amalgam always contains a substantial amount of mercury, some release of this toxic element is inevitable.

The favorable properties of dental amalgam, which have sustained its use despite numerous challenges and the development of alternatives, include low cost, ease of application, tolerance to variation in the placement procedure, and high longevity. The useful life of amalgam restorations varies widely, but amalgam restorations 30 or more years old are not uncommon. There are cases of premature failure, however. While some of them may be attributed to application errors, the cause of other failures can be traced to alterations of amalgam structure and properties under the service conditions.

Composition, Structure, and Types of Dental Amalgam

The two elements on which all true dental amalgams are based are mercury and silver. When mercury reacts with silver and the amount of mercury is more than about 50% by weight, the amalgamation reaction produces intermetallic compounds of silver and mercury of theoretically stoichiometric compositions Ag_2Hg_3 and $AgHg$. In dental amalgams, these phases are called γ_1 and β_1, respectively. When dental amalgam is prepared in the dental office, the product of the silver-mercury amalgamation reaction is mostly the γ_1 phase, and it becomes the matrix of the amalgam structure in which all the other phases are embedded. All dental amalgams, however, also contain tin to improve mechanical properties, to control the speed of amalgamation, and thus to provide a suitable working time for the dentist. Another essential element in modern amalgams is copper, which further improves the materials' properties. Among the minor alloying elements, zinc is most common, used as a "scavenger" to remove impurities during the melting of the elements in the preparation of the alloy for dental amalgam, which is used in powder form to prepare the amalgam. Other elements that have been used in some cases to improve the properties of dental amalgam include palladium and indium.

In dental practice, the amalgam is formed in small quantities, suitable for filling a cavity, by mixing the alloy powder with mercury in a process called *trituration*. Trituration in a mortar and pestle has been replaced by the use of mechanical amalgamators, in which the mixing of the alloy powder and mercury takes place in a plastic capsule that is shaken in a motorized device. The main purposes of trituration are to coat all of the powder particles with mercury and to remove some of the oxide from the alloy powder particles, which would prevent or impede the reaction with mercury. The amount of mercury used in trituration is always smaller than that required for complete amalgamation of the entire mass of the alloy.

To obtain the desired composition and phase structure within minutes after trituration, the major phase in all alloys for dental amalgam is a compound of silver and tin, Ag_3Sn, called the γ *phase*. A smaller amount of a silver-rich β Ag-Sn phase may be present in the alloy and participate in the reaction. Amalgamation of silver from the γ and β phases results in the formation of the γ_1 phase. Because the amount of mercury used in trituration is not sufficient for complete amalgamation of the alloy, the basic structure of dental amalgam is a matrix of mostly γ_1 phase, in which are dispersed the unreacted parts of the original alloy particles, typically about 30% by volume,[1] and other reaction products. An important characteristic of dental amalgam is its porosity, which has been estimated to occupy 5% to 7% of the amalgam material's volume.[2,3]

A small amount of tin from the amalgamated γ phase dissolves in the γ_1 reaction product. The fate of the remaining tin depends on the other elements present, mainly copper. The copper content of the alloy and the form in which it is introduced have resulted in the categorization of dental amalgams into two major types: low copper and high copper.

Low-copper amalgams containing less than 5% copper in the original alloy are also called "conventional" or γ_2-containing amalgams. In these amalgams, most of the tin combines with mercury in an intermetallic compound Sn_8Hg, called γ_2. Because tin is a soft, low-melting metal and mercury is liquid at room temperature, γ_2 is a soft phase that is easily corroded in the oral environment. Typically, the γ_2 phase constitutes about 10% of the amalgam by volume and often forms an interconnected network within the amalgam structure.[4] Alloys for low-copper amalgams are further divided into lathe-cut and spherical, depending on the manner of production or shape of the alloy particles. Cutting in a lathe results in irregular particles, whereas spraying the molten alloy in inert gas produces spherical particles. Figure 5-1 shows typical structures of lathe-cut and spherical low-copper dental amalgams, respectively.

Although low-copper dental amalgams are still used in some countries of the world, in many other countries they have been almost or completely replaced by high-copper amalgams. The alloy powder for high-copper dental amalgams usually contains more than 12% copper by weight. At this composition, most of the tin combines during amalgamation with copper to form another compound, Cu_6Sn_5, called η'. Because η' is stronger and more corrosion resistant than γ_2, better properties are obtained.

The larger amount of copper can be introduced in two fundamentally different ways, which yield the two major types of high-copper dental amalgams. In admixed amalgams, also called "blended" or "dispersed-phase" amalgams, two types of powder are mixed together. One type is usually similar to the powder for low-copper amalgams and contains mainly the γ phase (Ag_3Sn). The other powder is rich in copper: most admixed amalgams use an alloy of copper and silver or copper-silver-tin to facilitate amalgamation. In admixed amalgams, both powders may be spherical/irregular or one may be spherical (usually the high-copper alloy) and the other irregular. The second type of high-copper alloy for dental amalgam contains only one type of powder, and the resulting dental amalgam is called *single-composition-alloy amalgam*. This alloy is produced by melting the elements and usually spraying the molten alloy in an inert gas, resulting in spherical powder particles. The alloy structure then mainly consists of intermetallic compounds of silver-tin (Ag_3Sn, γ phase) and copper-tin (Cu_3Sn, ϵ phase).

Depending on the type of high-copper alloy powder, the structure of the amalgam varies. In

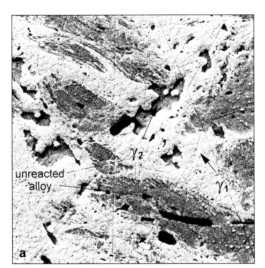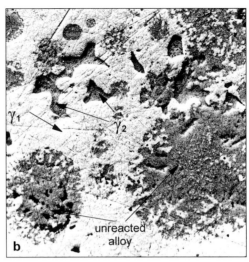

Fig 5-1 *(a)* Typical structure of a lathe-cut, low-copper dental amalgam (Velvalloy [SS White, Philadelphia, PA]), showing irregular unreacted alloy particles and the γ_2 reaction phase in a matrix of γ_1 phase (scanning electron micrograph [SEM], original magnification × 4,000). *(b)* Typical structure of a spherical, low-copper dental amalgam (Spheralloy [Kerr Manufacturing, Romulus, MI]), showing globular unreacted alloy particles and the γ_2 reaction phase in a matrix of γ_1 phase (SEM, original magnification × 4,000). (Courtesy of MB Butts, Medical College of Georgia, Augusta, GA.)

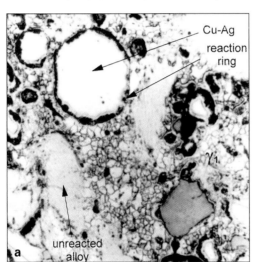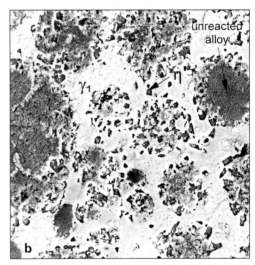

Fig 5-2 *(a)* Typical structure of an admixed, high-copper dental amalgam (Dispersalloy [Johnson & Johnson, East Windsor, NJ]), showing irregular unreacted alloy particles, spherical particles of the admixed Cu-Ag powder surrounded by reaction rings containing the η' reaction phase, and the γ_1 phase matrix (optical micrograph, original magnification × 2,000). *(b)* Typical structure of a single-composition-alloy, high-copper dental amalgam (Tytin [SS White]), showing spherical unreacted alloy particles and the η' reaction phase products in the γ_1 phase matrix (SEM, original magnification × 3,000). (Courtesy of MB Butts, Medical College of Georgia, Augusta, GA.)

single-composition-alloy amalgams, copper is released during amalgamation of the original alloy particles and combines with tin, resulting in the formation of a large number of small, irregular particles of the η' phase within the γ_1 matrix.[5] In admixed-type amalgams, the reaction of copper with tin takes place mainly at the periphery of the copper-rich particles, resulting in complex "rings" of fine particles of the γ_1 and η'[6,7] phases around them; small, rod-shaped η' particles can also be found throughout the γ_1 matrix.[5] Figure 5-2 shows typical structures of admixed and single-composition, high-copper amalgams, respectively.

Changes in Amalgam Structure and Properties in Service

The main conditions and variables that cause alteration in the amalgam structure and properties are time, temperature and temperature variation, mechanical forces, and the environment. Because all these forces act simultaneously or in a short time sequence, their effect on the amalgam and the amalgam restoration can be quite complex. It is possible, however, to examine each condition individually and describe its main effects before attempting to draw a complete picture of the interaction.

Time- and Temperature-Dependent Structural Changes

The structure and properties of dental amalgam change with time at room or body temperature. The reason for these changes is that the mixture of structural phases, which develops during amalgamation, is not at equilibrium, and lower energy can be achieved by further structural evolution. The changes are accomplished by diffusion and are possible at room or body temperature because of the relatively high diffusion rate of the elements, especially mercury, associated with the relatively low melting temperatures of the structural phases. The most substantial changes take place in the first hours and days after hardening; however, more subtle changes continue throughout the clinical life of the restoration.

Although most of the liquid mercury is used up within minutes after trituration as the amalgam hardens, it takes about two hours for the residual mercury to be consumed by reaction with the γ phase (Ag₃Sn).[8] The initial mercury-rich γ_1 phase (Ag-Hg-Sn) may then continue to react with the γ phase (Ag₃Sn) to produce more γ_1, or the β_1 phase. Marshall and Marshall[9] observed a substantial decrease of the γ-phase content in high-copper amalgams at 6 months, compared with 1 day, when aged at 37°C. The γ_1 phase in dental amalgams contains about 67% to 71% mercury by weight,[6,10] whereas the most commonly accepted formula for the γ_1 phase, Ag₂Hg₃,[11] would

indicate mercury content of 73.6% by weight. The β_1 phase (Ag-Hg) contains less mercury and more tin than the γ_1 phase, and a mixture of γ_1 and β_1 phases is thus a more stable state for the mercury contents used in dental amalgams. Transformation of γ_1 to β_1 was observed by Johnson[12,13] for both nonstoichiometric γ_1 and dental amalgams. The matrix of older amalgam restorations has been reported to consist of a mixture of γ_1 and β_1 phases.[14–17]

The γ_1-to-β_1-phase transformation appears to be affected by the amalgam composition. There is some evidence that the dissolved tin stabilizes the γ_1 phase.[18,19] In high-copper amalgams, most of the tin from the amalgamated γ phase reacts with copper to form a relatively stable η' phase (Cu₆Sn₅). The result is that less tin dissolves in the γ_1 phase of high-copper amalgams than in the same phase in low-copper amalgams,[20] where it coexists with the tin-rich, weak phase, γ_2 (Sn₈Hg). Therefore, the γ_1 phase matrix may convert more quickly to β_1 in high-copper amalgams than in low-copper amalgams. This was confirmed by analysis of retrieved restorations for admixed high-copper amalgams, but not for single-composition-alloy amalgams.[16] The mercury-poorer β_1 phase can be expected to have better mechanical properties than the γ_1 phase, which might contribute to better performance of high-copper amalgams. There is no empirical evidence, however, that this effect plays a significant role in the clinical performance of amalgam restorations.

In admixed high-copper amalgams, another type of phase change may occur over time, which significantly affects the amalgams' properties and behavior. In these amalgams, perhaps because of a less uniform initial copper distribution than in single-composition-alloy amalgams, a small amount of γ_2 phase may form during amalgamation even if the average copper content in the alloy is above 12%. The presence of this phase has been attributed to the room-temperature oxidation of the copper-rich component of the alloy, which hinders amalgamation.[21] The γ_2-phase content has been reported to decrease over time, becoming negligible after a year or two.[22,23] Curiously, a reappearance of the γ_2 phase has also been reported for various dental amalgams after two to eight years of dry storage, especially in amalgams with high copper content.[24]

Although the temperature difference between room temperature and body or oral temperature is relatively small, it is significant considering the high sensitivity of diffusion to temperature. The rate of phase changes in vivo may be further enhanced by temperature increases during the intake of hot foods or drinks. There are no data, however, showing how much the temperature variation in the oral cavity affects structural changes. The resulting effect of temperature variation appears to be a summation of the changes occurring at different rates at different temperatures.

Time- and Temperature-Dependent Property Changes

The properties of a set dental amalgam change rapidly during the first hour, but the rate of change rapidly decreases and becomes quite small after a day or two. The initial changes result from the development of the amalgam microstructure, including the consumption of all free mercury and precipitation of the reaction phases. As discussed above, however, some structural changes continue for many years and perhaps almost indefinitely, or at least until all the unreacted γ-phase particles are consumed or when the γ_1 phase is entirely converted into the β_1 phase.

The known short-term change is mainly an increase in strength. Dental amalgam is a brittle material, and its compressive strength is the major strength parameter. Since compressive strength is also the most easily measured mechanical property, an increase in compressive strength has been well documented.[25] There is little information available regarding other properties as a function of time after trituration, however, especially for long-term property changes such as those that could be attributed to specific developments in the amalgam microstructure.

The initial approach to structural stabilization is also accompanied by dimensional changes, which are of great clinical importance. While the short-term progress of the amalgamation reactions may be accompanied by complex dimensional variations, the final, overall dimensional change in commercial dental amalgams must be close to zero, with small tolerances in either expansion or contraction allowed by the specifications (eg, of the American National Standards Institute/American Dental Association [ANSI/ADA] or of the International Organization for Standardization [ISO]). The dimensional changes during setting of the amalgam, together with the surface texture of the amalgam at the tooth-amalgam interface, play a major role in the clinical problem of microleakage at this interface, which may cause postoperative sensitivity.[26,27] Because of the continuing solid-state reactions, slower changes in the specific volume of the amalgam are expected to continue even after the initial setting.

Mechanical Forces and Their Effect on Dental Amalgam

Amalgam restorations are subjected to a complex set of mechanical forces, mainly during chewing. Mastication involves large biting forces on the teeth, with maximal force ranging in adults from about 400 to 800 N for the first and second molars, where most amalgam restorations are placed.[28] Although the major forces are normal to the occlusal surfaces of the restorations, sizable shear forces also are involved. One result of the action of these forces is some permanent deformation, mainly in the occlusal surface layer. The deformation may occur in the form of instantaneous strain caused by large, fast-acting forces (eg, during biting on a hard piece of food) or as time-dependent strain resulting from prolonged application of stress.

Since dental amalgam is essentially a brittle material, a force that causes stress in excess of the critical value (fracture stress) initiates fracture of the amalgam. In amalgam restorations, the fracture may occur in the form of bulk fracture, ie, fracture propagating through a substantial cross section of the restoration. A more common fracture mode is *marginal fracture*, in which the edge of the restoration at the amalgam-tooth interface breaks off, resulting in "ditching" around the restoration margins. When a gap forms between the tooth and the restoration, the chewing force on the unsupported wedge of the margin generates a tensile stress, to which dental amalgam has low resistance. When fracture occurs by a sudden application of a stress exceeding the fracture stress, ie, at a relatively high strain rate, the fracture mode appears to be an intergranular separation as well as cleavage of the γ_1 grains, with the percentage of cleavage increasing with increasing strain rate.[25]

Fracture is facilitated by stress concentrations. In a multiphase and porous material, such as dental amalgam, numerous stress concentrations are likely at phase boundaries. Because of the brittle nature of amalgam, however, the most damaging are likely to be pores, scratches, and other sharp features at the surfaces subjected to tensile forces. Under these conditions fracture occurs when the stress-intensity factor exceeds the critical value, called the *fracture toughness*. Fracture toughness properties of various amalgams have been studied in the last two decades.[29–31]

Overloading, either in the bulk or at the margins, is not the only (perhaps not even the most common) cause of fracture of dental amalgam restorations. Because the stresses to which an amalgam restoration is subjected are not constant, fracture may occur due to metal fatigue. Fatigue is a form of failure caused by repetitive loading and unloading and is characterized by initiation and progressive extension of a crack as a function of the number of loading cycles. Such failure also occurs at stresses below the conventional fracture stress for a single loading to failure. Wilkinson and Haack[32] and Sutow et al[33] observed fatigue fracture of a low-copper amalgam at stresses much lower than compressive strength. Metal fatigue can be accelerated by a corrosive environment in the form of environment-induced cracking called *corrosion fatigue*.

The time-dependent strain, called *creep*, occurs rather readily in dental amalgam at body temperature because of the low melting temperatures of some of the phases and related high diffusion rates of elemental species. High-copper amalgams exhibit substantially lower creep rates than γ_2-containing low-copper amalgams.[34] When load-

ing takes place in the laboratory under creep conditions for an extended period of time, creep fracture may occur. Because the γ_1 phase, as well as the γ_2 phase in low-copper amalgams, exhibits plasticity at slow strain rates, ductile fracture may occur, characterized by a dimpled appearance of the fracture surfaces, resulting from microvoid coalescence. Both intergranular and transgranular modes of fracture have been observed at the slow strain rates of creep.[35]

Pure creep fracture seems unlikely under the loading conditions of dental amalgam restorations. A more probable cause of failure is a combination of time-dependent strain and repetitive loading, which may cause mechanical degradation called *creep fatigue* and will eventually result in rupture of the material. Williams and Hedge[36] and Williams and Cahoon[37] observed this form of failure in vitro using simulated amalgam restorations confined in metal dies and subjected either to thermal or mechanical cycling. They considered the appearance of intergranular fracture as evidence of low-stress, low-cycling-frequency creep fatigue.

In addition to deformation and fracture, mechanical forces affect dental amalgam restorations by abrasion, in which a small amount of the amalgam material is removed, mainly from occlusal surfaces, during mastication. Dental amalgam is relatively abrasion resistant compared to nonmetallic direct-filling materials, as evidenced by some restorations lasting several decades, and abrasion has not been a critical issue for dental amalgam restorations. Lutz et al[38] reported maximum in vivo wear in 180 days of about 16 μm in contact areas and 6 μm in contact-free areas of a high-copper amalgam. Considering average chewing frequency and duration, the difference between contact and contact-free wear rates represents an average loss per bite of about one tenth of an atomic layer, indicating that mastication is not a particularly severe abrasion process. Abrasion, however, may play a contributing role in conjunction with the corrosion processes, as discussed below.

Environmental Interactions and Effects on Dental Amalgam

Like any material suitable for permanent tissue replacement in the human body, dental amalgam exhibits relatively high corrosion resistance in the oral environment. Among the standard metallic restorative materials, however, dental amalgam ranks as one of the most corrosion susceptible. Most of the destructive force of the environment is due to electrochemical reactions. Tarnishing, ie, changes in surface appearance, is electrochemical or chemical in nature and may or may not be accompanied by degradation of other properties.

Corrosion, the degrading effect of electrochemical reactions on metals, generally involves conversion of some of the metal to dissolved ions or solid, nonmetallic corrosion products. The direct cause of this conversion is a reaction or reactions proceeding in the direction of oxidation, also called *anodic reactions*. For instance, copper from dental amalgams may dissolve in the oral liquids according to the reaction:

$$Cu \longrightarrow Cu^{++} \longrightarrow + 2e^-$$

and tin may oxidize to form tin oxide:

$$Sn + 2H_2O \longrightarrow SnO_2 + 4H^+ + 4e^-$$

Because of the presence of aggressive chloride ions in saliva and many foods, metallic chlorides are some of the most common corrosion products of dental amalgam, in addition to oxides and hydroxides.[39-47] The electrons released in the oxidation (anodic) reactions must be consumed in simultaneously occurring reduction (cathodic) reactions. For dental amalgam in the oral environment, the most common cathodic reaction is the reduction of dissolved oxygen:

$$O_2 + 4H^+ + 4e^- = 2 H_2O$$

The matrix of dental amalgam, the silver-mercury γ_1 phase, is thermodynamically very stable in saliva and suffers little corrosion. The small amount of tin dissolved in this phase oxidizes to form a solid oxide film on the surface.[23,48] This film plays an important role in slowing down the dissolution and evaporation of toxic mercury from dental amalgam restorations and also causes the γ_1 phase to react electrochemically as a less noble electrode than it would without tin. It does not, however, cause significant corrosion degradation of the γ_1 phase. The unreacted γ phase (Ag_3Sn) and ϵ phase (Cu_3Sn), although electrochemically more active than the γ_1 phase, are very stable compounds, which also are quite resistant to environmental degradation.[49-51] The two phases of the amalgam structure that are most susceptible to environmental degradation are thus the γ_2 phase (Sn_8Hg) in low-copper amalgams and the η' (Cu_6Sn_5) in high-copper amalgams.

The low corrosion resistance of low-copper dental amalgams was recognized in many early studies and attributed to the presence of the soft tin-mercury γ_2 phase.[52,53] Given the molecular ratio of Sn_8Hg, the electrochemical behavior of the γ_2 phase is dominated by tin rather than by the noble mercury. Tin exhibits good corrosion resistance in nearly neutral and minimally aggressive environments because it is not highly thermodynamically active and it is readily passivated when covered with a protective oxide film.[54] The γ_2 phase in dental amalgams, however, corrodes rather rapidly. This behavior is attributed to a combination of several factors. The presence of mercury in the phase probably makes the oxide film less stable than on pure tin. On the occlusal restoration surfaces, the protective film is easily disturbed by abrasion during mastication, and corrosion then occurs on the unprotected surface before the film reforms. Once the corrosion has penetrated deeper into the structure, the form of corrosion changes from uniform to crevice corrosion. In a crevice the localized chemistry of the electrolyte changes, resulting in a more aggressive solution than the bulk solution outside. The most important factors in this chemical change are acidification, due to hydrolysis of dissolved tin ions, and depletion of dissolved oxygen.[55]

Because the γ_2 phase often exists as a network throughout the structure[56] and may be associated with voids,[4] the corrosion attack can penetrate deep into the bulk of the restoration. The product of corrosion of the γ_2 phase appears to be a mixture of oxides, chlorides, and chloride hydroxides.[39,40,42,44–47] These products are poorly soluble in water, and if corrosion occurs within the structure, they remain in the space previously occupied by the γ_2 phase. Although crevice corrosion conditions eventually develop within the structure under the occlusal surfaces, the interface between the tooth and the restoration becomes a crevice cell as soon as oral fluids penetrate the space. Amalgam restorations not bonded to the tooth structure are thus inherently susceptible to crevice corrosion at the tooth-amalgam interface.

In high-copper dental amalgams, the soft, corrosion-prone γ_2 phase is replaced by the mercury-free η' (Cu_6Sn_5) phase. This phase is a much more stable compound, both chemically and mechanically, than the γ_2 phase,[51] and the difference is mainly responsible for the better mechanical and corrosion properties of high-copper dental amalgams compared with γ_2-containing amalgams. Still, the η' phase is the most corrosion-prone of the major phases in high-copper amalgams, and corrosion degradation of γ_2-free amalgams is characterized by conversion of the η' phase into corrosion products.[39,40,57,58] The η' phase appears to be electrochemically less stable in the amalgam structure than if prepared as an isolated copper-tin compound; the difference has been attributed to the presence of mercury in the amalgam and its destabilizing effect on the oxide film.[59]

When a binary compound, such as the γ_2 or η' phase, corrodes, the molecular structure disintegrates. In the corrosion of the γ_2 phase, the major part of tin converts selectively into the aforementioned solid corrosion products, leaving the noble mercury in the metallic state. Because the γ_2 phase corrodes while surrounded by phases containing mercury or capable of reacting with mercury, the liberated mercury is either readily absorbed into the γ_1 matrix or reacts with the γ phase, as during the original amalgamation. Conversion of tin in the η' phase into insoluble corrosion products, on the other hand, leaves copper, which is much less noble than mercury and much more soluble than tin. Copper from the corroded η' phase leaves the restorations mostly in the dissolved form,[39,40,60] although some solid products, such as chlorides, may also form.[41,43,47]

Because the η' phase appears dispersed within the amalgam structure and does not form a network, some penetration by the oxidizing species through the structure must occur and released copper must also be transported from the amalgam interior to the surface. Although some explanations have been offered, this aspect of high-copper amalgam corrosion has never been satisfactorily explained.

Potentially destructive corrosion reactions may occur when a zinc-containing dental amalgam is contaminated with water before or during insertion into the prepared tooth cavity. Because of the high thermodynamic activity of zinc, the reaction involves reduction of hydrogen ions into hydrogen gas and formation of voluminous solid corrosion products, causing "delayed expansion" and degradation of mechanical properties. These effects have been observed mostly in zinc-containing low-copper amalgams.[61–63]

When dental amalgam comes in contact with an object made of a different metal or alloy in the same electrolyte, redistribution of the electrochemical reactions causes a change in the corrosion potential and corrosion rate of both parts of the so-called *galvanic couple*. When dental amalgam contacts a more noble material, cathodic reactions occur preferentially on the noble metal while oxidation of the amalgam, which becomes the anode of the galvanic cell, is intensified. This interaction is potentially most severe for low-copper amalgams because an increase in the corrosion potential due to a galvanic contact may induce and accelerate the potential-dependent breakdown and dissolution of the γ_2 phase. In the range of metallic dental restorative materials, dental amalgam is anodic to most other dental alloys, but most significantly to noble casting alloys, such as alloys of gold or palladium.[64] A relatively low interaction occurs in contact with base metal alloys, such as Ni-Cr alloys or titanium.[64–67]

Tarnishing is a change, usually darkening, in the color of the restorations, attributable to the formation of surface films. Tarnishing of dental amalgam in vivo is one of the more complex phenomena of environmental interactions in the oral cavity. Although most attention has been focused on formation of sulfide tarnish films, other corrosion products, as well as carbonaceous organic biofilms, apparently play important roles.[68] Sulfide tarnishing has been attributed to reactions with sulfide ions, mainly present in some foods and drinks.[69,70] Silver and copper have particularly high affinity to sulfur, and the reaction products are insoluble, black, metal sulfides. Microorganisms have been reported to induce tarnish of some dental casting alloys.[71]

Aging of Dental Amalgam Restorations

While changes in the amalgam structure and properties due to time, temperature, mechanical forces, and environment can be individually observed and examined in the laboratory, a dental amalgam restoration is subjected to those effects simultaneously and over long periods of time. Complex and sometimes synergistic effects occur during the lifetime of a dental amalgam restoration. In the following discussion, an effort is made to outline these effects as they might occur in actual service. It must be recognized, however, that the published studies on which the description is based provide only brief snapshots of the conditions of dental amalgam restorations after specific in vivo or in vitro exposures, and thus many aspects of the described changes remain a matter of conjecture.

As the alloy for dental amalgam is triturated, the amalgamation reactions start, providing the dentist with a plastic mass that is inserted into the prepared tooth cavity, condensed, and carved. Within minutes, the reactions consume most of the free mercury and a large portion of the alloy powder, thus changing the plastic mass into a solid. Within a few hours, the more slowly continuing reactions generate a structure approaching a steady state. This structure exhibits sufficient strength for the restoration to withstand forces of mastication, although nearly full strength may take a day or two to develop. At this stage, the amalgam structure consists mainly of the matrix of the Ag-Hg-Sn γ_1 phase surrounding the unreacted particles of the original alloy and either the Sn-Hg γ_2 phase (in low-copper dental amalgams) or the Cu-Sn η' phase (in high-copper dental amalgams).

As soon as placement of the restoration in the prepared tooth cavity is complete, the dental amalgam is exposed to the environment and starts reacting with it. The initial environment for the external restoration surfaces consists of air, saliva, and usually some rinse used in the dental office. The immediate effect is the formation of oxide films, mainly tin oxide, on virtually all the surfaces of the amalgam exposed to the environment. A similar oxidation also occurs on the amalgam surfaces within the tooth cavity, where the dentinal fluid is the principal environment.

Within a relatively short time, usually a few hours, the restoration becomes subjected to food or drinks in addition to the continuing presence of saliva and to the mechanical forces of mastication. At the same time, temperature fluctuations occur. The restoration thus starts to experience the service conditions that will continue throughout its lifetime. One of these effects is partial removal of a very thin surface layer by abrasion due to chewing. Because the surfaces of the dental amalgam are now covered with a layer of oxide, it is this layer that is thinned and in some spots removed. Abrasion thus may result in exposure of a film-free surface of the phases of the amalgam microstructure to the environment, followed by repassivation when the abrasion forces cease. In the most severe abrasive situations, some of the metal also may be removed, exposing not only a fresh metal surface but also a surface that has been deformed and thus made even more susceptible to electrochemical attack. Because resistance to abrasion generally increases with increasing hardness, the phases most affected by the combination of abrasion and the environment are the softest phases of the amalgam microstructure, ie, the γ_1 matrix phase and, in low-copper amalgams, the corrosion-prone γ_2 phase.

Because the environment of the film-free surface is not only saliva but also the food involved in mastication, highly variable and complex reactions may occur. Once mastication stops, the amalgam slowly approaches the steady-state con-

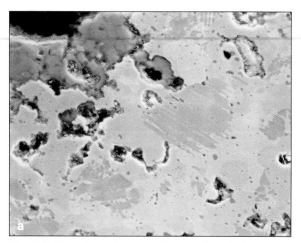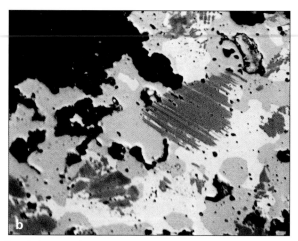

Fig 5-3 Scanning electron micrographs of the structure of a lathe-cut, low-copper dental amalgam (New True Dentalloy [SS White]) after 8 years of service in vivo. *(a)* Secondary electron image showing corrosion products of tin (upper left-hand corner and within porosities) (original magnification $\times$ 1,500). *(b)* Backscattered electron image of the same area as in *(a)*. The γ_1 and β_1 matrix phases are shown as darker gray (γ_1) and lighter gray (β_1) areas (original magnification $\times$ 1,500). (Courtesy of JD Adey and DB Mahler, Oregon Health Sciences University, Portland, OR.)

dition resulting from interaction with saliva, ie, the film grows back by electrochemical reactions to reach a thickness approaching the steady state. Although the abrasion rate per chewing event is very low, as discussed earlier, the frequent repetition of the abrasion/environment interaction events is important for the alterations of the amalgam restoration. In low-copper amalgams, the γ_2 phase on the surface is gradually both mechanically removed and electrochemically attacked, allowing the reactions to occur deeper and thus under more and more occluded conditions. Such occluded-cell corrosion conditions involve localized solution chemistry changes, which further intensify the corrosion attack in the form of pitting and crevice corrosion. If the γ_2 phase forms an interconnected network[56] and is associated with voids,[4] the corrosion attack continues to penetrate the structure. For the γ_1 phase, the abrasion/corrosion attack is much less severe; the removal and regrowth of the tin-oxide film, however, slowly depletes the tin content, possibly making this phase less stable and more prone to transformation to the β_1 phase, as discussed below.

With increasing time of service, more substantial environmental interaction takes place. Because the corrosion potential generally increases with time as the more active components are dissolved and some of the surface becomes covered with layers of reaction products and deposits, the potential may exceed the breakdown potential of the γ_2 phase still present on the surface in low-copper dental amalgams and thus may further accelerate its corrosion. Development of biofilms and production of metabolites of the microorganisms existing beneath biofilms are other sources of acidity, which enhance the corrosion process.[72] While the γ_2 phase in low-copper amalgams is the most corrosion-prone major phase of the amalgam microstructure, a much slower degradation of the Cu-Sn η' phase also occurs. In both cases the corroded phases are replaced with highly insoluble corrosion products of tin, which contribute virtually nothing to the strength of the material. The consequence is a loss of strength of the heterogeneously corroded amalgam. While mercury from the corroded γ_2 phase is absorbed by the γ_1 matrix or reacts with the residual original alloy, copper from the corroded Cu-Sn η' phase is mainly transported to the surface, where it is either dissolved in the oral liquids or forms solid corrosion products, such as chlorides.

The SEMs in Figs 5-3 and 5-4 illustrate some of the alterations of the amalgam microstructure in vivo for low-copper and high-copper dental amalgams, respectively. Figure 5-3a is a second-

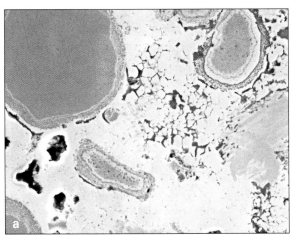 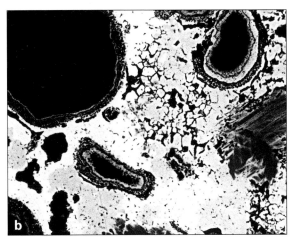

Fig 5-4 Scanning electron micrographs of the structure of an admixed, high-copper dental amalgam (Dispersalloy) after 5 years of service in vivo. *(a)* Secondary electron image (original magnification × 1,500). *(b)* Backscattered electron image of the same area as in *(a)*. The γ_1 and β_1 matrix phases are shown as darker gray (γ_1) and lighter gray (β_1) areas (original magnification × 1,500). (Courtesy of JD Adey and DB Mahler, Oregon Health Sciences University, Portland, OR.)

ary electron image of a lathe-cut, low-copper amalgam after 8 years of service, showing large amounts of tin corrosion products within the structure. Figure 5-3b is a backscattered electron image of the same area, showing that the matrix has become a mixture of γ_1 (darker gray) and β_1 (lighter gray) phases. Figure 5-4a is a secondary electron image of an admixed high-copper amalgam after 5 years of service, in which the η' phase in the reaction rings has been replaced with corrosion products of tin. A backscattered electron image in Fig 5-4b shows that the matrix of this amalgam also has become a mixture of the γ_1 and β_1 phases.

While the above changes affect the occlusal surface and to some extent all the external surfaces of a dental amalgam restoration, similar, but possibly even more rapid, corrosion occurs at the amalgam-tooth interface. Unless there is a bond between the tooth and the amalgam, oral liquids penetrate the interface by capillary action, and the dentinal fluid provides an additional environment for the corrosion process. In the resulting occluded corrosion cell, the corrosion reactions are accelerated by the acidic conditions and lack of oxygen. Consequently, degradation of the γ_2 or η' phase occurs initially more rapidly than at or below the external surface of the restoration. However, in low-copper amalgams,

and to a lesser degree in high-copper amalgams, the tooth-amalgam gap eventually becomes filled with solid corrosion products, which not only anchor the restoration in the cavity but also may slow down the corrosion process.

Because the dental amalgam surface within the prepared tooth cavity is initially exposed to a more aggressive environment than the saliva-exposed external surfaces, galvanic and concentration cell effects develop between the two regions, and the surface within the cavity becomes anodic with respect to a cathodic external surface. The result of this interaction is a decrease in the corrosion rate on the external surface and an increased rate of degradation at the regions adjacent to the walls of the prepared cavity. This effect, however, is likely to be rather small, and it diminishes even further when the tooth-amalgam gap fills with corrosion products, which increase the resistance in the current path between the two surface regions.

In all locations, the rate of corrosion is likely to decrease with time as the attack penetrates deeper into the structure. This effect is due to the growing length of the current path between the external surface and the corrosion sites and therefore a higher electrical resistance for this path. The external surfaces, which are exposed to an aerated electrolyte, are cathodic to the actively corroding sites and maintain a relatively high potential, which accelerates corrosion within the occluded cells. When electrical resistance decreases (an *ohmic drop*) between the external surface and the corrosion site, both the potential and the corrosion rate at the localized corrosion sites decrease.

While the corrosion reactions slowly consume the least resistant phases of the amalgam microstructure, continuing phase transformations change the surrounding phases. The most noticeable is the gradual replacement of the mercury-rich γ_1 phase with the more stable β_1 phase, as illustrated in Figs 5-3b and 5-4b. If tin stabilizes the γ_1 phase[19] and is removed from the γ_1 phase by electrochemical reactions with the environment, then the γ_1 to β_1 transformation should be accelerated. Corrosion enhancement of the γ_1 to β_1 transformation has been observed.[47,73,74] Because the β_1 phase contains less mercury and more tin than γ_1, it appears that the transformation also involves the consumption of some of the unreacted Ag-Sn γ phase and the Cu-Sn ϵ phase. The continuing amalgamation of the γ phase in low-copper amalgams theoretically results in the formation of some new γ_2 phase; this effect, however, is likely to be small enough to have negligible effect on the corrosion behavior.

In low-copper dental amalgams, some of the consumption of the γ phase also may be due to the liberation of mercury from the Sn-Hg γ_2 phase as this phase corrodes. The liberated mercury either reacts directly with the residual original alloy particles or dissolves in the γ_1 phase, thus increasing its mercury content and enhancing its reactivity with respect to the γ phase.

Although some opposing tendencies exist with regard to the effects of the environmental degradation and phase transformations on the mechanical properties, the overall result undoubtedly is a loss of strength. While the γ_1 to β_1 phase change is likely to contribute some strength increase, the decrease in the hard γ-phase content, which provides strengthening as it is dispersed in the much softer γ_1 matrix, results in a strength loss. Both major corrosion effects, ie, destruction of the γ_2 phase in low-copper dental amalgams and the slower oxidation of the η' phase in high-copper

amalgams, weaken the microstructure. In addition, formation of voluminous corrosion products within the microstructure may exert hydrostatic pressure on the surrounding metal. There is thus little doubt that, after a relatively short initial period, the strength of a dental amalgam decreases with the time of service, as observed in laboratory studies.[75,76]

After a long period of service, the bulk strength of the dental amalgam restoration may be reduced severely enough for bulk fracture to occur under the forces of mastication. Although bulk fracture may occur in any restoration simply because of excessive biting force, it is rare in a properly prepared new restoration. Most bulk fractures occur either because of incorrect cavity or amalgam preparation or because of long-term weakening of the amalgam structure by environmental effects. The most likely locations of bulk fracture are those of the smallest cross section, such as through the isthmus of Class II restorations.

Apart from abrasion and the extreme conditions that result in bulk fracture, chewing subjects the amalgam to stresses that may exceed the yield stress in more than just the thin surface layer and thus would cause permanent deformation. In view of the susceptibility of the amalgam to time-dependent strain, some of the deformation may occur by a mechanism of creep. In the initial service period, these deformation changes probably cause some rearrangement of the surface features of the restoration, thus altering slightly the restoration shape. The most important shape changes are those that contribute to the most visible and most common form of degradation of dental amalgam restorations, namely, marginal fracture. The breakdown of the margins is considered to be the most common cause of amalgam failure.[77]

The causes and mechanism of the fracture of the amalgam margins have been the subject of controversy and numerous studies, and both mechanical and corrosion processes have been implicated. Although the exact contribution of the various individual factors has not been fully elucidated, it appears reasonable to consider a mechanism or mechanisms in which mechanical forces, temperature fluctuation, time, and environmental effects all play some roles. It is also reasonable to consider that the relative contribution of the different forces may differ from patient to patient and from restoration to restoration.

One of the major steps in the breakdown of the margins is extrusion of the amalgam along the margins and formation or enlargement of the tooth-amalgam gap. Creep deformation of an amalgam restoration, as it is confined in the tooth cavity and subjected to the forces of mastication, may be the cause of extrusion of the restoration from the cavity and may contribute to the formation of a gap.[78,79] Dimensional changes due to the continuing reactions in the amalgam structure over time and the formation of voluminous corrosion products within the tooth-amalgam gap have also been proposed as potential causes of the creep-induced extrusion of restorations.[80,81] Another alternative mechanism proposes that thermal cycling within the oral environment results in stresses and creep deformation because of the difference in thermal expansion coefficients of tooth structure and dental amalgam.[82]

In reality, it is likely that all the above effects play some role, and only their relative contribution is uncertain, which may vary from patient to patient depending upon the properties of the amalgam, restoration shape and size, mastication forces, eating habits of the patient, and other factors. Regardless of the exact mechanism, the consequence of the extrusion and gap formation for the dental amalgam restoration is an unsupported layer (or wedge) of the amalgam at the margins. Although fracture at the margins can occur by thermocycling of an amalgam confined in a cavity even in the absence of this wedge, as demonstrated by Williams and Hedge,[36] the mechanical loading of an unsupported amalgam layer at the margin appears to be a more severe and thus more likely condition for fracture.

Just as there are numerous factors that may contribute to extrusion of the amalgam at the margins of the cavity, there are several possible modes of margin fracture as well. Under various conditions, the mode of fracture also varies, including a combination of effects acting in concert. The simplest and most obvious cause of frac-ture is overload, occurring when the force on the occlusal surface results in a stress exceeding the fracture stress. At an improperly prepared restoration containing an unsupported wedge of dental amalgam at the margin of a prepared tooth cavity, the normal force on the occlusal surface results in a bending load at the margin, which is associated with tensile stress in the overhanging wedge of amalgam. Because of the brittle nature and thus low tensile strength of dental amalgam, fracture occurs relatively easily. Under these conditions, fracture occurs when the stress intensity factor exceeds the fracture toughness of the amalgam.

As long as the tensile stress does not exceed the fracture stress, or the stress intensity factor remains below the fracture toughness value, sudden overload (*critical*) fracture does not occur. Fatigue fracture may occur gradually (*subcritically*), however, at stresses well below the fracture stress, as observed in dental amalgam in vitro by Sutow et al.[33] Evidence of fatigue failure in retrieved dental amalgam restorations has been reported.[83,84] Another fracture mode that has received substantial attention is creep fatigue; eg, fracture of dental amalgam in vitro as a result of thermocycling or mechanical loading has been attributed to this mode.[36,37]

Some controversy has developed with regard to the role and importance of corrosion in margin fracture of dental amalgam restorations. Sarkar,[82] Sarkar et al,[85] McTigue et al,[68] and others have emphasized the importance of corrosion damage in degradation. Hanawa et al,[86] on the other hand, observed marginal cracks in retrieved restorations even in the absence of significant corrosion attack. The evaluation of the role of corrosion is further complicated by the fact that low-copper dental amalgams, which generally are more susceptible to margin fracture than high-copper amalgams, also exhibit both higher creep rate[1] and higher corrosion susceptibility.[87]

Although fracture at the margins can occur under appropriate loading conditions for an uncorroded dental amalgam, it would defy logic and evidence to deny a significant role of corrosion in many, if not most, instances of margin breakdown. Dental amalgam corrodes in the oral environment, and corrosion results in the replacement of some of the microstructural phases with corrosion products lacking any load-bearing capacity. It is thus highly unlikely that resistance to fracture at the margins would not be reduced by the corrosion degradation. Although the documented improvement in the marginal integrity of high-copper dental amalgams compared with the γ_2-containing low-copper amalgams[34,77,88,89] has been correlated with their lower creep values,[34] there is every reason to believe that the better corrosion resistance of the high-copper amalgams also plays an important role.

The corrosion attack is especially intense in the amalgam-tooth gap at the margins due to crevice conditions; stress and strain resulting from mechanical loading of the margins also accelerate the corrosion attack. The loss of strength of dental amalgam due to corrosion has been documented.[75,90] Except for early fracture of those margins that are not subjected to the effects of the environment long enough to suffer corrosion damage, breakdown of the margins must be affected by the environmental degradation.

In addition to the direct lowering of the fracture strength, corrosion may accelerate degradation by a synergy with mechanical loading in the form of environment-induced cracking. Since the mechanical forces on a restoration fluctuate, corrosion fatigue rather than stress corrosion cracking is the more likely form of failure. Fatigue and creep fatigue of clinical restorations are thus likely to take the form of corrosion fatigue and creep-corrosion fatigue. The nature of these mechanisms, however, which are a matter of substantial controversy for other industrial metals and alloys, has not been determined for dental amalgam.

The electrochemical degradation of an amalgam restoration may be increased or decreased by direct contact with another metal, such as an adjoining metal crown or an endodontic post. A galvanic cell forms when the two metals have different individual corrosion potentials, as discussed earlier. Dental amalgam thus becomes the anode and is subjected to accelerated corrosion in contact with noble dental casting alloys, and possibly with some strongly passivating base metals, such as titanium.[65-67,91-93] Most base metals, such as the Ni-Cr dental alloys, however, do not inter-

act strongly with dental amalgams because of the closeness of the corrosion potentials. Despite the attention given to "oral galvanism" in the literature, a practical long-term effect on dental amalgam restorations is usually negligible because the rate of the galvanic interaction sharply decreases with electrical resistance in the current path between the dissimilar metals. In the case of adjoining restorations, even if in contact initially, corrosion of the more active metal usually results in the formation of nonmetallic corrosion products, which create an insulating layer at the previous contact points. Theoretically, a more damaging galvanic interaction occurs between restorations that come into contact only intermittently during chewing. This is because chewing also disturbs the surface films, thus both removing insulating layers and causing the anodic metal to corrode under the active condition of a film-free surface rather than in a passive state. Little is known, however, about the severity of such interaction in the long term. A galvanic interaction between endodontic posts and amalgam may not be significantly reduced by the development of a high-resistance contact. On the other hand, the surface area of a cathodic endodontic post is likely to be rather small compared with the surface area of the anodic amalgam, a galvanic situation that is much less detrimental than the opposite area ratio.

While phase changes and corrosion attack profoundly change the structure and properties of a dental amalgam restoration, tarnishing degrades the restoration's appearance without necessarily affecting its other functions. As discussed earlier, tarnishing in the oral cavity is a complex process, involving not only chemical and electrochemical interactions with sulfur (sulfide tarnishing) and formation of electrochemical corrosion products but also deposits of organic matter. Roughness of the amalgam surface then plays an important role in the retention of such deposits. A large part of the tarnishing films and deposits are probably continuously removed by chewing and tooth brushing. Corrosion and mechanical attack on a heterogeneous material, such as amalgam, is inherently nonuniform, however, and most amalgam restorations in time suffer roughening of the surface and some degree of tarnishing. Although tarnishing degrades the appearance of restorations, and in severe cases may itself be the cause of surface roughening, some insoluble solid films, such as metal sulfides, may provide a degree of protection against other electrochemical forms of attack.[64]

References

1. Mahler DB. Research on dental amalgam: 1982–1986. Adv Dent Res 1988;2:71–82.

2. Schoch P, Loebich O. Porosity of our amalgam fillings [in German]. Dtsch Zahnarztl Z 1955;10:785–790.

3. Jorgensen KD, Esbensen AL, Borring-Moller G. The effect of porosity and mercury content upon the strength of silver amalgam. Acta Odontol Scand 1966;24:535–553.

4. Wing G. Phase identification in dental amalgam. Aust Dent J 1966;11:105–113.

5. Boswell PG. Transmission electron metallography of non-gamma-2 silver dental amalgams. Scripta Metall 1979;13:383–388.

6. Mahler DB, Adey JD, Van Eysden J. Quantitative microprobe analysis of amalgam. J Dent Res 1975;54:218–226.

7. Okabe T, Mitchell R, Butts MB, Bosley JR, Fairhurst CW. Analysis of Asgar-Mahler reaction zone in Dispersalloy amalgam by electron diffraction. J Dent Res 1977;56:1037–1043.

8. Johnson LB Jr. Comparative rates of amalgam formation from tin, silver, and dental alloy powders. J Dent Res 1967;46:753.

9. Marshall SJ, Marshall GW Jr. Time-dependent phase changes in Cu-rich amalgams. J Biomed Mater Res 1979;13:395–406.

10. Mahler DB, Adey JD, Fleming MA. Hg emission from dental amalgam as related to the amount of Sn in the Ag-Hg (γ_1) phase. J Dent Res 1994;73:1663–1668.

11. Fairhurst CW, Cohen JB. The crystal structures of two compounds found in dental amalgam: Ag_2Hg_3 and Ag_3Sn. Acta Cryst 1972;B28:371–378.

12. Johnson LB Jr. Confirmation of the presence of β (Ag-Hg) in dental amalgam. J Biomed Mater Res 1967;1:415–425.

13. Johnson LB Jr. X-ray diffraction evidence for the presence of β (Ag-Hg) in dental amalgam. J Biomed Mater Res 1967;1:285–297.

14. Boyer DB, Edie JW. Composition of clinically aged amalgam restorations. Dent Mater 1990;6:146–150.

15. Mahler DB, Adey JD, Van Eysden J. Transformation of γ_1 in clinical amalgam restorations [abstract 190]. J Dent Res 1973;52:106.

16. Marshall SJ, Marshall GW, Letzel H, Vrijhoef MMA. β_1 content in amalgam restorations [abstract 36]. J Dent Res 1986;65:729.

17. Marshall SJ, Marshall GW Jr, Letzel H. γ_1 to β_1 phase transformation in retrieved clinical amalgam restorations. Dent Mater 1992;8:162–166.

18. Johnson LB Jr. Ag-Sn-Hg alloys as electron compounds. J Biomed Mater Res 1970;4:269–274.

19. Johnson LB Jr. The amount of tin in the γ_1 phase of dental amalgam. J Biomed Mater Res 1971;5:239–244.

20. Mahler DB, Adey JD. Sn in the Ag-Hg phase of dental amalgam. J Dent Res 1988;67:1275–1277.

21. Sarkar NK, Greener EH. Aging of Dispersalloy and its effect on the anodic behavior of its amalgams. Biomater Med Devices Artif Organs 1975;3:429–437.

22. Jensen SJ, Jorgensen KD. Stoichiometric and x-ray diffraction analysis on the γ_2 leads to η' transformation in a dispersant phase silver amalgam. Scand J Dent Res 1981;89:108–112.

23. Sarkar NK, Greener EH. In vitro chloride corrosion behaviour of Dispersalloy. J Oral Rehabil 1975;2:139–144.

24. Marshall GW. Reappearance of γ_2 in aged high Cu amalgams [abstract 33]. J Dent Res 1986;65:729.

25. Okabe T. Dental amalgams. In: Williams D (ed). Concise Encyclopedia of Medical and Dental Materials. Oxford: Pergamon Press, 1990:127–134.

26. Mahler DB, Nelson LW. Factors affecting the marginal leakage of amalgam. J Am Dent Assoc 1984;108:51–54.

27. Mahler DB, Nelson LW. Sensitivity answers sought in amalgam alloy microleakage study. J Am Dent Assoc 1994;125:282–288.

28. Craig RG (ed). Restorative Dental Materials, ed 10. St. Louis: Mosby, 1997:56.

29. Cruickshanks-Boyd DW, Lock WR. Fracture toughness of dental amalgams. Biomaterials 1983;4:234–242.

30. Hassan R, Vaidyanathan TK, Schulman A. Fracture toughness determination of dental amalgams through microindentation. J Biomed Mater Res 1986;20:135–142.

31. Lloyd CH, Adamson M. The fracture toughness (K_{Ic}) of amalgam. J Oral Rehabil 1985;12:59–68.

32. Wilkinson EG, Haack DC. A study of the fatigue characteristics of silver amalgam. J Dent Res 1958;37:136–143.

33. Sutow EJ, Jones DW, Hall GC, Milne EL. The response of dental amalgam to dynamic loading. J Dent Res 1985;64:62–66.

34. Mahler DB, Terkla LG, Van Eysden J, Reisbick MH. Marginal fracture vs mechanical properties of amalgam. J Dent Res 1970;49:1452–1457.

35. Mitchell RJ, Ogura H, Nakamura K, Hanawa T, Marker VA, Okabe T. Characterization of fractured surfaces of dental amalgams. In: International Symposium for Testing and Failure Analysis. Proceedings of the Advanced Materials Symposium. Materials Park, OH: ASM International, 1987:179–187.

36. Williams PT, Hedge GL. Creep-fatigue as a possible cause of dental amalgam margin failure. J Dent Res 1985;64:470–475.

37. Williams PT, Cahoon JR. Amalgam margin breakdown caused by creep fatigue rupture. J Dent Res 1989;68:1188–1193.

38. Lutz F, Phillips RW, Roulet JF, Setcos JC. In vivo and in vitro wear of potential posterior composites. J Dent Res 1984;63:914–920.

39. Brune D. Corrosion of amalgams. Scand J Dent Res 1981;89:506–514.

40. Espevik S. In vitro corrosion of dental amalgams with different Cu content. Scand J Dent Res 1977;85:631–636.

41. Lin JH, Marshall GW, Marshall SJ. Corrosion product formation sequence on Cu-rich amalgams in various solutions. J Biomed Mater Res 1983;17:913–920.

42. Marshall SJ, Marshall GW Jr. $Sn_4(OH)_6Cl_2$ and SnO corrosion products of amalgams. J Dent Res 1980;59:820–823.

43. Marshall SJ, Lin JH, Marshall GW Jr. Cu_2O and $CuCl_2 \cdot 3Cu(OH)_2$ corrosion products on copper rich dental amalgams. J Biomed Mater Res 1982;16:81–85.

44. Ravnholt G. Accelerated corrosion analysis of dental amalgams. Scand J Dent Res 1986;94:553–561.

45. Ravnholt G. Corrosion of dental alloys in vitro by differential oxygen concentration. Scand J Dent Res 1986;94:370–376.

46. Sarkar NK, Marshall GW, Moser JB, Greener EH. In vivo and in vitro corrosion products of dental amalgam. J Dent Res 1975;54:1031–1038.

47. Sutow EJ, Jones DW, Hall GC, Owen CG. Crevice corrosion products of dental amalgam. J Dent Res 1991;70:1082–1087.

48. Marek M, Hochman RF. Corrosion behavior of amalgam electrodes in artificial saliva [abstract 63]. IADR [International Association for Dental Research] Program and Abstracts, 1972.

49. Carter DA, Ross TK, Smith DC. Some corrosion studies on silver-tin amalgam. Br Corr J 1967;2:199–205.

50. Marek M, Hochman RF. The corrosion behavior of dental amalgam phases as a function of tin content [abstract 192]. J Dent Res 1973;52:106.

51. Marek M, Okabe T. Corrosion behavior of structural phases in high copper dental amalgam. J Biomed Mater Res 1978;12:857–886.

52. Wagner E. Beitrag zur klärung des korrosionsverhaltens der silber-zinn-amalgame [Contribution to clarification of the corrosion behavior of silver-tin amalgams]. Dtsch Zahnarztl Z 1962;17:99–106.

53. Jorgensen KD. The mechanism of marginal fracture of amalgam fillings. Acta Odontol Scand 1965;23:347–389.

54. Deltombe E, De Zoubov N, Vanleugenhaghe C, Pourbaix M. Tin. In: Pourbaix M (ed). Atlas of Electrochemical Equilibria in Aqueous Solutions. Houston: National Association of Corrosion Engineers (NACE), 1974:475–484.

55. Marek M, Hochman RF. Mechanism of crevice corrosion of dental amalgam [abstract L166]. J Dent Res 1975;54:L42.

56. Taylor DF. Porosity in silver-tin amalgams. J Biomed Mater Res 1972;6:289–304.

57. Holland GA, Asgar K. Some effects on the phases of amalgam induced by corrosion. J Dent Res 1974;53:1245–1254.

58. Otani H, Jesser WA, Wilsdorf HG. The in vivo and in vitro corrosion products of dental amalgams. J Biomed Mater Res 1973;7:523–539.

59. Ogletree RH, Marek M. Effect of mercury on corrosion of η´ Cu-Sn phase in dental amalgams. Dent Mater 1995;11:332–336.

60. Derand T, Johansson B. Corrosion of non-γ_2-amalgams. Scand J Dent Res 1983;91:55–60.

61. Yamada T. A study on high-copper amalgam: Effect of moisture contamination on dimensional changes of amalgams [in Japanese]. Kokubyo Gakkai Zasshi 1978;45:280–289.

62. Yamada T. A study on high-copper amalgam. Part II. Effect of moisture contamination on physical properties of amalgams [in Japanese]. Kokubyo Gakkai Zasshi 1979;46:202–210.

63. Yamada T. Effect of moisture contamination on copper amalgam [in Japanese]. Kokubyo Gakkai Zasshi 1980;47:399.

64. Marek M. The corrosion of dental materials. In: Scully JC (ed). Corrosion: Aqueous Processes and Passive Films. London: Academic Press, 1983:331–394.

65. Bumgardner JD, Johansson BI. Galvanic corrosion and cytotoxic effects of amalgam and gallium alloys coupled to titanium. Eur J Oral Sci 1996;104:300–308.

66. Horasawa N, Takahashi S, Marek M. Galvanic interaction between titanium and gallium alloy or dental amalgam. Dent Mater 1999;15:318–322.

67. Johansson BI, Bergman B. Corrosion of titanium and amalgam couples: Effect of fluoride, area size, surface preparation and fabrication procedures. Dent Mater 1995;11:41–46.

68. McTigue D, Brice C, Nanda CR, Sarkar NK. The in vivo corrosion of Dispersalloy. J Oral Rehabil 1984;11:351–359.

69. Swartz ML, Philips RW, el Tannir MD. Tarnish of certain dental alloys. J Dent Res 1958;37:837–847.

70. Sarkar NK, Fuys RA Jr, Stanford JW. The effect of copper on the sulfide tarnish resistance of dental amalgams [abstract 895]. J Dent Res 1976;55:B285.

71. Vaidyanathan TK, Vaidyanathan J, Linke HAB, Schulman A. Tarnish of dental alloys by oral microorganisms. J Prosthet Dent 1991;66:709–714.

72. Kleinberg I. Etiology of dental caries. J Can Dent Assoc 1979;45:661–668.

73. Lin JH, Marshall GW, Marshall SJ. Microstructures of Cu-rich amalgams after corrosion. J Dent Res 1983;62:112–115.

74. Lin JHC, Marshall GW, Marshall SJ. Phase changes in Cu-rich amalgams after corrosion in various solutions [abstract 65]. J Dent Res 1984;63:178.

75. Averette DF, Hochman RF, Marek M. The effects of corrosion in vitro on the structure and properties of dental amalgam [abstract 361]. J Dent Res 1978;57:165.

76. Chen CP, Greener EH. The effect of anodic polarization on the tensile strength of dental amalgam. J Oral Rehabil 1976;3:323–332.

77. Osborne JW, Binon PP, Gale EN. Dental amalgam: Clinical behavior up to eight years. Oper Dent 1980;5:24–28.

78. Derand T. Creep in amalgam Class V restorations. Odontol Revy 1976;27:181–186.

79. Derand T. Marginal failure of amalgam Class II restoration. J Dent Res 1977;56:481–485.

80. Osborne JW, Winchell PG, Phillips RW. A hypothetical mechanism by which creep causes marginal failure of amalgam restorations. J Indiana Dent Assoc 1978;57:16–17.

81. Paffenbarger GC, Rupp NW. Relation between clinical behavior and expansion of three amalgams [abstract 21]. J Dent Res 1983;62:172.

82. Sarkar NK. Creep, corrosion and marginal fracture of dental amalgams. J Oral Rehabil 1978;5:413–423.

83. Espevik S, Mjor IA. Topography and mechanism of marginal degradation of amalgam restorations [abstract 32]. J Dent Res 1979;58:100.

84. Mateer RS, Reitz CD. Corrosion of amalgam restorations. J Dent Res 1970;49:399–407.

85. Sarkar NK, Osborne JW, Leinfelder KF. In vitro corrosion and in vivo marginal fracture of dental amalgams. J Dent Res 1982;61:1262–1268.

86. Hanawa T, Ota M, Marker VA, Mitchell RJ, Okabe T. Crack initiation and propagation in retrieved amalgams [abstract 42]. J Dent Res 1988;67:118.

87. Marek M. Corrosion test for dental amalgam. J Dent Res 1980;59:63–69.

88. Letzel H, Vrijhoef MM. Long-term influences on marginal fracture of amalgam restorations. J Oral Rehabil 1984;11:95–101.

89. Mahler DB, Terkla LG, Van Eysden J. Marginal fracture of amalgam restorations. J Dent Res 1973;52:823–827.

90. Jorgensen KD. The strength of corroded amalgam. Acta Odontol Scand 1972;30:33–38.

91. Johansson BI. Electrochemical action due to short-circuiting of dental alloys: An in vitro and in vivo study. Swed Dent J Suppl 1986;33:1–47.

92. Johansson BI. An in vitro study of galvanic currents between amalgam and gold alloy electrodes in saliva and in saline solutions. Scand J Dent Res 1986;94:562–568.

93. Johansson BI, Lagerlof F. Integrated currents between amalgams and a gold alloy in saline solutions and natural saliva with different chloride content. Scand J Dent Res 1992;100:240–243.

6

AGING OF GLASS-IONOMER CEMENTS

Aphrodite I. Kakaboura, DDS, Dr Dent

Wilson and Kent[1] reported their development of glass-ionomer cements in 1972. The basic powder and liquid components that are mixed to yield glass ionomers consist of an aluminosilicate glass and a polycarboxylic acid, respectively. The main advantages of these cements, which set through an acid-base reaction, are an ability to bond chemically to enamel and dentin, a long-term fluoride release, and a coefficient of thermal expansion similar to tooth tissues.[2,3] However, the glass ionomers also exhibit several disadvantages: low strength and wear resistance, relatively poor esthetic appearance, and technique sensitivity associated with handling characteristics and sensitivity to moisture during the early setting phase. Various types of glass ionomers have been designed and used as restorative, luting, and base/liner materials.

Continuous modifications in conventional glass ionomers have led to introduction of new formulations. In 1985, the first report[4] of glass-cermet cements was published. Metal ions were incorporated into the glass particles to enhance the strength of the cements. The resin-modified glass ionomers represent the latest generation of glass ionomers,[5] in which the fundamental acid-base reaction is supplemented by a light-curing and/or chemical-curing polymerization reaction.[6] These cements were developed chiefly to provide improved mechanical strength, solubility, wear resistance, moisture sensitivity, and esthetic performance compared with conventional glass ionomers.

Structural Characteristics

Composition, Setting Reaction, and Structure

For conventional glass-ionomer cements, the powder component consists of ion-leachable glasses, which are based on the original SiO_2-AlO_3-CaF_2-$AlPO_4$-Na_3AlF_6 composition.[7] Several types of glasses with very complex structures have been used in commercial products. The glass controls the setting rate, strength, and translucency of the cement.[8] The particle size of the glass is of great importance for governing the setting time, film thickness, and essential powder-liquid ratio.[9] Fluoride glasses produce stronger cements than oxide glasses with improved handling properties and a potential cariostatic effect.[10] Small metallic particles, such as silver, may be incorporated into the glass during fusion, creating metal-reinforced glass-cermet cements.[4] The composition of the powder for resin-modified glass ionomers is basically similar to that for conventional glass ionomers. Strontium aluminosilicate or barium aluminosilicate glasses are used in some products to provide radiopacity.[11]

The liquid component of glass-ionomer cements is an aqueous solution of a homopolymer or a copolymer of mono-, di-, and tricarboxylic acids.[12] The polyacrylic, polymaleic, and itaconic acids are usually used. Tartaric acid is incorporated into the liquid to prolong the working time and increase the setting rate.[13] The type, molecular weight, and concentration of the polycarboxylic acid affect the acid reactivity, setting rate, and strength of the cement.[14] The polyacrylic acid may be in a vacuum-dried form incorporated into the glass powder to yield a water-hardening cement.[15] The basic composition of the liquid component for resin-modified glass ionomers is polycarboxylic acid, water, and 2-hydroxyethyl methacrylate (HEMA).[16] Some products contain methacrylate-based monomers or methyl methacrylate–modified polycarboxylic acids. Photoinitiators and/or chemical initiators of a free-radical polymerization mechanism are added to the liquid.

When the glass powder and the liquid of a conventional glass ionomer are combined, an acid-base reaction is induced.[17,18] Metal ions are released from the glass surfaces after attack by hydrogen ions of the polycarboxylic acid. Calcium polycarboxylate salts are formed, which are responsible for the initial set by gelation. Upon cement maturation, aluminum polycarboxylate salts are precipitated, resulting in the final set, and the glass particles are partially or totally degraded to a siliceous hydrogel.[9,18] The final set structure consists of unreacted and partially reacted glasses surrounded by a siliceous hydrogel and embedded in a mixture of ionic cross-linked calcium and aluminum polycarboxylate salts.

The setting reaction is based on a dual mechanism in the resin-modified glass ionomers.[6,19] The acid-base reaction is first induced after mixing the powder and liquid, followed by a free-radical polymerization reaction while the acid-base reaction is continued. Finally, a metal polycarboxylate salt hydrogel and a polymer network are formed. The polycarboxylate salt matrix plays a crucial role in strengthening the cement, while the poly-

mer matrix provides the initial set. Some resin-modified glass-ionomer products cannot be characterized as true glass-ionomer cements because an acid-base reaction has not been identified.[20]

Physicomechanical Properties

The physicomechanical properties of glass-ionomer cements vary widely among the different commercial products and among the types of cements. Variations in the powder-liquid ratio, glass powder, degree of cement hydration, and porosity all affect the properties of a cement.[2]

A remarkable increase in strength is apparent as the cement undergoes setting. However, the final strength of the set glass-ionomer cement remains low compared with resin composite and dental amalgam restorative materials.[21] In contrast, the glass-ionomer luting cements are stronger than the zinc phosphate and zinc polycarboxylate luting cements.[22]

Water has an important role in the integrity of the glass-ionomer cements.[23] Water absorption during the initial setting stage leads to deterioration of the cement and to loss of translucency. Simultaneously, dehydration of the cement causes surface crazing. Protection of the cement surface with a hydrophobic agent is suggested to prevent adverse effects of water upon cement maturation. The low resistance to wear and erosion of the glass-ionomer cements in various aqueous solutions causes rapid degradation.[24] The latter characteristic, together with the insufficient polishability of glass-ionomer cements, leads to an increasingly rough cement surface over time. The inclusion of metal ions in glass-cermet cements achieved no significant increase in strength or dissolution resistance of the cements.[25]

The resin-modified glass-ionomer cements exhibit more rapid development of strength and greater resistance to early moisture contamination than the conventional glass ionomers. The compressive strength, diametral tensile strength, flexural strength, and fracture toughness of the resin-modified cements have been dramatically improved compared with the conventional glass ionomers.[26,27]

Fluoride Release, Adhesion, and Biocompatibility

The glass particles in glass ionomers contain fluoride, which may be released mainly in the form of sodium fluoride.[28] Although the amount of fluoride released varies for the different glass-ionomer products, all cements have a similar release pattern.[29] A high rate of fluoride release is recorded during the first days, and a gradual continuous decline occurs thereafter. It has been shown that the cements can be recharged by fluoride uptake from the oral environment, thus acting as fluoride devices with slow release rates into the oral cavity.[30] The glass-ionomer cements are believed to exert a cariostatic effect due to this fluoride release. The resin-modified glass ionomers release a lower amount of fluoride than the conventional glass ionomers yet present essentially the same release-rate profile.[31]

The glass-ionomer cements can bond with enamel, dentin, and base metals. An ion-exchange process between the cement and the tooth substrate leads to the development of an ion-enriched intermediate layer of new material at the cement-tooth interface that is firmly attached to the tooth surface. Bond failures are located in the bulk of the cement rather than at the interface.[32] This means that the stronger the glass ionomer, the greater the adhesion. Thus, the significantly higher bond established between the resin-modified glass ionomers and the tooth tissues may be derived from the enhanced strength of the cements.

Residual polycarboxylic acid in the set cement may have an adverse effect on the pulp integrity. However, the high molecular mass of the acids and the dentin buffer capacity seem to cause only a mild irreversible pulpal inflammation in the absence of bacteria.[33]

Clinical Applications

Glass-ionomer cements are used in a variety of clinical applications. The poor esthetic appearance of these cements eliminates their use as restorative materials in esthetic anterior restorations. How-ever, the intrinsic adhesive properties of glass ionomers support their use for the restoration of cervical caries and for abrasion and erosion lesions. The low strength and wear resistance of the glass-ionomer cements, in addition to their brittle nature, prevent their use as restorative materials in occlusal and stress-bearing areas of the permanent teeth. On the other hand, these materials have been strongly recommended as alternatives to dental amalgam for posterior restorations in the primary teeth. Another recommendation for the clinical use of glass ionomers is as pit and fissure sealant in preventive dentistry because of their self-adhesive potential with enamel.

Fine-grained types of glass-ionomer cements have been used for luting of crowns, fixed partial dentures, and inlays. These materials are applied for orthodontic band cementation and bracket bonding as well. The adhesive capacity and the anticariogenic potential of the glass-ionomer cements are considered to be particularly beneficial properties for luting agents.

The clinical characteristics, importance, and extent of in vivo aging for the glass ionomers vary in relation to the aforementioned clinical applications. The in vivo aging performance of glass ionomers in restorations, in orthodontic practice, and in fixed prostheses will be described below.

Restorative Glass-Ionomer Cements

Degradation

The degree of degradation of restorative materials in the oral environment is directly related to the type of restoration and the biodynamic environment of the patient. Important clinical characteristics of restorations associated with material degradation are retention, marginal adaptation, marginal discoloration, anatomic form, color match, evidence of secondary caries, and surface texture. Restorative glass-ionomer cements are usually employed for Class I and II restorations of primary teeth, as well as in restorations of cervical lesions due to erosion/abrasion and of permanent teeth where caries has occurred.

Regardless of where glass-ionomer cements are used clinically, stresses arising from masticatory loads and frictional forces act upon the cement microstructure and lead to the formation of wear particles and detachment of cement material from the contacting surfaces.[34] Such surface pitting and chipping cause changes in surface texture and roughness. Changes in the anatomic form of the glass-ionomer restorations and marginal ditching arise from bulk material loss. Furthermore, fatigue, mechanical overloading, and corrosive actions of the oral fluids may also soften or degrade the glass ionomer.

In vivo assessment of material degradation in restorations involves direct and/or indirect evaluation methods. Various techniques of qualitative evaluation that have been employed, collectively described as *wear measurements*, are based on the preparation of replica models that are subsequently evaluated by ranking systems.[35,36] Reliable measurements can be performed with three-dimensional coordinate mapping of the surfaces, thus allowing quantitative determination of the material lost. However, these more sophisticated techniques principally have been used to investigate the wear degradation of resin composites, whereas there has been minimal application for the glass ionomers. Clinical evaluation of the latter restorations has been achieved only by qualitative observations, using the criteria and ranking system described by Cvar and Ryge.[37] The silicone impression/epoxy model method for the assessment of surface characteristics and wear patterns in glass-ionomer restorations has been used for more detailed examination.[36]

One hundred percent retention has been attained for both conventional glass-ionomer[38–43] and cermet cements[43–47] in Class II primary restorations for up to 5 years. Nevertheless substantial failure rates have been recorded due to bulk fracture of the cements. The low capacity of the glass ionomers to undergo strain without fracture, which presents a problem for the accurate measurement of the modulus of elasticity,[48] accounts for the bulk fractures that occur under chewing forces. These brittle fractures are located mostly at the isthmus of the glass-ionomer restorations.

The loss of anatomic form for posterior restorations prepared with the conventional glass ionomers and the cermets is a strong indication for cement deterioration and is already manifested during the first year in vivo. The loss of anatomic form that appears at an early postoperative time is more severe for the glass-cermet cements than for the conventional glass ionomers, both on the occlusal surface and along the proximal margins (Fig 6-1). At the same time, a pitted, rough surface with voids is created (Fig 6-2).

While the marginal quality of the glass-ionomer restoration is acceptable initially, it is found that progressive degradation in vivo leads to poor marginal adaptation (Fig 6-3). A time delay has been observed between the loss of marginal integrity and the loss of anatomic form. This phenomenon is probably due to differences in bonding of glass ionomers to enamel and dentin. The adhesive properties of glass ionomers are apparently sufficient to maintain marginal integrity despite the occlusal wear that occurs simultaneously. Nevertheless, a thin layer of glass ionomer remains attached to the cavity margins and undergoes fracture during the wear process, resulting in marginal problems at a later time.

Several intrinsic factors of conventional glass ionomers cause notable wear of cement restorations. These are related to the glass-ionomer structure and the cohesive properties of the cement. It has been calculated that the minimum stress imposed on a restoration by the opposing teeth is 40 MPa; the stress could be as high as 160 MPa during swallowing.[49] Yet the static strength of glass ionomers never exceeds 40 MPa.[48] This means that if the cyclic stress on the restoration in vivo exceeds the static strength of the glass ionomer, crack initiation and propagation can be induced. This is considered to be the basic failure mechanisms for brittle restorative materials. It is assumed that the structure of the glass ionomers does not permit the accumulation of internal stresses.[50] Concurrently, the presence of a siliceous hydrogel around the glass particles could function as a stress absorption mechanism. However, the absorption of water due to the

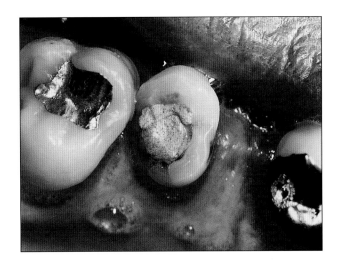

Fig 6-1 Glass-cermet restoration after 2 years of oral function *(center)*. Note the loss of anatomic form, the marginal fractures, and the pitted surface.

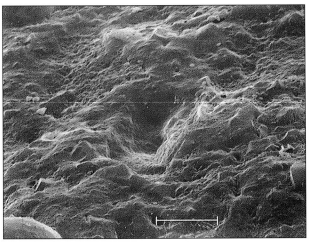

Fig 6-2 Secondary electron image of a silicone impression/epoxy model replica of the occlusal surface of a glass-cermet restoration following 10 months in the oral cavity. A wavy, rough surface where glass particles have been lost is apparent (bar = 20 μm).

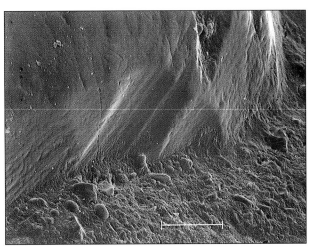

Fig 6-3 Secondary electron image of the marginal wear of the restoration in Fig 6-2 (bar = 100 μm).

hydrophilic nature of the cement may cause propagation of preexisting cracks. Wear of the glass ionomers could be additionally favored by the large, hard glass particles used as cement components.[34] Furthermore, chemical erosion is likely to have a decisive role in the initial matrix disruption. The wear pattern of conventional glass ionomers on the occlusal restoration surface is described as uniform, with no difference between occlusal contact (OCA) and contact-free (CFA) areas.[51] The latter may reflect the importance of chemical erosion in the cement failure process.

Clinically, wear of glass cermets appears to be substantially higher than that of conventional glass ionomers, in contrast to in vitro findings where laboratory wear machines were used.[52] This result implies the inability of the wear machines to simulate clinical conditions.

Improvement of flexural strength, modulus of elasticity, and resistance to dissolution of the resin-modified glass ionomers may be beneficial for their clinical performance in posterior restorations of primary teeth. However, wear also was shown to be the principal clinical problem for

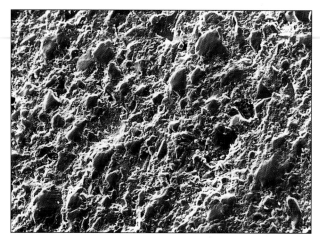

Fig 6-4 Secondary electron image of a silicone/epoxy replica of the outer surface of a resin-modified glass-ionomer cervical restoration after 7 months of oral service. Matrix dissolution and exposed glass fillers are evident (original magnification × 400; reproduced at 77%).

resin-modified glass ionomers, leading to loss of anatomic form similar to that exhibited by the glass-cermet cements.[47,53] Furthermore, the marginal adaptation of resin-modified glass-ionomer restorations is disrupted very rapidly, with the development of marginal integrity problems after the first year of oral function. The early slow wear rate that has been observed in vivo for the resin-modified glass ionomers can be attributed to the initial protection supplied by the polymer network.

Following water absorption from the oral environment, detachment of the filler particles from the cement matrix may occur (Fig 6-4) because the glass particles in resin-modified glass-ionomer cements are embedded in a multiphase matrix. In addition, the cyclic wear pattern of the resin-modified glass ionomers,[54] in contrast to the uniform wear of conventional glass-ionomer cements, results in the "pluck-out" effect on the glass fillers.[51] Thus, from a clinical viewpoint, all types of glass ionomers have been proved to exhibit levels of wear resistance that are unsuitable for high-stress-bearing restorations.

The poor degree of complete retention of conventional glass-ionomer sealants is in contrast to their low loss rate.[55–57] While the partial retention shows their adhesive capacity to enamel, their rapid degradation renders them inappropriate even as preventive materials. Similar performance was found in resin-modified glass ionomers applied as sealants, where a high degradation rate of the cement and marginal discoloration of the restorations were observed.[58,59]

Glass-ionomer deterioration also is responsible for clinical problems in cervical restorations where stress is much lower than on occlusal tooth surfaces. Although there appears to be negligible loss of anatomic form in cervical restorations (Fig 6-5), poor marginal integrity (Fig 6-6) and the resulting marginal discoloration (Fig 6-7) are common occurrences.[60–64] While the low flexural fatigue limit of the glass ionomers might be expected to induce marginal microfractures or complete loss in cervical restorations, the gradual overall dissolution seems to create marginal ditching, apparently protecting the cement from fracture (Fig 6-8). The continuous loss of the cement matrix exposes fillers, which, along with voids, leads to surface roughness (Fig 6-9). Additionally, changes in cement composition were found at the outer surface of several glass-ionomer restorations, which may be attributed to reactions induced between saliva elements and the cement (Fig 6-10).

The self-bonding capacity of glass ionomers has been demonstrated in cervical restorations as well. Retention rates of 93% to 100% [60–62,65] and 93% to 95% [61,64,66,67] have been reported for over 3.5 years in vivo with conventional and resin-modified glass ionomers, respectively. The maintenance of cement adaptation to the cavity walls during oral function may cause the high degree of retention (Fig 6-11). It should be pointed out that these retention rates have been achieved commonly on high-caries-risk patients and under particularly difficult circumstances, eg, where adhesion to a dentin substrate is involved without cavity preparation.

Darkening of resin-modified glass ionomers in vivo reflects a principal characteristic of the aging process.[58,68–71] This type of cement is not normally protected by a hydrophobic agent during the early setting stages. Thus, it is possible for a sub-

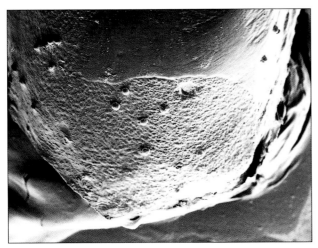

Fig 6-5 Secondary electron image of a silicone/epoxy replica of a Class V conventional glass-ionomer cement restoration 4 years after placement. Despite the marginal defects and the rough surface, loss of anatomic form cannot be observed (original magnification × 20; reproduced at 77%).

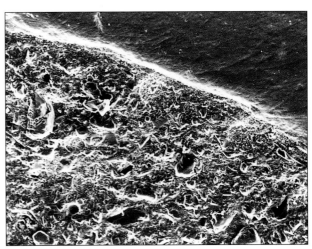

Fig 6-6 Secondary electron image of cement dissolution along the incisal margins of the restoration shown in Fig 6-5, resulting in the creation of marginal defects (original magnification × 300; reproduced at 77%).

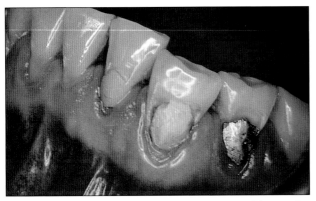

Fig 6-7 Marginal discoloration and integrity problems of a 3-year-old conventional glass-ionomer cement restoration.

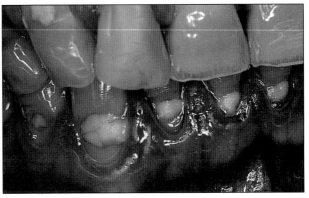

Fig 6-8 Cement loss in 2-year-old conventional glass-ionomer restorations, presenting problems at the margins and the bulk of the restorations.

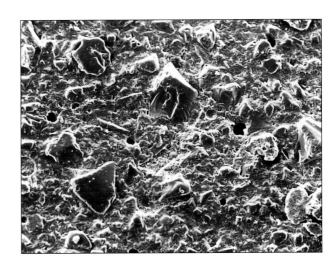

Fig 6-9 Secondary electron image of a silicone/epoxy replica of the outer surface of a conventional glass-ionomer cervical restoration following 6 months in vivo. Disruption of the matrix, large unsupported glass particles, and voids are evident (original magnification × 400; reproduced at 77%).

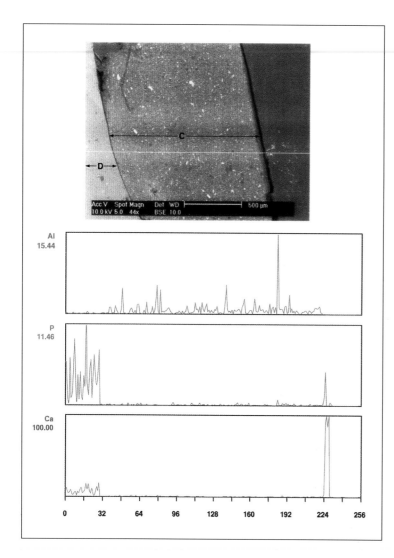

Fig 6-10 Secondary electron image of a longitudinal section of an extracted tooth with a 6-month-old Class V conventional glass-ionomer cement restoration and radiographic linescan images of aluminum, phosphorus, and calcium. The white line in the secondary electron image shows the position of the radiographic linescan analysis (D: dentin; C: cement). The aluminum linescan image indicates the glass-ionomer cement area. Note the increase in the intensities of the calcium and phosphorus peaks at the outer cement surface.

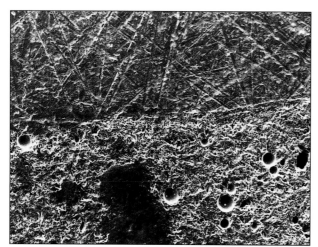

Fig 6-11 Secondary electron image of a silicone/epoxy replica of a longitudinal section of an extracted tooth with a 6-month-old Class V conventional glass-ionomer restoration. Perfect adaptation is depicted at the cement-incisal surface interface (original magnification × 250; reproduced at 77%).

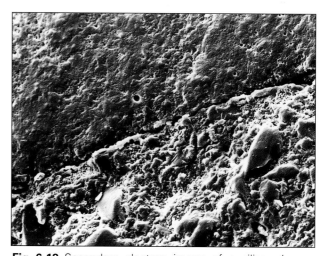

Fig 6-12 Secondary electron image of a silicone/epoxy replica of the incisal margin of a 6-month-old Class V resin-modified glass-ionomer cement restoration. The gap formation is obvious (original magnification × 300; reproduced at 77%).

stantial amount of water to be absorbed from the oral environment, which ultimately leads to the observed color change.[62,65,68,70]

Furthermore, aging of resin-modified glass ionomers in Class V restorations appears to be mainly manifested by an increase in marginal discrepancies during a particularly short postinsertion time (Fig 6-12). This behavior is considered to be due to aggravation of the marginal discrepancy that existed when the cement was originally placed in the prepared tooth cavity; it has been stated that only 85% of these restorations are gap-free immediately after placement of the glass ionomer.[71] The maintenance of a relatively smooth outer surface and original anatomic form characterizes resin-modified glass ionomers even after 2 years in Class V restorations.

Anticariogenic Behavior

The anticariogenic potential of glass ionomers, which arises from their fluoride-releasing property, has been emphasized for these cements. In vitro measurements indicate that the fluoride release seems to occur at a high rate during postsetting maturation and then undergoes a subsequent reduction to that expected from equilibrium diffusion processes.[72] In addition, dissolution of these cements, as a result of aging in vivo, may cause further fluoride elution, reinforcing their antimicrobial properties both in the microenvironment of the restoration and in the whole oral environment.

It is known that fluoride inhibits the bacterial activity of *Streptococcus mutans*,[73] which has been identified as one of the most important microorganisms in the etiology of caries and has been suggested to have significance in the etiology of recurrent caries. The fluoride ions are thought to interfere with initial bacterial adhesion and colonization, and they may alter the ecology of the dental plaque by removing the competitive advance induced by microorganisms such as *S mutans*. The most important effect of fluoride on bacterial plaque is believed to be the reduction of acid production because these ions appear to inhibit the glycolytic enzyme enolase that adversely affects the ability of the bacteria to survive.[73]

The antimicrobiologic/anticariogenic behavior of glass-ionomer restorations in vivo has been evaluated by various methods, such as measurement of the fluoride concentration in the whole saliva or in the dental plaque accumulated on the restoration and adjacent teeth. Another method is evaluation of the potential of enamel and dentin for fluoride uptake along the cavity walls. Furthermore, the assessment of the cariogenic ecology of dental plaque and carious dentin flora in glass-ionomer restorations has been used. Although these methods may indicate the anticariogenic potential of glass ionomers, true clinical documentation is achieved when there is a reduction of the incidence of secondary caries in glass-ionomer restorations.[74–80]

The possibility of fluoridation of the oral environment from the action of glass-ionomer restorations is based upon the results of only two studies. In the first study, the fluoride-ion concentration in unstimulated saliva was monitored for 2 to 6 weeks posttreatment by Koch and Hatibovic-Kofman.[74] A significant increase was observed immediately after placement of the glass ionomer, followed by a continuous gradual reduction. At the final measurement, the fluoride percentage in saliva was 10 times higher than the baseline value. This pattern of changing fluoride-ion concentration in saliva showed the same profile as that previously found in in vitro studies.

In the second study, Rezk-Lega et al[75] recorded particularly high (0.2 to 0.3 ppm) fluoride-ion concentrations in saliva for up to 1 year, which surprisingly were generated by only two glass-ionomer restorations in each mouth. This level of fluoride, which is higher than the initial fluoride content of the cements, is probably due to the fluoride supplement taken by children throughout the study. Thus, studies to date demonstrate that the glass-ionomer restorations provide an increase in the in vivo fluoride-ion concentration at early postoperative times. However, additional research in needed to assess the duration of this concentration increase.

Even if the efficiency of glass ionomers for early saliva enrichment with fluoride is accepted, no fluoride uptake by the enamel of teeth adjacent to the restorations has been demonstrated during that period.[76] Fluoride uptake by enamel and dentin is believed to result in higher caries resistance. However, the evidence of in vivo fluoride uptake by the cavity walls for glass-ionomer restorations has been examined in only two investigations. Both studies[77,78] found significant amounts of fluoride uptake, although it decreased with increasing depth from the interface. However, Skartveit et al[77] tested a product with a high fluoride content (11.3% by weight), and Mukai et al[78] used a resin-modified glass-ionomer liner as the restorative material.

Controversy has arisen over the accuracy of the analytical techniques used to detect fluoride diffusion into the hard dental tissues of the cavity walls, and possible errors that may occur in the elemental analysis have been described.[79,80] For example, the high-vacuum conditions required cause cohesive failures of the cement. Thus, a thin layer of the cement remains on the dental tissues, causing interference in the elemental analysis. Moreover, the various grinding techniques that have been employed cannot ensure complete removal of the cement from these dental tissues. Because of these problems, unambiguous evidence has not been obtained to support the hypothesis that glass ionomers have the ability to enrich the dental tissues adjacent to the restorations with fluoride.

The fluoride concentration in the dental plaque of 3-year-old glass-ionomer restorations was found to be slightly greater than that in the plaque accumulated in vivo on the other teeth,[81] the only investigation providing such results for realistic clinical conditions. In addition, contrary to in vitro results, no increase in the plaque fluoride concentration was measured 3 days after topical application of fluoride gel, which implies no recharge effect for old glass-ionomer restorations. The claim that glass-ionomer restorations have the potential to act as a fluoride source for adjacent dental plaque originates from an in situ model using bonded brackets, which reduces the study's value for considering the in vivo aging of glass-ionomer restorations under true clinical conditions.[82]

Although possible fluoride enrichment of the dental plaque occurred in the Forss et al study,[81] no long-term significant decrease in the levels of *S mutans* and lactobacilli was found. There was a temporary reduction in the amounts of these pathogens only in the first week after placement of the glass-ionomer restoration.[81,83-85] The lack of correlation between the plaque fluoride and an antibacterial effect could be attributed to various factors. For example, the fluoride level in dental plaque adjacent to the glass-ionomer restoration may not be sufficiently high to inhibit the cariogenic flora. It also is possible that the ionized form of fluoride, which is the active state,[86] is present at low levels in saturated dental plaque. The speculation over the causes is due to the fact that the mechanism for the inhibition of acid in plaque by fluoride is still unknown.

In contrast, a reduction in the prevalence of *S mutans* has been verified in mature plaque sampled from the margins of old restorations[87] and from interproximal tooth sites adjacent to glass-ionomer restorations.[88] However, in the latter case, the restorative material was a glass-cermet cement, and it is known that silver ions released from the glass cermet enhance the antibacterial activity of the cement.[89]

The mostly contrasting findings between in vivo and in vitro studies of the antimicrobiological activity of glass ionomers may indicate the inability of the in vitro environment to resemble the clinical situation. It is possible that during a long period of service in vivo, compounds derived from saliva and plaque may be absorbed by the glass-ionomer surface. Thus, the inward and outward diffusion pathways can be blocked, with a subsequent reduction in the migration rate of the metal ions. Moreover, no inhibition effect of the glass ionomers on pellicle formation after contact with saliva has been detected,[90] and thus further interference on the diffusion of the ions is expected. Consequently, there is a need to evaluate the long-term anticariogenic potential of glass ionomers at the clinical sites recommended for their application.

No differences were observed in the microbacterial ecology of carious dentin in restorations enclosed with a glass ionomer or a resin composite after 7 to 24 days in vivo.[91-93] Additionally, no changes in the color or hardness of the carious dentin were assigned using clinical evaluation criteria. However, the validity of these findings may be questioned because there was no assessment of possible microleakage in the restorations. Thus, the microorganisms detected in the carious dentin may have penetrated through the restorations from the oral environment.

Until recently, the efficiency of glass ionomers to inhibit secondary caries in restorations in vivo had been considered well documented by clinical trials. It also had been considered proven in a substantial number of in vitro studies using the experimental caries model. However, a systematic assessment, carried out by Randall and Wilson,[94] of a large number of clinical studies presenting evidence of inhibition of secondary caries in glass-ionomer restorations showed that few fulfilled the criteria of a proper clinical study. In addition, neither a positive nor a negative effect of glass ionomers on the occurrence of secondary caries was established by the studies assessed. Moreover, two epidemiologic investigations have confirmed that the most common cause for the replacement of glass-ionomer restorations is secondary caries.[95,96]

In summary, there is no strong evidence from in vivo research that supports the anticariogenic properties of glass-ionomer restorations aged in the oral environment.

Pulp Responses

In general, pulpal injury associated with restorations is principally caused by bacteria from the oral cavity in cases where the marginal adaptation is poor and by cytotoxic reactive components released from immature restorative materials. Pulp reactions can range from pulpitis to necrosis. The impact of the two foregoing causes cannot be assessed in protocols that employ clinical criteria to assess pulp sensitivity.

Histologic examination of the pulp tissue is necessary to verify any bacterial influence as well as the type and the extent of pulp deterioration. The study of pulp reactions caused by restorations in vivo requires well-designed prospective follow-up clinical investigations, along with monitoring of other symptoms displayed by the patients over

a sufficient period of time.[97] The experimental sample should include various types of restorations in deep and shallow cavities in patients of various age groups. All of these parameters affect dentin permeability, which determines the penetration of toxic and nontoxic bacterial components to the pulp.

Few studies of glass-ionomer cements using well-designed experimental models have been conducted. Demirci et al[98] detected slightly adverse pulp response but no necrotic pulps from a resin-modified glass ionomer placed in Class V cavities of intact teeth. Two other clinical trials from over two decades ago, using conventional glass-ionomer cements, demonstrated a nonappreciable irritating reaction over an 8-month period.[99,100]

Current knowledge of the pulp risk during early setting of glass ionomers and after in vivo aging has been acquired largely from animal studies.[101,102] It is obvious that such models cannot provide reliable findings for human teeth under conditions appropriate for clinical usage of glass ionomers. There are major differences between the anatomy, structure, and composition of animal teeth and human teeth.[103] Also, the usual approach of preparing small and shallow cavities in intact, caries-free teeth with healthy pulp does not represent standard in vivo operative dentistry conditions. Moreover, the short observation time commonly used in animal studies, which does not exceed 3 months, cannot attribute pulp complications to degradation of the glass ionomers.

In summary, the in vivo pulp response to young and old glass-ionomer restorations aged in the oral environment has been evaluated by clinical criteria rather than thorough scientific study.

Luting Glass-Ionomer Cements in Orthodontics

Zinc phosphate cements and resin composites were used routinely for many years in cementation of orthodontic bands and bonding of brackets to tooth enamel, respectively. The requirements for an orthodontic cement include a sufficiently low film thickness, the capacity to ensure appliance retention throughout the treatment period, and easy removal at the end of treatment with the least possible damage to the tooth structure. Inhibition of enamel demineralization around bands and brackets during treatment is a particularly desired characteristic for an orthodontic cement or adhesive.

For the zinc phosphate cements used to cement bands, clinical problems include band dislodgment due to gradual cement degradation and demineralization during fixed-appliance therapy, which has been reported to be as high as 50%.[104] The glass-ionomer cements have become an attractive substitute for zinc phosphate cements in band cementation because of several advantages: chemical adhesion to enamel and dentin, superior physicomechanical properties, and antimicrobial potential for the reduction of demineralization defects. The glass ionomers have been suggested for bracket bonding as an alternative to resin composites because, in addition to the preceding advantageous characteristics, the cement is easily removed during the debonding procedure. Furthermore, replacement of the conventional luting glass-ionomer cements with the more recently developed resin-modified glass ionomers has provided the potential for wider use in bracket bonding.

Retention

The materials used for band cementation should exhibit sufficient cohesive strength to resist the dynamic stresses imposed on teeth during orthodontic therapy and degradation in oral fluids. Band retention failure in clinical studies conducted in the late 1980s, where the conventional glass-ionomer cements had been utilized, did not exceed 2.3% over 2 years of treatment.[105–107] A high failure rate (9.5%) was observed only with an experimental product.[108] These results suggest superior retention capacity of the glass ionomers compared to the zinc phosphate cements.

The reason for the relatively low failure rate of bands luted with glass ionomers is particularly interesting. Examination of the failed bands revealed that the major part of the cement remained attached to the enamel, whereas only a thin layer of cement, if any, covered the inner sur-

face of the metal band. The latter feature of the failure pattern indicates that the bulk glass-ionomer cement is not the weak link in the band-cement-tooth system. The relatively weak bond of the cement with the metal band is the major cause of the band failure. This supports in vitro results that find the ability of glass ionomers for bonding to base metals, such as those used for bands, is inferior to their ability for bonding with enamel.[109]

The long-term clinical efficiency of glass ionomers for bracket bonding is unacceptable. Bond failure rates up to 36%[110–112] have indicated that these materials are unsuitable for this application. The vast majority of bond failures in brackets bonded with glass ionomers occurred cohesively within the cement. Stronger mechanical retention (interlocking) of the glass ionomer provided by the bracket's base design may result in a bond strength that is superior to the cohesive strength of the cement under dynamic loading. Thus, the bulk glass-ionomer cement is the weakest component of the enamel-cement-bracket system.

In vitro observations of the higher bond strength for resin-modified glass ionomers, compared with conventional glass ionomers, have been verified by clinical results. Significant reduction of the bond failure rate relative to that of conventional glass ionomers, which is comparable to that of resin composites, has been reported for up to 1 year after the onset of the treatment.[113–116] In addition, the in vivo bond failures were predominantly found at the enamel-cement interface. Long-term clinical trials should confirm the effectiveness of resin-modified glass ionomers for bracket bonding.

Anticariogenic Behavior

Orthodontic fixed appliances hinder tooth cleaning and favor plaque accumulation because there is a much greater number of potential retention sites. An increase in the number of S mutans and lactobacilli has been reported after the placement of orthodontic bands and brackets.[117] Their presence increases the caries challenge, and visible incipient caries lesions are developed adjacent to brackets within 1 month. The overall incidence of white spot formation during fixed orthodontic therapy is 11% to 22%, and demineralization of the labial surfaces of the teeth around orthodontic brackets and bands can be as high as 50%.[118] The potential of the glass ionomers for long-term fluoride release in various buffered solutions has been well established in vitro. Simultaneously, various mechanisms underlying the caries-preventing effects of fluoride are known. This background is the basis for the observed decrease in the frequency of enamel demineralization when glass-ionomer cements are used as bonding agents in orthodontic appliances.

In vivo studies have been designed to verify the cariostatic activity of the glass-ionomer cements in patients wearing fixed orthodontic appliances. The amounts of caries-associated microorganisms such as *S mutans* and lactobacilli, as well as the fluoride concentration in dental plaque adjacent to brackets bonded with glass ionomers, have been determined following specific periods of orthodontic treatment. The fluoride level in the whole saliva of the patients is considered to be an important factor in the assessment of the anticariogenic property of the glass ionomers. Clinical investigations also have examined the incidence and the extent of the enamel demineralization around orthodontic appliances.

It is of special importance that no causative correlation has been established between the fluoride level and the prevalence of caries-associated microorganisms in plaque accumulated on brackets bonded with glass ionomers. The high fluoride release rate from glass ionomers during the post-setting maturation process resulted in a significantly high fluoride concentration in plaque around the brackets over a 2-day period.[82] Although the elevated level of fluoride in vivo decreased over a period of 6 months, it was still higher than that found in plaque with the use of a resin composite luting cement that was tested simultaneously. No significant long-term inhibition effect was manifested on the growth of *S mutans* and lactobacilli in these plaque samples.[114,119,120]

The clinical consequences of caries-associated microorganisms such as *S mutans* and lactobacilli on caries are difficult to estimate, and additional investigations are needed. The presence of these

bacteria does not necessarily indicate that active caries is present. Other microorganisms such as *Streptococcus sobrinus* may be implicated in the caries process, particularly in young children, where it was shown that caries activity was more closely related to the oral levels of *S sobrinus* than other prevalent species of *S mutans*.[121] *S sobrinus* also was detected at incipient lesions around resin-retained brackets, but not *S mutans* or lactobacilli as expected.[120] The volume of plaque examined is an experimental variable that may interfere with interpretation of these experimental results with respect to the ecology of bacteria in plaque. Although it is known that the microbial composition changes with increasing thickness of dental plaque, this parameter was not determined in these investigations (cited in Hallgren et al[119]).

Elevated fluoride levels were found in the whole saliva of patients 1 day after the bonding of orthodontic appliances, whereas these levels returned to the baseline value within 28 days postinsertion.[122] Calculation of the first-day amount of saliva fluoride per daily production of saliva showed that 0.02 mg fluoride was added to the oral cavity. Compared with the systematic administration of fluoride, this dose is a negligible amount. It is interesting to speculate why a significantly lower amount of fluoride is released in saliva in vivo than that measured in various buffered solutions in vitro. The most likely reason for this reduction may be the different mechanisms governing the fluoride release from glass-ionomer cements aged in the oral environment. Immediately after cement placement, the fluoride concentration is increased in the fluid around the cement, the pellicle, and the plaque, after which the fluoride diffuses into the saliva. With an increase in plaque thickness, the fluoride diffusion rate into the saliva is decreased, and the level in the plaque attains a saturation condition.

In summary, from the evidence currently available, it may be argued that luting glass ionomers cannot act as fluoride devices for the whole oral environment over a long-term orthodontic treatment period.

The occurrence of incipient enamel lesions adjacent to bands and brackets attached by glass ionomers has been established by direct clinical observation, evaluation of color slides obtained clinically, and use of microradiography on extracted teeth that had been aged in vivo. The tooth surfaces bonded with a resin-reinforced glass ionomer exhibited a short-term tendency to be less affected by demineralization, compared with those bonded with the resin luting agent.[123] The demineralization resistance was limited to a narrow zone, not wider than 0.5 mm around the bracket base.[120,123,124]

The beneficial cariostatic influence of the glass ionomers was further reduced at tooth sites that favored plaque accumulation and where the access to oral hygiene was difficult. Thus, a relatively high frequency of incipient caries (24%) was noted at tooth surfaces cervical to the brackets during a 2-year period of treatment and seemed to be affected by the local ecologic conditions of each tooth. Therefore, differences in the distribution of white spots were observed at various locations adjacent to the orthodontic brackets.[125] However, the amount of white spot formation is lower than that found with the use of resin-composite luting agents.[124] Band cementation with glass ionomers decreased considerably the evidence of white spots, compared with that observed with the use of zinc phosphate luting cements.[105,108]

In conclusion, it can be suggested that the use of glass ionomers as luting cements in orthodontic practice does not provide the desired long-term caries protection. Nevertheless, these cements present an advantage over the resin composites and zinc phosphate cements.

Luting Glass-Ionomer Cements in Fixed Prosthodontics

Luting cements provide the link between the fixed prosthesis and the prepared tooth structure, thus playing an important role in the longevity of the restorations. The major drawbacks of the most commonly used luting agents, zinc phosphate cements, are associated with a lack of adhesion and a low resistance to dissolution in oral fluids. Despite these disadvantages, an overall survival rate of 74.0 ± 2.1% was found for fixed partial dentures after 15 years in the oral cavity.[126] However, alternative materials have been introduced because of increased esthetic demands, along with an attempt to improve clinical performance over that achieved with use of the zinc phosphate cements.

The conventional glass-ionomer luting cements were introduced in the mid-1980s, and resin-modified glass ionomers have been available since 1995. The in vitro performance of the glass-ionomer luting cements has been assessed in terms of their mechanical properties, wear resistance, solubility and water sorption, adhesive efficiency, biocompatibility, and color stability.[127] However, there is concern that these in vitro evaluations cannot predict the clinical outcome when the glass-ionomer luting cements are subjected to clinical conditions, particularly for metal and ceramic inlays/onlays, full crowns, and multiunit prostheses.

Although glass ionomers have been used as luting cements for over 15 years, no reliable long-term investigations on the in vivo aging of these cements is presently available. The retention rates of various fixed prostheses cemented with glass ionomers have been selected as criteria to define the in vivo longevity of the cements as luting agents.[128–130] However, the luting agent may have only a minimal impact on the resulting retention rates achieved. Moreover, the inherent difficulties in standardization of the in vivo assessment do not allow valid conclusions. Furthermore, the clinical success of a fixed prosthesis is influenced by a wide range of variables, including the shape and position of the crowns and the occlusion of the patient, in addition to the properties of the luting agent.

One shortcoming in use of glass ionomers as luting cements is the occurrence of tooth sensitivity. Studies found that within the first 2 weeks, postcementation hypersensitivity was manifested in 11% to 34% of the teeth that received crowns.[131,132] It is assumed that this postoperative sensitivity may be induced by tooth desiccation during crown preparation, bacterial contamination, or irritation from the cement per se. The absence of evidence for in vivo bacterial leakage in cemented crowns for up to 3 months post-cementation excludes bacterial penetration as a possible cause of tooth sensitivity in the early stages of oral function. In addition, a remarkable reduction (2.1% to 4.0%) in the occurrence of pulp sensitivity was noted over a 5- to 8-year follow-up period.[128,129,133,134] Thus, tooth sensitivity seems to be eliminated during the aging of the glass-ionomer cement. These observations suggest that the tooth sensitivity that has been characterized as irreversible pulpitis is instead a short-term phenomenon related to the setting characteristics of glass-ionomer cements. The prolonged setting time of the cements, which is necessary for optimum fitting of the prostheses, is likely to maintain the low acidity of the cements for a long time, thus causing the sensitivity presented.

Glass-ionomer luting cements, apart from the cementation of fixed partial dentures, also have been used recently for cementation of ceramic inlays. In order to prevent bulk fracture of the brittle ceramic inlays, adhesive cementation is necessary to ensure good adaptation to the prepared tooth structure. Because of the adhesive capacity of glass ionomers, these cements are the materials of choice, along with traditional resin cements. A series of controlled clinical studies has examined the aging performance of the glass-ionomer luting cements at the margins of ceramic inlays.[135–138] The cement seems to be subjected to gradual degradation vertically and horizontally, which leads to marginal ditching. Consequently, partial fracture or total loss of the ceramic inlay may be caused by adhesive bond failure, which mostly occurs at the ceramic-cement interface. The cement is separated from the inlay and remains at the interface with the prepared tooth structure. The brittle nature of the cements, their high dissolution rate and low wear resistance, and the relatively poor bond between the cement and the rough ceramic surface, account for the cement deterioration at the occlusal margins of the restorations, where there is substantial stress from functional forces in vivo. The high prevalence of fractures at the cement-ceramic interface for inlays luted with glass ionomers confirms the in vitro results found with different prosthesis

designs. The in vivo performance of the glass ionomers was determined from clinical criteria or by evaluating casts of the ceramic inlay restorations with the scanning electron microscope. However, the use of retrieval analysis of teeth to assess the margins and interfaces in restorations luted with glass ionomers after specific periods of oral service should offer the possibility for the most reliable and detailed characterization.

Identification of the glass-ionomer cement adaptation at crown margins, using a dye to reveal microleakage for extracted teeth that had been aged in vivo,[139] is a questionable approach because it is not clear whether the observed leakage is due to a gap at the margins or to diffusion through the glass ionomer. The hydrophilic nature and porosity of the glass-ionomer cements strongly favor the dye absorption mechanism, suggesting that the findings of White et al[139] for use of a resin-modified glass-ionomer luting agent are not valid. The short time (6 months) that the crowns were in the oral cavity further limits the validity of the study. The marginal integrity of cast crowns cemented with a resin-modified glass ionomer was verified on extracted teeth after 6 months in vivo, and the origin of the marginal discrepancies was found to be degradation of the cement.[140] However, the short time period of the study and the high standard deviations obtained do not permit conclusions about the clinical performance of the glass-ionomer cement.

The potential longevity of a prosthesis is, to a large extent, determined by the solubility of the cement and its resistance to disintegration in the oral cavity. From a clinical point of view, long-term solubility is a crucial factor that leads to marginal ditching and microbial penetration. As has already been pointed out, in vitro solubility tests cannot resemble the dynamic and complex in vivo conditions. On the other hand, in vivo assessment of solubility has been obtained only with the use of in situ models consisting of intraoral appliances that can be removed from the mouth for subsequent measurement of material loss. The results obtained by the in situ models have two important limitations: First, the dissolution is determined as a result of physicochemical erosion, not mechanical fatigue in crowns and fixed partial dentures; and second, a large cement surface is exposed directly to the oral fluids, whereas a thin layer of cement is subjected to the oral environment under clinical conditions.[141–143]

In summary, glass-ionomer luting cements seem to undergo homogeneous dissolution of their elements upon aging. Their resistance to dissolution is higher than for the zinc phosphate and polycarboxylate cements used commonly as luting materials. It should be pointed out that, despite the cement dissolution found, no incidence of secondary caries has been detected over an 8-year period in cast restorations luted with a glass ionomer.[129] However, the results of this one study, where the extent of secondary caries was assigned using clinical criteria, cannot substantiate the in vivo anticariogenic activity of the glass-ionomer luting cements.

References

1. Wilson AD, Kent BE. A new translucent cement for the dentistry. The glass ionomer cement. Br Dent J 1972;132: 133–135.

2. Walls AG. Glass polyalkenoate (glass-ionomer) cements: A review. J Dent 1986;14:231–246.

3. Mount GJ. Glass ionomers: A review of their current status. Oper Dent 1999;24:115–124.

4. McLean JW, Gasser O. Glass-cermet cements. Quintessence Int 1985;16:333–343.

5. Mitra SB [inventor]. Photocurable ionomer cement systems. European patent 323,120. 1988.

6. Kakaboura A, Eliades G, Palaghias G. An FTIR study on the setting mechanism of resin-modified glass-ionomer restoratives. Dent Mater 1996;12:173–178.

7. Wilson AD, Kent BE [inventors]. Surgical cement. UK patent 1,316,129. 1973.

8. Smith DC. Composition and characteristics of glass-ionomer cements. J Am Dent Assoc 1990;120:20–22.

9. Hatton PV, Brook IM. Characterization of the ultrastructure of glass-ionomer (poly-alkenoate) cements. Br Dent J 1992;173:275–277.

10. Wilson AD, Nicholson JW. Polyalkeonate cements. In: Wilson AD, Nicholson JW (eds). Acid-Base Cements: Their Biomedical and Industrial Applications. Cambridge, UK: Cambridge University Press, 1993:90–196.

11. Smith DC. Development of glass-ionomer cement systems. Biomaterials 1998;19:467–478.

12. Crisp S, Kent BE, Lewis BG, Ferner AJ, Wilson AD. Glass-ionomer cement formulations. II. The synthesis of novel polycarboxylic acids. J Dent Res 1980;59:1055–1063.

13. Crisp S, Lewis BG, Wilson AD. Characterization of glass-ionomer cements. 5. The effect of tartaric acid in the liquid component. J Dent 1979;7:304–312.

14. Wilson AD, Crisp S, Abel G. Characterization of glass-ionomer cements. 4. Effect of molecular weight on physical properties. J Dent 1977;5:117–120.

15. McLean JW, Wilson AD, Prosser HJ. Development and use of water-hardening glass ionomer luting cements. J Prosthet Dent 1984;52:175–181.

16. Sidhu SH, Natson TF. Resin-modified glass ionomer materials. A status report for the American Journal of Dentistry. Am J Dent 1995;8:59–67.

17. Matsuya S, Maeda T, Ohta M. IR and NMR analyses of hardening and maturation of glass-ionomer cement. J Dent Res 1996;75:1920–1927.

18. Nicholson JW. Chemistry of glass-ionomer cements: A review. Biomaterials 1998;19:485–494.

19. Wilson AD. Resin-modified glass ionomer cements. Int J Prosthodont 1990;3:425–429.

20. McLean JW, Nicholson JW, Wilson AD. Proposed nomenclature of glass ionomer dental cements and related materials. Quintessence Int 1994;25:587–589.

21. Mitra S, Kedrowski B. Long-term mechanical properties of glass ionomer. Dent Mater 1994;10:78–82.

22. Oilo G. Luting cements: A review and comparison. Int Dent J 1991;41:81–88.

23. Wilson AD, Paddon JM. Dimensional changes occuring in a glass-ionomer cement. Am J Dent 1993;6:280–282.

24. Kunzelmann K. Glass-ionomer cements, cermet cements, "hybrid" glass ionomers and compomers—Laboratory trials—Wear resistance. Trans Acad Dent Mater 1996;9:89–129.

25. Williams JA, Billington RW, Pearson GJ. The comparative strengths of commercial glass-ionomer cements with and without metal particles. Br Dent J 1992;172:279–282.

26. Gladys S, Van Meerbeek B, Braem M, Lambrechts P, Vanherle G. Comparative physico-mechanical characterization of new hybrid restorative materials with conventional glass-ionomer and resin composite restorative materials. J Dent Res 1997;76:883–894.

27. el Hejazi AA, Watts DC. Creep and visco-elastic recovery of cured and secondary-cured composites and resin-modified glass-ionomers. Dent Mater 1999;15:138–143.

28. Wilson AD, Groffman DM, Kuhn AT. The release of fluoride and other chemical species from a glass-ionomer cement. Biomaterials 1985;6:431–433.

29. Forsten L. Fluoride release of glass ionomers. J Esthet Dent 1994;6:216–222.

30. Creanor SL, Carruthers LM, Saunders WP, Strang R, Foye RH. Fluoride uptake and release characteristics of glass ionomer cements. Caries Res 1994;28:322–328.

31. Levallois B, Fovet Y, Lapeyre L, Gal JY. In vitro fluoride release from restorative materials in water versus artificial saliva medium (SAGF). Dent Mater 1998;14:441–447.

32. Watson TF. Bonding glass-ionomer cements to tooth structure. In: Davidson CL, Mjör IA (eds). Advances in Glass-Ionomer Cements, ed 1. Chicago: Quintessence, 1999: 121–135.

33. Sasanaluckit P, Albustany KR, Doherty PJ, Williams DF. Biocompatibility of glass ionomer cements. Biomaterials 1993;14:906–916.

34. Mair LH, Stolarski TA, Vowels RW, Lloyd CH. Wear: Mechanisms, manifestations and measurements. Report of a workshop. J Dent 1996;24:141–148.

35. Taylor DF, Bayne SC, Sturdevant JR, Wilder AD. Correlation of M-L, Leinfelder and USPHS clinical evaluation techniques for wear. Dent Mater 1990;6:151–153.

36. Kreulen CM, van Amerongen WE. Wear measurements in clinical studies of composite resin restorations in the posterior region: A review. ASDC J Dent Child 1991;58: 109–123.

37. Cvar JF, Ryge G. Criteria for the Clinical Evaluation of Dental Restorative Materials. San Francisco: United States Public Health Service, 1971:1–6.

38. Walls AW, Murray JJ, McCabe JF. The use of glass polyalkenoate (ionomer) cements in the deciduous dentition. Br Dent J 1988;165:13–17.

39. Forsten L, Karjalainen S. Glass ionomers in proximal cavities of primary molars. Scand J Dent Res 1990;98:70–73.

40. Hickel R, Voss A. A comparison of glass cermet cement and amalgam restorations in primary molars. ASDC J Dent Child 1990;57:184–188.

41. Hung TW, Richardson AS. Clinical evaluation of glass ionomer–silver cermet restorations in primary molars: One year results. J Can Dent Assoc 1990;56:239–240.

42. Welbury RR, Walls AW, Murray JJ, McCabe JF. The 5-year results of a clinical trial comparing a glass polyalkenoate (ionomer) cement restoration with an amalgam restoration. Br Dent J 1991;170:177–181.

43. Kilpatrick NM, Murray JJ, McCabe JF. The use of a reinforced glass-ionomer cermet for the restoration of primary molars: A clinical trial. Br Dent J 1995;179:175–179.

44. Croll TP, Riesenberger RE, Miller AS. Clinical and historic observation of glass ionomer–silver cermet restorations in six human primary molars. Quintessence Int 1988;19: 911–919.

45. Stratmann RG, Berg JH, Donly KJ. Class II glass-ionomer–silver restorations in primary molars. Quintessence Int 1989;20:43–47.

46. Smales RJ, Gerke DE, White IL. Clinical evaluation of occlusal glass ionomer, resin and amalgam restorations. J Dent 1990;18:243–249.

47. Espelid I, Tveit AB, Tornes KH, Alvheim H. Clinical behaviour of glass ionomer restorations in primary teeth. J Dent 1999; 27:437–442.

48. Braem MA. Physical properties of glass-ionomer cements: Fatigue and elasticity. In: Davidson CL, Mjör IA (eds). Advances in Glass-Ionomer Cements, ed 1. Chicago: Quintessence, 1999:67–84.

49. Hagberg C. Assessment of bite force: A review. J Craniomandib Disord 1987;1:162–169.

50. Maeda T, Mukaeda K, Shimohira T, Katsuyama S. Ion distribution in matrix parts of glass-polyalkenoate cement by SIMS. J Dent Res 1999;78:86–90.

51. McKinney JE, Antonucci JM, Rupp NW. Wear and microhardness of glass ionomer cements. J Dent Res 1987;66: 1134–1139.

52. de Gee AJ. Physical properties of glass-ionomer cements: Setting shrinkage and wear. In: Davidson CL, Mjör IA (eds). Advances in Glass-Ionomer Cements, ed 1. Chicago: Quintessence, 1999:51–65.

53. Donly KJ, Segura A, Kanellis M, Erickson RL. Clinical performance and caries inhibition of resin-modified glass ionomer cement and amalgam restorations. J Am Dent Assoc 1999;130:1459–1466.

54. Sidhu SK, Sherriff M, Watson TF. In vivo changes in roughness of resin-modified glass ionomer materials. Dent Mater 1997;13:208–213.

55. Boksman L, Gratton DR, McCutcheon E, Plotzke OB. Clinical evaluation of a glass ionomer cement as a fissure sealant. Quintessence Int 1987;18:707–709.

56. Mejàre I, Mjör JA. Glass ionomer and resin-based fissure sealants: A clinical study. Scand J Dent Res 1990;98: 345–350.

57. Övrebö RC, Raadal M. Microleakage in fissures sealed with resin or glass ionomer cement. Scand Dent J 1990;98: 66–69.

58. Smales RJ, Lee YK, Lo FW, Tse CC, Churg MS. Handling and clinical performance of a glass ionomer sealant. Am J Dent 1996;9:203–205.

59. Winkler MM, Deschepper EJ, Dean JA, Moore BK, Cochran MA, Ewoldsen N. Using a resin-modified glass ionomer as an occlusal sealant: A one-year clinical study. J Am Dent Assoc 1996;127:1508–1514.

60. Powell LV, Gordon GE, Johnson GH. Clinical evaluation of direct esthetic restorations in cervical abrasion/erosion lesion: One-year results. Quintessence Int 1991;22:687–692.

61. Tyas MJ. The effect of dentine conditioning with polyacrylic acid on the clinical performance of glass ionomer cement: 3-year results. Aust Dent J 1994;39:220–221.

62. Neo J, Chew CL, Yap A, Sidhu S. Clinical evaluation of tooth-colored materials in cervical lesions. Am J Dent 1996; 9:15–18.

63. de Araujo MA, Araujo RM, Marsilio AL. A retrospective look at esthetic resin composite and glass-ionomer Class III restorations: A 2-year clinical evaluation. Quintessence Int 1998;29:87–93.

64. Brackett WW, Gilpatrick RO, Browning WD, Gregory PN. Two-year clinical performance of a resin-modified glass-ionomer restorative material. Oper Dent 1999;24:9–13.

65. Brackett WW, Browning WD, Ross JA, Gregory PN, Owens BM. 1-year clinical evaluation of Compoglass and Fuji II LC in cervical erosion/abfraction lesions. Am J Dent 1999; 12:119–122.

66. Maneenut C, Tyas MJ. Clinical evaluation of resin-modified glass-ionomer restorative cements in cervical "abrasion" lesions: One-year results. Quintessence Int 1995;26: 739–743.

67. Wilder AD, Boghosian AA, Bayne SC, Heymann HO, Sturdevant JR, Roberson TM. Effect of powder/liquid ratio on the clinical and laboratory performance of resin-modified glass-ionomers. J Dent 1998;26:369–377.

68. Abdalla AI, Alhadairy HA. Clinical evaluation of hybrid ionomer restoratives in Class V abrasion lesions: Two-year results. Quintessence Int 1997;28:255–258.

69. Abdalla AI, Alhadainy HA, Garcia-Godoy F. Clinical evaluation of glass ionomers and compomers in Class V carious lesions. Am J Dent 1997;10:18–20.

70. Duke ES, Trevino DF. A resin-modified glass ionomer restorative: Three-year clinical results. J Indiana Dent Assoc 1998;77:13–16.

71. Ferrari M, Davidson CL. Sealing capacity of a resin-modified glass-ionomer and resin composite placed in vivo in Class 5 restorations. Oper Dent 1996;21:69–72.

72. De Moor RJ, Verbeek RM, De Maeyer EA. Fluoride release profiles of restorative glass-ionomer formulations. Dent Mater 1996;12:88–95.

73. Shellis RP, Durkworth RM. Studies on the cariostatic mechanisms of fluoride. Int Dent J 1994;44:263–273.

74. Koch G, Hatibovic-Kofman S. Glass ionomer cements as a fluoride release system in vivo. Swed Dent J 1990;14: 267–273.

75. Rezk-Lega F, Ogaard B, Rolla G. Availability of fluoride from glass-ionomer luting cements in human saliva. Scand J Dent Res 1991;99:60–63.

76. Seppa L, Salmenkivi S, Forss H. Enamel and plaque fluoride following glass ionomer application in vivo. Caries Res 1992;26:340–344.

77. Skartveit L, Tveit AB, Tötdal B, Övrebö R, Raadal M. In vivo fluoride uptake in enamel and dentin from fluoride-containing materials. ASDC J Dent Child 1990;57:97–100.

78. Mukai M, Ikeda M, Yanagihara T, et al. Fluoride uptake in human dentine from glass-ionomer cement in vivo. Arch Oral Biol 1993;38:1093–1098.

79. Duschner H, Ernst CP, Götz H, Rauscher M. Advanced techniques of micro-analysis and confocal microscopy: Perspectives for studying chemical and structural changes at the interface between restorative materials and cavity walls. Adv Dent Res 1995;9:355–362.

80. Eliades G. Chemical and biological properties of glass-ionomer cements. In: Davidson CL, Mjör IA (eds). Advances in Glass-Ionomer Cements, ed 1. Chicago: Quintessence, 1999;85–101.

81. Forss H, Näse L, Seppä L. Fluoride concentration, mutans streptococci and lactobacilli in plaque from old glass ionomer fillings. Caries Res 1995;29:50–53.

82. Hallgren A, Oliveby A, Twetman S. Fluoride concetration in plaque adjacent to orthodontic appliances retained with glass ionomer cement. Caries Res 1993;27:51–54.

83. Forss H, Jokinen J, Spets-Happonen S, Seppa L, Luona H. Fluoride and mutans streptococci in plaque crown on glass ionomer and composite. Caries Res 1991;25:454–458.

84. van Dijken J, Persson J, Sjöström S. Presence of Streptococcus mutans and lactobacilli in saliva and on enamel, glass ionomer cement, and composite resin surfaces. Scand J Dent Res 1991;99:13–19.

85. van Dijken JW, Kalfas S, Litra V, Oliveby A. Fluoride and mutans streptococci levels in plaque on aged restorations of resin-modified glass ionomer cement, compomer and resin composite. Caries Res 1997;31:379–383.

86. Jenkins NG. The Physiology and Biochemistry of the Mouth, ed 4. Oxford, UK: Blackwell, 1978:486–487.

87. Svanberg M, Mjör IA, Orstavik D. Mutans streptococci in plaque from margins of amalgam, composite, and glass-ionomer restorations. J Dent Res 1990;69:861–864.

88. Svanberg M, Krasse B, Ornerfeldt HO. Mutans streptococci in interproximal plaque from amalgam and glass ionomer restorations. Caries Res 1990;24:133–136.

89. Froward GC. Non-fluoride anticaries agents. Adv Dent Res 1994;8:208–214.

90. Hannig M. Transmission electron microscopy of early plaque formation on dental materials in vivo. Eur J Oral Sci 1999;107:55–64.

91. Weerheijm KL, de Soet JJ, van Amerongen WE, de Graaff J. The effect of glass-ionomer cement on carious dentine: An in vivo study. Caries Res 1993;27:417–423.

92. Kreulen CM, de Soet JJ, Weeheijm KL, van Amerongen WE. In vivo cariostatic effect of resin modified glass ionomer cement and amalgam on dentine. Caries Res 1997; 31:384–389.

93. Weerheijm KL, Kreulen CM, de Soet JJ, Groen HJ, van Amerongen WE. Bacterial counts in carious dentine under restorations: 2 year in vivo effects. Caries Res 1999;33: 130–134.

94. Randall RC, Wilson NH. Glass-ionomer restoratives: A systematic review of a secondary caries treatment effect. J Dent Res 1999;78:628–637.

95. Mjör IA. Glass-ionomer cement restorations and secondary caries: A preliminary report. Quintessence Int 1996;27: 171–174.

96. Wilson NH, Burke FJ, Mjör IA. Reasons for placement and replacement of restorations of direct restorative materials by a selected group of practitioners in the United Kingdom. Quintessence Int 1997;28:245–248.

97. Bergenholtz G. In vivo pulp responses to bonding of dental restorations. Trans Acad Dent Mater 1998;12:123–147.

98. Demirci M, Ucok M, Kucukkeles N, Soydan N. Pulp reaction to a tri-cure resin-modified glass ionomer. Oral Surg Oral Med Oral Pathol Oral Radiol Endod 1998;85:712–719.

99. Tobias RS, Browne RM, Plant CG, Ingram DV. Pulpal response to a glass ionomer cement. Br Dent J 1978; 144:345–350.

100. Nordenvall KJ, Bannstrom M, Torstensson B. Pulp reactions and microorganisms under ASPA and Concise composite fillings. ASDC J Dent Child 1979;46:449–453.

101. Plant CG, Browne RM, Knibbs PJ, Britton AS, Sorhan T. Pulpal effects of glass ionomer cements. Int Endod J 1984;17:51–59.

102. Mjör IA, Nordahl I, Tronstad L. Glass ionomer cements and dental pulp. Endod Dent Traumatol 1991;7:59–64.

103. Lin CP, Douglas WH. Structure-property relations and crack resistance at the bovine dentin-enamel junction. J Dent Res 1994;73:1072–1078.

104. McComb D. Luting in orthodontic practice. In: Davidson CL, Mjör IA (eds). Advances in Glass-Ionomer Cements, ed 1. Chicago: Quintessence, 1999:171–182.

105. Fricker JP, McLachlan MD. Clinical studies on glass-ionomer cements. Part 2: A two year clinical study comparing glass-ionomer cement with zinc phosphate cement. Aust Orthod J 1987;10:12–14.

106. Fricker JP. A 12-month clinical study comparing four glass-ionomer cements for the cementation of orthodontic molar bands. Aust Orthod J 1989;11:10–13.

107. Stirrups DR. A comparative clinical trial of a glass ionomer and a zinc phosphate cement for securing orthodontic bands. Br J Orthod 1991;18:15–20.

108. Maijer R, Smith DC. A comparison between zinc phosphate and glass ionomer cement in orthodontics. Am J Orthod Dentofacial Orthop 1988;93:273–279.

109. Zumstein TA, Strub JR. Adhesion of cement. Quintessence Int 1983;14:1–8.

110. Miller JR, Mancl L, Arburkle G, Baldwin J, Phillips RW. A three-year clinical trial using a glass ionomer cement for the bonding of orthodontic brackets. Angle Orthod 1996;66:309–312.

111. Norevall LI, Marcusson A, Persson M. A clinical evaluation of glass ionomer cement as an orthodontic bonding adhesive compared with an acrylic resin. Eur J Orthod 1996;18:373–384.

112. Miguel JA, Almeida MA, Chevitarese O. Clinical comparison between a glass ionomer cement and a composite for direct bonding of orthodontic brackets. Am J Orthod Dentofacial Orthop 1995;107:484–487.

113. Fricker JP. A 12-month clinical evaluation of a light-activated glass polyalkenoate (ionomer) cement for the direct bonding of orthodontic brackets. Am J Orthod Dentofacial Orthop 1994;105:502–505.

114. Wright AB, Lee RT, Lynch E, Young KA. Clinical and microbiologic evaluation of a resin modified glass ionomer cement for orthodontic bonding. Am J Orthod Dentofacial Orthop 1996;110:469–475.

115. Cacciafesta V, Bosch C, Melsen B. Clinical comparison between a resin-reinforced self-cured glass ionomer cement and a composite resin for direct bonding of orthodontic brackets. Part I: Wetting with water. Clin Orthod Res 1998;1:29–36.

116. Fricker JP. A new self-curing resin-modified glass-ionomer cement for the direct bonding of orthodontic brackets in vivo. Am J Orthod Dentofacial Orthop 1998;113:384–386.

117. Lundstrom F, Krasse B. Streptococcus mutans and lactobacilli frequency in orthodontic patients; The effect of chlorhexidine treatments. Eur J Orthod 1987;9:109–116.

118. Ogaard B. Prevalence of white spot lesions in 19-year-olds: A study on untreated and orthodontically treated persons 5 years after treatment. Am J Orthod Dentofacial Orthop 1989;96:423–427.

119. Hallgren A, Oliveby A, Twetman S. Caries associated microflora in plaque from orthodontic appliances retained with glass ionomer cement. Scand J Dent Res 1992; 100:140–143.

120. Örtendahl T, Thilander B, Svanberg M. Mutans streptococci and incipient caries adjacent to glass ionomer cement or resin-based composite in orthodontics. Am J Orthod Dentofacial Orthop 1997;112:271–274.

121. Hirose H, Hirose K, Isogai E, Miura H, Ueda I. Close association between Streptococcus sobrinus in the saliva of young children and smooth-surface caries increment. Caries Res 1993;27:292–297.

122. Hallgren A, Oliveby A, Twetman S. Salivary fluoride concentrations in children with glass ionomer cemented orthodontic appliances. Caries Res 1990;24:239–241.

123. Czochrowska E, Ogaard B, Duschner H, Ruben J, Arends J. Cariostatic effect of a light-cured, resin-reinforced glass-ionomer for bonding orthodontic brackets in vivo: A combined study using microradiography and confocal laser scanning microscopy. J Orofac Orthop 1998;59:265–273.

124. Marcusson A, Norevall LI, Persson M. White spot reduction when using glass ionomer cement for bonding in orthodontics: A longitudinal and comparative study. Eur J Orthod 1997;19:233–242.

125. Twetman S, McWilliam JS, Hallgren A, Oliveby A. Cariostatic effect of glass ionomer retained orthodontic appliances. An in vivo study. Swed Dent J 1997;21:169–175.

126. Creugers NH, Kayser AF, van't Hof MA. A meta-analysis of durability data on conventional fixed bridges. Community Dent Oral Epidemiol 1994;22:448–452.

127. Rosentiel SF, Land MF, Crispin BJ. Dental luting agents: A review of the current literature. J Prosthet Dent 1998;80: 280–301.

128. Brackett WW, Metz JE. Performance of a glass ionomer luting cement over 5 years in a general practice. J Prosthet Dent 1992;67:59–61.

129. Metz JE, Brackett WW. Performance of a glass ionomer luting cement over 8 years in a general practice. J Prosthet Dent 1994;71:13–15.

130. Pameijer CH, Nilner K. Long term clinical evaluation of three luting materials. Swed Dent J 1994;18:59–67.

131. Bebermeyer RD, Berg JH. Comparison of patient-perceived postcementation sensitivity with glass-ionomer and zinc phosphate cements. Quintessence Int 1994;25:209–241.

132. Kern M, Kleimeier B, Schaller HG, Strub JR. Clinical comparison of postoperative sensitivity for a glass ionomer and a zinc phosphate luting cement. J Prosthet Dent 1996; 75:159–162.

133. Fitzgerald M, Heys RJ, Heys DR, Charbeneau GT. An evaluation of a glass ionomer luting agent: Bacterial leakage. J Am Dent Assoc 1987;114:783–786.

134. Johnson GH, Powell LV, DeRouen TA. Evaluation and control of post-cementation pulpal sensitivity: Zinc phosphate and glass ionomer luting cements. J Am Dent Assoc 1993;124:38–46.

135. Höglund C, van Dijken J, Olofsson AL. A clinical evaluation of adhesively luted ceramic inlays: A two-year follow-up study. Swed Dent 1992;16:169–171.

136. Aberg CH, van Dijken J, Olofsson AL. Three-year comparison of fired ceramic inlays cemented with composite resin or glass ionomer cement. Acta Odontol Scand 1994; 52:140–149.

137. Zuellig-Singer R, Bryant RW. Three-year evaluation of computer-machined ceramic inlays: Influence of luting agent. Quintessence Int 1998;29:573–582.

138. van Dijken JW, Ormin A, Olofsson AL. Clinical performance of pressed ceramic inlays luted with resin-modified glass ionomer and autopolymerizing resin composite cements. J Prosthet Dent 1999;82:529–535.

139. White SN, Yu Z, Tom JF, Sangsurasak S. In vivo microleakage of luting cement for cast crowns. J Prosthet Dent 1994;71:333–338.

140. White SN, Yu Z, Tom JF, Sangsurasak S. In vivo marginal adaptation of cast crowns luted with different cements. J Prosthet Dent 1995;74:25–32.

141. Pluim LJ, Arends J, Havinga P, Jongebloed WL, Stokroos I. Quantitative cement solubility experiments in vivo. J Oral Rehabil 1984;11:171–179.

142. Phillips RW, Swartz ML, Lund MS, Moore BK, Vickery J. In vivo disintegration of luting cements. J Am Dent Assoc 1987;114:489–492.

143. Hersek NE, Canay S. In vivo solubility of three types of luting cement. Quintessence Int 1996;27:211–216.

7

DEGRADATION MECHANISMS OF DENTAL RESIN COMPOSITES

Karl-Johan Söderholm, DDS, MPhil, Odont Dr

Knock and Glenn[1] patented the first particulate-filled ceramic-polymer composite for dental use in 1951. Bowen[2] improved this material by developing a new resin, bisphenol glycidyl dimethacrylate (bis-GMA), that formed a strongly cross-linked polymer matrix in which silane-treated ceramic filler particles could chemically bond to the curable resin matrix. The material group that fell under Bowen's original patent[2] was called *dental composites*, a term that may not be ideal for this particular group of materials. The term *composite material* refers to any combination material in which the individual components may be clearly distinguished from one another.[3] The individual components may have different shapes (eg, three-dimensional networks, fibers, or particles) and consist of different materials (eg, ceramics, polymers, or metals). The individual components of a material may also be of the same material type, but if they are distinguishable, the material may still be called *composite*. An example of such a composite is the regular heat-cured polymethyl methacrylate (PMMA) used in dentistry, which consists of prepolymerized PMMA beads surrounded by a heat-cured PMMA matrix. Such a composite is an example of a particulate polymer-polymer composite or a truly resinous composite. A material like the one introduced by Knock and Glenn[1] and later by Bowen[2] is an example of a polymer filled with ceramic particles and should thus be called a *particulate-filled ceramic-polymer composite*. In the text that follows, the terms *composite*, *dental resin composite*, *dental composite*, and *resin composite* are used to describe these particulate-filled ceramic-polymer composites. This usage replaces the more cumbersome *particulate-filled ceramic-polymer composite* with simpler terms that have traditionally been associated with this type of material in dentistry.

During the early use of the first dental composites, it was noticed that restorations made of these materials lost their original shapes[4] and surface properties[5] over time (Fig 7-1). The mechanism for the degradation initially was related to a purely mechanical wear process, but research revealed that chemical processes also could be involved.[6] The nature of the degradation process is therefore either mechanical or chemical or a combination of both. During the degradation of dental composites, small volumes of material components leave the surface of the restoration. These material species are either identical to the components of the resin composite or consist of components formed by various chemical degradation mechanisms. After the different degradation products have left the surface of the resin composite restoration, they may continue degrading as they are transported through the body[7] (Fig 7-2). Consequently, compounds different from

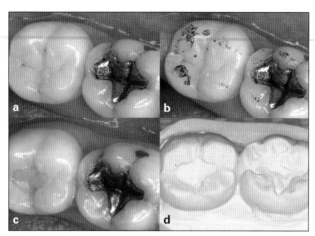

Fig 7-1 Degradation of a Class II occlusal restoration during a three-year period. *(a and b)* Initial conditions after placement. *(c)* Condition after 3 years of clinical service. *(d)* Gypsum model of the 3-year-old composite restoration shows quite well the magnitude of the occlusal wear.

the original ones may form and be transported to remote locations in the body (see Fig 7-2), where they participate in various biologic reactions[8,9] (Fig 7-3). These reactions can cause health problems, which may show up in regions located far away from the original restoration site.[10] It can be extremely difficult to link these health problems to the composition of the resin composite, particularly since we still know very little about the degradation mechanisms that occur when the different components of the resin composite are transported through the body. To avoid speculating too much about these remote degradation mechanisms, this chapter will focus on reviewing existing knowledge dealing with different mechanical and chemical degradation processes of dental resin composites in the oral cavity. We will start with different mechanical wear mechanisms and finish with different chemical degradation processes.

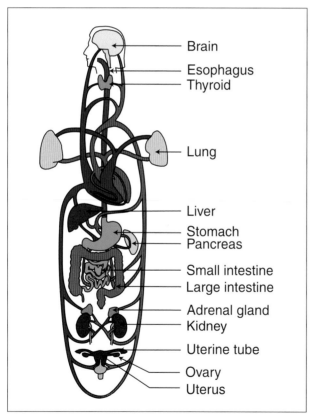

Fig 7-2 Schematic drawing of a female showing the key organs that may participate in the degradation process of components released from dental materials, including dental composites. For example, a monomer molecule such as triethylene glycol dimethacrylate (TEGDMA), released from a dental composite restoration, can be absorbed by the digestive tract and degraded further as it passes the liver and leaves the body via the lungs.[7]

Fig 7-3 *(opposite page)* (a) Different active and inactive receptor proteins exist inside cells. (b) A contaminant or a degradation product such as bisphenol A can act as a steroid hormone and bond to the hormone binding site. (c) When such bonding occurs, the receptor protein becomes activated after releasing its inhibitor protein complex. (d) The exposed DNA binding sites of the receptor protein then bond to a specific site along the DNA molecule, and RNA polymerase is released. (e) The polymerase separates the two DNA helices, and RNA transcription is initiated and continues until the polymerase reaches the stop signal for RNA polymer transcription. (f) The steroid hormone-simulating compound is released and metabolized while the inhibitory protein complex bonds to the DNA binding domain of the receptor protein (g). The released RNA chain (e) starts biologic processes that under certain circumstances can cause harm to the host.

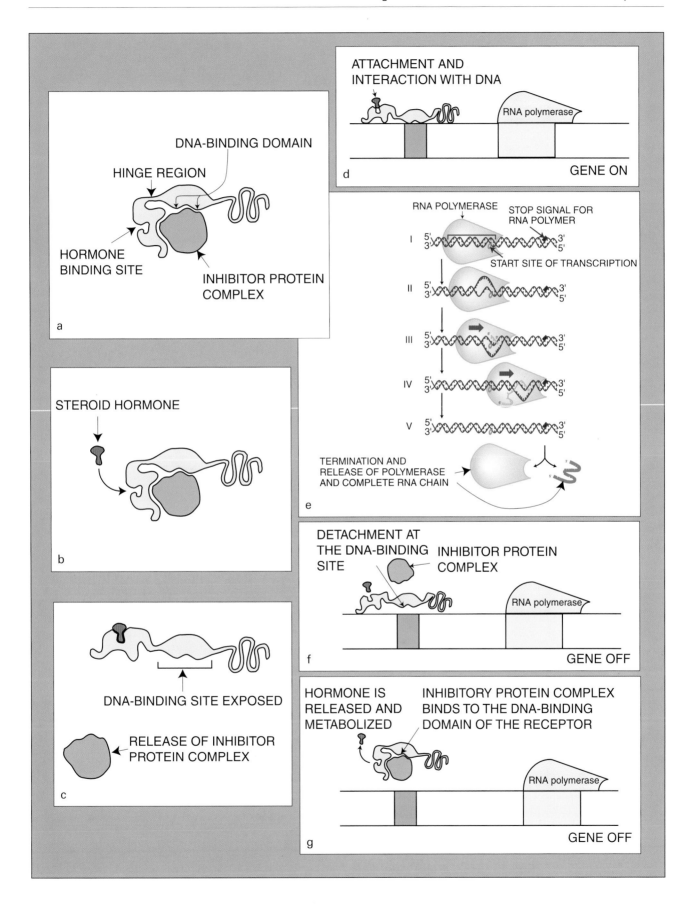

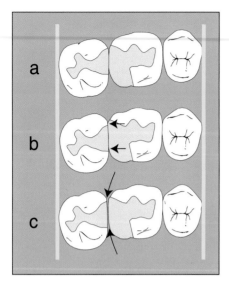

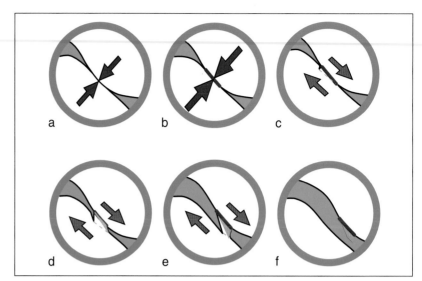

Fig 7-4 Proximal composites placed on the first and second molars *(a)*. As proximal wear progresses, the two teeth either move closer to each other *(b)* or lose their contact *(c)*. In the first case *(b)*, the proximal tissue will not be sufficiently stimulated or cleaned by sliding food or oral hygienic procedures, but in the second case *(c)*, food will become impacted between the teeth and cause periodontal problems.

Fig 7-5 The mechanism of adhesive wear. When two surfaces are forced against each other, high localized pressure can be generated at small contact regions *(a)*. The high pressure can cause localized adhesion *(b)*. When the two surfaces then slide against each other, cracks develop in the weaker material *(c)*, yet some material remains adhered to the stronger surface *(d)*. When the sliding has proceeded a certain distance *(e and f)*, the adhered material is torn away from its original surface *(f)*. (Adapted from Söderholm and Richards[11] with permission.)

Wear

Wear Mechanisms

The degradation process of dental resin composites is complex and includes various wear mechanisms.[11] It was the high wear rate of early composites that triggered a growing interest in different degradation mechanisms of dental resin composites.[4] As the interest in different wear mechanisms increased, it also became clear that wear is still incompletely understood. Wear of teeth and restorations causes changes in function and esthetics over time. Excessive wear can cause pathologic conditions, such as changes in vertical dimensions and traumatic contacts with soft tissues, while proximal wear can result in mesial tooth migration, food impaction, and malocclusion (Fig 7-4). Currently, no experimental studies have proven that swallowed wear particles cause

any biologic problems, but the possibility should not be excluded that future research might prove that some adverse biologic reactions may occur from these particles.

Because of the biologic implications of excessive wear, both local and remote, the clinician must develop a good understanding of different wear mechanisms and how these mechanisms may affect the surrounding tissues and/or materials. At the present time, the different mechanisms involved in the wear process of posterior resin composites are of primary interest, but as the population ages, wear of other materials, including the natural dentition, will become equally important. This chapter will address the wear problem generally in an attempt to make the information applicable to other materials as well.

Wear of dental resin composites is the unwanted removal of solid material from the surfaces of the composite restoration. Such a definition sounds simple, but it includes many diverse phenomena such as sliding, abrasion, chemical degradation, and fatigue, just to mention the most common ones.[12] Any one of these mechanisms may operate by itself or in combination with other mechanisms. In the clinical environment, the wear process of dental materials can become very complex. Variables such as chewing load, chewing frequency, occlusal contact area, and type of food intake will affect the wear rate. In addition to these patient-related variables, the way the clinician manipulates the resin composite material during and after preparing the restoration will affect the clinical wear rate. Air incorporation, efficiency of curing, grinding and polishing procedures, and occlusal design of the restoration are some of the operator-related variables that will affect the clinical wear rate.

Because of the complex nature of composite degradation, one must realize that *wear* is a general term for material loss. The several mechanisms that cause different types of wear (adhesion, abrasion, fatigue, corrosion, and others) are discussed below.

Adhesive wear

Adhesive (or sliding) wear may be distinguished as the most fundamental of the several types of wear. This type of wear arises in the following way. When two flat surfaces, no matter how smoothly and finely they are finished, are brought into solid contact, they will only touch at a relatively few isolated points (Fig 7-5). These contact areas will resist further approach and become compressed. These very small areas carry the entire load between the two surfaces. It follows, then, that because of the generally very small size of the true contact area, the local pressures are extremely high, even under low load, and usually exceed the yield strength of the softer of the two materials in contact.[13] As a result of these high local pressures, minute "welds" are formed at each of the contact areas. When the two surfaces are displaced in relation to each other, these welds are sheared, resulting in failures in the "welded" regions[14–16] (see Fig 7-5). The failure will occur within the weakest region, generally in the softer of the two contacting materials. The galled wear particle

may initially remain adhered to the harder surface, but it is often loosened during subsequent sliding. In either case, the softer of the two surfaces has suffered wear according to the original definition of adhesive wear.

Cleanliness of the surfaces greatly facilitates adhesive wear; saliva, on the other hand, insulates the two surfaces from each other and interposes a layer of foreign material that may prevent the weld from forming.[17] Although the presence of saliva greatly reduces the amount of adhesive wear, it does not eliminate it completely. A few welds are always present that can be the starting points for incipient large-scale galling, if the conditions become sufficiently severe.

Studies of adhesive wear under constant pressure have shown that the volume of the material removed is proportional to the true contact area of the two solid surfaces and the distance of sliding.[18–21] The true area, however, will depend on the hardness of the softer material and the pressure on the surface, such that the true area increases as the hardness decreases and the pressure increases.[18] Because the initial contact points may be smaller than the worn-in ones, the average initial contact pressure may be several times the average contact pressure for the worn-in surface. Consequently, the initial wear rate will be many times the final wear rate. As the wear progresses, it generally results in an increase in the contact area and, as a result, the wear rate will decrease. Finally, when the contact area stabilizes, the average pressure becomes constant, and the wear rate reaches its final steady-state value. This behavior has also been shown to occur in posterior dental composites.[22] That such behavior is related to adhesive wear alone is unlikely because most wear mechanisms are pressure dependent, and as wear continues and the contact areas increase, the pressure consequently tends to decrease.

To conclude, the adhesive wear of dental resin composites should be minimal after initial wear-in and probably much lower than either abrasive or corrosive wear, the other two major types of sliding wear. Because adhesive wear requires contact between occluding surfaces, it cannot occur in contact-free regions. In most instances, therefore, adhesive wear can be ignored as a signifi-

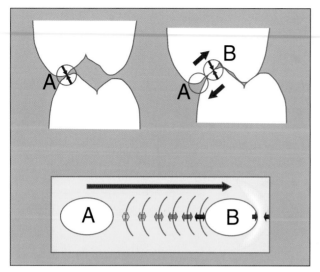

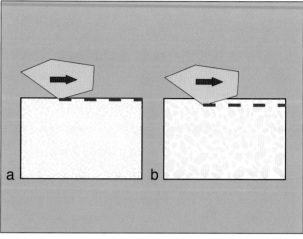

Fig 7-6 Two-body wear occurs when two bodies are forced against each other and slide in contact from point A to point B. During the sliding movement, material in the maxillary tooth is compressed in front of the mandibular cusp when the mandibular cusp slides toward central occlusion. At the same time, the material left behind the cusp as it slides toward central occlusion is stretched, at which point tensile stresses are induced in those regions. These tensile stresses may be sufficient to induce cracks perpendicular to the direction of the sliding cusp. (Adapted from Söderholm and Richards[11] with permission.)

Fig 7-7 During two-body wear, abrasive particles are forced into the surface of a softer material, where they plow furrows. The surface of a composite with short interparticle distance *(a)* is harder than the surface of a composite with longer interparticle distance *(b)*. The harder surface of the material in *(a)* results in a more shallow indentation and wear furrow, which explains why a composite with shorter interparticle spacing is more wear resistant than a composite with longer interparticle spacing. (Adapted from Söderholm and Richards[11] with permission.)

cant wear mechanism of dental resin composites. However, there are certain important situations in which adhesive wear may lead to noticeable results. These include wear-in and continuous wear of occlusal contact regions throughout the lifetime of the composite restoration, for the occlusion of a patient typically undergoes continuous changes.

Abrasive wear

In abrasive wear, the removal of solid material from a resin composite surface is accomplished by a much harder surface or body that plows along it. There are two general situations for this type of wear. In one case, the hard surface is the harder of the two rubbing surfaces (two-body wear or cutting wear). In the other case, the hard surface is a third body, generally a small particle of grit or abrasive, caught between the two surfaces and sufficiently hard to abrade either one or both of the surfaces (three-body wear). These will be discussed in turn.

Two-body wear Two-body wear occurs when two bodies slide against each other.[12] During such a sliding movement, compressive and tensile stresses are developed in the surfaces (Fig 7-6). If these stresses, particularly the tensile stresses, reach a critical level, cracks develop perpendicular to the direction of the sliding body. As the sliding process is repeated, the cracks grow, causing local material chipping and material loss, a process that is called *two-body wear*. This type of two-body wear is reminiscent of the adhesive wear process described above.

Another more commonly seen two-body wear process is so-called *cutting wear*, in which the plowing or abrasive removal of material is produced by one of the two rubbing surfaces[23] (Fig 7-7). This is the simplest and most easily under-

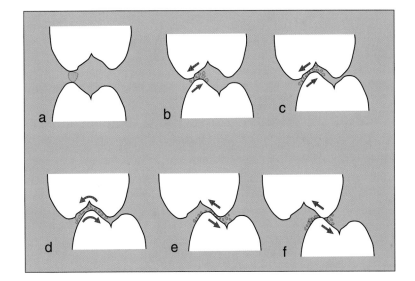

Fig 7-8 Three-body wear occurring during mastication. In the first step *(a)*, the food particle is compressed to failure between opposing cusps. The smaller particles are then forced along the occlusal surfaces during mastication *(b–f)*. The particles may rotate over the surface during the wear process, which explains why a three-body wear process is less efficient than a similar two-body wear process. (Adapted from Söderholm and Richards[11] with permission.)

stood situation of wear. The primary requirements for its occurrence are a great dissimilarity in hardness between the two rubbing surfaces and a certain amount of roughness in the harder of the two surfaces. Of the latter, asperities under the normal load dig into the softer surface and literally plow furrows that break loose into wear particles. A typical example of cutting wear is when a diamond bur cuts along the surface of a posterior resin composite. During such a cutting process, the diamond grains move in a direction parallel to each other and form straight lines along the surface.

Three-body wear The removal of material through the abrasive mechanism by a small, hard particle of grit caught between the two rubbing surfaces, called *three-body wear*,[12] is an extremely important factor in the total overall wear of resin composites and probably is responsible for the largest amount of clinical wear, for mastication involves the generation of fine food particles that slide over the occlusal table (Fig 7-8). However, food is not the only source of such hard particles; filler particles released from the resin composite surface itself during wear also will contribute to abrasive wear. Hence, filler particles released from the resin composite surface through adhesive or corrosive wear will cause abrasive wear if the particles remain between the surfaces. As men-

tioned above, the latter is an example of interaction between different types of wear and contributes to the complexity of separating the effects of the factors responsible in a particular case.

In attempting to understand the influence of various factors on abrasive wear, both the resin composite surface and the abrasive element itself must be considered. As for the resin composite surface, the common wisdom is that the most important approach to increase its abrasive wear resistance is to increase the surface hardness of the resin composite. Such an increase can be achieved by shortening the interparticle filler spacing by using finer filler particles (see Fig 7-7) or by improving the degree of cure of the resin. Such an increase in hardness results in more shallow indentations left by the abrasive particles, which results in less material loss during "plowing" (see Fig 7-7).

It has been shown that certain physical characteristics of the abrasive particles have a pronounced effect on their ability to wear surfaces. These include particle size, ie, coarse particles produce rougher surfaces and generally more wear than fine particles. The hardness of the abrasive particles is obviously important and must be significantly greater than the hardness of the softer of the two rubbing surfaces. Their hardness, relative to that of each of the two rubbing surfaces, will determine whether the abrasive particles will be loose and moving around between the two rubbing surfaces or whether they will become embedded in the softer of the two surfaces. If the abrasive particles become embedded, they form something of a polishing disk acting on the opposing surface. The shape or degree of angularity of the abrasive particles is also important in that angular particles of a soft material produce more wear than rounded, harder ones. Considering these aspects, one should expect that large variations in clinical wear of composite restorations will exist among patients due to considerable variations regarding their abrasive food particles.

The effect of hardness of the resin composite surface undergoing wear has already been noted. Probably more important for abrasive wear resistance is the amount of elastic deformation that the composite surface can sustain. In the presence of a harder abrasive particle, the surface in question deforms elastically, but after the particle has passed on, the surface returns to its original configuration with no plastic deformation or permanent damage. Consequently, the flexibility of the surface would be another important variable in considering its ability to resist wear from an abrasive or an opposing harder surface. For instance, a tire offers an excellent example of the importance of flexibility as a property for wear resistance. One way to understand the wear resistance of a tire is to consider the amount of elastic energy that can be stored in the surface region of the wearing surface; the ability to store elastic energy is a measure of its abrasive wear resistance. Thus, the greater the amount of this stored energy, the greater the tire's wear resistance. The modulus of resilience, which is equal to the square of the elastic limit of stress divided by twice the elastic modulus for a linearly elastic material and which measures the elastic energy that can be stored per unit volume in a solid body, should therefore be considered an important variable in predicting abrasive wear resistance.

To conclude, abrasive wear of dental composites is most likely the mechanism that dominates the wear process of composites. However, because abrasive wear is determined by the properties of the wear particles, and insofar as the wear particles are patient dependent due to food and

chewing habits, one should expect that patient-related factors determine this type of wear. Considering that, these variables must always be included in the selection of restorative materials, not only dental composite materials. An interesting aspect, however, is that an increase in modulus of resilience should reduce the abrasive wear rate. That finding, linked to clinical claims that placement of an unfilled resin on the surface of a composite restoration reduces wear, may suggest that the longevity of posterior composites may be significantly improved by a yearly reapplication of the unfilled resin.

Fatigue wear

The adhesive and abrasive wear types are the principal ones associated with sliding motion between solid surfaces. To them must be added one more distinct type of wear, which occurs primarily when surfaces are in contact with cyclic compression and sliding but in which the friction is generally low. In the engineering field, wear of ball bearings belongs to this group. In dentistry, chewing to some extent resembles the ball-bearing situation, though some plowing also occurs. Food particles tumble over the surface during mastication in a rotational movement similiar to that of a ball bearing. Under extreme conditions, ie, when no plowing occurs, only surface cold working and fatigue take place. This type of wear results in a pattern that is characterized by local pitting or flaking of the surface and occurs rather suddenly without prior visible warning after a relatively long life and many cycles of revolution. However, when it does occur, the particle, and the pit left after it is removed, is relatively large, many times larger than the typical wear particle produced by the other types of wear mechanisms. This pitting is the result of surface fatigue due to the repeated stresses.

Surfaces in direct contact during chewing withstand higher loads than occlusal surfaces that are not in direct contact. When two surfaces are in contact under load, elastic stresses are distributed in the material of each body in the vicinity of the contact area (Fig 7-9). Application of the Hertz equations for the elastic deformation of solid bodies shows that the maximum shear stress does

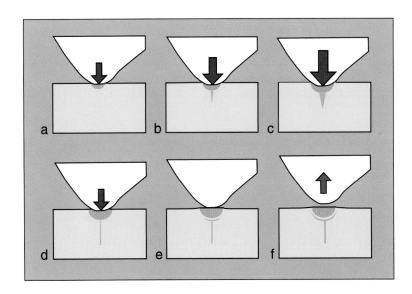

Fig 7-9 The mechanism of fatigue wear. As localized force increases, plastic deformation and densification occurs locally *(a)*. As the plastic deformation region grows, a vertical crack develops *(b and c)*. When the load decreases *(d)*, the crack closes because of elastic relaxation, and the compressed region is "lifted up" as a result of stress relief in the surrounding region. During that process, horizontal cracks develop *(e and f)*. Initially, none of these cracks is seen on the occlusal surface. (Adapted from Söderholm and Richards[11] with permission.)

not occur immediately at the surfaces of the two bodies, but at a small, finite distance beneath the surface. As these contact regions are continuously exposed to a significant fraction of their elastic limit of stress, fatigue failures may occur in these regions. When a fatigue crack does develop, it occurs in the general vicinity of the maximum shear stress just below the surface.[24] Once initiated, like all fatigue cracks, it propagates, generally parallel to the surface, until a region of material is separated from the bulk of the restoration. This region ultimately becomes detached and falls out. The net result of one or more such flaked-out regions is a badly pitted surface.

In cases of combined chewing and sliding, an additional tangential stress induced by the sliding accelerates the pitting. The result is that the maximum value of the total stress is increased over that for pure chewing alone, but its location is raised nearer to the surface. As a result, the tendency to pitting failure is somewhat increased, but the pits when formed are shallower. In the limit of principally sliding motion with only a minor component of chewing, the point of maximum stress may be so near the surface that the wear particles resulting from surface fatigue become indistinguishable from those produced by the other sliding types of wear.

To conclude, surface fatigue of dental resin composites can only occur in primary contact regions. Because dental resin composites seem to experience general wear, and that wear is higher in contact regions, one may question whether surface fatigue is a wear mechanism of significant concern for most resin composites. The reason such a question should be raised is that surface fatigue implies a catastrophic failure, something that is rarely seen in modern resin composites.

Corrosive wear (chemical wear)

The fourth important wear mechanism under sliding conditions is *corrosive* or *chemical wear*.[12] As the name implies, it takes place when chemicals from the environment degrade the matrix,[25] the filler, or the matrix-filler interface.[26,27] It also could be a result of formation of precipitates in the oral cavity, whereby these precipitates are transferred to one or both of the rubbing surfaces from which they are subsequently removed by the rubbing process. In the oral environment, chemicals from drinks, food, microorganisms, and body fluids, including saliva, can easily induce chemical wear. For example, it is known that alcohol can plasticize resins,[28] that water causes filler leaching, that some enzymes produced by microorganisms cause resin degradation,[29] and that ketones produced during some general disease processes can dissolve resins. In other words, chemical degradation processes of dental resin composites do occur in the oral environment.

From the above it can be concluded that corrosive (or chemical) wear requires the presence of both chemical degradation and rubbing to occur.

The component that usually dissolves materials and induces corrosive wear in the oral environment is saliva. The composition of saliva, however, also determines the type of film formed on the surface of the resin composite. As in the other types of wear, the presence of a film may act either as a lubricant or as a corrosive agent. Therefore, the role of saliva on the wear process becomes quite complex, particularly considering the variations in saliva composition and viscosity found among patients.

To conclude, chemical wear of dental composites is a wear mechanism that interacts strongly with the previously described types of wear. However, since chemical wear is strongly dependent on patient variables such as saliva composition and food and drink intake, on interactions of these variables, and on adhesive and abrasive wear, chemical wear and its effect on overall wear is difficult to determine. However, from a clinical point of view, the practitioner should consider chemical wear when selecting materials, for certain patients (eg, alcoholics, diabetics) may be more prone to chemical wear than others.

Minor types of wear

The four wear mechanisms discussed so far cover the principal types of mechanical wear that probably account, singly or collectively, for most wear experienced in present-day dental resin composites. There are, however, a number of minor types of wear mechanisms, at least insofar as we presently understand them, that should be distinguished from the major types. These minor types may explain some extreme wear situations.

Erosive wear One example of a minor type of wear mechanism is erosive wear, a wear process that is caused by high-velocity liquids. The wearing away of material by liquid erosion may be a distinct type of phenomenon because it may be a combination of chemical wear (solubility), increased transportation rate (liquid velocity), and adhesive wear between liquid and solid. Erosive wear also can be classified as a form of three-body wear. In the latter case, abrasive particles hit the surface and are forced along it by gas pressure or a liquid. Wear occurs during both the impact phase and the sliding phase. An example of erosive wear is found in the use of a water pick.

Impact chipping Another minor type of wear is so-called *impact chipping*. Under the high impact involved in cutting teeth and composites, a certain amount of local fracturing of the surface takes place. It is found to increase with increasing hardness of the surface and suggests that failure by brittle fracture under impact is the key failure mechanism. Figure 7-9 shows that as the localized force increases, plastic deformation and densification occur locally. This process results in a vertical crack. As the load decreases, the crack closes and the compressed region is lifted up because of stress relief. During that process, horizontal cracks develop. This mechanism occurs during air abrasion. During ultrasonic scaling, both erosive wear and impact chipping occur.

Clinical Wear

Occlusal wear

Of the foregoing wear mechanisms, abrasive wear mechanisms (see Figs 7-6 to 7-8) dominate the occlusal surface wear of posterior resin composites. In regions with primary cusp contacts, the opposing cusp introduces localized stresses in the region where food particles are crushed between the occlusal table and the opposing cusp. When the food particles are crushed, there is an instantaneous reduction in the localized stress levels at the site of the crushed particles while other particles that now carry the load generate localized stresses at their occlusal-table-to-cusp contact. The smaller of the newly crushed particles now can slide over the surface as the food is forced along the escape routes. These particles induce three-body wear when they escape. At the same time, plastic deformation may occur locally as the stress levels increase in regions adjacent to the food particles forced against the resin composite surface at the occlusal contact points. This in turn will initiate a fatigue wear process (see Figs 7-6 to 7-9).

As the chewing process proceeds, the cusps will reach the resin composite surface, and elastic/plastic deformation will occur at the site of the cusp-composite contact. If the cusp then slides away from the originally compressed contact point, a submicroscopic "wave" of resin composite will move in front of the cusp in the sliding direction (see Fig 7-6). The material in that wave is under compression, whereas the material in the region behind the sliding cusp will be in tension. As the cusp slides along the surface, the stress levels in the resin composite will change from compression to tension in the sliding direction. These changes in stress may become more or less cyclic, depending upon the chewing pattern of the patient. Over time, these cyclic changes can cause fatigue wear in that region. During such a sliding movement and associated changes in stresses, protruding filler particles may tilt and be pulled away from the resin composite surface. The larger the filler particles, the longer the tilt arms become and the more readily the particles will tilt and become dislodged. If such a large particle is lost, a correspondingly large volume of the resin composite will be lost. That mechanism may explain why the first generations of resin composites, containing filler particles that averaged 20 to 40 µm in size, were not wear resistant. By reducing the particle sizes, the surface friction and the length of the tilt arm decrease, with a concomitant decrease in the wear rate.

Jørgensen et al[30] presented a breakthrough in understanding clinical wear in 1979. They showed that adding a small amount of pyrogenic silica particles (particle sizes ranging from 0.02 to 0.04 µm) to a sealant had a profound effect on increasing its wear resistance. These fine particles were much more efficient in decreasing the wear rate than were larger filler particles. Based on these findings, Jørgensen et al[30] proposed that decreasing the interparticle spacing, which is best achieved with the smallest filler particles, was the key to improving the wear resistance of composites (see Fig 7-7). Their explanation is easy to accept, particularly if it is assumed that three-body wear is the dominant wear mechanism of dental resin composites. Thus, by assuming that most food particles passing through the oral cav-

ity exceed a minimal particle size, an interparticle spacing that is shorter than the minimal food particle size would protect the resin matrix between the filler particles from three-body wear generated by food particles. From the clinical research data currently available, it seems that the critical interparticle spacing is around 1 µm.

Based upon the claim by Jørgensen et al[30] and supporting clinical results, it may be concluded that the use of finer particles for a fixed filler volume fraction results in decreased interparticle spacing and reduced wear. That conclusion is correct, but a complicating factor is that the total filler surface area increases as the particle size decreases. That increase in total filler surface area results in more resin being bonded to the filler particles, and to retain a certain workable viscosity of the composite, more resin matrix is needed. Because of this increase in the amount of resin matrix, the filler-volume fraction decreases as the filler particles become smaller. The decrease in filler-volume fraction required for retaining a suitable viscosity becomes particularly obvious after the particle sizes become smaller than a few tenths of a micron. Because a high filler volume fraction reduces polymerization shrinkage and thermal expansion/contraction and also improves mechanical properties such as modulus of elasticity and strength, there is an optimal particle size that should be used in a posterior resin composite. Therefore, it is not surprising to find that the commercial posterior resin composite products with the best wear resistance have average particle sizes near 1 µm. For particles of this size, interparticle spacing is sufficiently short to give good wear resistance, and maximal filler loading can be attained while achieving reasonably smooth resin composite surfaces.

Another key factor in strengthening a resin composite is to have good stress transferability at the resin-filler interface. Such stress transfer can be enhanced by either improving the bond between the filler and the matrix or by increasing the filler surface area. Smaller particles increase the total filler surface area, as do filler particle shapes that favor mechanical retention. It is also known that fibers are more efficient as reinforcing agents than spheres, so long as the fibers are oriented in the force direction. However, it is important to emphasize that fibers oriented perpendicular to the force direction can decrease strength. The more efficient strengthening capacity of a fiber may be understood by analyzing potential differences between a sphere and a fiber used as reinforcing fillers. If a fiber is pulled out from a resin, frictional stresses develop along the fiber surface. As the fiber length increases, these frictional forces (ie, shear stresses) become so high that the strength of the fiber sets the limit of how much stress the material can bear without failure. For the sphere, the situation is different. As the sphere-filled composite is subject to tensile strain, all stress is transferred to the filler-resin interface that now provides much less frictional resistance. As seen from this discussion, there is a certain critical fiber length above which optimal stress-bearing ability is attained. It is plausible that below a certain size, the fiber-reinforcing effect of a particulate filler is limited. That may also explain why clinical studies have shown that resin composites containing particles with average sizes below 1 μm are associated with an increased risk of marginal ditching.

The foregoing discussion may explain existing clinical results regarding the performance of posterior resin composite restorations. In one meta-analysis,[31] the outcome revealed that the most wear-resistant posterior resin composite was Clearfil Posterior (Kuraray, Kashima, Japan), followed by P-50 (3M, Dental Products Division, St. Paul, MN) and Z-100 (3M). These three materials have two characteristics in common: their mean filler particle size is around 1 μm and their filler volume fractions are high. A closer comparison reveals that Clearfil Posterior contains more irregular particles, some of which are also larger than the filler particles in P-50 and Z-100. The better reinforcing effect that these particles contribute within marginal regions may explain why Clearfil Posterior was found to be the most wear-resistant posterior resin composite of the products studied.

To summarize, it seems that the ideal posterior resin composite should have a mean particle size close to 1 μm in diameter. The particle size distribution should include a small fraction of larger particles (around 3 to 5 μm) and a small amount of submicron-size particles. The filler volume fraction should exceed 60%. With these criteria, the main drawback of such a resin composite would be the larger particles and their effect on surface roughness. However, that drawback would be compensated for by reduced tendency for marginal breakdown.

To understand the wear processes that occur clinically, it is important to use reliable wear evaluation methods. Several evaluation systems have been described for the assessment of changes in anatomical form of resin composite restorations. Unfortunately, reliable quantitative determinations are still rare, and when they are used, they are resource demanding, reducing their usefulness for the average clinical evaluator. In addition, it is also known that major discrepancies exist between in vivo and in vitro wear-rate determinations of posterior resin composites and that attempts to correlate in vitro results with long-term in vivo performance have not always been completely successful. Therefore, long-term quantitative in vivo wear measurements are still essential to determine the clinical performance of new posterior composite materials.

In clinical studies, Willems and colleagues[32–34] measured the wear of 52 Class II restorations placed in mandibular and maxillary first and second molars. The five resin composites that were evaluated were Exp LF (an ultrafine experimental composite with intermediate filler volume fraction), P-30 (3M), P-30 APC (3M), P-50 APC (3M), and Marathon (Den-Mat, Santa Maria, CA). The measurements were made on epoxy replicas at baseline; 6 months; and 1, 2, and 3 years using a measuring microscope and a technique described elsewhere.[35] The occlusal contact area (OCA) and contact-free occlusal area (CFOA) wear values were averaged at each recall session and used to calculate the general wear of each resin composite. The mean wear and standard deviation for OCA and CFOA wear were measured in microns.

The resin composites P-30, P-30 APC, and P-50 APC showed OCA wear rates ranging from 110 to 149 μm after 3 years of clinical service (Fig 7-10). The Exp LF and Marathon resin composites had much higher OCA wear rates of 215 and 242 μm, respectively, after 3 years of in vivo function (see Fig 7-10). Exp LF also showed an exceptionally high CFOA wear value of 151 μm after 3 years. The resin composites P-30, P-30 APC, and P-50 APC had approximately the same OCA wear, and all three composites showed significantly lower OCA wear than Marathon, whereas the OCA wear for Exp LF and Marathon was not significantly different during the 3 years of this study.

These results may seem high compared with other studies. The wear results presented in Fig 7-10 are high because they are referred to fixed standard points, whereas most other clinical studies refer the wear rate to surrounding enamel margins. Because the enamel wears over time (Fig 7-11), wear values referred to the surounding enamel margins (Fig 7-12) underestimate the true composite wear. A comparison of Figs 7-10 and 7-12 illustrates this important point.

Finally, it is necessary to emphasize that the large standard deviations for the wear results in these figures are due to the multifactorial aspect of the wear process and biologic variation. Tooth wear is a very complex phenomenon that depends upon several extrinsic and intrinsic factors.[36-38] Obviously, all of these factors can cause a large biologic spread among individuals. These natural variations are translated into large standard deviations, which are inherent with in vivo studies (see Figs 7-10 to 7-12).

Proximal wear

There is no doubt that there have been major improvements in the occlusal wear resistance of posterior resin composites during the past 20 years. Currently, the occlusal wear rates of many posterior resin composites are reported to be 10 to 50 μm/year (Fig 7-12); during the early 1980s, the occlusal wear rates were 80 to 100 μm/year. However, despite numerous clinical wear studies that have been conducted over the years, very few studies are available that have measured the proximal wear of posterior composites. In studies conducted by Wendt et al,[39] using a technique previously described by Ziemiecki et al,[40] the proximal wear rate of posterior resin composites was found to be substantially higher than the occlusal wear rate. According to Wendt et al,[39]

the resin composite wear on a single proximal surface was several times higher than that on the occlusal surface (Fig 7-13). Such a dramatic wear rate could cause potential long-term problems by facilitating mesial tooth movement and changes in the occlusal relationships (see Fig 7-4). Because very few proximal wear studies are currently available, there is a strong need to verify or reject the above claims.

Considering the claims discussed in the preceding paragraph, how can the proximal wear of posterior resin composites be substantially higher than occlusal wear? A possible explanation is that proximal restoration surfaces might not be as well light-cured as occlusal surfaces. During light-curing, the use of a metal matrix band may prevent the light from reaching the contact region as much as it reaches the occlusal surface. Also, the distance from the light tip to the proximal region is longer than the distance from the light tip to the occlusal surface, and this difference in distance will result in more efficient curing of the posterior composite at the occlusal surface than at a proximal surface. In addition, a proximal surface is essentially in continuous contact with the adjacent surface on the next tooth (Fig 7-14), whereas an occlusal contact with the opposing surface only occurs when the restoration contacts a food bolus or the occlusal surface of the opposing tooth. Consequently, the contact time between proximal surfaces is longer than it is between occlusal contacts. Because of the longer contact time, more total wear may occur even when the wear rate per active wear time unit is lower on the proximal surface.

Another explanation is that different wear mechanisms cause occlusal and proximal wear. Environmental variations such as differences in bacterial colonization and retention on the two surfaces may also explain some of the differences in wear. For example, some microorganisms produce esterase, which facilitates resin degradation by breaking ester linkages present in the resin composites. Because microorganisms are also more easily retained on proximal surfaces, enzymatic degradation may be an important component to consider when trying to explain the higher proximal wear rate.

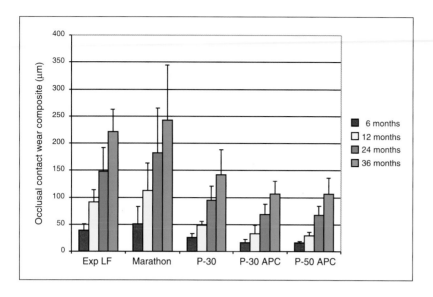

Fig 7-10 Occlusal contact wear of 5 dental composites during a 3-year period. The wear shown in this figure is the total composite wear measured (µm) from a fixed reference plane. (Data from Willems.[32])

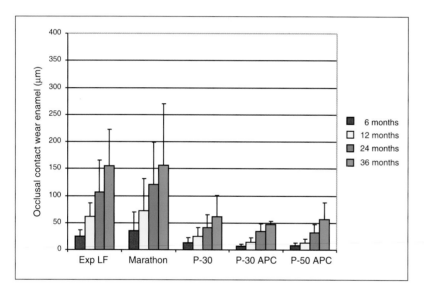

Fig 7-11 Occlusal contact wear of enamel adjacent to the composite materials shown in Fig 7-10. The wear shown here is again measured (µm) in relationship to a fixed reference plane. (Data from Willems.[32])

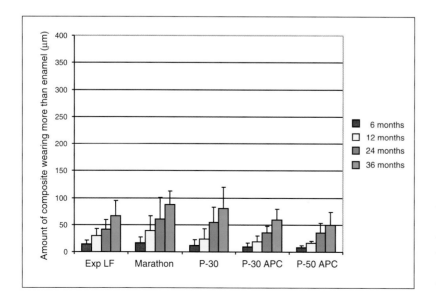

Fig 7-12 Wear of five dental composites when the surrounding enamel margins are used as reference points. Comparison with Fig 7-10 shows that the measuring technique (in µm) strongly affects the results presented in the literature. (Data from Willems.[32])

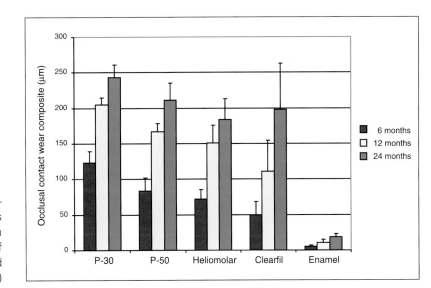

Fig 7-13 Proximal wear of four composites and enamel during a 2-year period. As seen from this figure, the proximal wear (in µm) after 2 years is higher than the wear of the same materials shown in Figs 7-10 and 7-12 after 2 years. (Data from Wendt et al.[39])

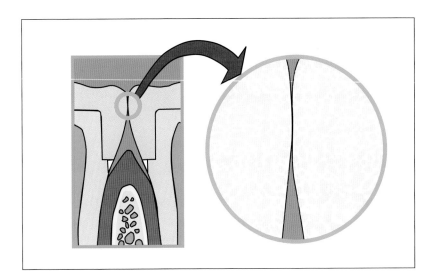

Fig 7-14 Two teeth in contact with each other. The greater proximal wear may be explained by assuming that the two proximal surfaces rub against each other during normal mastication and that this rubbing motion induces either two-body or three-body wear. Other wear mechanisms, such as corrosive wear, also may be involved in proximal wear. (Adapted from Söderholm and Richards[11] with permission.)

Chemical Degradation

From the preceding discussion, it is obvious that in addition to different mechanical processes, chemical processes are also involved in the degradation of dental composites and that the dominant resin composite degradation process is abrasive wear, with corrosive wear playing a less significant role in most cases. The abrasive wear process is a purely mechanical interaction between two or three bodies, whereas corrosive wear includes one or more chemical degradation mechanisms. Mechanical wear processes that remove corrosion products accelerate chemical degradation. Important components of any chemical degradation process are not only how reactive compounds are transported to the surface layer but also how degradation products are transported away from the reactive site. Thus, chemical degradation of dental resin composites is strongly influenced by diffusion of molecules and the speed with which different molecules react while cusps, food particles, and fluids remove the corrosion products from the polymer surface.

Consequently, the diffusion properties of the resin composite material, particularly the matrix material, play a key role in the chemical degradation process. Because variables such as composition of the resin, degree of conversion, filler-matrix bonding, and filler volume fraction are all variables that affect diffusion, they also all affect the chemical degradation process. Components present in the oral environment may change the diffusion conditions by causing swelling of the resin matrix, which would then change the degradation rate.

Because dental resin composites consist of filler particles that are bonded to a resin matrix via a coupling agent, the following degradation mechanisms are discussed in the next sections: degradation of the filler particles, degradation of the filler-silane interface, and degradation of the matrix.

Degradation of the Filler Particles

Different chemicals can degrade the filler surfaces. Filler degradation occurs either on a resin composite surface with exposed filler particles or inside a resin composite after diffusion of chemicals through the resin matrix. The most abundant chemical in the mouth is saliva with its high water content. Water by itself may cause hydrolytic breakdown of the filler surface.[26,41,42] That breakdown is caused by two main mechanisms. Elemental leaching from the filler provides the first mechanism. After water diffuses through the matrix and reaches the filler surface, it starts attacking the glass surface and, as that attack proceeds, the surface breaks down. The hydrolytic degradation of glass was first identified by Charles,[43] who tried to explain why virgin glass was much stronger than glass that had been exposed to humidity in the air. He discovered that as a result of exposure of the glass to water, sodium ions leached from the glass surface and were replaced by hydrogen ions from the water. Because of the smaller size of the hydrogen ions, a tensile stress was induced in the outer layer of the glass, which contributed to a process that Charles termed *stress corrosion*.[43]

Charles[43] also discovered that as the hydrogen ions were absorbed by the glass surface, the OH^- ion concentration of the water adjacent to the glass surface increased. When the pH of that water exceeded 9.5, the OH^- ions started to rupture the siloxane bonds of the glass surface. During that process, the broken siloxane bond also absorbed a hydrogen ion. Thus, breaking the siloxane bond resulted in the formation of two SiOH groups, along with the formation of a new OH^- ion that was free to participate in the next siloxane bond breakage (Fig 7-15). The reaction becomes autocatalytic by continuously producing new OH^- ions as the existing ones are consumed in the siloxane-bond-breakage reaction. As the autocatalytic reaction proceeds, the surface expands and becomes weaker. When this happens, a failure may occur in the surface layer of the glass. In 1981, the same degradation mechanism was reported to occur in a glass-filled PMMA model material simulating a dental resin composite.[26] In studies that followed,[27,41,44] similar degradation mechanisms were identified for commercial dental resin composites (Figs 7-15 and 7-16).

The foregoing results were obtained for resin composites that had been stored in distilled water, but it was important to determine whether the hydrolytic degradation reaction also occurred in saliva. To answer this question, leaching patterns were compared for experimental resin composites stored in either distilled water or artificial saliva.[45,46] Each month, the resin composite samples were transferred to freshly mixed artificial saliva or freshly distilled water. That process was repeated over a 3-year period, and each month the silicon, barium, and aluminum contents of the water or artificial saliva were determined. One experimental composite contained a quartz filler and the other contained a barium-glass filler. Storage of these resin composite materials in a saliva-simulating solution resulted in significantly higher filler leaching than when the same resin composites were stored in distilled water. A possible explanation for the increased leaching ability is that the presence of different ions at the interface results in a charge balance that may not form as easily when distilled water is used (an

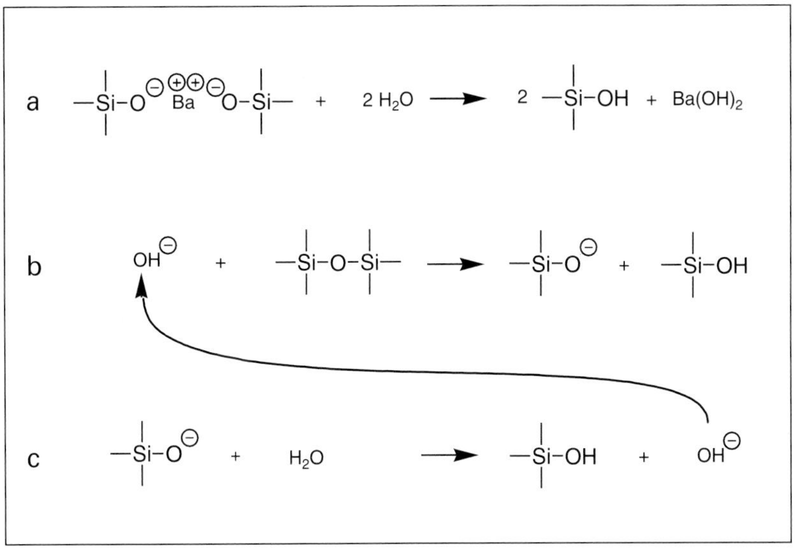

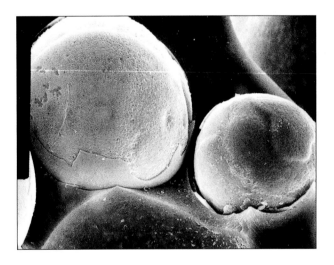

Fig 7-15 Hydrolytic degradation of a glass that contains glass-modifying ions (in this case barium ions). *(a)* When such a glass is stored in water, water molecules substitute the glass-modifying ions with H⁺ ions. As more and more hydrogen ions are tied up by the glass structure, the pH of the water at the glass surface increases. *(b)* When a critical pH value has been reached, the OH⁻ ions break some of the siloxane linkages forming Si-OH and ⁻O-Si. *(c)* These ⁻O-Si groups then react with more H⁺ ions, which results in the release of more OH⁻ ions. The latter ions can then react again with the siloxane bonds and the reaction becomes autocatalytic *(c to b)*.

Fig 7-16 Scanning electron micrograph of unsilanated soda-lime glass beads used as ceramic filler particles in a polymer matrix. After 32 days of storage in water at 60°C, the surface of the beads has degraded. The degradation resulted in a weak layer that separated from the glass sphere when the composite was tested in diametral compression. Diameters of the glass sphere range from 10 to 15 μm.

ion-exchange mechanism). For example, a decrease in surface-charge density may facilitate the migration of a positive ion from the filler surface because another positive ion from the salt solution can enter the surface and neutralize potential charge differences. This scenario suggests that the ion-exchange mechanism, at least to some extent, causes the glass surface to degrade slower than might be expected from the leaching of barium. The experimental observation that filler leaching was constant over time further suggests that the ion release rate at the filler-matrix interfaces inside the material is faster than the rate of ion migration through the matrix (Fig 7-17).

Another filler degradation mechanism of clinical interest is the reaction between different filler particles and fluoride compounds (Fig 7-18). It has been known for some time that fluoride treatments, particularly when a gel tray treatment is used, can induce surface changes in dental resin composites.[47] These changes are caused by filler degradation, debonding, and filler dislodgment.[48] The mechanism is based upon the interaction of fluorine ions with the silicon atom of the silica structure. When that reaction occurs, the siloxane bond is broken, and hydrogen ions react with the SiO⁻ to form SiOH. In vitro wear studies have shown that topical acidulated phosphate fluoride

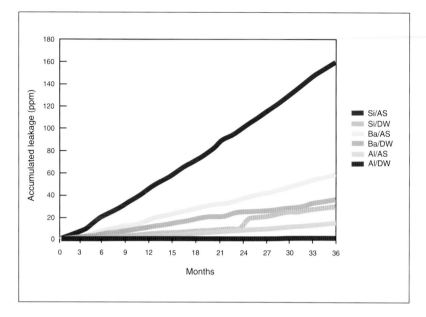

Fig 7-17 Linear plot of amounts of different elements leached into either artificial saliva (AS) or distilled water (DW) from filler particles containing silicon (Si), barium (Ba), or aluminum (Al). It can be seen that leaching in artificial saliva is clearly higher than in distilled water and that the rate of leaching remains constant, at least over a 3-year period. (Data from Söderholm et al.[46])

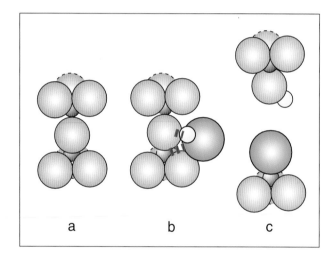

Fig 7-18 Schematic illustration of hydrofluoric acid attack of the siloxane bond. A simplified silica structure is shown in *(a)*, where the small red spheres represent the silicon atoms and the blue spheres the oxygen atoms. As the HF molecule approaches, the strongly negative fluorine ion *(green sphere)* interacts with the strongly positive silicon atom while the positive hydrogen *(yellow sphere)* interacts with the oxygen atom *(b)*. These interactions break the siloxane bond, and the adjacent silicon atoms will separate after the formation of an SiOH group and an SiF group *(c)*.

(APF) agents cause extensive loss of filler from the resin composite specimens, whereas 1.1% NaF causes less damage.[49]

Degradation of the Filler-Silane Interface

A very important component of a dental resin composite is the coupling agent.[2,42,50] This agent most often consists of γ-methacryloxypropyl-trimethoxy silane (MPS). At one end of that molecule, the silane molecule reacts with the filler surface and forms a siloxane bond; at the other end of the MPS molecule, the methacrylate group polymerizes with the resin matrix and forms another covalent bond. In addition, the carbonyl group of MPS forms a hydrogen bond with the filler surface, a bond that is capable of breaking and reforming[51] (Fig 7-19). The filler-silane-resin region can fail in two ways. The first failure mechanism may be initiated by filler-surface degradation. As the filler surface degrades, stress transfer will tear away the coupling agent from the filler surface, causing complete debonding. This mode of failure is known to occur in the field of fiber-reinforced plastics, but whether it plays a

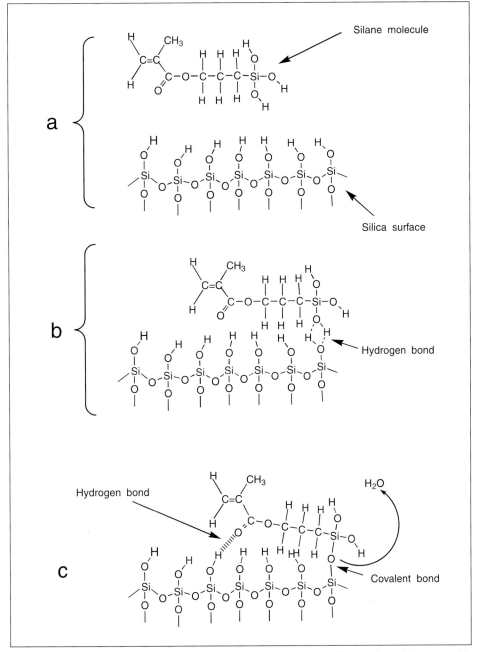

Fig 7-19 The reaction between a silane such as MPS and a silica surface *(a)* starts with hydrogen-bond formation *(b)*. *(c)* Water is then released through a condensation reaction from that bond site, and a covalent bond forms. Hydrogen bonding occurs between the carbonyl group of the MPS and an OH group of the silica surface at the same time, causing the MPS molecule to orient itself parallel to the silica surface.

significant role in the wear process of dental resin composites has not yet been proven. The second failure mechanism is enzymatic degradation of the silane molecule itself.

Previous studies have shown that filler-surface degradation is much more pronounced on glass filler particles that have not been silane coated than on those that have been silane coated.[26] That difference can be related to the hydrophobic nature of the silane-coated filler surface. However, despite the slower reaction rate of the silane-treated glass surfaces, it is still clear that elements leach from the filler surface over time.[46] It is also well known that water exposure decreases the mechanical properties of most resin composites. Such a decrease is strongly affected by the plasticizing effect of water on most resins, but it can also be caused by attack of water at the filler-resin interface. During such attacks, the filler surfaces are weakened and siloxane bonds between the glass surface and the silane are ruptured. Because of the latter, a key factor in the filler-silane interface breakdown is how easily water can penetrate the silane coating and reach the filler surface. As mentioned earlier, the silane-coated filler particles used in dental composites are hydrophobic, which implies that water will not reach the glass surface as readily as it will for unsilanated filler particles. Consequently, the breakdown of the silane-treated filler surface should be a rather slow degradation process.

As for the silane molecule itself and its breakdown, it is ordinarily a quite stable molecule. However, the MPS molecule has an ester linkage that could degrade under certain conditions. That ester linkage is most degradable at low pH values and, as the water-filler interaction raises the pH, the ester linkage should not be a key concern in the degradation that might occur in this region. A much bigger concern is the bond between the silane and the polymer matrix and how well that bond forms during polymerization. In the literature, the silane coating is often shown as a monolayer (Fig 7-20), where one of the ends of the silane molecule bonds to the filler surface and the other to the resin. But such a picture is an oversimplification of the real situation, for it suggests that silane forms a monolayer between the filler surface and the resin. Instead, the filler surface is coated with many monolayers of silane molecules during silane treatment (Fig 7-21). The hydroxylated silane molecules condense to oligomeric siloxanols that initially are soluble and fusible but ultimately condense to rigid cross-linked structures. Contact of a treated surface with a monomer is facilitated while the siloxanols still have some degree of solubility. Bonding with the resin can then take several forms. The oligomeric siloxanol layer may be compatible in the liquid matrix resin and form a true copolymer during the resin cure. Alternatively, the oligomeric siloxanol may only have partial solution compatibility with the matrix resin and form an interpenetrating polymer network, as the siloxanols and matrix resin cure separately with a limited amount of copolymerization.[50]

A very important factor that determines the quality of the silane treatment is the thickness of the silane film. The monolayer closest to the filler surface is chemically bonded to this surface while, as the silane thickness increases, the layers become more and more physicosorbed and disorganized (see Fig 7-21). As the disorganization increases, the risk of forming a weaker bond increases, as the wrong end of the silane molecule may be in contact with the curable matrix material. Because of these inherent problems, the quality of the silane treatment could have a significant effect on the filler-matrix coupling.

Degradation of the Matrix

Degradation of the resin matrix material is influenced by the degree of cure. In addition, both the filler-silane degradation mechanism and the poor silane-resin bond are influenced by the degree of cure. An increased degree of cure influences degradation at the filler surface by increasing the resin density and decreasing the diffusion rate through the matrix material, which thereby slows the reaction rate at the filler surface. Also, a higher degree of cure is likely to produce a more efficient silane-resin cure and thus a better filler-resin bond.

When different degradation mechanisms of the resin matrix are considered, monomer leaching and molecular substitution should be included. When a resin composite is placed in ethanol, more monomer is leached during a shorter time interval than if it were placed in water. When monomer molecules leach into alcohol, alcohol molecules diffuse into the resin. During this process, the matrix will swell and retain alcohol molecules within the resin network. Because of the space the alcohol molecules occupy, they will increase the

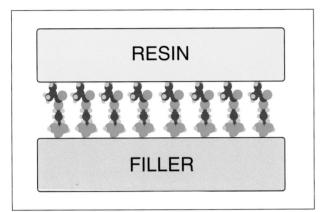

Fig 7-20 Drawing representing the commonly held belief that silane molecules form a direct link between the silica surface and the resin by forming a monolayer where the silane molecules are oriented perpendicular to the silica surface. The yellow and blue spheres at the filler surface represent the OH groups of the MPS; the red spheres at the resin surface represent the carbon atoms adjacent to the C=C bonds of the MPS. This molecular orientation, which is often presented in the literature, is not consistent with results from spectroscopic studies.

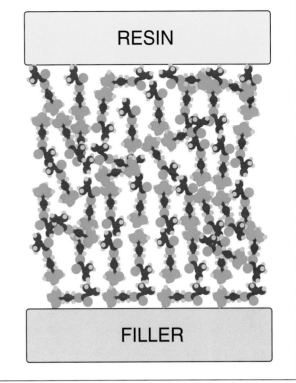

Fig 7-21 Rather than forming a monolayer, the silane molecules in general form multilayers of silane molecules that are more or less randomly oriented. It is only the silane molecules closest to the silica surface that are chemically bonded to the silica surface, while most silane molecules are physically retained on the silica surface.

distance between the polymer chains. The increase in chain spacing results in weaker polar interactions between the separated chains (Fig 7-22), which results in a softer and more wear-susceptible matrix. In vitro studies have also shown that alcohol decreases the wear resistance of dental composites,[28] a result that is expected. Similar results have also been claimed to occur in vivo.

Degradation of dental resin composites can also occur as a result of overheating during polishing. If the frictional heat locally exceeds 200°C, methyl methacrylate–based resins start depolymerizing and form monomer segments.[52] These segments can in turn leach out from the surface, leaving the surface more porous and less dense.

Such a decrease in density can in turn facilitate diffusion and degradation caused by other compounds.

It has been shown that oxygen can interact with the methacrylate group and produce formaldehyde.[53] This reaction occurs according to the formula:

$$H_2C=CCH_3-OOR + O_2 \rightarrow HCHO + CH_3COCOOR$$

Øysaed et al[53] found that formaldehyde was released from the resin composite surface and could be detected even after 115 days of immer-

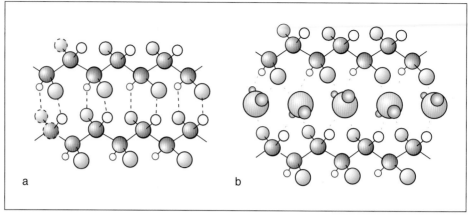

Fig 7-22 Polymer chains held together by weak intermolecular bonds *(a)*. If this material is stored in a medium containing molecules that can diffuse into the polymer, the diffusing molecules, here shown as water molecules *(orange and green spheres)*, will separate the polymer chains *(b)*. When such a separation occurs, the strength of the intermolecular bonds decreases and the polymer becomes plasticized.

sion in water. The highest quantity of released formaldehyde occurred in resin composites having surfaces that had not been cut after polymerization in contact with air. The thickness of the oxygen-inhibited layer increased with increased TEGDMA content. Covering the surface with a matrix strip seemed to have the same effect as cutting it away. Formaldehyde formed either through direct oxidation of the methacrylate group (see the preceding formula) or through decomposition of oxygen-methacrylate copolymers. The highest quantities were released initially. Increased porosity of the resin composite may also increase the formaldehyde content because of the increased retention of oxygen. The amount of formaldehyde release from a resin composite surface without an oxygen-inhibition layer was in the range of 0.1 $\mu g/cm^2$.

In addition to the above degradation mechanisms, it has also been shown that enzymes, such as esterase, present in the oral cavity may hydrolyze and break the ester linkages found in different resins. Munksgaard and Freund[29] examined how different dental resins were attacked by porcine liver esterase and found that the order of breakdown was bis-GMA < TEGDMA < urethane ethylene dimethacrylate (UEDMA) < diethylene glycol dimethacrylate (DEGDMA). They also

determined the esterase activity of saliva in 43 individuals and found that the conversion rate was 4.54 ± 3.24 mmol methacrylic acid/hour. The esterase activity of human saliva was capable of softening resin composites. Studies conducted by de Gee et al[25] have also shown that enzymes are capable of accelerating the in vitro wear of resin composites.

Conclusions

From the foregoing presentation it should be clear that there are several mechanisms that can cause in vivo degradation of dental resin composites. The major contribution to this degradation arises from well-understood wear mechanisms, particularly two-body and three-body wear. A third type of wear that affects resin composites is corrosive wear. Corrosive wear is a combination of chemical degradation and two- and three-body wear. All of these wear mechanisms are strongly influenced by the degree of cure. A higher degree of cure results in a stronger resin, through which solvents will not diffuse as easily as through a resin with a lower degree of cure. A slower diffusion rate will also decrease the reaction rate between different environmental components and different material components, such as the filler surface and/or the matrix. A higher degree of conversion can be achieved with more efficient curing systems as well as by minimizing exposure of the uncured resin to oxygen.

Based on available information about resin composites and what is known about the amount of degradation products released from such restorations over time, it does not seem that the amounts are high enough to cause any toxic effects. However, the released components could act as antigens that may cause allergic reactions. Because of the rather limited knowledge currently available about the different degradation mechanisms, particularly after worn particles have been swallowed, more research is needed in this field. Such studies should target enzymatic degradation mechanisms because enzymatic processes might form compounds that are more bioactive than the original components used in the resin composite. Until all possible degradation mechanisms for resin composites and their resulting compounds are thoroughly known, it is not possible to be certain that these materials are completely safe.

Acknowledgment

Portions of the section on wear were previously published in Söderholm KJ, Richards ND. Wear resistance of composites: A solved problem? Gen Dent 1998;46:256–263.

References

1. Knock FE, Glenn JF [inventors]. Dental material and method. US patent 2,558,139. 26 June 1951.

2. Bowen RL [inventor]. Dental filling material comprising vinyl-silane treated fused silica and a binder consisting of the reaction product of bisphenol and glycidyl methacrylate. US patent 3,066,112. 27 Nov 1962.

3. Holliday L. Composite Materials. Amsterdam: Elsevier, 1966.

4. Phillips RW, Avery DR, Mehra R, Swartz ML, McCune RJ. Observations on a composite resin for Class II restorations: Three-year report. J Prosthet Dent 1973;30: 891–897.

5. Weitman RT, Eames WB. Plaque accumulation on composite surfaces after various finishing procedures. J Am Dent Assoc 1975;91:101–106.

6. Draughn RA. Fatigue and fracture mechanics of composite resins. In: Vanherle G, Smith DC (eds). Posterior Composite Resin Dental Restorative Materials. Utrecht: Peter Szulc, 1985:299–316.

7. Reichl FX, Durner J, Muckter H, et al. Effect of dental materials on gluconeogenesis in rat kidney tubules. Arch Toxicol 1999;73:381–386.

8. Olea N, Pulgar R, Perez P, et al. Estrogenicity of resin-based composites and sealants used in dentistry. Environ Health Perspect 1996;104:298–305.

9. Söderholm KJ, Mariotti A. Bis-GMA–based resins in dentistry: Are they safe? J Am Dent Assoc 1999; 130:201–209.

10. Mariotti A, Söderholm KJ, Johnson S. The in vivo effects of bisGMA on murine uterine weight, nucleic acids and collagen. Eur J Oral Sci 1998;106: 1022–1027.

11. Söderholm KJ, Richards ND. Wear resistance of composites: A solved problem? Gen Dent 1998;46:256–263.

12. Burwell JT. Survey of possible wear mechanisms. Wear 1957/58;1:119–141.

13. Briscoe BJ, Tabor D. Friction and wear of polymers. In: Clark DT, Feast WJ (eds). Polymer Surfaces. New York: Wiley, 1978:1–23.

14. Green AP. Friction between unlubricated metals: a theoretical analysis of the junction model. Proc Roy Soc 1955;A228:191–204.

15. Greenwood JA, Tabor D. Deformation properties of friction junctions. Proc Phys Soc (London) 1955;66B: 609–619.

16. Greenwood JA, Tabor D. The properties of model friction junctions. In: Proceedings of the Conference on Lubrication and Wear. London: Institution of Mechanical Engineers, 1957:314–317.

17. McFarlane JS, Tabor D. Adhesion of solids and the effect of surface films. Proc Roy Soc 1950;A202:224–317.

18. Holm R. Electric Contacts. Stockholm: Almqvist and Wiksells, 1946.

19. Archard JF. Contact and rubbing of flat surfaces. J Appl Phys 1953;24:981–988.

20. Burwell JT, Strang CD. On the empirical law of adhesive wear. J Appl Phys 1952;23:18–28.

21. Rabinowicz E, Tabor D. Metallic transfer between sliding metals: An autoradiographic study. Proc Roy Soc 1951;A208: 455–475.

22. Lambrechts P, Braem M, Vanherle G. Accomplishments and expectations with posterior composite resins. In: Vanherle G, Smith DC (eds). Posterior Composite Resin Dental Restorative Materials. Utrecht: Peter Szulc, 1985:521–540.

23. Spurr RT, Newcomb TP. The friction and wear of various materials sliding against unlubricated surfaces of different types and degrees of roughness. In: Proceedings of the Conference on Lubrication and Wear. London: Institution of Mechanical Engineers, 1957: 269–275.

24. Lawn BR, Swain MV. Microfracture beneath point indentations in brittle solids. J Mater Sci 1975;10: 113–122.

25. de Gee AJ, Wendt SL, Werner A, Davidson CL. Influence of enzymes and plaque acids on in vitro wear of dental composites. Biomaterials 1996;17:1327–1332.

26. Söderholm KJ. Degradation of glass filler in experimental composites. J Dent Res 1981;60:1867–1875.

27. Söderholm KJ, Zigan M, Ragan M, Fischlschweiger W, Bergman M. Hydrolytic degradation of dental composites. J Dent Res 1984;63:1248–1254.

28. Wu W, McKinney JE. Influence of chemicals on wear of dental composites. J Dent Res 1982;61:1180–1183.

29. Munksgaard EC, Freund M. Enzymatic hydrolysis of (di)methacrylates and their polymers. Scand J Dent Res 1990;98:261–267.

30. Jørgensen KD, Hørsted P, Janum O, Krogh J, Schultz J. Abrasion of Class I restorative resins. Scand J Dent Res 1979;87:140–145.

31. Taylor DF, Bayne SC, Leinfelder KF, Davis S, Koch GG. Pooling of long-term clinical wear data for posterior composites. Am J Dent 1994;7:167–174.

32. Willems G. Multi-standard Criteria for the Selection of Potential Posterior Composites [dissertation]. The Netherlands: University of Leuven, 1992.

33. Willems G, Lambrechts P, Braem M, Vanherle G. Three-year follow-up of five posterior composites: in vivo wear. J Dent 1993;21:74–78.

34. Willems G, Lambrechts P, Lesaffre E, Braem M, Vanherle G. Three-year follow-up of five posterior composites: SEM study of differential wear. J Dent 1993;21:79–86.

35. Lambrechts P, Vanherle G, Vuylsteke M, Davidson CL. Quantitative evaluation of the wear resistance of posterior dental restorations: A new three-dimensional measuring technique. J Dent 1984;12:252–267.

36. Braem M, Lambrechts P, Van Doren V, Vanherle G. In vivo evaluation of four posterior composites: Quantitative wear measurements and clinical behavior. Dent Mater 1986;2:106–113.

37. Lambrechts P, Braem M, Vanherle G. Evaluation of clinical performance for posterior composite resins and dentin adhesives. Oper Dent 1987;12:53–78.

38. Lambrechts P, Braem M, Vuylsteke Wauters M, Vanherle G. Quantitative in vivo wear of human enamel. J Dent Res 1989;68:1752–1754.

39. Wendt SL Jr, Ziemiecki TL, Leinfelder KF. Proximal wear rates by tooth position of resin composite restorations. J Dent 1996;24:33–39.

40. Ziemiecki TL, Wendt SL, Leinfelder KF. Methodology for proximal wear evaluation in posterior resin composites. Am J Dent 1992;5:203–207.

41. Söderholm KJ. Leaking of fillers in dental composites. J Dent Res 1993;62:126–130.

42. Söderholm KJ. Filler systems and resin interface. In: Vanherle G, Smith DC (eds). Posterior Composite Resin Dental Restorative Materials. Utrecht: Peter Szulc, 1984; 139–159.

43. Charles RJ. Static fatigue of glass, Part I. J Appl Phys 1958;29:1549–1553.

44. Söderholm KJ. Filler leachability during water storage of six composite materials. Scand J Dent Res 1990; 98:82–88.

45. Söderholm KJ, Mukherjee R, Longmate J. Filler leachability of composites stored in distilled water or artificial saliva. J Dent Res 1996;75:1692–1699.

46. Söderholm KJ, Yang MCK, Garcea I. Filler particle leachability of experimental dental composites. Eur J Oral Sci 2000;108:555–560.

47. Yaffe A, Zalkind M. The effect of topical application of fluoride on composite resin restorations. J Prosthet Dent 1981;45: 59–62.

48. Papagiannoulis L, Tzoutzas J, Eliades G. Effect of topical fluoride agents on the morphologic characteristics and composition of resin composite restorative materials. J Prosthet Dent 1997;77:405–413.

49. Kula K, McKinney JE, Kula TJ. Effects of daily topical fluoride gels on resin composite degradation and wear. Dent Mater 1997;13:305–311.

50. Plueddemann EP. Silane Coupling Agents. New York: Plenum, 1982.

51. Söderholm KJ, Shang SW. Molecular orientation of silane at the surface of colloidal silica. J Dent Res 1993; 72:1050–1054.

52. Davidson CL, Duysters PPE, De Lange C, Bausch JR. Structural changes in composite surface material after dry polishing. J Oral Rehabil 1981;8:431–439.

53. Øysaed H, Ruyter IE, Sjøvik Kleven IJ. Release of formaldehyde from dental composites. J Dent Res 1988;67:1289–1294.

Section IV

ORTHODONTICS

8

DISINTEGRATION OF ORTHODONTIC APPLIANCES

Arne Hensten-Pettersen, DDS, MS, Dr Odont, Odont Dr HC (Lund)

Nils Jacobsen, DDS, MS, Dr Odont

Although low, the prevalence of materials-related side effects is probably higher in orthodontics than in other areas of dental treatment.[1] Specific attention has been paid to the role of nickel derived from orthodontic appliances in the manifestation of hypersensitive reactions and in the development of tolerance.[2] The prevalence of adverse reactions may be regarded as the result of the physical and chemical conditions characteristic of orthodontic appliances. Unlike dental restorations, orthodontic devices are never an integrated part of the natural dentition, having a relatively large material surface in close contact with mobile mucosal tissues and open to attack in the aggressive oral environment. In addition, the extraoral parts of orthodontic appliances are in contact with skin, adding another biologic factor.

Orthodontic appliances are intended to function for a limited period of time. The chemical composition of orthodontic materials, such as base metal alloys or chemically cured (cold-cured) resins, may facilitate the release of metal ions, unreacted monomers, and degradation products, in contrast to their restorative counterparts. Otherwise, orthodontic materials comprise many of the biomaterial categories of restorative dentistry.

The durability of any biomaterial is dependent on its chemical stability. The material should resist dissolution, erosion, and corrosion at an accept-able level and not release unreacted components. Orthodontic appliances are exposed in vivo to a variety of microbial products, temperature differences, pH variations caused by intrinsic or extrinsic factors, abrasion forces from chewing and brushing, friction between wires and slots, material strain connected with force activation, and electrochemical/electrolytic processes facilitated by saliva. In addition, airborne agents such as sulfur dioxide may add to the corrosive environment. The result of (or more accurately, the process of) exposure of materials to natural conditions such as the oral environment for a prolonged period of time is called *aging*. Aging may be mimicked and accelerated by simulated environmental factors (artificial aging).

This chapter summarizes the main characteristics of in vivo aging of orthodontic biomaterials as judged by retrieval studies and release of components after in vivo use or artificial aging, presents an overview of chemical substances released from orthodontic materials into the oral cavity, and discusses their biologic significance.

Aging of Metallic Appliances

Archwires, brackets, molar bands, facebows, and other orthodontic appliances are available in a variety of shapes and chemical compositions. The

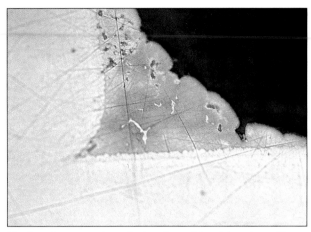

Fig 8-1 Cross section of a bracket with soldered steel base and slot parts. The silver solder is inhomogeneous and may be susceptible to corrosion processes.

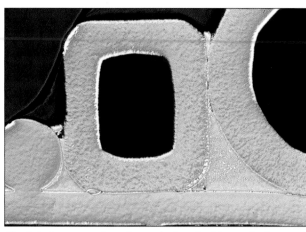

Fig 8-2 Cross section of a molar band with steel tubes and pin joined by silver-based solder. The combination of different alloys and complex geometry facilitates corrosion processes.

most common alloys are austenitic stainless steel (18% chromium, 8% nickel), Co-Cr, Ni-Ti (54% nickel, 46% titanium), and beta-titanium (11% molybdenum, 6% zirconium, 2% to 4% zinc). Brackets and molar bands are often made of stainless steel. Metallic parts of removable appliances are manufactured from stainless steel or Co-Cr alloys. Different components of fixed appliances may be soldered or brazed together. Most solders are composed of silver, copper, and zinc. Some solders are based on gold.[3]

Attachment System

The attachment system contains many corrosion-facilitating factors. Metallic brackets are complex devices, including slots and wings for archwire attachment and a bracket base adapted for bonding to enamel. The bracket base may be an integral part of the bracket system and may be machined or cast with various degrees of roughness. Otherwise, the bracket system may be a layered complex of alloys differing in composition and welded or soldered together (Fig 8-1). Foil mesh welded to the bonding pad or base is common. Stainless steel of varying quality is the alloy of choice, although one-piece pure-titanium brackets are available. Miniaturization of brackets has required the addition of increased amounts of

heavy metals such as chromium and nickel for strengthening, reducing the corrosion resistance.[4] Stainless steel molar bands may have soldered fixtures for archwire attachment (Fig 8-2).

Retrieval Studies

Examination of removed appliances has often focused on issues associated with repeated use of brackets or archwires in which aging is one of several factors. Although corrosion may not be visible during use (Fig 8-3), clinical observations and visual inspection of removed appliances have shown the presence of surface tarnishing and fretting corrosion located at areas of archwires that slide through bracket slots, presumably representing a continuous disruption of the passivating oxide film. Bracket/base detachment and surface reactions observed in contact areas bordering bonding adhesives and elastomerics have been interpreted as the result of bimetallic galvanic corrosion and crevice corrosion.[5] Scanning electron microscopic (SEM) observations of bands, brackets, and metallic parts of removable appliances composed of stainless steel, Co-Cr, and Ni-Cr alloys showed crevice, stress, and pitting corrosion after 3 to 50 months of use, whereas stainless steel archwires showed no corrosive surface reactions.[6]

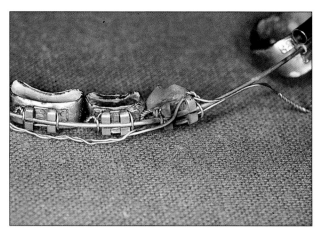

Fig 8-3 Corrosion processes may not be visible during the use of appliances. This complex appliance was bright and shiny after 2 years intraorally but showed localized corrosion when stored in saline solution for 4 weeks.

Corrosion of type 304 stainless steel bracket bases and mesh structures was observed by SEM in cases where black stains were visually seen on debonded tooth surfaces. It was argued that the black stain was caused by oxides of nickel and chromium after exposure to corrosive salivary factors penetrating a porous bonding material.[7] X-ray energy-dispersive spectroscopic analysis of the bonding material adjacent to the sites of base and mesh corrosion demonstrated the presence of chromium, nickel, iron, and chlorine. Indications of the presence of microorganisms also were reported.[8]

Experimental Studies

Experimental setups simulating bracket bonding in artificial saliva indicated base and mesh corrosion in eight out of nine stainless steel bracket brands as judged by stereomicroscopy. The exception was an American Iron and Steel Intitute (AISI) type 316L brand with a nickel content higher than the usual AISI 304 types. Certain commercial recycling procedures increased the liability that brackets would undergo corrosion, including the 316L type.[9]

The integrity or deterioration of archwires has also attracted considerable attention on the basis of their role as an active force-delivery agent in orthodontics. Potentiodynamic polarization experiments and SEM observations of archwires composed of stainless steel, Co-Cr, Ni-Cr, Ni-Ti, and beta-titanium exposed to electrochemical corrosion in artificial saliva showed surface corrosion of all iron- and nickel-containing wires, whereas beta-titanium wires demonstrated excellent corrosion resistance. Variations between samples of nominally identical composition were attributed to different surface roughness.[10]

Corrosion of Ni-Ti archwires has been of particular interest because of their large nickel content. Early electrochemical studies indicated that pitting corrosion of Ni-Ti archwires took place in a 1% saline solution.[11] However, later investigations indicated that surface irregularities observed in Ni-Ti archwires may be the result of manufacturing, not of clinical use,[12] although clinical use may lead to surface discoloration by contaminants such as KCl. It has been argued that the surface irregularities are favorite sites for selective dissolution of nickel.[13] Recent studies employing potentiostatic anodic dissolution in 0.9% NaCl, accompanied by complementary SEM observations, showed that stainless steel and Ni-Ti archwires were susceptible to pitting and localized corrosion, whereas the corrosion potential of beta-titanium wires was very low. Epoxy coating of Ni-Ti wires reduced the corrosion, but the use of a nitride coating had minimal effect. The corrosion potential differed for wires from several vendors.[14] Polishing reduced the corrosion rate of Ni-Ti and other archwire types significantly.[15]

In vitro investigations indicate that no metallic orthodontic alloy, however metallurgically advanced, completely avoids surface reactions in some form and to some degree. Retrieval observations reveal the tracks of similar corrosive activities in vivo. However, the potential importance of these phenomena for clinical performance of orthodontic appliances will not be considered in the present context, where attention will be focused on the released substances.

Simulated In Vivo Ion Release

Full-mouth orthodontic appliances exposed to 0.05% saline solution exhibited release of about 40 μg nickel and 36 μg chromium per day.[16] A similar release of these ions occurred from standard fixed appliances for the maxillary arch immersed in artificial saliva at 37°C. More nickel than chromium was released, reaching a maximum after 1 (nickel) and 2 weeks (chromium), then decreasing. There was no significant difference in release of nickel and chromium between appliances containing Ni-Ti or stainless steel archwires.[17] This observation may be explained by the results from release studies using separate parts of orthodontic appliances, such as molar bands, brackets, facebows, and archwires, in 0.9% saline solution. The release of nickel and chromium from stainless steel archwires was negligible, and the release of nickel ions from Ni-Ti archwires was zero, although these archwires contain 54% nickel by weight. The largest ion release was found from soldered stainless steel appliances, such as facebows and molar bands, implicating the bimetallic contact as an important corrosive factor.[3] A recent experiment exposing a fixed appliance, which contained 2 molar bands (types 304 and 316 stainless steel), 10 type 316 stainless steel brackets, 1 Ni-Ti archwire, and 1 Ag-Cu-Pd–brazing alloy, to inorganic or organic acids confirmed the nickel and chromium release by atomic absorption spectrophotometry. In addition, copper ions and some silver and palladium ions were released from the brazing alloy. Low pH favored the release. The daily release of nickel, copper, and chromium from the orthodontic appliance decreased after the first day and was considered "well below that ingested with a normal daily diet."[18]

Intraoral Ion Release

In vivo investigations indicated an increased salivary concentration of nickel and iron immediately after the insertion of a fixed orthodontic appliance containing an average of 13 stainless steel bands or brackets and 1 nickel-based archwire per person. However, large individual variations were seen, and no increased salivary nickel concentra-

tion could be demonstrated after 3 weeks.[19] Similar investigations to determine the amounts of nickel and chromium in saliva did not reveal increased concentrations of these ions in a 1-day to 1-month period after insertion of fixed appliances, when compared with data before insertion.[20] Other investigations confirm that the nickel released from orthodontic appliances may not be measurable in saliva after 1 week and is insufficient to affect the level of nickel in the blood.[21]

General Remarks on Metallic Appliances

Clinical and microscopic observations of surface phenomena indicate that intraoral aging of the attachment system takes place. However, similar aging phenomena at the free surfaces of archwires or the inner surfaces of facebows are not obvious. Titanium-containing archwire alloys can be considered relatively inert. However, slot and tube contact areas of brackets and bands may contribute to reciprocal corrosive effects on wires and attachments. Aging phenomena of this kind are associated with the complex mosaic of shapes and parts of fixed orthodontic appliances, facilitating corrosion by a reduced redox potential and increased plaque accumulation at grooves, crevices, and border areas. The contact between base metal alloys with different galvanic potentials, such as solders or brazing materials on brackets and bands, as well as the wire-slot contact, is a factor that enhances corrosion processes.

Obviously, the large variation in orthodontic alloys prevents general statements regarding corrosion susceptibility for groups of alloys. While stainless steels are susceptible to corrosion, aging phenomena vary significantly among these alloys. The fact remains that release of one particular metal ion is not dependent on the relative content of that particular metal in the orthodontic alloy. Bimetallic contact or the metallurgic characteristics of other metals of the alloy may be more decisive.[22]

In summary, the studies referred to above demonstrate that chemical factors in the oral environment have a corrosive effect on metallic orthodontic appliances, releasing ions such as nickel, chromium, iron, manganese, copper, silver, and palladium when the brazing alloys are included. Studies on removable partial dentures containing Co-Cr alloys indicate that cobalt ions may also be released from Co-Cr-containing metallic parts of orthodontic appliances.[23,24] In addition, disruption of passivating oxide films may contribute to the release of additional metal ions such as titanium, molybdenum, zirconium, and zinc.[25] A common feature is that the oxidation level and the concentration of released metals are largely unknown.[26]

Aging of Resin-Based Orthodontic Appliances

Organic Leachants

The repertoire of resin-based materials used in orthodontics comprises removable appliances, brackets, and bonding systems involving resin composites, polyacid-modified composites (compomers), and resin-modified glass ionomers. With the exception of chemically cured removable appliances, there is no significant difference between resin-based polymers for prosthodontic or restorative use and the corresponding orthodontic products. Hence, the intraoral deterioration mechanisms are similar.

Metal ions in saliva may derive from nonbiomaterial sources,[27] whereas the probability of other sources for organic components associated with resin-based polymers is low. The identification of certain organic components in saliva by analytical methods, such as chromatographic/mass spectrometry and high-performance liquid chromatography, is therefore interpreted as indicative of released biomaterial components. The aim of this section is to present an overview of organic components that may appear after aging of resin-based orthodontic biomaterials. Similar to metallic alloys, information on leaching from polymer materials is obtained from in vitro experiments using different organic solvents, from in vivo measurements, or from in vivo–simulating conditions.[28]

In principle, resin-based orthodontic materials are polymerization products from a series of methacrylate monomers and comonomers that open up the vinyl double linkage for polymerization with the aid of chemical activators or external energy (light or heat). Polymethyl methacrylate (PMMA) is used here to illustrate general principles for curing and deterioration. The production of PMMA-based removable appliances involves the use of prepolymerized PMMA beads, a methyl methacrylate (MMA) monomer system, cross-linking agents, initiators (eg, benzoyl peroxide), plasticizers (eg, dibutyl phthalate), stabilizers (eg, phenyl salicylate or 2-hydroxy 4-methoxy benzophenone), and inhibitors (eg, hydroquinone). In chemical-curing systems, a redox initiator-accelerator system (eg, benzoyl peroxide/tertiary aromatic amine) or a barbiturate-based system with copper ions is used. The degree of monomer conversion is lower for chemically cured PMMA than its heat-cured counterpart, although both materials contain residual unreacted monomer. Chemically cured PMMA is often employed for the production of removable appliances in orthodontics.

Aging of resin-based polymers occurs by oxidation and hydrolization processes in unreacted monomers, comonomers, and additives.[29] The resulting single components could be a mixture of residual monomers, small molecular additives, and degradation products, with varying degrees of solubility in aqueous media such as saliva. However, food and beverages acting as organic solvents may facilitate the release of large, lipophilic molecules as well.

PMMA-Based Removable Appliances

Elution experiments in saline solutions, artificial saliva, and organic solvents have confirmed that leaching does take place from PMMA-based materials, depending on the medium. Organic solvents facilitate the leaching of the lipophilic substances in vitro, giving an exaggerated impression of the behavior of potential leachants. Chemically curing resins release more MMA monomer, methacrylic acid, benzoic acid, and formaldehyde than their heat-curing counterparts.[30,31] The release of residual monomers in aqueous solvents takes place at a faster rate during the first 24 hours.[32] Such resins have also shown the release of aromatic additives and degradation products, such as phenyl benzoate (PB), phenyl salicylate (PS), biphenyl (BP), and 2-methoxy 4-hydroxy benzophenone in ethanol, whereas only the amounts of PB and PS could be quantitatively measured in Ringer's solution.[33]

Saliva from orthodontic patients using chemically cured PMMA-based removable appliances showed the presence of PB and PS. These substances were interpreted as derived from the benzoyl peroxide initiator. Other organic additives such as dibutyl phtalate and dicyclohexyl phthalate softeners have been found in saliva from patients with new PMMA dentures.[34]

Orthodontic Bonding Adhesives

Specific data on chemical components released into the oral cavity by the aging of orthodontic bonding materials are not available. Bond failure statistics provide an indirect parameter to describe bonding adhesives, reflecting deterioration processes to some extent. However, the role of adhesive aging regarding the ability to resist tensile, shear, torque, and peel functional stresses is difficult to distinguish from other factors such as the influence of the operator, etching techniques, moisture control, patient age, and other patient variables.[35] In addition, the aging processes vary for different bonding systems, such as the chemically cured two-paste systems, "no-mix" adhesives, light-activated direct-bonding systems, precoated brackets, resin-modified glass ionomers, and compomers. This variability prevents any statements beyond referring to aging processes of these materials in general. However, when information associated with the corresponding restorative materials is considered, orthodontic adhesives release a series of methacrylates and dimethacrylates, initiators, accelerators, and inhibitors resembling those mentioned previously, and decomposition products such as methacrylic acid, benzoic acid–methyl ester, ethylene glycol, and formaldehyde.[28]

Apart from organic compounds, resin-composite materials may release silicon and boron from hydrolyzed fillers, along with remnants of coupling agents. Degradation of glass-ionomer-containing bonding cements is a complex process involving the release of glass particles, along with fluoride and aluminum ions accompanied by traces of other ions such as boron, barium, strontium, silicon, sodium, and potassium.[36]

One potentially important aspect of the adhesive issue should be noted: the possibility of enzymatic breakdown of resin-based bonding materials as part of the aging phenomena. Nonspecific esterases and hydrolases are present in saliva at different concentrations as the result of cell and microbial activity. Experimentally, enzymatic degradation of bisphenol glycidyl methacrylate (bis-GMA) and triethylene glycol dimethacrylate (TEGDMA) polymers and resin-modified glass-ionomer cements has been demonstrated.[28,37,38] If enzymatic activities are genuine components of the aging processes for resin-based materials in general, they are also highly relevant for orthodontic adhesives.

Some interesting observations about this effect on direct-bonding materials have been obtained from studies on used bracket samples with retained adhesives on their bases.[39] On average, one in five collections of brackets from orthodontic practitioners contained some brackets with channels or pockets, interpreted to be microbial decay of the adhesive, and yellow-green discoloration. The deterioration phenomena were noticed for adhesives on both ceramic and metallic brackets. It was suggested that the organic ingredients of bonding resin composites were consumed by opportunistic aerobic and anaerobic microorganisms introduced during orthodontic treatment, for brackets from some clinics showed this characteristic while others did not. Whatever the explanation for these observations, the possibility remains that microbial enzymatic activity may contribute to an enhanced deterioration of resin-based adhesives, combined with other factors such as inferior polymerization techniques.

Table 8-1 Some potential leachants from orthodontic appliances

INORGANIC IONS*	ORGANIC COMPOUNDS
From base-metal alloys and solders:	From cold-curing acrylic resins:
22 Titanium	Compounds such as:
24 Chromium	MMA (residual monomer)
25 Manganese	MA (degradation product)
26 Iron	EGDMA (cross-linking agent)
27 Cobalt	Other monomers
28 Nickel	Phenyl benzoate (from initiator)
29 Copper	Phenyl salicylate (from initiator)
46 Palladium	Phthalate softeners
47 Silver	Formaldehyde (from MMA)
From glass ionomers, inorganic part of composite adhesives, and ceramics:	From bonding adhesives, mono-, and dimethacrylate monomers:
5 Boron	Residual monomers:
9 Fluorine	Bis-GMA
11 Sodium	UDMA
12 Magnesium	TEGDMA
13 Aluminum	EGDMA
14 Silicon	HEMA
19 Potassium	MMA
30 Zinc	Initiators/photoinitiators
38 Strontium	Accelerators
40 Zirconium	
50 Tin	Reaction and decomposition products of the above, such as:
55 Cesium	
56 Barium	Bisphenol A
58 Cerium	Ethylene glycol
	Other

*Numbers given are atomic numbers.

Degradation Products from Ceramic Brackets

Ceramics are more resistant than most other dental materials to the chemical environmental factors of the oral cavity and are degraded only because of mechanical forces or chemical attack by strong acids. Apart from occasional observations of black stains, in vivo aging of ceramic brackets is limited to mechanical failures, such as wing fracture, associated with the brittle characteristics of the ceramic material.[40] Under unusual circumstances, traces of principal elements such as aluminum, magnesium, tin, zinc, zirconium, cesium, and cerium could be released.[41]

Summary of Released Substances

Based upon this background information, it is concluded that the released substances from orthodontic appliances are a mixture of unreacted material components and deterioration products of largely unknown concentration (Table 8-1). Elution experiments have shown that a large part of the

Table 8-2 Potential biologic interactions

TOXICITY (DOSE DEPENDENT)	ALLERGY (DOSE INDEPENDENT)
General toxicity, target organs	Type I, immediate reactions
Local toxicity, entrance tissue	Type IV, delayed reactions (contact dermatitis)
	Tolerance development?

release takes place within 24 hours, and a smaller part continues over time as the result of true material aging. The released substances comprise a long list of metallic ions, often with unknown oxidation states, together with their oxidation products. Glass ionomers and/or other ceramic/polymer combination products contribute remnants from the inorganic fillers and coupling agents. Resin-based removable appliances and bonding adhesives release monomers and oxidation products, chemical species associated with polymerization, and other additives.

The wide array of released substances has few common characteristics, usually a mixture of inorganic ions and compounds together with organic compounds. Some products are surface precipitates in the form of discoloration, and some are soluble compounds released into the neighboring mucosa or salivary flow. The released molecules have very different characteristics of dissolution behavior. Most are of small molecular weight, and their concentration is difficult to assess because many components cannot be distinguished from similar components derived from nutrients, cooking utensils, or the respiratory environment. Their biologic significance therefore is not easily assessed.

Biologic Aspects

Uptake of Xenobiotics

Any biologic effect of a foreign substance is dependent on its passage through a cellular membrane to reach the intracellular environment. The foreign substance may interfere with the functions of central biochemical molecules in a number of ways within this environment, resulting in an increased risk of toxic reactions or activation of the immune system, eliciting hypersensitive reactions (Table 8-2).

In principle, substances introduced into the oral cavity can be absorbed by the gastrointestinal tract after swallowing, by inhalation (if volatile), and by the oral mucosa. In addition, dermal uptake is of importance for substances from extraoral appliances. All uptake routes imply passive diffusion guided by general biophysical principles, ie, depending on molecular size, lipophilicity/hydrophilicity, polarity, and concentration. Passage through the oral mucosa or skin adjacent to the orthodontic appliance is of primary interest because the concentration gradient is higher at these sites and because (subclinical) mechanical injury may facilitate the passage of foreign substances. The oral mucosa and the skin are similar structures with similar functions. However, the protective principles are different: a nonkeratinized epithelial layer covered by a mucinous lining for the former and a multilayered, keratinized epithelial skin surface for the latter. Unoccluded, intact skin is therefore considered to represent a larger obstacle for diffusion than the mucosal counterpart, although the constant renewal of the mucinous layer of the oral mucosa represents an important mode of clearance for foreign substances released into the oral cavity. When all of the relevant factors are considered, it is thought that foreign molecules are more readily absorbed by the oral mucosa than by the skin.[42] However, skin is believed to contain a larger concentration of the antigen-presenting Langerhans cells, which may be important for immunologic sensitization.

Toxicity

A majority of the released metal ions are well-known toxicants. Cytotoxic data indicate similar properties for the polymer-associated ingredients.[28] However, although cytotoxic data are excellent for study of toxic mechanisms at the cellular level, such data may well be irrelevant for the clinical situation. All toxicodynamic reasoning is based on the dose concept, ie, the amount of a substance to which an organism is exposed is expressed as the quotient of the weight of the substance and the body weight of the organism, which allows comparison of the toxic potential of different substances. Toxic effects on vital target organs are possible only if the concentration of a toxicant exceeds a threshold level that cannot be taken care of by the toxicokinetic repair and elimination mechanisms. Given the minute concentrations of toxicants associated with orthodontic biomaterials, a general toxic reaction would be inconceivable.

Local toxic effects at entrance locations are more plausible, although these have not been demonstrated in the orthodontic clinic. Over the years, animal studies have shown inflammatory reactions to experimental resin-based implants, and gingival biopsies adjacent to cast dental restorations have shown an increased concentration of relevant metals.[43,44] Subdermal implantation of Fe-Cr-Ni and Co-Cr-Ni wires showed no tissue reactions different from the reference material, except for tissue surrounding soldered areas.[45] Other parallel information is scarce for orthodontic materials, but gingival inflammatory reactions are occasionally observed with attachment systems. The role of released substances for these reactions is unclear. Observations of this kind could be explained by an increased accumulation of bacterial plaque, enhanced by increased free surface energy of the adjacent metal bands or brackets. However, experimental evidence does not support this theory conclusively.[46] Another explanation could be associated with increased plaque retention following impaired hygienic procedures caused by intricate fixed appliances, implicating appliance construction rather than material aging.

Allergy

Allergy is an acquired condition resulting in an immunologic overreaction following contact with a foreign substance, provided the individual has the necessary genetic disposition and previous contact (sensitization) with the substance. Although the modern approach tends to downplay the differences between various modes of allergic reaction, it may be useful to employ the traditional concepts of immediate reaction (Type I) and delayed reaction (Type IV) for the present discussion.[47]

In the immediate reaction, the absorbed antigen combines with immunoglobulin E (IgE) antibodies located in mast cells or basophilic leukocytes, leading to cell disintegration and release of mediators, which causes increased capillary permeability and contraction of smooth muscles and ultimately urticaria, asthmatic seizures, or decreased blood pressure, depending on the organ involved. The immediate reaction is associated with complete antigens, although there is increasing evidence that haptens also may cause IgE-mediated Type I allergic reactions.[48] A Type I reaction related to residual latex proteins on naural latex gloves is a risk for dental practice in general.[49] The latex problem also includes delayed reactions associated with other latex-related chemicals. The latex issue is common to all clinical health professions and is not further discussed here. However, the orthodontist treating young individuals who have had previous contact with latex through repeated surgical interventions should keep in mind the possibility of allergic reactions to natural latex gloves and elastomerics.

In the delayed Type IV reaction, incomplete antigens (haptens) derived from biomaterials are absorbed by the oral mucosa or skin and are attached to surface molecules at the Langerhans cells to form complete allergens. After transport to the regional lymph nodes, a series of immuno-

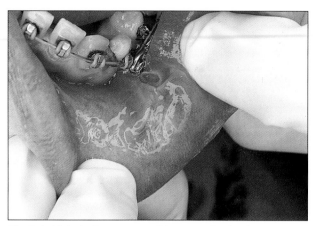

Fig 8-4 Nickel allergy caused by an orthodontic appliance on the lower left lip. (Courtesy of S Kumar, Kongsvinger, Norway.)

logic reactions take place, resulting in the production of activated, "custom-made" T cells, provided that a previous contact with the particular allergen has taken place. The allergen–T cell encounter results in the release of inflammatory mediators and the formation of diffuse, intraoral red zones, blisters, and ulcerations, accompanied by pain and a burning sensation that is sometimes extended to the perioral area (Fig 8-4). Reactions of this kind are referred to as *allergic contact mucositis* or *dermatitis*. Clinically, reactions of this kind may be difficult to distinguish from irritant reactions. Because the activated T cells may be present in areas distant from the exposure site and because the allergen is circulated by the Langerhans cells, eczematic and urticarial reactions may occur on the face or elsewhere, resulting in what is termed *systemic contact dermatitis*.[50]

Testing and Sensitization

Identification of substances causing adverse reactions of this kind is attempted by interpretation of epicutaneous reactions after placing samples of suspected allergens on the skin, usually for 48 hours. Commercial epicutaneous test kits for use by allergists or dermatologists are available for a number of problem areas. Similar intraoral tests have proven less reliable, requiring larger concentrations of allergens. Intraoral sensitization is also more difficult to obtain. One reason may be the number of Langerhans cells in the mucosa is smaller than in the skin.[51] For such reasons, sensitization by extraoral appliances may be more likely than by their intraoral counterparts. However, an orthodontic patient may have been sensitized after contact with a relevant allergen in other ways, leading to an allergic contact reaction to orthodontic appliances.

Thus, although released substances from orthodontic appliances are not toxic in the usual sense, the orthodontist may be challenged with fundamental biologic phenomena related to immunologic reactions that are not fully understood. The following section is an attempt to discuss these factors in relation to potential allergens released from orthodontic biomaterials. Specific emphasis will be placed on the role of nickel.

Potential Sensitizers and Observed Reactions

All organic leachants listed in Table 8-1 are characterized as potential sensitizers, as are a majority of the metals, depending on their oxidation state or compound. The metal ions from base metal alloys (upper left column in Table 8-1) are assumed to be of the most importance. Of these, nickel, chromium, and cobalt have been associated with hypersensitive reactions in orthodontics. Confirmed nickel allergy in a 14-year-old boy led to severe gingival swelling and to painful erythematous macular lesions of the oral and labial mucosa following the insertion of Ni-Ti archwires.[52] Similar reactions were seen in a 14-year-old-girl judged by circumstantial evidence to be allergic to nickel.[53] In both cases, the archwires had to be removed. Nickel, cobalt, and chromium have been implicated in other case reports.[50,54] Reactions to bonding materials have included gingival and labial reactions and facial rashes.[55]

A survey of Norwegian orthodontists showed that dermal reactions such as redness, itching, eczema, fissuring, and desquamation most often could be attributed to metal parts of extraoral appliances. Such reactions were more frequent than intraoral reactions. The incidence of intra-oral reactions was approximately equal for metallic appliances and resin-based removable appliances or bonding material.[56] The general incidence of patient reactions was estimated to be about 1:100, including bearable nuisances. Parallel information on adverse reactions among orthodontic personnel was not metal related but was associated with the handling of resin-based materials for removable appliances and bonding techniques. The incidence was about 12% among orthodontists.[56] In both cases, the proportion of true allergic reactions was unknown. An updated estimate would probably be lower for patients and personnel today, considering the availability of coatings for extraoral metal parts and other material improvements, as well as the increased use of "no-touch" techniques in the handling of bonding materials.

Sensitization and Tolerance

The relationship between sensitization by a potential allergen at an early age and the reaction obtained after a new contact is not always straightforward and predictable. Many observations indicate that early contact with potential allergens may actually lead to a diminished probability for allergic reactions at a later date, ie, an increased tolerance level. This phenomenon has been proposed by immunologists in discussing the overuse of hygienic measures that prevent children from having "natural" contact with potential pathogenic allergens. In orthodontics, the tolerance concept has been introduced to explain observations associated with nickel reactions, where sensitization through nickel-containing costume jewelry and other articles for everyday use is well known, particularly among the young female population. The piercing fad has aggravated this tendency and also shown that the sensitization is not a biologically gender-dependent phenomenon.[57] However, large-scale clinical studies have indicated that oral exposure to nickel-containing orthodontic appliances at an early age actually induces a partial tolerance for nickel-containing piercing items that would otherwise have sensitization capacity.[2,58]

Sensitization Through Orthodontic Appliances

The tolerance concept does not prevent the possibility of allergic reactions following orthodontic treatment after a previous sensitizing contact with antigens such as nickel has taken place. Some information also indicates that conversion to a nickel-positive reaction may be elicited by orthodontically derived nickel,[59] particularly from nickel-containing extraoral appliances. However, a recent review on this subject concludes that the risk is extremely low for patients who are not nickel hypersensitive at the start of the orthodontic treatment.[60]

Conclusions

In summary, aging and release phenomena occurring in orthodontic appliances result in the oral tissues being exposed to a large number of different components derived from metallic and resin-based materials. The presence of certain metal ions and organic components has been demonstrated in saliva, whereas the presence of other ingredients is based on in vitro experimental evidence and reasoning associated with microscopic observations of aged materials. The released ingredients have few common characteristics and their concentration is low, but many are biologically active substances in toxicity and allergenic potential.

It is assumed that a portion of these substances diffuse through the oral mucosa and are distributed in the blood and lymph circulation. However, the concentrations are too low to have any toxic effect on target organs, and local tissue reactions are difficult to distinguish from reactions associated with differences in free surface energy and microbiologic plaque formation. The risk evaluation therefore is concentrated on the possibility of sensitizing individuals through orthodontic appliances, or more probably, of eliciting allergic reactions in previously sensitized individuals. Most information on this subject has focused on metal ions such as chromium, cobalt, and nickel, whereas patient reactions to resin-based bonding ingredients and removable appliances are more scattered. With this reservation, a fair conclusion would be that, despite aging phenomena related to base metal alloys and resin-based materials in orthodontics, the safety of orthodontic biomaterials is high, and the risk of a materials-related hazard causing harm is correspondingly low.

References

1. Jacobsen N, Hensten-Pettersen A. Adverse reactions to biomaterials in dental specialty practice. Trans Soc Biomater 1990;12:263.

2. Kerosuo H, Kullaa A, Kerosuo E, Kanerva L, Hensten-Pettersen A. Nickel allergy in adolescents in relation to orthodontic treatment and piercing of ears. Am J Orthod Dentofacial Orthop 1996;109:148–154.

3. Grímsdóttir MR, Gjerdet NR, Hensten-Pettersen A. Composition and in vitro corrosion of orthodontic appliances. Am J Orthod Dentofacial Orthop 1992;101:525–532.

4. Hamula DW, Hamula W, Sernetz F. Pure titanium orthodontic brackets. J Clin Orthod 1996;30:140–144.

5. Matasa CG. Attachment corrosion and its testing. J Clin Orthod 1995;29:16–23.

6. Kratzenstein B, Weber H, Geis-Gerstorfer J, Koppenburg P. In vivo corrosion investigations of orthodontic appliances [in German]. Dtsch Zahnärztl Z 1985;40:1146–1150.

7. Maijer R, Smith DC. Corrosion of orthodontic brackets. Am J Orthod 1982;81;43–48.

8. Gwinnett AJ. Corrosion of resin-bonded orthodontic brackets. Am J Orthod 1982;82:441–446.

9. Maijer R, Smith DC. Biodegradation of the orthodontic bracket system. Am J Orthod Dentofacial Orthop 1986;90:195–198.

10. Kappert HF, Jonas I, Liebermann M, Rakosi TH. Corrosion circumstances of different orthodontic wires [in German]. Fortschr Kieferorthop 1988;49:358–367.

11. Sarkar, NK, Redmond W, Schwaninger B, Goldberg AJ. The chloride corrosion behaviour of four orthodontic wires. J Oral Rehabil 1983;10:121–128.

12. Grimsdottir MR, Hensten-Pettersen A. Surface analysis of nickel-titanium archwire used in vivo. Dent Mater 1997;13:163–167.

13. Oshida Y, Sachdeva RC, Miyazaki S. Microanalytical characterization and surface modification of TiNi orthodontic archwires. Biomed Mater Eng 1992;2:51–69.

14. Kim H, Johnson JW. Corrosion of stainless steel, nickel-titanium, coated nickel-titanium, and titanium orthodontic wires. Angle Orthod 1999;69:39–44.

15. Hunt NP, Cunningham SJ, Golden CG, Sheriff M. An investigation into the effect of polishing on surface hardness and corrosion of orthodontic archwires. Angle Orthod 1999;69:433–440.

16. Park HY, Shearer TR. In vitro release of nickel and chromium from simulated orthodontic appliances. Am J Orthod 1983:84:156–169.

17. Barrett RD, Bishara SE, Quinn JK. Biodegradation of orthodontic appliances. Part I: biodegradation of nickel and chromium in vitro. Am J Orthod Dentofacial Orthop 1993;103:8–14.

18. Staffolani N, Damiani F, Lilli C, et al. Ion release from orthodontic appliances. J Dent 1999;27:449–454.

19. Gjerdet NR, Erichsen ES, Remlo HE, Evjen G. Nickel and iron in saliva of patients with fixed orthodontic appliances. Acta Odontol Scand 1991;49:73–78.

20. Kerosuo H, Moe G, Hensten-Pettersen A. Salivary nickel and chromium in subjects with different types of fixed orthodontic appliances. Am J Orthod Dentofacial Orthop 1997;111:595–598.

21. Bishara SE, Barrett RD, Selim MI. Biodegradation of orthodontic appliances. Part II: Changes in the blood level of nickel. Am J Orthod Dentofacial Orthop 1993;103:115–119

22. Metallic medical and dental materials. In: IARC Monographs on the Evaluation of Carcinogenic Risks to Humans, vol. 74. Geneva and Lyon: World Health Organization and the International Agency for Research on Cancer, 1999.

23. Stenberg T. Release of cobalt from cobalt-chromium constructions in the oral cavity of man. Scand J Dent Res 1982;90:472–479.

24. de Melo JF, Gjerdet NR, Erichsen ES. Metal release from cobalt-chromium partial dentures in the mouth. Acta Odont Scand 1983;41:71–74.

25. Schmalz G. Biological interactions of dental cast alloys with oral tissues. Trans Acad Dent Mater 1999;13:97–114.

26. Øysæd H, Ruyter IE. Water sorption and filler characteristics of composites for use in porsterior teeth. J Dent Res 1986;65:1315–1318.

27. Wirz J, Dilenna P. Metals in saliva [in German]. Quintessenz 1992;43:869–874.

28. Geurtsen W. Biological interactions of non-metallic restorative materials with oral tissues. Trans Acad Dent Mater 1999;13:75–93.

29. Ruyter IE, Øysæd H. Analysis and characterization of dental polymers. CRC Crit Rev Biocompatibility 1988;4:247–279.

30. Koda T, Tsuchiya H, Yamauchi M, Ohtani S, Takagi N, Kawano J. Leachability of denture-base acrylic resins in artificial saliva. Dent Mater 1990;6:13–16.

31. Tsuchiya H, Hoshimo Y, Tajima K, Takagi N. Leaching and cytotoxicity of formaldehyde and methyl methacrylate from acrylic resin denture base materials. J Prosthet Dent 1994;71:618–624.

32. Vallittu PK, Miettinen, V, Alakuijala P. Residual monomer content and its release into water from denture base materials. Dent Mater 1995;11:338–342.

33. Lygre H, Klepp KN, Solheim E, Gjerdet NR. Leaching of additives and degradation products from cold-cured orthodontic resins. Acta Odontol Scand 1994;52:150–156.

34. Lygre H, Solheim E, Gjerdet NR, Berg E. Leaching of organic additives from dentures in vivo. Acta Odontol Scand 1993;51:45–51.

35. Millett DT, Cattanach D, Robertson M. A 5-year clinical review of bond failure with a light cured adhesive. Angle Orthod 1998;68:351–356.

36. Øilo G. Biodegradation of dental composites/glass ionomer cements. Adv Dent Res 1992;6:50–54.

37. Freund M, Munksgaard EC. Enzymatic degradation of BIS-GMA/TEGDMA-polymers causing decreased microhardness and greater wear in vitro. Scand J Dent Res 1990;98: 351–355.

38. Geurtsen W, Bubeck P, Leyhausen G, Garcia-Godoy F. Effects of extraction media upon fluoride release from a resin-modified glass-ionomer cement. Clin Oral Invest 1998; 2:143–146.

39. Matasa CG. Microbial attack of orthodontic adhesives. Am J Orthod Dentofacial Orthop 1995;108:132–141.

40. Karamouzos A, Athanasiou AE, Papadopoulos MA. Clinical characteristics and properties of ceramic brackets: A comprehensive review. Am J Orthod Dentofac Orthop 1997; 112:34–40.

41. Anusavice KJ. Degradability of dental ceramics. Adv Dent Res 1992;6: 82–89.

42. Squires CA, Johnson NW. Permeability of oral mucosa. Br Med Bull 1975;31:169–175.

43. Wennberg A, Mjør IA, Hensten-Pettersen A. Biological evaluation of dental restorative materials: A comparison of different test methods. J Biomed Mater Res 1983;17:23–36.

44. Schmalz G, Garhammer P, Hiller KA, Reitinger T. Metal content of biopsies from the neighborhood of casting alloys [abstract 1048]. J Dent Res 1999;78(special issue):236.

45. Gjerdet NR, Kallus T, Hensten-Pettersen A. Tissue reactions to implanted wires in rabbits. Acta Odontol Scand 1987;45: 163–169.

46. Øgaard B. Oral microbiological changes, long-term enamel alterations due to decalcification, and caries prophylactic aspects. In: Brantley WA, Eliades T (eds). Orthodontic Materials: Scientific and Clinical Aspects. Stuttgart: Thieme, 2001: 123–142.

47. Kanerva L, Estlander T, Jolanki R. Occupational skin allergy in the dental profession. Dermatol Clin 1994;12:517–531.

48. Roitt I, Brostoff J, Male D. Immunology, ed 5. London: Mosby, 1998:302–317, 341–352.

49. Warshaw EM. Latex allergy. J Am Acad Dermatol 1998; 39:1–24.

50. Veien NK, Bochhorst E, Hattel T, Laurberg G. Stomatitis or systemically-induced contact-dermatitis. Contact Dermatitis 1994;30:210–213.

51. Kaaber S. Allergy to dental materials with special reference to the use of amalgam and polymethylmethacrylate. Int Dent J 1990;40:359–365.

52. Al-Waheidi EM. Allergic reaction to nickel orthodontic wires: a case report. Quintessence Int 1995;26:385–387.

53. Dunlap CL, Vincent SK, Barker BF. Allergic reaction to orthodontic wire: Report of case. J Am Dent Assoc 1989;118: 449–450.

54. Hensten-Pettersen A, Gjerdet NR, Kvam E, Lyberg T. Nickel allergy and orthodontic treatment [in Norwegian]. Nor Tannlaegeforen Tid 1984;94: 567–572.

55. Malmgren O, Medin L. Hypersensitivity reactions by using bonding materials in orthodontics [in Swedish]. Tandläkartidningen 1981;73:544–546.

56. Jacobsen N, Hensten-Pettersen A. Occupational health problems and adverse patient reactions in orthodontics. Eur J Orthod 1989;11:254–264.

57. Nielsen NH, Menné T. Nickel sensitization and ear piercing in an unselected Danish population. Contact Dermatitis 1993;29:16–21.

58. Van Hoogstraten IM, Andersen KE, von Blomberg BM, et al. Reduced frequency of nickel allergy upon nickel contact at an early age. Clin Exp Immunol 1991;85:441–445.

59. Bass JK, Cisneros GJ. Nickel hypersensitivity in the orthodontic patient. Am J Orthod Dentofacial Orthop 1993;103: 280–285.

60. Lindsten R, Kurol J. Orthodontic appliances in relation to nickel hypersensitivity: A review. J Orofac Orthop 1997;58: 100–108.

9

CHARACTERISTICS OF USED ORTHODONTIC BRACKETS

Claude G. Matasa, D Chem Eng, D Tech Sci

In the United States, the Food and Drug Administration of the federal government considers metallic orthodontic brackets to be Class I, low-risk medical devices; in Europe, these brackets benefit from a similar classification, IIa. These designations justify in part the lack of interest that the metallic brackets present to both governmental authorities and clinicians. In the United States, plastic brackets have been classified as showing a higher risk (Class II), whereas bioinert ceramic brackets, which have led to many enamel fractures, are not even classified. The risk factor related to these noninvasive orthodontic appliances pales in comparison with that of many other medical devices that are commonly employed in hospitals, such as pacemakers, angioplasty balloons, and catheters.

Even when orthodontic brackets are subjected to tests, they are always performed on new samples that are not representative of the actual brackets used during the treatment of patients. The orthodontic brackets in the mouth of the patient at some point during therapy behave much closer to the used, rather than to the new, condition.

Fabricated by three basic methods (milling, casting, and injection molding) from at least 10 types of stainless steel, 2 oxides (alumina [Al_2O_3] and zirconia [ZrO_2]), and various polyesters (filled and unfilled), modern orthodontic brackets vary in quality and price.[1] Used brackets may dif-

fer from new brackets either because the former were subjected to debonding, their chief cause of bracket damage, or because they were altered by wear during orthodontic therapy. The alteration may be twofold: mechanical (change of shape and strength) and chemical (corrosive attack).

Characteristics of Used Metallic Brackets

There are tens of thousands of different brackets on the market, as well as over 30 bracket manufacturers and as many prescriptions.[2] While the tremendous number of recommended values for torque and angulation during orthodontic treatment may be debatable, manufacturers claim to adhere to them strictly for their marketed brackets.

The surfaces of debonded brackets may vary from almost invisible alterations to relatively heavy, uniform corrosion (Fig 9-1) and to a partial covering of materia alba. Despite distortions due to debonding, which vary according to the manner in which the debonding pliers have been applied, the metallic brackets are usually recovered intact after completion of orthodontic treatment. Exceptions are those brackets that were subjected to galvanic corrosion especially due to dissolution of the material used for brazing the base to the body of the bracket. To avoid the dis-

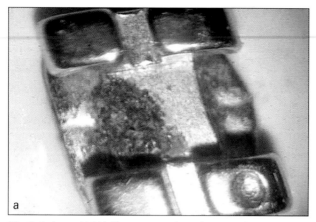
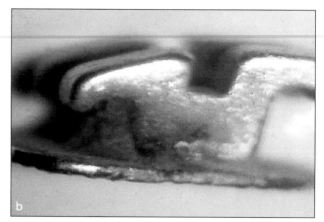

Fig 9-1 *(a and b)* Uniform corrosion of two stainless steel brackets.

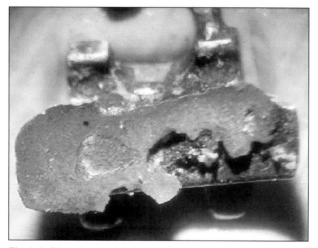

Fig 9-2 Dissolved solder on a clinically used stainless steel direct-bonding tube.

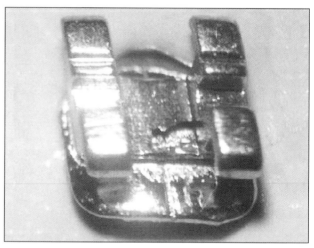

Fig 9-3 Galvanic corrosion of a stainless steel bracket due to gold-alloy brazing.

solution of solder on brackets during clinical use (Fig 9-2), several manufacturers are now using gold-based brazing materials. However, this approach may lead to dissolution of the stainless steel, which is less noble than the gold alloys (Fig 9-3). With the exception of gold-plated brackets, worn metallic brackets that have been coated with TiN or ZrN lose their pleasant goldlike appearance, and titanium brackets become even more grayish and rough.

A thorough inspection of clinically used brackets (after discarding the distorted ones) shows that the brackets that are in the best condition have mesh bases and individually cut slots, ie, not having the slots formed with the use of a mold. (Such an inspection also demonstrates that some clini-

cians do not adequately question the quality of the brackets purchased.) It is common knowledge that inspections of brackets by the manufacturers are performed statistically during quality-control procedures, ie, only a certain fraction of the brackets are examined, usually 10 to 100 out of 1,000. Typically, a relatively large proportion of the brackets (up to 2%, depending upon the manufacturer and product line) are found to have defects for which only the manufacturer is responsible. While certain defects (slight flaws for the in-and-out areas of the slots, minor double angulations, and improper base stamping or marking) do not hinder use of the brackets for patient treatment, other defects (reversed angulations and torques) may wreak havoc for orthodontic thera-

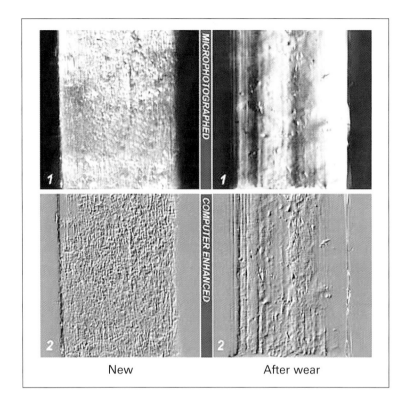

Fig 9-4 Slot bottoms of two similar stainless steel brackets, before and after in vivo wear.

New   After wear

py. Some defects (insufficient slot depth, totally missing slots, and filled tie-wings) render clinical use of the brackets impossible.[3,4]

Physical Characteristics and Properties of Brackets

Bracket Shape

Recently introduced brackets combine a large number of features and are quite complex in design.[2] Considering the number of mechanisms that have been suggested for self-engagement, a bracket providing such mechanisms would be even more complex, greatly increasing the difficulty of manufacturing an appliance in which all of the intended functions are performed. Accordingly, selection of appliances by the orthodontist should take into consideration the proper functionality, integrity, and mechanical resistance of all parts of the brackets. During clinical removal, a bracket is often altered by the common methods of debonding[5] and, as a result, distortions in the

dimensions often occur. While distortions in the overall shape of the bracket may be readily observed, changes in the clinically important slot size dimensions, which can significantly affect archwire-bracket friction, are not evident visually.

Slot Smoothness

As the archwire slides through the bracket slot during orthodontic therapy, friction between the surfaces of the wire and bracket is of major importance. With few exceptions, there is less friction when the two sliding surfaces are smooth than when the surfaces are rough. A bracket slot that has been continuously subjected to the fretting and sliding of several archwires will provide less resistance to their movement.

Counterintuitively, Kapur et al[6] found a trend for the mean frictional force to increase with repeated use of the brackets. Comparative micrographs of slot bottoms obtained for the same type of bracket have shown, however, that clinically worn brackets exhibit far smoother surfaces than their brand-new counterparts[7] (Fig 9-4). In addition, atomic force microscopy (AFM) measure-

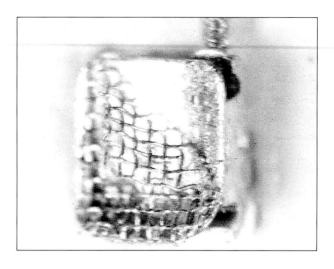

Fig 9-5 Mesh detachment from a bracket due to differences in the stainless steels used.

ments applied to the slot bottoms of new and used brackets of similar types have confirmed these observations by showing a reduction of about 1 μm between the highest peaks and the lowest valleys on the bracket surfaces.[8] The recently introduced titanium brackets have static and kinetic frictional coefficients against stainless steel, nickel-titanium (Ni-Ti), and beta-titanium archwires comparable to those for stainless steel brackets.[9]

Bracket Strength

When a metallic bracket material experiences stress greater than the elastic limit (yield strength) of the alloy, permanent deformation occurs as a result of the movement of very large numbers of line defects in the crystal structure, which are known as *dislocations*.[10] The addition of other elements to a metal, ie, alloying, increases the strength and hardness because these solute atoms (or the resulting precipitates in some cases) impede the movement of the dislocations.[10] The mechanisms for the strengthening imparted by the alloying elements are discussed in engineering materials textbooks.[11] For example, for the stainless steel alloys used for fabrication of orthodontic brackets, the addition of carbon, copper, and niobium to the alloy composition (the latter two of which form precipitates) provides strengthening. In recent years, because of the trend toward miniaturization, the original, corrosion-resistant austenitic stainless steels used for the manufacture of orthodontic brackets have been replaced with martensitic or precipitation-hardened (PH) stainless steels with lower corrosion resistance.

Because the slot walls (tie-wings) of orthodontic brackets are relatively thin, only the strongest alloys can be used for these appliances. Conventional methods to determine the tensile strength of metals cannot be used for the brackets because of their very small sizes. However, microhardness measurements using the Vickers indenter can be employed, for the Vickers hardness and the tensile strength are proportional for a given alloy.[12] The Vickers hardness of the stainless steel alloy will vary from the pad to the bracket and even for different sites or different grains in the same region of the bracket. Such measurements have shown that there is an increase in hardness of about 5% to 10% for clinically used brackets, compared with new brackets of the same type.[13] The corresponding increase in strength of the stainless steel is attributed to cold working from the mastication to which the brackets were subjected over the 2-year period of orthodontic treatment.

Bracket Integrity

Extensive observations by the author have shown that some 50% to 70% of the debonded metallic orthodontic brackets are not damaged by wear, chemical attack, or debonding. Aside from mechanically induced alterations, mesh detachment may occur from the use of different stainless steels in the fabrication of the bracket (Fig 9-5). Consequently, consideration of the in vivo corrosion behavior of the bracket alloys is important.

Chemical Properties of the Oral Environment and Types of Corrosion

Oral Environment

The oral environment is considered to be a harsh regime that promotes the corrosion of dental alloys.[14] Saliva, which contains over 500 mg/L of Cl⁻ ions,[15] is considered to attack stainless steels aggressively. Chloride ions are known to be capable of destroying the passivity that provides the corrosion resistance of stainless steels.[16] Most types of stainless steel, such as American Iron and Steel Institute (AISI) types 304 and 316, which are important for orthodontic use,[17,18] are not resistant to HCl at any concentration or temperature.[16] Organic acids, which result from food decomposition, and the sulfur-containing compounds found in saliva also can strongly promote corrosion. In addition, an urban mouth breather inhales in 2 hours approximately 1 cubic meter of air with a potential sulfur dioxide intake of about 2.3 mg.[19] The presence of these corrosive agents is compounded by the existence of microbiologically influenced corrosion (MIC), which arises from a variety of microorganisms. These include the sulfate-reducing *Bacteriodes corrodens*, *Desulfovibrio desulfuricans*, and *Desulfotomaculum*; the sulfur-oxidizing *Thiobaccilum ferroxidans*, *Beggiatoa*, and *Thiotrix*; and the acid-producing *Streptococcus mutans*, the latter known to attack dental alloys in the mouth.[20] Another category of aggressive species in vivo consists of the "iron bacteria," microorganisms known to assimilate iron, typified by *Sphaerotilus*, *Hyphomicrobium*, and *Gallionella*.[21,22]

The oral environment, which negatively affects the brackets, also affects the tissues. During orthodontic treatment, direct-bonding brackets are subjected to the agents previously mentioned and

behave according to their composition, metal treatment, and design. Although minimizing corrosion is important for the integrity and performance of brackets, it is also highly desirable from the viewpoint of the health of the patient. Besides causing allergic reactions, heavy-metal ions can generate a host of other afflictions that culminate in tissue necrosis.[23] In addition, metal ions released from brackets due to corrosion processes can stain teeth. Hydroxyapatite (HA), the principal component of tooth enamel, is capable of ion exchange and can incorporate metal ions released from the brackets, such as Cr^{3+} and Ni^{2+}. The Cr^{3+} ions are colored and can generate green spots on the enamel.[24] In a survey of 800 orthodontists, approximately 25% reported stains present on the teeth after the resin was removed, a portion of which was attributed to corrosion.[25]

It has been demonstrated that the harmful nickel ion release reaches a maximum within the first 2 weeks following bracket placement,[23] after which it decreases to a low level.[26] This result was observed in vitro in a nonagitated medium. Examination of corroded stainless steel brackets indicates that several types[27] of corrosion that cause the release of metal ions can occur. These corrosion processes have a variety of causes, as discussed in the following sections.

Superficial Uniform Corrosion

Under normal conditions, stainless steel orthodontic alloys are protected against chemical attack by a thin, passivating chromium oxide layer that prevents the penetration of corrosive agents into the underlying bulk alloy.[11,17,27] In some cases, this surface oxide layer is damaged by exposure of the bracket to chlorides. To repassivate stainless steel parts, ie, to regenerate the protective film, immersion for a relatively brief period of time in oxidizing agents, such as diluted nitric acid, which may or may not contain sodium or potassium dichromate, usually suffices.[28]

Pitting Corrosion

Usually caused by the uneven attack of chloride ions on randomly distributed sites, pitting corrosion is rather common but not spectacular.[27] Although the potential for pitting corrosion can be tested with the aid of salt-fog cabinets used in industrial practice, an industrial method may also be used on brackets. Following the American Society for Testing and Materials (ASTM) standard for ferrous alloys,[29] approximately equal weights of different brands of brackets are immersed for 4 and 72 hours in a dilute aqueous solution of iron chloride ($FeCl_3$) and HCl. After rinsing and drying, the weight loss is reported as a fraction of the initial weight of the test sample (group of brackets). Comparison of results obtained by the author for new and used brackets, after the adhesive was removed, showed no significant differences. The weight loss for stainless steel bracket products decreased in the following order: Diamond (Ormco, Orange, CA) > Glance (3M Unitek, Monrovia, CA) > Speed (Orec, San Marcos, CA) > Miniature and Dynalock (3M Unitek) > Twins and Cat (Lancer, San Marcos, CA) > Smile and Style (Ormco) > Dynabond (3M Unitek) > Straight Arch (Forestadent, Pforzheim, Germany) > Twins (RMO, Denver, CO) > Mini Diamond (Ormco) > Ultratrim (Dentaurum, Ispringen, Germany) > Accuarch and Microarch (GAC, Islandia, NY) > Triple Action and Master Series (American Orthodontics, Sheboygan, WI). The most resistant brackets to the chloride ion test medium were the Attract and Standard Edgewise products (Ormco/A-Company).[30] The weight loss observed was corroborated by an obvious difference in the color of the test solutions.

When a bracket is subjected to HCl attack, the most heavily cold-worked parts of the bracket undergo less dissolution (Fig 9-6). A convenient method was developed by the author[31] to investigate the corrosion behavior of brackets in a chloride-ion environment, based upon the principle that a proportional volume of hydrogen is released along with the dissolution of the alloy when the bracket undergoes corrosive attack. The test can be easily performed by immersing the brackets in a tray containing a 5% aqueous HCl solution and placing them under a test tube filled with this corrosion medium. It has been found with this test that measurements of the volume of hydrogen released from the different brands of corroding brackets have an almost identical order to the values of weight loss measured according to the ASTM standard.[29]

Accelerated corrosion tests have been developed in Germany and Japan for the detection of nickel released by dental alloys, using dilute lactic acid for the test medium rather than HCl and measuring the nickel released by atomic absorption spectroscopy. The German standard, adopted by the International Organization for Standardization (ISO standard 6871-2, 1996) uses a solution of 1.1% lactic acid and 0.6% NaCl. Recommended for stainless steel alloys, this standard cannot be employed directly for brackets because of the required dimensions of the test specimens. In contrast, the Japanese standard,[32] which utilizes 50 mL of an aqueous solution containing 0.1 mol lactic acid, has been designed to test a single bracket, regardless of size or shape, which provides direct information about the nickel released from a specific product. A comparison of the amounts of nickel released per unit area of the various brackets is not feasible because of their complex geometries.

In a similar test procedure developed by the author, various used bracket products were immersed in the German solution, which was converted to a gel form and contained a reagent that changed color in response to the ions released. The release of nickel was correlated to the size of the spot generated around each bracket using gel chromatography. Of the 20 brands and product lines tested, little or almost no spots corresponding to nickel release were displayed by the following: Miniature Twin and Twin Torque (3M Unitek), Elite Mini Twin (Ortho Organizers, San Marcos, CA), Mini Diamond (Ormco), or Mini Twin (Ormco/A-Company).

Crevice Corrosion

The procedure for acid etching and direct bonding to tooth enamel exposes brackets to crevice corrosion conditions at the interfaces between the bracket and adhesive and between the bracket and the elastomeric ligatures,[27] as shown in Fig 9-7. Under clinical conditions, the depth of the crevice may reach 2 to 5 mm, perforating the base

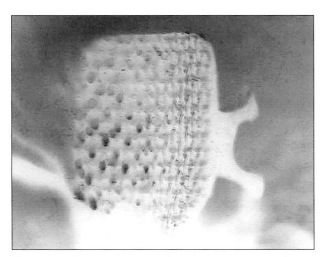

Fig 9-6 Uniform dissolution of a stainless steel bracket in an aqueous hydrochloric acid (HCl) solution.

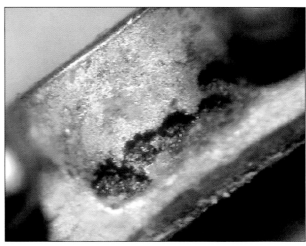

Fig 9-7 Corrosion under the tie-wing of a stainless steel bracket at the elastomer-metal interface.

in one-piece brackets, and the amount of metal dissolved from the bracket can be relatively high. The attack is principally due to an insufficient concentration of oxygen in these areas to regenerate the passive chromium-oxide layer on the surface of the stainless steel bracket. It was found that this type of attack arose from the use of a stainless steel with inferior corrosion resistance,[31] such as AISI type 303 (which contains sulfur to reduce the amount of cutting energy and blade wear), and attack also occurred for another stainless steel (AISI type 304) with better corrosion resistance.[33] Even a stainless steel with excellent free-standing corrosion resistance, AISI type 316L, may not be resistant to crevice corrosion conditions.[34] Further research in this area would be worthwhile.

Galvanic Corrosion

Galvanic corrosion[27] can occur when two different metals (or even two specimens of the same alloy that have been subjected to different treatments) are joined. The less noble metal (or the less noble region on the surface of a metal specimen) undergoes oxidation (loss of electrons) and becomes anodic, with release of soluble cations into the surrounding medium (electrolyte). The more noble metal (or the more noble region on the surface of a metal specimen) becomes the cathodic portion of the electrochemical cell and does not undergo corrosion. Galvanic series tables[27] are available that provide some guidelines about which of two coupled metals or alloys would undergo corrosion in the oral environment. Depending upon the environment,[35] a stainless steel can be in either an active or passive state for corrosion. In the active state the protection from the surface layer of chromium oxide ceases to exist, and the stainless steel can become less corrosion resistant than copper.

In brackets, the stainless steels are galvanically coupled to the brazing fillers, which have evolved from the use of solder to silver-alloy brazing and recently to gold-alloy brazing. With soldering or silver-alloy brazing, stainless steel is more noble than the alloy used for joining, leading to detachment between the bracket and the base, whereas with gold-alloy brazing, the stainless steel is less noble than the brazing alloy, which leads to attack of the latter (see Fig 9-3).

Intergranular Corrosion

As will be discussed later, stainless steel brackets are subjected to a range of temperatures during

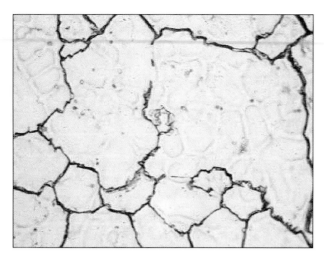

Fig 9-8 Grain boundary deposition of chromium-carbide precipitates during the intergranular corrosion of a stainless steel bracket.

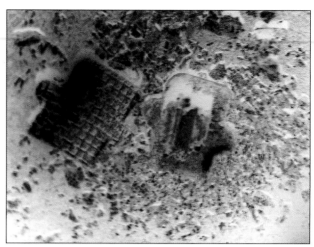

Fig 9-9 Severe nitric acid attack of a stainless steel bracket.

manufacturing at which sensitization[27,35] of the alloy to intergranular corrosion can occur. At elevated temperatures, chromium and carbon in the stainless steel react to form chromium carbide precipitates at the grain boundaries (Fig 9-8). This carbide, soluble even in weak acids, and the depletion in chromium render these areas of the alloy susceptible to intergranular corrosion after prolonged exposure of the bracket alloy to the sensitization temperature range (approximately 500°C to 800°C) during manufacturing or subsequent clinical procedures. In contrast to uniform or pitting corrosion, where a larger portion of the bracket surface undergoes dissolution, only the regions of the alloy near the grain boundaries are removed, which can result in separated grains. Figure 9-9 shows the effect of severe nitric acid attack on a stainless steel bracket, where the detached metal grains have formed a powder. The portions of the bracket that have experienced more cold working during processing (the mesh and the foil) have remained intact because cold working hinders chromium carbide precipitation at the grain boundaries.[36] Tests in accordance with an ASTM method[37] (exposure for 48 and 96 hours to boiling 65% nitric acid) performed on used brackets, where the adhesive had been previously removed, showed that the weight loss decreased in the following order[30]: Dynalock (3M Unitek) > Accuarch (GAC) > Lewis (3M Unitek) > Twins (RMO) > Lewis (Ormco) > Diamond (Ormco). As with the previously described pitting test, the Attract and MiniTwin brackets (Ormco/A-Company), fabricated from AISI type 316L stainless steel, were the least attacked.

Microbiologically Influenced Corrosion

Interestingly, among several brackets made of fiber-reinforced polycarbonate, polycrystalline alumina, and stainless steel, the latter have shown the highest capacity for plaque retention.[38,39]

For many years, engineers concerned with leaking stainless steel tanks and pipes have found that a number of microorganisms actually feed on the metal; the same phenomenon has been described as occurring on used brackets.[40,41] The microorganisms generated cone-shaped craters in the base (Fig 9-10) and preferentially attacked along the grain boundaries of brackets that had been previously sensitized by welding. While such phenomena were often encountered years ago, today they are infrequent, probably due to better oral hygiene by patients. The product that was most subject to this mode of attack was found by the

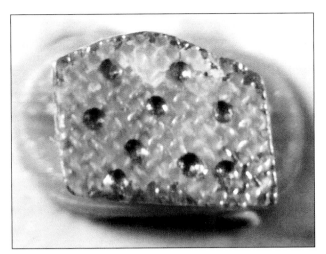

Fig 9-10 Attack of the mesh base of a stainless steel bracket by microorganisms.

author to be the most corrosion resistant in the previously described corrosion test methods, namely, the Standard Twin brackets (Ormco/A-Company) fabricated from AISI type 316L stainless steel.

Factors Influencing Properties of Brackets

Manufacturing

The processes currently used to manufacture brackets are milling, casting, and injection molding. The milling process uses blades to cut bars or tubes (Adenta, Gilching, Germany; CEOSA, Madrid, Spain; Advanced Orthodontics, New York, NY). To fabricate brackets by casting (Ormco/A-Company and Ortho Organizers), molten stainless steel alloy is poured into refractory investment molds using the lost-wax process; then a "tree" is cast, with branches that end in brackets. In the manufacture of brackets by injection molding, fine particles of the steel are mixed with plastics and lubricants. The resulting mass is then extruded into molds, after which this "green material" is subjected to high temperatures. In the first step, the organic materials are carefully volatilized to maintain the desired proportions of the bracket dimensions. (The green material is approximately 20% larger than the final product.) In the second step, the metal is heated to remove all organic material, and in the third step the metal particles coalesce, leading to brackets that have a density of up to 96% of the milled brackets.

The brackets obtained using these three manufacturing processes are either commercially released as such or are subjected to further processing steps. Thus, some cast brackets have their slots milled, after which they are brazed to mesh bases (Standard Edgewise, Ormco/A-Company), but other molded brackets (Prestige, Pyramid Orthodontics, San Marcos, CA) have the protrusions of their injection-molded bases coined to provide retention.

Comparing manufacturing processes, the most expensive is casting and the least expensive is injection molding. It is very likely that in time, as initial problems are solved for new manufacturers using this technique, most brackets will be made by injection molding, which has the important advantage of allowing the use of any alloy, not always the case with the other processes. Both casting and injection molding expose the stainless steel to temperatures at which the bracket becomes susceptible to intergranular corrosion,[11,27,35] which also leads to reduced strength.

Alloy Composition

As noted previously, there are at least 10 types of stainless steel of known composition currently used to manufacture brackets.[1] While earlier stainless steels were selected for their chemical resistance, today's applications demand improved bonding (brazed mesh), greater mechanical strength (miniaturization), versatile processing (casting or injection molding), and increased biocompatibility (less nickel). As will be discussed, each of these demands has desirable consequences.

Although the original stainless steel alloy for brackets (AISI type 304), which contained 8% nickel, was designed to withstand chemical attack, it was suggested[33] nearly two decades ago that voids at the resin-bracket interface, along with poor oral hygiene by patients, led to crevice corrosion of the stainless steel in vivo, which caused enamel stains. Chemical analysis of these colored corrosion products indicated the presence of chromium compounds. A contemporary in vitro study[42] found that the daily release of nickel and chromium from a full-mouth appliance into an aqueous NaCl solution was much less than the normal dietary intake of these elements, but it was also noted that hypersensitivity reactions may occur in some patients who had prior hypersensitivity to these elements. More recently, the rates of in vitro release of nickel and chromium from full-mouth appliances, containing brackets, bands, and either stainless steel or Ni-Ti archwires, into an artificial saliva were measured over a 4-week period.[26] Although it has been noted earlier in this chapter that relevant experimental measurements of elemental release must be made under the complex conditions that exist in vivo, no significant increases in nickel content were found in the blood of patients undergoing initial orthodontic therapy with fully banded and bonded orthodontic appliances, including those with Ni-Ti archwires.[43]

Many bracket manufacturers use a stainless steel with improved corrosion resistance (AISI type 316L) that contains up to 14% nickel, but concern about the well-known allergen nature of nickel has led manufacturers to decrease the amount of nickel in bracket alloys to 4% (PH 17-4 stainless steel) and even to almost zero (Mezanium, Scheu Dental, Iserlohn, Germany; Noninium, Dentaurum; Ni-Free, Forestadent; NoNi, Pyramid Orthodontics). In these stainless steels, nickel has been replaced with other elements such as cobalt, molybdenum, and manganese. To provide the desired homogeneous austenitic structure for the brackets, manganese has been added in amounts as high as 18%. Unfortunately, while the addition of nickel increases the stability of the austenitic phase, improving the corrosion resistance of the stainless steel alloy, the addition of high amounts of manganese lowers it.[28,44] Practitioners thus have to choose between brackets made of nickel-containing stainless steels that are more corrosion resistant and brackets made of nickel-free stainless steels that may corrode and release other heavy-metal ions.

To withstand the same torque as a bracket of standard size, a miniaturized bracket (ie, one with a thinner wall) must be manufactured from a stronger stainless steel than the AISI types 304 and 316L.

Some manufacturers have used precipitation-hardening stainless steels to fabricate stronger brackets while others have used martensitic stainless steels. In contrast, other manufacturers add sulfur to the stainless steel alloy composition to provide greater ease of milling; as a result, these brackets have less corrosion resistance.

Brazing

Most practitioners prefer brackets with mesh bases, being convinced that these offer the best resin adhesion between the bracket and etched tooth enamel. To attach the mesh to the base, the bracket must either be welded (now considered obsolete) or brazed. It has been observed that silver-alloy brazing yielded a weak and corrosion-susceptible union between the bracket and base. Many silver-brazed brackets detached during wear or debonding either due to improper wetting of the stainless steel substrate by the brazing alloy or to the high corrosion susceptibility of the latter, which was less noble than stainless steel and experienced galvanic corrosion.

Several manufacturers (GAC, Orec, Ormco, and RMO) have replaced silver brazing alloys with gold alloys, which is evident from the yellow line separating the brackets and bases. While gold brazing alloys provide a good joint, their greater nobility than stainless steel leads to galvanic corrosion of the latter, as previously discussed (see Fig 9-3).

To avoid such problems, 3M Unitek introduced the first one-piece (monoblock) brackets in the late 1980s. Initially bulky and rough compared with their combined counterparts (joined bracket and base), the one-piece brackets were easier to manufacture and therefore less expensive, in addition to being less prone to errors during manufacturing.[3,4] The starting material was a round bar (later replaced by a tube), from which the brackets were cut in a series of successive operations using a lathe. Because the process for manufacturing one-piece brackets is not patentable, it has been duplicated by other companies, notably Adenta, Advanced Orthodontics, and CEOSA. The manufacturing process rapidly dulls cutting blades, and softer (and more corrosion-susceptible) stainless steels are sometimes used for fabrication of the brackets.

Characteristics of Used Ceramic Brackets

While brackets made of silicates (glass) or other inorganic compounds, such as various borides, carbides, silicides, or nitrides obtained by elevated-temperature sintering, would have acceptable strength for clinical applications, there are only two types of ceramic brackets in widespread commercial use: aluminum oxide (alumina) and zirconium oxide (zirconia). A comprehensive review article[45] is available that presents the clinical characteristics of ceramic brackets and information about adhesive bond strength, frictional resistance to sliding archwires, base surface characteristics, debonding techniques and enamel fracture risks, enamel abrasion and wear, and bracket fracture. The article also contains guidelines and criteria concerning specific clinical applications.

Mechanical Properties

A recent study has shown that the properties of used ceramic brackets were essentially indistinguishable from those of their new counterparts, employing measurements of impact resistance and a new testing protocol based on ophthalmic lens standards.[46]

The predominantly ionic bonding character and the crystalline structures of alumina and zirconia account not only for their high hardness and compressive strength but also for their low flexural strength.[10,18] As will be discussed further, stresses introduced during ligation and archwire activation, forces of mastication and occlusion, and scratches applied during finishing or bracket removal are all capable of creating stress concentrations that may cause crack propagation from existing flaws in the ceramic brackets and ultimately fracture. To obtain information from practitioners about the resistance to fracture of commercial ceramic brackets, the American Association of Orthodontists (AAO) conducted a survey of orthodontists, which found that significant problems were encountered with the clinical fracture of these brackets. The AAO recommended disclosure to patients regarding the difficulties encountered with ceramic brackets.[47]

A study performed on eight different ceramic bracket products has shown that all of these products were sufficiently strong to withstand the commonly accepted magnitudes of archwire torquing forces.[48] Another in vitro study, investigating the influence of second-order archwire activations, found it unlikely that these could be a significant cause of ceramic bracket failure, despite a significant difference in fracture resistance not only between brands but also between central and lateral incisors.[49]

Zirconia brackets are not widely used in orthodontics because their color varies between ivory and yellowish, attributed to the addition of other metal oxides to achieve a sought-after tetragonal structure. In principle, when the zirconia brackets are subjected to the stress fields at the tips of advancing cracks, the partially stabilized zirconia (PSZ) structure undergoes a martensitic transformation from the metastable tetragonal structure to the equilibrium monoclinic structure. This phase transformation causes a local volume increase that can stop the propagation of the cracks; the compressive stresses at the edge of the crack front require further energy for crack propagation.[18] Direct measurements using the Vickers microindentation technique have indicated that the fracture toughness of one brand of zirconia brackets is much smaller than desired and is similar to that reported for some brands of polycrystalline alumina brackets. This result was explained by x-ray diffraction analyses and scanning electron microscopy observations, which showed that that specific brand of zirconia brackets did not possess the desired PSZ structure.[18]

Chemical Properties

Alumina and zirconia are barely soluble; therefore, their interaction with the environment is almost nil. After heating above 800°C during processing, alumina is not subsequently affected by exposure to strong acids, such as sulfuric acid. Deposits on the bracket surface may result in an unattractive stained appearance, and continuous contact with the oral environment may result in some decrease in strength of alumina brackets. A study of dense alumina rods showed a penetration of saline solution during in vitro testing.[50] Although zirconia is reported to be biocompatible,[51] its poorer light-transmission characteristics compared with alumina, which reduces the generation of free radicals needed for polymerization, may result in less complete curing of light-activated adhesives.[52]

Factors Influencing Properties of Ceramic Brackets

Manufacture

The two methods currently used to obtain ceramic brackets are based on milling the rods obtained from a melt or on injecting a dough containing various ingredients and the ceramic powder particles into a mold that is subsequently heated to temperatures at which the ceramic particles are sintered.[53] The majority of ceramic bracket products are fabricated from alumina, for which the ceramic processing technology is mature. The first method leads to the production of clear ceramic brackets from (nominally) single-crystal alumina, often termed *monocrystalline*, whereas the second method yields polycrystalline brackets, which have a translucent appearance due to optical scattering by the alumina grain boundaries.

Alumina and other dental ceramics, unlike ductile metals such as the gold alloys and stainless steels used in dentistry, are highly brittle. These ceramics are particularly weak under tensile stress or bending conditions. Crack propagation occurs when the local magnified stress at structural defects such as surface cracks and internal porosity or at grain boundaries exceeds the strength of the material.[10,18]

The process of alumina rod cutting for the preparation of single-crystal brackets leads to sites of potentially high local stress concentration whenever sharp corners are generated. To alleviate this problem, some manufacturers, such as Dentaurum, subject their alumina brackets to a supplementary heat treatment to eliminate such residual stresses. Because the subsequent sintering never entirely eliminates porosity, injection-molded polycrystalline alumina brackets always have bulk and surface imperfections, which may result in stress concentrations that cause fracture when tensile or bending forces are too high.

Scanning electron micrographs of clinically fractured single-crystal alumina brackets showed that the principal causes of failure were internal defects in the ceramic (47.5%) and external defects produced by machining (42.5%); the cause of 10% of the failures could not be determined.[54] The fracture resistance of the polycrystalline alumina brackets is superior to that of the single-crystal alumina brackets because crack propagation in the former follows an irregular path along the grain boundaries, whereas no such obstacles to crack propagation exist in the latter.[55] (Even if commercial single-crystal alumina brackets in reality consist of a few crystals, ie, relatively large grains of alumina, their resistance to crack propagation would still be much lower than that of the polycrystalline alumina used in conventional ceramic brackets, which have grain sizes typically in the 10 to 20 μm range.[18])

The most discouraging aspect for the use of ceramic brackets, ie, enamel breakage during debonding, led to the replacement of chemical adhesion (with which these brackets were initially provided[55]) with mechanical interlocking. As a result, the formerly flat, silanated bracket bases are now seldom used; base designs with indentations (Allure, GAC), grooves (Signature, RMO), or sintered ceramic particles (Transcend 6000, 3M Unitek) are currently popular.

Geometry

The bulk of material used and the shape of the ceramic bracket strongly influence its structural integrity. Rather than carefully considering the implications of the brittle nature of alumina brackets, many manufacturers appear to have copied the designs of metal brackets, resulting in products that too often fracture during treatment or debonding. A simple test, borrowed from the optical lens industry, has confirmed that a single bracket is more resistant to fracture than a reinforced twin bracket, that the latter is more resistant to fracture than a twin bracket, and that a bracket with residual tensile stresses relieved by heat treatment is more resistant than ceramic brackets that have not received this stress-relief annealing.[46]

Staining

In the as-received condition from the manufacturer, both single-crystal and polycrystalline alumina brackets have good to excellent esthetic appearance that matches well the natural shade range of tooth enamel.[53] Single-crystal alumina brackets (Starfire, Ormco/A-Company) usually remain transparent, even after years of in vivo use, but the rough surfaces (corresponding to individual grains[18]) of polycrystalline alumina brackets become covered and stained with various substances from the oral environment and typically have a yellowish appearance. In some cases, used ceramic brackets may have a yellow-pinkish or green hue, arising from contact with a corroding stainless steel archwire.

The inclusion of common oxides, such as magnesia (MgO), in the composition of zirconia brackets (and perhaps the presence of impurities) causes new zirconia brackets to have an unattractive ivory or yellowish appearance, which has hindered widespread adoption of these ceramic brackets for clinical use. It may be possible that ingenious future manufacturing strategies (eg, cubic zirconia) will result in the fabrication of zirconia brackets that match the shade of natural tooth enamel more closely or are nearly transparent.

Friction

The roughness of ceramic bracket slots varies with the manufacturing technique. A slot cut with a diamond wheel is more uniform in surface topography than a slot that was fabricated by a molding process. Commonly, ceramic brackets are considered not only to have increased sliding friction with archwires but also to create nicks in metallic archwires (which have lower hardness) and thus decrease the time of clinical use for the archwires.[56] The roughness of the slots for polycrystalline alumina brackets is associated with the surface topography of the individual grains of the ceramic.[18]

Atomic force microscopy examination of the slot bottoms of used ceramic brackets shows leveling of the surface topography and deposition of metal debris from archwires.[8] The AFM observations suggest that archwire-bracket sliding friction should decrease with clinical use of the alumina brackets, although further research is needed to determine the rate at which such reduction would occur in vivo. These preliminary results also suggest that clinically relevant evaluations of archwire-bracket friction should be performed with used ceramic brackets rather than with the as-received brackets that have been typically used for such studies.

Characteristics of Used Plastic Brackets

After several decades of relatively limited clinical use,[18] (unfilled) plastic brackets are currently in sharp decline because esthetic ceramic brackets have superior properties. Fabricated principally from polycarbonates (polyesters having a structure similar to bisphenol glycidyl methacrylate [bis-GMA]), as well as from polysulfones and polyurethanes, the unfilled plastic brackets not only discolor in vivo but also creep under torque imposed during orthodontic treatment due to inadequate strength to withstand all intraoral and extraoral orthodontic forces.[57,58] As was the case for ceramic brackets, clinical problems encountered with the unfilled plastic brackets also have arisen in part from manufacturers apparently following the earlier designs of metallic brackets rather than carefully considering the properties of polymeric bracket materials in terms of the demands imposed by clinical conditions of orthodontic therapy. In addition to permanent deformation occurring during treatment, these plastic brackets often deform during debonding and fracture at the tie-wings. Even if fracture does not occur during debonding, permanent deformation of the plastic brackets is common.[58,59]

Under stress, most polycarbonates experience an internal change of structure, which is evidenced by transformation from a transparent appearance to a more opaque white appearance. Another concern is that polycarbonate brackets typically have poor affinity to resin adhesives. To remedy these problems, manufacturers have developed new composite brackets, in which other materials are incorporated into the plastic.

Characteristics of Composite Brackets

Available for almost two decades, clinical use of brackets fabricated from two different types of materials is becoming more widespread, offering perhaps the safest solution for esthetic treatments. While there are patents on coating metal brackets, most efforts to design composite products were directed toward improving the adherence or resistance to fracture of the ceramic brackets.

Ceramic whiskers inserted into ceramic structures have been found to increase the fracture toughness by a factor of five,[60] although the author is not aware of its current application to improve ceramic orthodontic brackets. Ceramic brackets with comparable increases in fracture toughness over that available with current products[18] would greatly allay concern about bracket fracture during debonding. Furthermore, the use of exterior coatings made of alumina, zirconia, magnesia, and titania (TiO_2) have been disclosed as increasing the resistance to crack propagation for ceram-

ics.[61] The most common ceramic-matrix composite brackets currently in use (Clarity, 3M Unitek) are those with a stainless steel slot liner that allows larger archwire activations and a nonceramic interface with the tooth that prevents enamel fracture during debonding. Efforts have been made both to increase the strength of the plastic materials used for the fabrication of brackets and to improve the resistance of these plastics to staining and discoloration.[1]

Mechanical Properties

Because these products are relatively new, few investigations on composite brackets have been published. Crow[62] has found the shear bond strength of plastic-reinforced brackets to be clinically acceptable. Guan et al[63] have examined the bond strength of several composite brackets (plastic brackets containing ceramic fillers in the matrix) and suggest that the exposed fillers on the base surfaces may have a more important role for the adhesion to tooth enamel than the undercuts on the bracket bases that were designed by the manufacturers for this purpose. Bishara et al[64] have found that the previously described Clarity bracket (3M Unitek), which has been designed to have a consistent failure mode during debonding, exhibits a shear bond strength comparable to that of conventional ceramic brackets.

Feldner et al[65] have investigated four types of polycarbonate brackets for their torque-deformation characteristics. Of these four types (pure polycarbonate, ceramic-reinforced polycarbonate, metal-slot-reinforced polycarbonate, and metal-slot/ceramic-reinforced polycarbonate), only the metal-slot-lined brackets were found to be strong enough to withstand clinically desired levels of torque. Due to the large range of possibilities offered, it is very likely that there will be an increasing clinical use of these composite brackets in the future.

Chemical Properties

Composite brackets, which combine the properties of at least two of the three major classes of dental materials (metals, ceramics, and polymers), may have problems associated with their individual material components and interactions between the different types of materials. However, while metal liners currently may still corrode and the plastic matrix may still suffer some discoloration, future developments may yield a proper combination of the components with substantially improved products for orthodontic patients. Future studies to evaluate the properties of such composite brackets as a result of clinical use will be a highly important area of orthodontic materials research.

References

1. Matasa CG. Biomaterials in orthodontics. In: Graber TM, Vanarsdall R (eds). Orthodontics, Current Principles and Techniques, ed. 3. St. Louis: Mosby, 2000:305–338.

2. Matasa CG. Direct bonding metallic brackets: Where are they heading? Am J Orthod Dentofacial Orthop 1992;102: 552–560.

3. Matasa CG. Flaws in bracket manufacturing. J Clin Orthod 1990;24:149–152.

4. Matasa CG. Defend yourself against faulty appliances. I. Faults due to poor manufacturing J Gen Orthod 1991;2:5–9.

5. Oliver RG, Pal AD. Distortion of edgewise orthodontic brackets associated with different methods of debonding. Am J Orthod Dentofacial Orthop 1989;96:65–71.

6. Kapur R, Sinha PK, Nanda RS. Frictional resistance in orthodontic brackets with repeated use. Am J Orthod Dentofacial Orthop 1999;116:400–410.

7. Matasa CG. The friction between bracket-ligation and archwire: State of the art [in German]. Inf Orthod Kieferorthop 1995;27:523–534.

8. Matasa CG. Bracket slot friction examined through atomic force microscopy [in Portuguese]. Rev Dent Press Ortod Ortoped Maxilar (Brazil) 1997;2:60–75.

9. Kusy RP, Whitley JQ, Ambrose WW, Newman JG. Evaluation of titanium brackets for orthodontic treatment. Part I: The passive configuration. Am J Orthod Dentofacial Orthop 1998;114:558–572.

10. Brantley WA. Structures and properties of orthodontic materials. In: Brantley WA, Eliades T (eds). Orthodontic Materials: Scientific and Clinical Aspects. Stuttgart: Thieme, 2001:1–25.

11. Brick RM, Pense AW, Gordon RB. Structure and Properties of Engineering Materials, ed. 4. New York: McGraw-Hill, 1977.

12. Dieter GE. Mechanical Metallurgy, ed. 3. New York: McGraw-Hill, 1986.

13. Matasa CG. Metal strength of direct bonding brackets. Am J Orthod Dentofacial Orthop 1998;113;282–286.

14. Mueller HJ. Tarnish and corrosion of dental alloys. In: Korb LJ, Olson DL (eds). Corrosion. ASM Handbook, vol. 13. Materials Park, OH: ASM International, 1987:1338–1366.

15. McCann HC. Inorganic components of salivary secretions. In: Harris RS (ed). Art and Science of Dental Caries Research. New York: Academic Press, 1968:55–70.

16. Degnan TF. Corrosion by hydrochloric acid. In: Korb LJ, Olson DL (eds). Corrosion. ASM Handbook, vol. 13. Materials Park, OH: ASM International 1987:1162–1166.

17. Brantley WA. Orthodontic wires. In: Brantley WA, Eliades T (eds). Orthodontic Materials: Scientific and Clinical Aspects. Stuttgart: Thieme, 2001:77–103.

18. Eliades T, Eliades G, Brantley WA. Orthodontic brackets. In: Brantley WA, Eliades T (eds). Orthodontic Materials: Scientific and Clinical Aspects. Stuttgart: Thieme, 2001: 143–172.

19. Barton K. Protection Against Atmospheric Corrosion. New York: Wiley, 1973.

20. Palaghias G. Oral corrosion and corrosion inhibition processes: An in vitro study. Swed Dent J Suppl 1985;30:1–72.

21. Tatnall RE. Microbial corrosion of metals. Mater Perform 1981;20:32–40.

22. Pope DH, Stoecker JD. Microbiologically influenced corrosion. In: Moniz BJ, Pollock WI (eds). Process Industries Corrosion. Houston: National Association of Corrosion Engineers, 1986:235–246.

23. Gjerdet NR. Clinical and biological aspects of orthodontics materials. In: Mjör IA (ed). Dental Materials, Biological Properties and Clinical Evaluations. Boca Raton, FL: CRC Press, 1985:165–176.

24. Ceen RF, Gwinnett AJ. Indelible iatrogenic staining of enamel following debonding. J Clin Orthod 1980;15:713–715.

25. Gwinnett AJ. Corrosion of resin-bonded orthodontic brackets. Am J Orthod Dentofacial Orthop 1982;81:441–446.

26. Barrett RD, Bishara SE, Quinn JK. Biodegradation of orthodontic appliances. Part I: Biodegradation of nickel and chromium in vitro. Am J Orthod Dentofacial Orthop 1993; 103:8–14.

27. Fontana MG. Corrosion Engineering, ed. 3. New York: McGraw-Hill, 1986.

28. Davis JR (ed.) ASM Specialty Handbook: Stainless Steels. Atmospheric and Aqueous Corrosion. Materials Park, OH: ASM International, 1994.

29. American Society for Testing and Materials. Standard 48-76/ G-31-10, Method A. West Conshohocken, PA: ASTM, 1976.

30. Matasa CG. Stainless steels and direct-bonding brackets. II. Chemical behavior [in German]. Inf Orthod Kieferorthop 1993;25:147–166.

31. Matasa CG. Attachment corrosion and its testing. J Clin Orthod 1995;29:16–23.

32. Ministry of Health and Welfare of Japan. Nickel evaluation in orthodontic brackets. Standard 1985.3.30, No. 294.

33. Maijer R, Smith DC. Corrosion of orthodontic bracket bases. Am J Orthod Dentofacial Orthop 1982;81:43–48.

34. Ailor WH. Handbook of Corrosion Testing and Evaluation. New York: Wiley, 1970.

35. Franks R. Corrosion of stainless steels. In: Uhlig HH (ed). Corrosion Handbook. New York: Wiley, 1948.

36. Anusavice KJ. Phillips' Science of Dental Materials, ed. 10. Philadelphia: Saunders, 1996.

37. American Society for Testing and Materials. Standard A 262-90, Method C. West Conshohocken, PA: ASTM, 1990.

38. Palaghias G, Eliades G. Characterization of oral films adsorbed on surfaces of dental materials in vivo [abstract 668]. J Dent Res 1992;71:599.

39. Eliades T, Eliades G, Brantley WA. Microbial attachment on orthodontic appliances. I. Wettability and early pellicle formation on bracket materials. Am J Orthod Dentofacial Orthop 1995;108:351–360.

40. Matasa CG. Stainless steels and direct-bonding brackets. III. Microbiological behavior—Adhesive included [in German]. Inf Orthod Kieferorthop 1993;25:269–285.

41. Matasa CG. Corrosion of brackets: A challenge for the orthodontist [in French]. Actual Odontostomatol 1994;187;401–409.

42. Park HY, Shearer TR. In vitro release of nickel and chromium from simulated orthodontic appliances. Am J Orthod Dentofacial Orthop 1983;83:156–159.

43. Bishara SE, Barrett RD, Selim MI. Biodegradation of orthodontic appliances. Part II: Changes in the blood level of nickel. Am J Orthod Dentofacial Orthop 1993;103:115–119.

44. Sedriks AJ. Corrosion of Stainless Steels, ed. 2. New York: Wiley, 1996.

45. Karamouzos A, Athanasiou AE, Papadopoulos MA. Clinical characteristics and properties of ceramic brackets: A comprehensive review. Am J Orthod Dentofacial Orthop 1997; 112:34–40.

46. Matasa CG. Impact resistance of ceramic brackets according to ophthalmic lenses standards. Am J Orthod Dentofacial Orthop 1999;115;158–165.

47. Holt MH, Nanda RS, Duncanson MG Jr. Fracture resistance of ceramic brackets during arch wire torsion. Am J Orthod Dentofacial Orthop 1991;99:287–293.

48. Aknin PC, Nanda RS, Duncanson MG Jr, Currier GF, Sinha PK. Fracture strength of ceramic brackets during archwire torsion. Am J Orthod Dentofacial Orthop 1996;109:22–27.

49. Lindauer SJ, Macon CR Browning H, Rubenstein LK, Isaacson RJ. Ceramic bracket fracture resistance to second order archwire activations. Am J Orthod Dentofacial Orthop 1994;106:481–486.

50. Krainess FE, Knapp WJ. Strength of a dense alumina ceramic after aging in vitro. J Biomed Mater Res 1978;12:241–246.

51. Bortz SA, Onesto EJ. Biocompatibility of zirconia. Bull Am Ceram Soc 1973;52:898–912.

52. Winchester LJ. Bond strengths of five different ceramic brackets: An in vitro study. Eur J Orthod 1991;13:293–305.

53. Swartz ML. Ceramic brackets. J Clin Orthod 1988;22:82–88.

54. Viazis AD, Chabot KA, Kucheria CS. Scanning electron microscope (SEM) evaluation of clinical failures of single crystal ceramic brackets. Am J Orthod Dentofacial Orthop 1993; 103:537–544.

55. Eliades T, Lekka M, Eliades G, Brantley WA. Surface characterization of ceramic brackets: A multi-technique approach. Am J Orthod Dentofacial Orthop 1994;105:10–18.

56. Bishara SE. Ceramic brackets and the need to develop national standards. Am J Orthod Dentofacial Orthop 2000; 117:595–597.

57. Dooley WD, Hembree JH Jr, Weber FN. Tensile and shear strength of Begg plastic brackets. J Clin Orthod 1975;9: 694–697.

58. Alkire RG, Bagby MD, Gladwin MA, Kim H. Torsional creep of polycarbonate orthodontic brackets. Dent Mater 1997; 13:2–6.

59. Rains MD, Chaconas SJ, Caputo AA, Rand R. Stress analysis of plastic bracket configurations. J Clin Orthod 1977;11: 120–125.

60. Dogan R. Reinforced ceramics. Chem Eng News 1988;66: 7–14.

61. Olson WL, Karasek KR [inventors]. Alumina composite reinforced by zirconia. US patent 4,732,877. 1988.

62. Crow V. Ex vivo shear bond strength of fibreglass reinforced aesthetic brackets. Br J Orthod 1995;22:325–330.

63. Guan G, Takano-Yamamoto T, Miyamoto M, Hattori T, Ishikawa K, Suzuki K. Shear bond strengths of orthodontic plastic brackets. Am J Orthod Dentofacial Orthop 2000;117: 438–443.

64. Bishara SE, Olsen ME, Von Wald L. Evaluation of debonding characteristics of a new collapsible ceramic bracket. Am J Orthod Dentofacial Orthop 1997;112:552–559.

65. Feldner JC, Sarkar NK, Sheridan JJ, Lancaster DM. In vitro torque-deformation characteristics of orthodontic polycarbonate brackets. Am J Orthod Dentofacial Orthop 1994; 106:265–272.

10

AGING OF ORTHODONTIC UTILITIES AND AUXILIARIES

Theodore Eliades, DDS, MS, Dr Med, PhD

George Eliades, DDS, Dr Dent

William A. Brantley, PhD

David C. Watts, PhD

A wide range of auxiliaries and utilities are frequently used in routine orthodontic practice. These materials present an ideal model for the study of material alterations in vivo, because the practitioner may remove them during patients' regular visits without affecting the progression of treatment. Wires, elastomeric modules, and other utilities are changed periodically during therapy, so their retrieval necessitates no special procedures.

However, used materials from some appliances, such as brackets and bands, can be collected only after the full term of treatment because of ethical concerns over intentional debonding and rebonding of the appliances and the associated undesirable, irreversible effects on enamel. The use of brackets or bands recovered after completion of treatment imposes minor temporal limitations on the study of the effect of the oral environment, because treatment usually exceeds 18 months. Most important, the surface integrity of brackets recovered after debonding may be altered significantly by scratches and bending of bracket bases, as well as by defects in the area underneath the tie-wings, where the debonding force is usually applied using pliers.[1]

Retrieval of orthodontic materials may furnish crucial information on the effects of intraoral conditions on the materials' performance. The main factor that distinguishes the oral environment from in vitro media is the presence of complex oral flora and their by-products, as well as the accumulation of plaque on the material. This milieu cannot be simulated under current in vitro research approaches, most of which involve exposure of materials to various electrolytes, artificial saliva, water, and other media. The literature has a notable lack of data on the actual intraoral aging pattern of orthodontic materials and associated phenomena such as ionic release, leaching of substances, and the effect of in vivo aging on mechanical properties (see chapter 1). These effects may arise from the interaction of the material constituents or components with the oral environment. Thus, possible surface alterations of the material may have unpredictable effects on its biologic performance.

Retrieval analysis, which investigates the performance of materials in the environments in which they were intended to function, recently has begun to be used in the analysis of dental materials. This method has furnished new information, such as specific microbial species that can attack orthodontic adhesives.[2] Retrieval analysis has been used for some decades in biomedical applications of materials, including arthroplasty materials,[3] and a significant portion of the published studies on orthopedic materials deals with retrieved materials. Furthermore, the development of international standards for the retrieval analysis of orthopedic materials shows the significance of this method in studying their performance.[4,5] However, retrieval studies have some disadvantages; eg, they lack a sequential description of the alterations induced, and they are unable to derive quantitative data.

The main alterations induced during intraoral service of orthodontic wires occur on nickel-titanium (Ni-Ti) archwires, because the practitioner usually changes stainless steel and cobalt-chromium-nickel archwires as treatment progresses according to an escalating stepwise process starting with wires of smaller diameters. Thus, the duration of intraoral exposure of the latter two groups of wires is usually less than 2 months, provided that there is full engagement of each wire size. (The fourth major group of archwires, those fabricated from beta-titanium, would not be expected to undergo significant surface alterations in vivo.[6]) In contrast, Ni-Ti wires, which offer the advantage of full bracket slot engagement from the early stages of treatment, may be retained in the intraoral cavity up to a year and analyzed later.

Although stainless steel archwires are rarely used longer than 2 months, aging of headgear inner bows fabricated from stainless steel may be of interest, because treatment with extraoral appliances may last for up to a year. Thus, the wire segment exposed to the oral environment is expected to function for an extended period.

Because the expected period of performance of brackets or bands and archwires is long, the in vivo alteration of the material and its possible effects on mechanical properties and biologic behavior are important. Materials made of elastomeric chains, in contrast, are changed periodically (every 3 to 4 weeks). These viscoelastic materials undergo a time-related decrease of the force they exert on activation, with a rapid loss during the first 24 hours.[7] Thus, their aging pattern is char-acterized by a very rapid onset of maturation and intraoral alteration, a fact that makes the study of the aging of these products interesting from both materials science and clinical orthodontics perspectives.

In this chapter, the term *aging* does not refer to the actual structural and mechanical alteration of the bulk material induced by the intraoral service. To include the wide variety of surface alterations, *aging* describes the wide range of phenomena that accompany exposure of the material to the oral cavity. Further research should address the potentially complex structural changes and mechanical property alterations associated with the actual use of the materials.

Chapters 8 and 9 discuss the major effects on brackets of aging in the oral environment and describe corrosion and degradation. This chapter explores and classifies the surface alterations of the materials used in the majority of orthodontic cases: Ni-Ti archwires, stainless steel inner face-bow wires, and polyurethane elastomeric chains.

Nickel-Titanium Archwires

Although much research has focused on the detailed study of the mechanical properties and phase transformation changes of Ni-Ti wires,[6] information on the effects of the intraoral environment on surface structural and compositional alterations is scarce. As emphasized above, in vivo conditions may alter the anticipated outcome of several treatment-related parameters of materials performance. As previously noted, Ni-Ti wires are used for prolonged periods, perhaps up to 1 year. There are three critical aspects of materials performance for Ni-Ti orthodontic wires aged in vivo: the corrosion behavior and biocompatibility, the mechanical response (mainly superelastic or shape-memory properties), and the effects on archwire-bracket friction. Also important are potential hypersensitivity reactions and biocompatibility concerns arising from the nickel dissolution documented to occur in vivo,[8] along with tribological considerations involving the presumably increased friction from sliding of the roughened surfaces of wires on bracket slots.[9] Corrosion

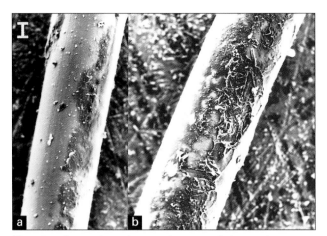

Fig 10-1 Secondary electron images of the surface morphology of Ni-Ti wires retrieved from the same patient after 1 week *(a)* and 1 month *(b)* of intraoral exposure. Note the extent of fixed intraoral integuments on the surface (original magnification × 60; bar = 100 μm).

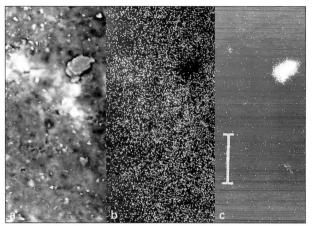

Fig 10-2 Backscattered electron image *(a)* of an intraoral integument formed on the surface of an Ni-Ti wire after 1 week of intraoral exposure, with corresponding x-ray maps of sodium *(b)* and calcium *(c)*. Distributions of potassium and chlorine were similar to the distribution for sodium, whereas the phosphorus distribution was identical to that of calcium (original magnification × 400; bar = 50 μm).

fatigue cracking or stress corrosion cracking also may arise at the pits or other roughened areas that have been observed[6,10] on the surfaces of these archwires in the as-manufactured condition.

A search of the literature reveals few published reports analyzing wires aged in vivo.[11–13] Moreover, past studies have focused on corrosion resistance and surface morphology using microscopic examination of retrieved archwire surfaces.

A recent study of the material surface composition relative to topographic features revealed a severe aging pattern affecting the structure and surface reactivity of the wire alloy.[14] This study found that retrieved wire specimens were covered with regional accumulations of microcrystalline particles (Fig 10-1) that exhibit birefringence under polarized light. In addition, Fourier transform infrared (FTIR) spectroscopy of as-received and retrieved wire surfaces provided evidence of an aging pattern involving irreversible adsorption of proteinaceous matter consisting of amide complexes with concentrations that increased with time. Exposure of the wire specimens to the oral cavity for 2 months induced formation of a well-organized integument largely covering the wire,

leaving free only small areas of exposed wire surface (Fig 10-2). Wire striations on retrieved specimens were smoothened, and surface porosity had increased, whereas the biofilm region was dominated by widely scattered granular particles embedded in an amorphous substrate. Electron probe microanalysis of the surfaces demonstrated a uniform distribution of sodium, potassium, and chlorine, whereas the distribution of calcium and phosphorus showed well-defined high-intensity islands corresponding to the regions of the surface covered by the biofilm (Fig 10-3). Prolonged intraoral exposure of the wires in the same patient usually resulted in the formation of well-organized and heavily calcified solid integuments compared with shorter exposure times. No difference in the extent of the changes induced was noted between the incisor and molar regions, and round, square, and rectangular archwires from different manufacturers had identical aging patterns.

This study[14] also revealed that wire surfaces engaged in bracket slots demonstrated material loss and various modes of corrosion, such as delamination and crevice and pitting corrosion (Fig 10-4).

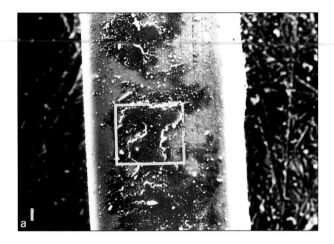

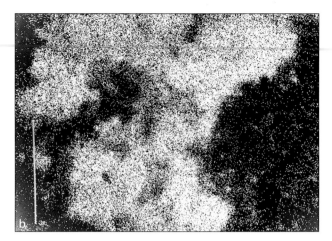

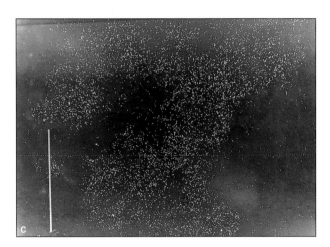

Fig 10-3 Secondary electron image *(a)* of a heavily calcified region formed on an Ni-Ti archwire retrieved after 2 months of intraoral exposure. X-ray maps of calcium *(b)* and phosphorus *(c)* are shown for the region inside the rectangle (original magnification of *(a)* × 100, bar = 1 mm; original magnification of *(b)* and *(c)* × 400, bar = 100 μm).

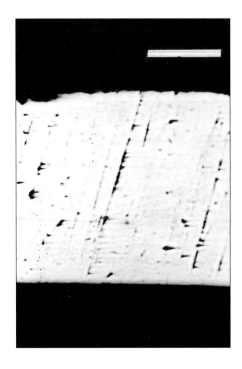

Fig 10-4 Reflected light microscope image of a cross-sectioned Ni-Ti wire after 3 weeks of intraoral service. Note the wear pattern of the wire surface engaged in the bracket slot *(top)* relative to the other wire surface *(bottom)* (original magnification × 50).

The sites of the retrieved wires engaged in the brackets often exhibited much smaller grain size compared with the etched reference wires. Surface regions engaged in the bracket slot demonstrated excessive wear, and characteristic patterns of delamination were observed. The increased deterioration of this region may be attributed to compressive forces accompanying wire activation through ligation and possible frictional damage produced inside the slot. Alternatively, this effect may arise from a plowing action that occurs during sliding of the Ni-Ti archwire in the stainless steel bracket slot. The titanium-containing Ni-Ti and beta-titanium wire alloys are most likely to exhibit this effect, because their adherence to the rollers or die walls during the wire-drawing process creates rough surfaces on the archwires.[6] An increased frequency of cracks and crevices can be found at the wire edge opposite that engaged in the bracket due to the presence of local tensile forces.[14] These force vectors apparently induce changes in the microstructure of the Ni-Ti alloy, leading to a reduction in grain size at the locations of compressive forces, which extend beyond the near-surface region.[14] Further research is needed to verify this observation. Changes in the microstructure of shape-memory alloys that arise from stress-induced martensite formation have been described[15]; the martensitic transformation occurs above the transition temperature range[16] when external stress is applied. (The phase transformations in Ni-Ti orthodontic alloys are most conveniently studied by differential scanning calorimetry.[17])

As discussed in chapter 1, biofilm formation and mineralization on materials placed intraorally are considered nonspecific mechanisms, the initial steps of which are governed by the surface properties of the material[18–20]; in contrast, the extent of mature plaque formation is influenced predominantly by individual intraoral conditions.[21] These integuments substantially modify the morphology, surface composition, and electrochemical reactivity of wires. Nevertheless, mineralized regions may protect the alloy substrate, especially under low-pH conditions, where the corrosion rate of Ni-Ti wires increases.[12]

On a clinical level, these described alterations may affect the roughness of the archwire and have detrimental effects on the efficacy of certain mechanotherapeutic approaches, such as sliding mechanics. The alterations also introduce the potential for leaching of nickel from the Ni-Ti alloy.

Possible Implications of Nickel-Titanium Alloy Aging on Archwire-Bracket Friction

The role of archwire surface roughness on bracket friction during sliding has not been unequivocally defined. In vitro studies have shown that friction increases with increased roughness of the wire and bracket surfaces.[1,6,22,23]

The studies have indicated that in general, the roughened surfaces arising from the manufacture of beta-titanium and Ni-Ti wires and ceramic brackets increase friction. Kusy and Whitley[24] measured the coefficients of friction of orthodontic wires having root-mean-square (RMS) surface roughness ranging from 0.04 (stainless steel) to 0.23 μm (Ni-Ti) on stainless steel and polycrystalline alumina flats having 0.03 and 0.26 μm RMS roughness, respectively. Their results showed that the beta-titanium wire (RMS roughness = 0.14 μm) exhibited the highest coefficient of friction, although the Ni-Ti wire had the roughest surface (RMS roughness = 0.23 μm). These authors reported mass transfer from the beta-titanium wire to the stainless steel and polycrystalline alumina contact flats, which they thought might arise from the relatively low compressive yield strength of the beta-titanium wire alloy. Because the coefficient of friction depends on the roughness of the surfaces and the yield strength of the involved materials,[25,26] further clarification is needed of the role of surface roughness on archwire-bracket friction employing an experimental configuration in which these two parameters will not vary simultaneously. Another possible explanation for the observed results is that the surface roughness differences may not actually affect friction in vivo and that greater differences in roughness may be required to produce a measurable effect. More-

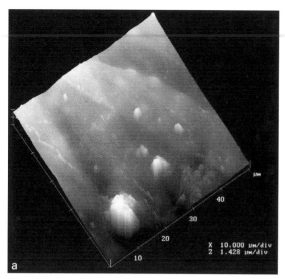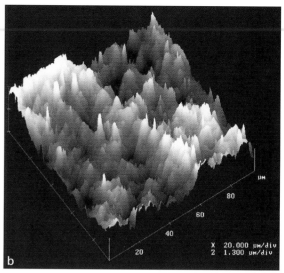

Fig 10-5 Tapping mode three-dimensional atomic force microscope (AFM) images of a retrieved Ni-Ti wire surface before *(a)* and after *(b)* intraoral exposure for 6 months. The increased surface roughness of the retrieved sample is evident in *(b)*. (Courtesy of N Silkas, University of Manchester, UK.)

over, Kusy and Whitley[24] performed their frictional test on dry and relatively clean sample surfaces, so no biofilm or calcified regions[14] were included. The adsorption of these intraoral integuments may greatly reduce the coefficient of friction by producing a boundary lubrication effect (through salivary protein adsorption and plaque accumulation); alternatively, calcified integuments may increase the surface roughness and resistance to shear forces (Fig 10-5).

These considerations, along with the complexity of the oral environment, may explain the results of a study[27] investigating the effect of using different archwires on the rate of space closure in vivo. This study showed no statistically significant difference in average space closure in vivo between conventional and ion-implanted beta-titanium wires; the rate of closure obtained was similar to that reported for stainless steel archwires in laboratory studies. Thus, further in vivo studies are needed to determine the effect of archwire surface roughness on bracket friction and how these important factors affect the efficacy of orthodontic therapy.

Nickel Leaching from Nickel-Titanium Orthodontic Wire Alloys

Leaching of nickel and other elements from Ni-Ti or stainless steel alloys has attracted considerable interest from investigators during the past two decades because of possible serious consequences of archwire alloy corrosion.[28–42] Research studies have attempted to reliably simulate the intraoral environment and assess the amount of nickel leached from orthodontic alloys.

For implanted nickel-containing alloys, such as the alloys used in orthopedic surgery for arthroplasty applications, the rate of nickel release may range from 0.8100 to 0.0081 µg/h per body weight, totaling 5 to 500 mg/y for a 70-kg individual.[43] However, the orthopedic model, in which the biomedical device is implanted in tissues, is irrelevant for orthodontic applications, in which the nickel-containing alloy is placed in the oral environment. Thus, the frequently used medical tests involving implantation of nickel-containing alloys have no relevance for the clinical use of nickel-containing alloys in orthodontics.

Although the implantation procedure may be considered more invasive than the intraoral placement of a wire alloy, the reactivity of the implanted alloy with the environment is actually decreased because of the formation of a connective tissue capsule surrounding the foreign body. In contrast, intraorally placed archwires continuously react with the environment the open oral cavity. Moreover, the large weight percentage of nickel in the Ni-Ti orthodontic alloys, ranging from 50% to 54%, may enhance the potential for release of this element.[2]

A study has shown that full-mouth orthodontic appliances exposed to a 0.05% saline solution released nickel and chromium ions amounting to about 40 µg nickel and 36 µg chromium per day.[44] Another in vitro study[45] examined the release of nickel and chromium into an artificial saliva from standard fixed appliances for the maxillary arch. The nickel release reached a maximum after approximately 1 week; then the rate of release decreased over the next 3 weeks. In contrast, chromium release increased during the first 2 weeks and remained at nearly the same level during the next 2 weeks. For both stainless steel and Ni-Ti archwires, the release of nickel, on average, was 37 times greater than that of chromium. However, the release rates of each element from these two archwire alloys did not differ significantly.

Table 10-1 assesses the clinical applicability and scientific validity of the evidence in the literature. In general, studies on nickel release from nickel-containing alloys can be classified into three major categories based on the environment: in vitro, retrieval (ex vivo investigation of samples aged in vivo), and in vivo.

In vitro studies may have several flaws arising from their necessarily simplified methodology. For example, assessing the weight of a specimen prior to and following exposure to various organic acids or other potent factors, as well as assigning the weight difference to the amount of nickel leached, could yield inconclusive evidence about the composition and kinetics of the eluted substances, as well as the reactive state of the leached species (see Table 10-1). Moreover, assuming that the leached species are in the form of nickel ions—a hypothesis that cannot be verified—there is no information on the binding state or composition of nickel-containing complexes. This parameter may modulate the biologic performance of the nickel-containing alloy, because nickel in particulate form presents a fraction of the adverse effects of its counterpart in a soluble condition, as will be discussed in chapter 12.

There are significant concerns with the common research technique of estimating release by using of storage media composed of nonagitated, nonreplenished solutions. Because the solution is saturated rapidly, the release rate rapidly reaches a plateau as equilibrium is established between the metal ions in the solution and the metal ions at the metal-solution interface. This situation leads to the erroneous conclusion that the release rate increased initially and subsequently remained constant, an observation at variance with research showing that aging of the alloy during corrosion fatigue results in increased ion release.[29] The results from such protocols should not be used to establish hypotheses for the kinetics of nickel leaching from alloys or their biologic performance.

Retrieval analyses of used samples are reliable and present no ethical concerns. However, characterization of used materials samples is indirect; it makes an inference about the processes that occurred in vivo. Therefore, retrieval procedures and handling of test specimens are critically important to obtain reliable information. Several protocols for proper retrieval procedures and maintenance of specimens prior to and during testing have been established by international organizations.[4]

The most clinically relevant methods to evaluate nickel release estimate its concentration in biologic fluids (saliva, blood, and urine). In orthodontic applications, saliva is the first diluting pool for the released nickel, and the results are directly associated with the amount leached. A study of the salivary content in orthodontics patients indicated an increased concentration of nickel and iron during the immediate 3 weeks following placement of fixed orthodontic appliances.[46] However, large individual variations, deriving from the variability in the number of

Table 10-1 Classification of methods to study nickel release from nickel-containing alloys

ENVIRONMENT	METHOD	RELIABILITY AND CLINICAL RELEVANCE
In vitro	Weighing of specimens before and after immersion in solvent solutions or acids (eg, hydrochloric acid or lactic acid)	Yields no information on what is actually released or on the mechanism. Lacks clinical relevance (oral flora, plaque, and calcification processes are not integrated in the model).
	Same as above, but detection of the leached nickel in the solution using spectroscopic methods	Like the previous method, lacks clinical relevance. Yields no information on the state of the nickel released (free or compounds), which largely affects its reactivity.
	Estimation of nickel leached from alloys in nonagitated, nonreplenished storage media	Like the previous methods, lacks clinical relevance. The nickel leached rapidly reaches a plateau because of the establishment of equilibrium between ions present in the solution and the alloy-solution interface. False description of release kinetics.
Retrieval (ex vivo study of specimens aged in vivo)	Elemental x-ray analysis of nickel in retrieved specimens after intraoral placement, as well as in as-received specimens	It is hypothesized that the nickel missing has been leached. Yields no information on the mechanism. Is clinically relevant.
In vivo	Determination of salivary nickel levels in patients before and after initiation of treatment or relative to a control population	Provides information about nickel levels in the first "diluting pool" of the human body. The sample must be in treatment for 18 months to allow study of the effect of material aging and fatigue on nickel release. Sequential sampling is suggested to ensure continuity of data. Is clinically meaningful.
	Determination of urinary or blood nickel levels in patients before and after initiation of treatment or relative to a control population	Provides information about nickel levels following excretory clearance. Decreased values mistakenly may be assigned to low release levels rather than to low nickel excretory clearance associated with accumulation in an organ.

bands and brackets bonded to each patient, precluded the determination of statistically significant differences in nickel concentration. The same study also could not compare statistically the increases in nickel and chromium levels in saliva for 1-day and 1-month periods after placement of the fixed appliances with the levels prior to placement. Another investigation confirmed that the nickel released from orthodontic appliances may not be measurable in saliva or blood after 1 week.[47]

The foregoing in vivo studies may have failed to determine the true potential of nickel release because the testing conditions differed greatly from the routine clinical situation. Not only were the time periods for in vivo aging of the materials relatively short; the saliva sampling periods also did not exceed 1 month, which is almost 20 times less than the duration of typical orthodontic treatment. As a result, the studies could not determine the effects of corrosion processes accompanied by mechanical phenomena such as wear and fatigue, which may affect ion release.[29] Moreover, these studies sampled saliva[46,47] at specific intervals, resulting in an absence of continuous and cumulative data over an adequately long time. The protocol for saliva collection, which involved stimulation though chewing a piece of paraffin wax or gum, inevitably restricted collection to saliva secreted almost directly from the salivary gland. A general lack of wetting of the oral cavity, including the teeth, limited exposure of the brackets to salivary flow.

Furthermore, short-term release patterns from dental alloys have proven to be poor predictors of long-term release potential. Recent evidence has shown that in multiple-phase alloys, long-term release may be higher than release within the first week, whereas single-phase alloys present various release patterns with increasing or decreasing rates, depending on the element released.[48] Interpretation of these findings is difficult because of the complex compositions typical of dental alloys. Therefore, release studies employing time intervals in the range of 1 month should be viewed with skepticism.

The examination of the metal content of biologic fluids may present additional difficulties. The metal concentration in urine or blood may depend on various metabolic functions, such as the infusion or excretory rates of the metal, which vary among individuals. Excretory rates are usually derived from mathematical modeling of the infusion of a metal in an organism.[43] Because of ethical considerations, metal infusion cannot be performed on human subjects, and thus its associated reactions cannot be determined; the information currently available derives from animal models. This limitation greatly limits the clinical applicability of the data, because equations to predict the total body metal content do not take into account the presence of multicompartment components in the organism (which may differ depending on the animal model employed), as

well as the selective binding of metals to organs. In rabbits, for example, nickel shows a high affinity for kidneys, whereas molybdenum is selectively accumulated in the spleen.[43] Therefore, in addition to the inaccuracy of the actual rates presented in various studies, there is a fundamental error in the logic of interpreting the information obtained. Despite the observation that the levels of some substance—eg, nickel—in the blood or urine of orthodontic patients are no different from the levels in untreated individuals, one cannot exclude the possibility that the substance has been accumulated in an organ or that its excretory rate is low.

Stainless Steel Inner Facebow Wires

Aging of stainless steel inner facebow wires may be important in clinical practice because of possible wire fracture and nickel release. Although evidence of nickel release in orthodontics has been published extensively,[49–60] release from facebow wires has received little attention.[59–61] The literature contains no evidence suggesting different nickel release rates from Ni-Ti wires and stainless steel wires, but it may be postulated that facebow wires do not leach significant amounts of nickel, based on the following considerations: (1) intraoral placement is limited to 6 to 9 months; (2) patients are instructed to wear these appliances for 9 to 13 hours daily; and most important, (3) patients do not wear facebows while masticating or drinking.

In a recent study[61] of inner facebow wire components, the aging pattern was almost identical to that of Ni-Ti archwires aged in vivo. Microscopic examination showed that the surfaces of retrieved specimens were partially covered by islands of an amorphous material with a regional accumulation of microcrystalline particles (Figs 10-6 and 10-7). This finding supports the nonspecific nature of the in vivo maturation process. Moreover, aging patterns similar to the patterns reported for orthodontic wires have been described in retrieved

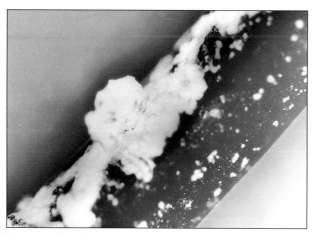

Fig 10-6 Calcified integument formed on the buccal surface of a retrieved headgear inner bow, close to the molar tube (bright-field, reflected light microscope image; original magnification × 20).

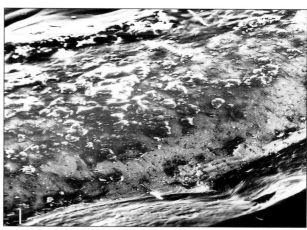

Fig 10-7 Secondary electron image of a headgear inner bow component engaged in a molar buccal tube. Only granular deposits are observed. The stainless steel wire surface demonstrated cracks that are probably attributable to frictional forces developed during insertion of the bow into the molar tube (original magnification × 100; bar = 100 μm).

polyethylene acetabular sockets and bone cements from revised total hip arthroplasties.[62,63]

As with Ni-Ti wires, prolonged exposure of stainless steel facebow wires to the oral cavity resulted in increased intensities of N–H, amide I–III, and –CH–OH groups detected by FTIR, implying a higher concentration of irreversibly adsorbed proteinaceous matter on wire surfaces and its possible contribution to a more densely precipitated film.[62–66] The major difference between the aging of facebow and Ni-Ti wires seems to be the film thickness of the species precipitated on the wire surfaces; in facebow wires the thickness of the biofilm locally exceeded 300 μm.[61] The latter study[61] noted no differences among the areas sampled on a given facebow wire, and identical aging patterns with an acquired biofilm were observed for facebow wire specimens from different manufacturers.

The previously described mineralized regions on the surfaces of Ni-Ti wire alloys exposed to the oral environment during orthodontic treatment may protect the bulk wire, especially under low-pH conditions, where the corrosion rate of alloys is increased.[29] However, such a protective role has not been described for stainless steel and

needs to be verified by further research on headgear wires.

The clinical significance of the previously described alterations induced in vivo is related to the fatigue and fracture behavior of the alloy, as well as to its biologic performance. Exposure to the oral environment, coupled with the application of complex loads due to the engagement of the inner wire to the molar tube, may lower the amount of stress at which fracture of the wire occurs because of corrosion fatigue.

Biofilm adsorption and calcification on stainless steel facebow wires may provide a protective inert film, thereby reducing the incidence of host immune response through decreased exposure of the alloy surface to the oral environment. Alternatively, the intraoral aging process described in the previous study[59] on facebow wires, involving adsorption of ions and the associated reactions, may accelerate corrosion and disintegration in the oral cavity, which is generally considered a severe environment (Fig 10-8).[67]

Further research should be performed to clarify the effects of aging on the biocompatibility and fracture strength of facebow wires. It is noteworthy that despite the extensive use of headgear

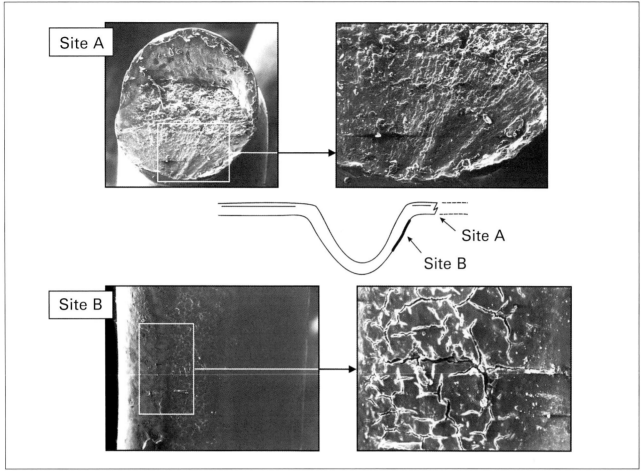

Fig 10-8 Secondary electron images of an intraorally fractured stainless steel inner facebow wire. Site A: *(left)* Fracture surface demonstrating three distinct zones, the fracture initiation zone *(bottom)*, the region of ductile fracture *(middle)*, and the shear lip zone for final fracture *(top)* (original magnification × 75). *(right)* Higher-magnification photomicrograph of the fracture initiation zone and a portion of the ductile fracture zone shown in the rectangle (original magnification × 225). Site B: A region on the facebow wire that was remote from the site of fracture. Regions of apparent deposits and intergranular fracture at low magnification *(left)* (original magnification × 100) are evident at higher magnification *(right)* (original magnification × 340). Note that Site B was on the side for tensile strain in the plastically deformed wire.

as an integral part of orthodontic treatment, information on the aging process and associated cohort phenomena for the alloy is lacking. This shortage of information may derive from the fact that in standard orthodontic therapy, each stainless steel wire is commonly used for only 2 to 3 months. Nevertheless, the period of use may exceed 3 to 4 months for some applications, such as the quad-helix appliance or the rapid maxillary expansion screw type of appliance, and headgear may be worn as long as 9 months.

Polyurethane Elastomeric Chains

Polyurethane elastomers are produced by the condensation polymerization of di-isocyanates and polyols.[68] Their main constituents are a di-isocyanate (Ar–NCO); a long-chain hydroxy-terminated polyol; either a polyester or a polyether (R–OH); and a chain extender, which is some short-chain structural group such as a diamine. These polymers have short, rigid portions (the aromatic rings and the ureas) joined by short, flexible "hinges" (the diamine linker and the CH_2 group between the aromatic ring), as well as long, very flexible portions (the polyether) whose lengths can be adjusted. The polymer is easily stretched and regains its shape on relaxation. (Hence, it is an elastomer.)

The aging of elastomeric chains has received considerable attention in the orthodontic literature because the force degradation of these materials would have clinical significance.[69–77] Although a more appropriate term for this effect would be *force relaxation*, the literature has used *force degradation* because it represents the consequence of this effect, which arises from structural degradation of the polymer chain. Investigators have used several protocols to induce aging and assess how it alters the force exerted by the elastomer. These protocols include dry or wet testing states, the latter using water, artificial saliva, or fluoride media of acidic or neutral pH[78]; various testing temperatures; and the application of steady or decreasing force. However, these in vitro protocols cannot reliably simulate intraoral conditions because of the many complex variables present in vivo, including the action of oral flora and their by-products and the possible synergistic effect of these variables.[75]

Moreover, polyurethanes are not inert materials; they are strongly affected by heat, moisture, and prolonged contact with enzymes.[72] Water acts as a plasticizer of the polyurethanes by weakening intermolecular forces, which leads to chemical degradation. Analysis of leached substances from stretched elastomeric modules intended for orthodontic applications has shown increased leaching following 1 week of loading for specimens immersed in water. This effect is evidently due to the presence of ester or ether backbone linkages, which are highly susceptible to hydrolysis and are the first structural groups in the polyurethanes to be affected by water attack. Thus, intruding water molecules may weaken the material and reduce the load required to maintain a fixed extension (force relaxation).

Figure 10-9 depicts the microscopic appearance of elastomeric modules under polarized light; Fig 10-9a shows the as-received condition and Fig 10-9b, the condition after stretching in vitro. Stretching induced the formation of isochromatic (color) and isoclinic (dark) fringes related to the stress intensity and stress direction vectors, respectively. The large number and closer arrangement of isochromatic fringes at the intermodular links imply that this region exhibits a high intensity and high gradient of residual stress. Although the direction of the applied in vitro tensile force was along the axis of the module, the residual stresses that developed at the links and rings were directed vertically to the material margins, as noted from the symmetric direction of the isoclinic fringes.[79]

Retrieved specimens have demonstrated similar residual stress distribution patterns. However, the interaction of the elastomers with the oral environment strongly modified the optical transmission characteristics of the modules, diminishing polarized light resolution. The original structure of the elastomeric module, consisting mainly of partially oriented fissures and ridges, as shown in Fig 10-10a, was transformed to a smooth structure. This structure was highly oriented to the direction of the applied force following stretching or intraoral exposure. Retrieved specimens contained a considerable number of microscopic fractures, as shown in Fig 10-10b, and there was irreversible adsorption of numerous intraoral integuments, as shown in Figs 10-11a and 10-11b. The chain rings of retrieved materials always show evidence of permanent deformation, which is associated with the engagement of the material underneath the bracket wings (Fig 10-12).

Increased intraoral exposure of the polyurethane elastomers results in organization of the thick deposits and a roughened surface morphology, as demonstrated in Fig 10-13. The distribution patterns of potassium, sodium, and chlorine followed those of the deposits but had a considerably lower intensity than the 1-week intraoral exposure group shown in Fig 10-11b. Based on the much higher relative x-ray signal intensity, the concentration of calcium in these deposits was greater than that of phosphorus. The aging pattern of elastomerics resembles that of the Ni-Ti wires and facebow wires discussed previously.[75]

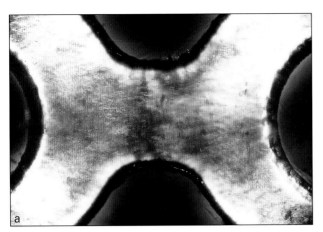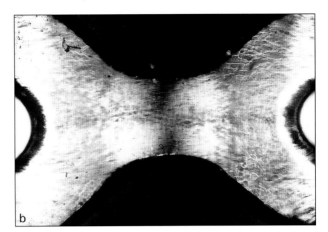

Fig 10-9 Transmittance polarized light images of an intramodular link region of an elastomeric chain before *(a)* and after *(b)* 50% elongation relative to the initial length for 24 hours in air. Note the permanent deformation and the formation of an isoclinic fringe (dark band), which implies the development of residual stress vectors perpendicular to the coaxially applied load (bright-field microscope image; original magnification × 12.5).

Phase-contrast imaging using polarized light optical microscopy confirmed that the stress adsorption mechanism in these materials seems to be macromolecular chain orientation and elongation coaxial to the applied load. However, regional discontinuities emanating from the design of chains may locally exaggerate stress effects, leading to a microtearing pattern and the establishment of microfractures that propagate from margins to bulk material. This failure pattern follows the orientations of the residual stress, which was demonstrated from the direction of the isoclinic fringes in the polarized light images (Fig 10-14).

An FTIR spectroscopic analysis of untreated elastomeric modules revealed variations in their molecular composition, implying the use of different (polyester) urethane raw materials in fabrication.[79] These variations were mainly assigned to differences in the peak intensity between free urethane ester and hydrogen-bonded ester stretching vibrations. Minor changes in the intensity of some groups were found in spectra obtained from specimens stretched in vitro relative to untreated controls; this finding may be attributed to macromolecular orientation effects due to plastic deformation of the chain. However, the most prolonged changes in molecular composition occurred after intraoral exposure of these materials. The role of

hydrogen bonding is very important in polyurethanes, because these materials may act as both hydrogen donors through –HN groups or hydrogen acceptors through C=O groups.

The different pattern of materials aged in vitro and in vivo may be reflected in the differences between elastomers aged in artificial environments and those retrieved from patients undergoing treatment, as described previously. A study (Eliades et al, unpublished data, 2002) examining chains aged in vitro showed remarkable differences. The study compared *(1)* specimens treated by 3 weeks of immersion in a solution of 75% ethanol and 25% water (volume per volume) to induce accelerated aging, *(2)* specimens stretched for 3 weeks in air at 50% extension relative to their original length, and *(3)* specimens immersed in the 75% ethanol–25% water solution in the 50% stretched condition. Elongated (stretched) specimens in air underwent molecular orientation attributed to poly(methylene glycol) soft segments and chain extruders such as butanediol. Aging in air occurred through an oxidative degradation of alpha-methylene groups by the formation of ester, carboxylic acid, or aldehyde groups due to hydrogen abstraction from alpha-methylene groups. The study found no major differences between stretched and nonstretched chains immersed in

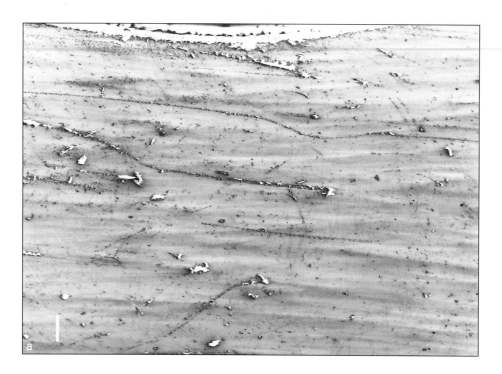

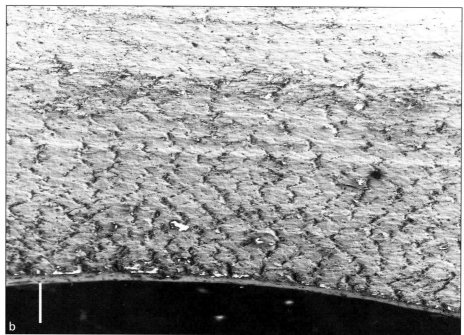

Fig 10-10 Secondary electron images of an elastomeric orthodontic chain in the as-received condition *(a)* and following 50% elongation relative to the initial length in air *(b)*. Note the orientation of the macromolecular chains parallel to the applied load in both *(a)* and *(b)*, as well as the wavy dark features in *(b)*, which are cracks perpendicular to the applied load caused by permanent deformation and failure of some macromolecular chains (bar = 100 µm).

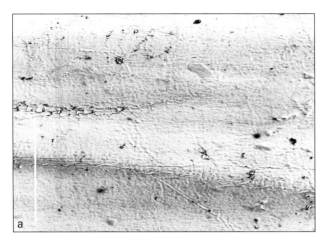 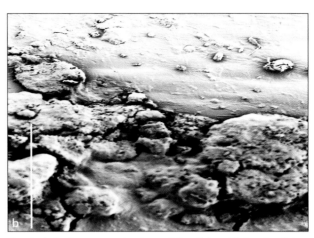

Fig 10-11 Secondary electron images of an elastomeric orthodontic chain in the as-received condition *(a)* and following intraoral exposure for 1 week *(b)*. Intraoral exposure resulted in adsorption of macromolecular integuments, which were initially mineralized by potassium and sodium and later by calcium and phosphorus, establishing a well-organized calcified region (original magnification × 400; bar = 100 μm).

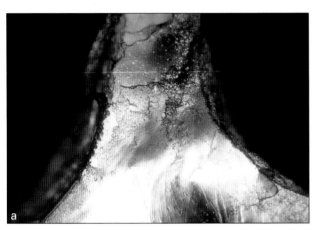 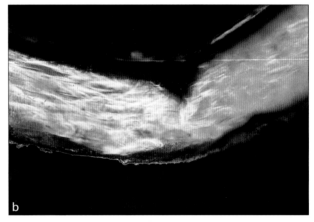

Fig 10-12 Reflected light microscope images of retrieved elastomeric chains after 3 weeks of intraoral exposure. Note cracks and permanent deformation of the ring-shaped modular unit at the region engaged to the bracket wings (bright-field microscope images; original magnification × 20). *(a)* Intermodular link. *(b)* Cracks and built-up deposits.

the ethanol-water bath, whereas FTIR analysis of the extracts revealed high concentrations of alcohol and alkene in stretched chains.

Thus, it appears that aging of polyurethane elastomeric modules in vitro involves initial degradation of ether groups, followed by loss of free urethane, hydrogen-bonded urethane, and urea (Eliades et al, unpublished data, 2002). The changes in the non-hydrogen-bonded and hydrogen-bonded polyurethane carboxyls during testing in air support this model of chain reorientation, where there is rearrangement of the intramolecular hydrogen bonding between NHCO groups due to the greater kinetic flexibility of the polymer chains.

Oxidative degradation reactions of alpha-methylene groups by formation of ester, carboxylic acid, or aldehyde groups due to hydrogen abstraction from alpha-methylene groups have been shown to accompany aging in air, although this process is slow.

The analysis of chain extracts following immersion in water for 3 weeks has shown the presence of alcohol and alkene extracts at high concen-

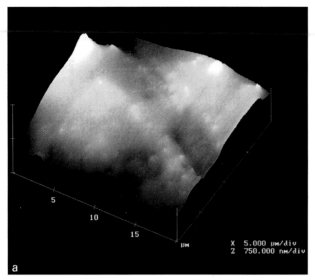 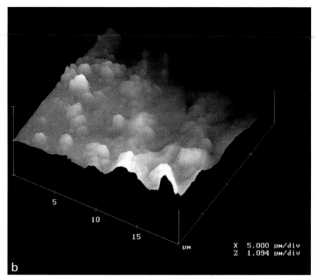

Fig 10-13 Tapping mode three-dimensional atomic force microscope images of the surface of an elastomeric chain before *(a)* and after *(b)* intraoral exposure for 1 week. Note the increased surface roughness following intraoral exposure, which is due to the adsorption of granular integuments. The sensitivity of the vertical scale has been expanded in *(a)* compared with *(b)*. (Courtesy of N Silikas, University of Manchester, UK.)

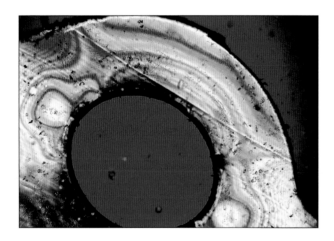

Fig 10-14 Transmitted polarized light image of a ring-shaped elastomeric modular unit after 50% elongation relative to initial length for 24 hours in air. Note the distribution of the isochromatic fringes, which demonstrate the residual stress intensity and stress gradient in this region (bright-field microscope image; original magnification × 8; λ/2 filter).

tration, which suggests a degradation mechanism involving hydrogen abstraction from beta-methylene groups. Although alpha-methylene abstraction is considered the predominant degradation mechanism of polyurethanes,[80] under strain the activation energy of hydrogen abstraction from beta-methylene groups is reduced and this species is preferentially attacked, resulting in the loss of alcohol, alkene, or ketone groups.

References

1. Eliades T, Eliades G, Brantley WA. Orthodontic brackets. In: Brantley WA, Eliades T (eds). Orthodontic Materials: Scientific and Clinical Aspects. Stuttgart: Thieme, 2001:143–173.

2. Matasa CG. Microbial attack of orthodontic adhesives. Am J Orthod Dentofacial Orthop 1995;108:132–141.

3. Witkiewicz H, Deng M, Vidovszky T. A differential scanning calorimetry study of retrieved orthopedic implants made of ultra high molecular weight polyethylene. J Biomed Mater Res 1996;33:73–82.

4. International Standardization Organization. Draft International Standards 12891-1: Retrieval and Analysis of Implantable Medical Devices. Geneva, Switzerland: International Organization for Standardization, 1996.

5. American Society for Testing and Materials. Standard practice for analysis of retrieved metallic orthopaedic implants, designation F 561-87 (reapproved 1994). In: 1997 Annual Book of ASTM Standards, sec 13. Vol 13.01: Medical devices. West Conshohocken, PA: American Society for Testing and Materials, 1997:65–69.

6. Brantley WA. Orthodontic wires. In: Brantley WA, Eliades T (eds). Orthodontic Materials: Scientific and Clinical Aspects. Stittgart: Thieme, 2001:78–105.

7. Eliades T, Eliades G, Watts DC, Brantley WA. Elastomeric ligatures and chains. In: Brantley WA, Eliades T (eds). Orthodontic Materials: Scientific and Clinical Aspects. Stuttgart: Thieme, 2001:173–189.

8. Veien NK, Borchorst E, Hattel T, Laurberg, G. Stomatitis or systemically-induced contact dermatitis from metal wire in orthodontic materials. Contact Dermatitis 1994;30:210–213.

9. Tselepis M, Brockhurst P, West VC. The dynamic frictional resistance between orthodontic brackets and arch wires. Am J Orthod Dentofacial Orthop 1994;106:131–138.

10. Edie JW, Andreasen GF, Zaytoun MP. Surface corrosion of nitinol and stainless steel under clinical conditions. Angle Orthod 1981;51:319–324.

11. Grímsdóttir MR, Hensten-Pettersen A. Surface analysis of nickel-titanium archwires used in vivo. Dent Mater 1997;13: 163–167.

12. Oshida Y, Sachdeva RCL, Miyazaki S. Microanalytical characterization and surface modification of TiNi orthodontic archwires. Biomed Mater Eng 1992;2:51–69.

13. Mohlin B, Muller H, Odman J, Thilander B. Examination of Chinese NiTi wire by a combined clinical and laboratory approach. Eur J Orthod 1991;13:386–392.

14. Eliades T, Eliades G, Athanasiou AE, Bradley TG. Surface characterization of retrieved orthodontic NiTi archwires. Eur J Orthod 2000;22:317–326.

15. Weyman CM. Shape memory alloys. Mater Res Soc Bull 1993;18(4):49–56.

16. Andreasen GF, Heilman H, Krell D. Stiffness changes in thermodynamic nitinol with increasing temperature. Angle Orthod 1985;55:120–126.

17. Bradley TG, Brantley WA, Culbertson B. Differential scanning calorimetry (DSC) analyses of superelastic and non-superelastic nickel-titanium orthodontic wires. Am J Orthod Dentofacial Orthop 1996;109:589–597.

18. Baier RE, Meyer AE, Natiella RR, Carter JM. Surface properties determine bioadhesive outcomes: Methods and results. J Biomed Mater Res 1984;18:337–355.

19. Glantz P-O. Alteration of the surfaces of teeth. In: Leach SA (ed). Dentin, Plaque and Surface Interactions in the Oral Cavity. London: IRL, 1980:95–100.

20. Baier RE, Glantz P-O. Characterization of oral in vivo films found on different types of solid surfaces. Acta Odontol Scand 1978;46:289–301.

21. Quirynen M, Marechal M, Busscher HJ, et al. The influence of surface free-energy on planimetric plaque growth in man. J Dent Res 1989;68:796–799.

22. Downing A, McCabe JF, Gordon PH. The effect of artificial saliva on the frictional forces between orthodontic brackets and archwires. Br J Orthod 1994;22:41–46.

23. Eliades T, Brantley WA. Friction: On the edge of friction: A critique of bracket-archwire friction research protocols and their clinical relevance. Hel Orthod Rev 1999;2:17–29.

24. Kusy RP, Whitley JQ. Effect of surface roughness on the coefficients of friction in model orthodontic systems. J Biomech 1990;23:913–925.

25. Ashby MF, Jones DRH. Engineering Materials. New York: Pergamon, 1998:35–40.

26. Sears FW, Zamansky MW, Young HD. University Physics, ed 6. New York: Addison-Wesley, 1982:134–144.

27. Kula K, Phillips C, Gibilaro A, Proffit WR. Effect of ion implantation of TMA archwires on the rate of orthodontic sliding space closure. Am J Orthod Dentofacial Orthop 1998;114: 577–580.

28. Pereira MC, Pereira ML, Sousa JP. Histological effects of iron accumulation on mice liver and spleen after administration of a metallic solution. Biomaterials 1999;20:2193–2198.

29. Fontana MG. Corrosion Engineering, ed 3. New York: McGraw-Hill, 1986:105–142, 452–454, 469–473.

30. Torgersen S, Moe G, Jonsson R. Immunocompetent cells adjacent to stainless steel and titanium miniplates and screws. Eur J Oral Sci 1995;103:46–54.

31. Vreeburg KJJ, de Groot K, von Blomberg BME, Scheper RJ. Induction of immunological tolerance by oral administration of nickel and chromium. J Dent Res 1984;63:124–128.

32. Wataha JC, Lockwood PE, Marek M, Ghazi M. Ability of Ni-containing biomedical alloys to activate monocytes and endothelial cells in vitro. J Biomed Mater Res 1999;45: 251–257.

33. Wataha JC, Sun ZL, Hanks CT, Fang DN. Effect of Ni ions on expression of intercellular adhesion molecule 1 by endothelial cells. J Biomed Mater Res 1997;36:145–151.

34. Zhou D, Salnikow K, Costa M. Cap43, a novel gene specifically induced by Ni^{2+} compounds. Cancer Res 1998;58: 2182–2189.

35. Salnikow K, Su W, Blagosklonny MV, Costa M. Carcinogenic metals induce hypoxia-inducible factor-stimulated transcription reactive oxygen species-independent mechanism. Cancer Res 2000;60:3375–3378.

36. Chen CY, Sheu JY, Lin TH. Oxidative effects of nickel on bone marrow and blood of rats. J Toxicol Environ Health 1999;58: 475–483.

37. Salnikow K, Gao M, Voitkun V, Huang X, Costa M. Altered oxidative stress responses in nickel-resistant mammalian cells. Cancer Res 1994;24:6407–6412.

38. Madden MC, Thomas MJ, Ghio AJ. Acetaldehyde production in rodent lungs after exposure to metal-rich particles. Free Radic Biol Med 1999;26:1569–1577.

39. Ghio AJ, Carter JD, Dailey LA, Devlin RB, Samet JM. Respiratory epithelial cells demonstrate lactoferrin receptors that increase after metal exposure. Am J Physiol 1999;276: 933–940.

40. Liang R, Senturker S, Shi X, Bal W, Dizdaroglu M, Kasprzak KS. Effects of Ni (II) and Cu (II) on DNA interaction with the N-terminal sequence of human protamine P2: Enhancement of binding and mediation of oxidative DNA strand scission and base damage. Carcinogenesis 1999;20:893–898.

41. Lloyd DR, Phillips DH. Oxidative DNA damage mediated by copper, iron and nickel fenton reactions: Evidence for site-specific mechanisms in the formation of double-strand breaks, 8-hydroxydeoxyguanosine and putative intrastrand cross-links. Mutat Res 1999;424:23–36.

42. Lee YW, Broday L, Costa M. Effects of nickel on DNA methyltransferase activity and genomic DNA methylation levels. Mutat Res 1998;415:213–218.

43. Black J. Biological Performance of Materials: Fundamentals of Biocompatibility. New York: Marcel Decker, 1999:28–44.

44. Park HY, Shearer TR. In vitro release of nickel and chromium from simulated orthodontic appliances. Am J Orthod 1983; 84:156–159.

45. Barrett RD, Bishara SE, Quinn JK. Biodegradation of orthodontic appliances, I. Biodegradation of nickel and chromium in vitro. Am J Orthod Dentofacial Orthop 1993;103:8–14.

46. Kerosuo M, Moe G, Hensten-Pettersen A. Salivary nickel and chromium in subjects with different types of fixed appliances. Am J Orthod Dentofacial Orthop 1997;111:595–598.

47. Gjerdet NR, Erichsen ES, Remlo HE, Evjen G. Nickel and iron in saliva of patients with fixed orthodontic appliances. Acta Odontol Scand 1991;49:73–78.

48. Wataha JC, Lockwood PE, Nelson SK. Initial versus subsequent release of elements from dental casting alloys. J Oral Rehabil 1999;10:798–803.

49. Kanerva L, Estlander T, Jolanki R. Occupational skin allergy in the dental profession. Dermatol Clin 1994;12:517–531.

50. Bass JK, Fine H, Cisneros GJ. Nickel hypersensitivity in the orthodontic patient. Am J Orthod 1993;103:280–285.

51. Hensten-Pettersen A. Nickel allergy and dental treatment procedures. In: Maibach HI, Menne T (eds). Nickel and the Skin: Immunology and Toxicology. Boca Raton, FL: CRC Press, 1989:195–205.

52. Dunlap CL, Vincent SK, Barker BF. Allergic reaction to orthodontic wire: Report of a case. J Am Dent Assoc 1989; 118:449–450.

53. Van Hoogstraten IM, Andersen KE, Von Blomberg BM, et al. Reduced frequency of nickel allergy upon oral nickel contact at an early age. Clin Exp J Immunol 1991;85:441–445.

54. Lindsten R, Kurol J. Orthodontic appliances in relation to nickel hypersensitivity: A review. J Orofac Orthop 1997;58: 100–108.

55. Staerkjaer L, Menné T. Nickel allergy and orthodontic treatment. Eur J Orthod 1990;12:284–289.

56. Marcusson JA, Lindh G, Evengård B. Chronic fatigue syndrome and nickel allergy. Contact Dermatitis 1999;40: 269–272.

57. Wataha JC, Lockwood P, Erek M, Ghazi M. Ability of Ni-containing biomedical alloys to activate monocytes and endothelial cellls in vitro. J Biomed Mater Res 1999;3: 251–257.

58. Wataha JC, Sun ZL, Hanks CT, Fang DN. Effect of Ni ions on expression of intercellular adhesion. J Biomed Mater Res 1997;36:145–151.

59. Greig DGM. Contact dermatitis reaction to a metal buckle on a cervical headgear. Br Dent J 1983;155:61–62.

60. Hensten-Pettersen A, Jacobsen N, Grímsdóttir MR. Allergic reactions and safety concerns. In: Brantley WA, Eliades T (eds). Orthodontic Materials: Scientific and Clinical Aspects. Stuttgart: Thieme, 2000:287–299.

61. Eliades T, Eliades G, Watts DC. Intaroral aging of the inner headgear component: A potential biocompatibility concern? Am J Orthod Dentofacial Orthop 2001;119:300–306.

62. Magnissalis E, Eliades G, Eliades T. Multitechnique characterization of articular surfaces of retrieved ultrahigh molecular weight polyethylene acetabular sockets. J Biomed Mater Res 1999;48:365–373.

63. Eliades T. Degree of Carbon-Carbon Double Bond Conversion and Chemical Composition of Retrieved Bone Cement from Revised Total Hip Arthroplasties, and Effect of Moisture During Polymerization on the Mechanical Properties of Bone Cement [dissertation]. Athens, Greece: University of Athens, 2002.

64. Leininger RI, Hutson T, Jakobsen R. Spectroscopic approaches to the investigation of interactions between artificial surfaces and protein. Ann NY Acad Sci 1987;516:173–183.

65. Baier RE, Glantz P-O. Characterization of oral in vivo films found on different types of solid surfaces. Acta Odontol Scand 1978;46:289–301.

66. Vasin M, Rosanone J, Sevastianov V. The role of proteins in the nucleation and formation of calcium containing deposits on biomaterial surfaces. J Biomed Mater Res 1998;39: 491–497.

67. Greene ND. Corrosion of surgical implant alloys: A few basic ideas. In: Fraker AC, Griffin CD (eds). Corrosion and Degradation of Implant Materials. [Proceedings of the Second Symposium, American Society for Testing and Materials, Philadelphia, 1985]. Philadelphia: ASTM, 1985:5–7.

68. Billmeyer F W Jr. Thermosetting resins. In: Textbook of Polymer Science. New York: Wiley, 1984:361–390.

69. Brooks DG, Hershey HG. Effect of heat and time on stretched plastic orthodontic modules [abstract 363]. J Dent Res 1976;55(special issue B):B152.

70. Chau Lu T, Wang WM, Tarng TH, Chen JW. Force decay of elastomeric chains. Am J Orthod Dentofacial Orthop 1993; 104:373–377.

71. De Genova DC, McInness-Ledoux P, Weinberg R, Shaye R. Force degradation of orthodontic elastomeric chains: A product comparison study. Am J Orthod 1985;87:377–384.

72. Ferriter JP, Meyers CE, Lorton L. The effect of hydrogen ion concentration on the force-degradation rate of orthodontic polyurethane chain elastics. Am J Orthod Dentofacial Orthop 1990;98:404–410.

73. Huget EF, Patrick KS, Nunez LJ. Observations on the elastic behavior of a synthetic orthodontic elastomer. J Dent Res 1990;69:496–501.

74. Kuster R, Ingervall B, Buergin W. Laboratory and intraoral tests of the degradation of elastic chains. Eur J Orthod 1986;8:202–208.

75. Phua SK, Castillo E, Anderson JM, Hiltner A. Biodegradation of a polyurethane in vitro. J Biomed Mater Res 1987;21: 231–246.

76. Rock WP, Wilson HJ, Fisher SE. A laboratory investigation of orthodontic elastomeric chains. Br J Orthod 1985;12: 202–207.

77. Rock WP, Wilson HJ, Fisher SE. Force reduction of orthodontic elastomeric chains after one month in the mouth. Br J Orthod 1986;13:147–150.

78. von Fraunhofer JA, Coffelt MTP, Orbell GM. The effect of artificial saliva and topical fluoride treatments on the degradation of the elastic properties of orthodontic chains. Angle Orthod 1992;62:265–274.

79. Eliades T, Eliades G, Watts DC. Structural conformation of in vitro and in vivo-aged orthodontic elastomeric modules. Eur J Orthod 1999;21:649–658.

80. Stokes K, Coury AJ, Urbanski P. Autooxidative degradation of implanted polyether polyurethane devices. Biomater Appl 1987;1:411–448.

Section V

ENDODONTICS

11

AGING OF ENDODONTIC INSTRUMENTS AND MATERIALS

Spiros Zinelis, PhD

John Margelos, DDS

A variety of materials, instruments, and devices (eg, rubber dam clamps, files, reamers, silver and gutta-percha points, and sealers) are used in current endodontic therapy. Despite the many improvements that have occurred in these materials, instruments, and devices in recent years, clinical failures such as clamp or instrument fracture, corrosion of silver points, disintegration of sealers, and microleakage may jeopardize the outcome of endodontic therapy. Numerous causes related to the physical properties and manipulative characteristics of endodontic materials and the design of endodontic instruments and devices have been associated with these failures. Although conclusive clinical evidence is still unavailable about the implications of in vivo aging of endodontic materials on clinical treatment failures, an understanding of the likely major causes can provide insight into failure prevention and can increase the efficacy of endodontic therapy.

Many experimental and clinical studies have been conducted to elucidate the failure process. In vitro studies have been performed under controlled laboratory conditions to determine clinically relevant physical and mechanical properties, such as corrosion resistance, modulus of elasticity, and hardness of materials used in fabrication of endodontic instruments and devices. Results from this type of study are extensively used to classify commercial products according to specific material properties. Other studies have been used to determine the behavior of materials in vivo or to predict an approximate failure time by simulating clinical conditions. The last approach is widely used in nondental industries to predict the service time of components that are vulnerable to fatigue, corrosion, or other detrimental processes or to establish appropriate criteria for selection of structural materials.

Unfortunately, current simulation models for dental materials and products often yield information that is not relevant to clinical practice because the controlled laboratory conditions for in vitro tests typically do not properly account for variables existing clinically that can yield entirely different in vivo failure mechanisms. Despite the inability of current laboratory tests to describe the clinical behavior of endodontic materials, these tests nonetheless can be successfully used to determine important properties of materials and instruments or devices. In addition, an important aspect of such in vitro tests is their ability to compare experimental materials or devices with their counterparts that have a history of successful clinical performance. On the basis of these considerations, the requirements of the International Organization for Standardization (ISO, Geneva, Switzerland) should be regarded as rejection cri-

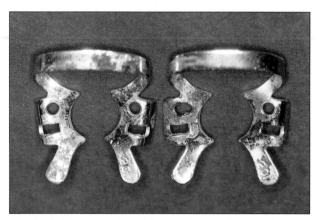

Fig 11-1 Macroscopic evidence of corrosion on the surfaces of clinically used rubber dam clamps. The dark areas arise from the formation of corrosion products on the base and the bow of each device.

teria and not as proof that ideal clinical performance will be achieved by the endodontic materials and instruments or devices.

In vivo studies of endodontic instruments and devices have been based upon clinical observations, such as estimation of the percentages of broken and deformed or discarded files of certain types, or an analysis of instruments retrieved after clinical use. The latter type of study aims to determine factors relevant to the aging of instruments and devices during clinical service by using materials characterization techniques. Although the validity of results from these investigations is widely accepted, in vivo studies of endodontic instruments, devices, and materials have been limited.

This goal of this chapter is to present and analyze the results of a variety of investigations concerning the effects of intraoral use on a wide array of materials, instruments, and devices currently used in endodontic practice.

Rubber Dam Clamps

The rubber dam is used in root canal therapy to isolate a tooth or teeth and to prevent patients from inhaling or swallowing irrigants, medicaments, or instruments. The rubber dam also provides a clean and dry field and prevents contami-

nation of the working area by saliva. Although rubber dam clamps have been used for many years, there are no ISO or American National Standards Institute/American Dental Association (ANSI/ADA) standards for the production or laboratory testing of these devices.

Current commercial clamps are classified in two types according to the materials used in their fabrication. The first type is a plain carbon martensitic steel containing approximately 0.8% carbon (wt %), with Vickers hardness ranging from about 600 to 650.[1] The carbon steel clamps are electroplated in a nickel solution to provide a coating thickness of about 6.5 μm. The nickel coating is applied to promote corrosion resistance of the device. The second material is a martensitic stainless steel containing approximately 13.5% chromium, 1.0% molybdenum, 0.38% carbon, 0.55% manganese, and 0.40% silicon, with a Vickers hardness of about 525.[2] A United States government document[3] specifies a type 420 martensitic stainless steel[4] with minor differences in composition (12% to 14% chromium, a minimum 0.15% carbon, 1% manganese, 1% silicon, 0.04% phosphorus, and 0.03% sulfur).

Although the technique of applying these devices in the mouth is straightforward, the infrequent intraoral fracture of rubber dam clamps is of great concern, for the broken fragments tend to spring out of the mouth with considerable velocity and unpredictable direction. Previous studies[1,2,5] have proposed stress corrosion cracking (SCC) as the most likely fracture mechanism based upon the simultaneous occurrence of stress and corrosion observed in these devices during repeated clinical use. While this mechanism is a plausible source of failure, clinical evidence for the validity of this hypothesis does not currently exist. Nonetheless, the simultaneous effects of corrosion and relatively low stresses (which might be expected under typical clinical conditions) can lead to mechanically accelerated uniform corrosion.[6]

Macroscopic examination of clinically failed rubber dam clamps has shown that corrosion is the most detrimental process under clinical conditions and that the most frequently corroded area is the base, which is in direct contact with

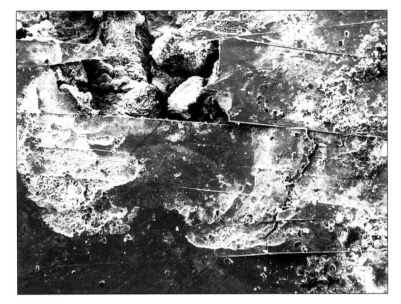

Fig 11-2a Scanning electron microscope (SEM) photograph showing a representative area from the base of a corroded rubber dam clamp after multiple uses in vivo. Corrosion is extensive on some areas of the nickel coating, which has been totally removed from the region in the upper left corner. Parallel fractured segments due to barrel plating when the coating was deposited are also evident (original magnification × 70).

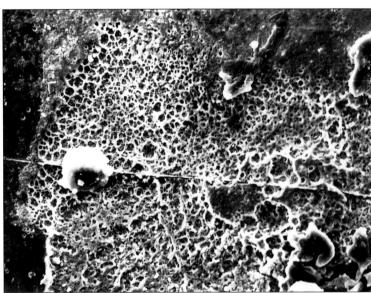

Fig 11-2b Higher-magnification SEM photograph of the corrosion pattern. The presence of an integument from the oral environment is evident (original magnification × 600).

irrigants, bleaches, detergents, and other fluids used in dentistry. This finding is in accordance with clinical observations,[1] where 17 to 21 rubber dam clamp fractures occurred when the acid-etch technique was used. Discoloration also is found on the bow surface of more extensively corroded clamps (Fig 11-1). Figure 11-2a shows corrosion on some areas of the coating on the base. The coating is totally removed from the upper left corner; the corrosion pattern in Fig 11-2b appears at higher magnification.

In endodontics, corrosive fluids mainly consist of H_2O_2, NaOCl (sodium hypochlorite), and ethylenediaminetetraacetic acid (EDTA). However, much more corrosive inorganic acids, such as H_3PO_4, used in restorative dentistry for etching tooth enamel, may cause significant corrosion of rubber dam clamps. Although nickel plating is used to improve the corrosion performance of carbon steel clamps, nickel is not resistant to environments containing chloride ions; additionally, nickel and its reaction products are toxic.[7]

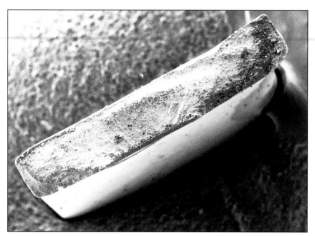

Fig 11-3 Scanning electron microscope photograph of the fracture surface of a rubber dam clamp that failed during its first clinical use. In the center of the figure, a pattern of cracks radiates from the groove mechanically engraved when this device was labeled (original magnification × 28).

Despite these disadvantages, nickel is widely used with organic additives to produce a very bright finish, even though these coatings are much more brittle than semibright finishes.[7] This brittle character may explain the cracks observed in the coatings of clinically fractured clamps.[1]

Although the use of stainless steel for fabricating these clamps has greatly improved corrosion resistance, compared to that of carbon steel clamps, the presence of chloride ions is considered the primary cause of pitting. However, it is not possible to establish a single critical chloride ion limit for each type of stainless steel because the corrosiveness of a particular concentration of chloride ions may be greatly affected by the presence or absence of other chemical species.[8] Therefore, keeping fluids as far as possible from the surface of a rubber dam clamp is recommended to minimize corrosion. A precaution against fracture would be instant replacement of a clamp when there is macroscopic evidence of discoloration. The strength of the clamp may be greatly reduced by the corrosive in vivo environment, but the decrease in strength with each clinical use of the device is as yet unknown.

Another type of failure found in rubber dam clamps appears in Fig 11-3, where a clamp with no evidence of corrosion fractured in a brittle manner during its first use. The cracks originated from the grooves produced by the mechanical engraving used to label the device. The labeling technique was previously implicated[9] in crack initiation and subsequent fatigue fracture of forged cobalt-chromium-molybdenum femoral stems. This behavior was attributed to residual stresses produced by thermal alterations in the alloy around the labeled region. The magnitude of these stresses is unknown, but brittle fracture has often occurred[10] in welded parts under external stresses far below the yield strength of the alloy. It is suggested that the use of mechanical engraving to label rubber dam clamps should be replaced by other techniques, such as electrochemical processes, that do not adversely affect the mechanical properties of the material.

Endodontic Files

R-type root canal rasps and barbed broaches are endodontic instruments dating from the nineteenth century, although their use in today's endodontic practice is limited. In 1901, carbon steel K-type files and reamers were introduced by the Kerr Manufacturing Company (currently Kerr Corporation, Division of Sybron International, Romulus, MI). These carbon steel instruments were progressively replaced by stainless steel instruments[11] for superior ductility and corrosion resistance. The aim of the K-type instrument manufacturing process was to promote endodontic cutting efficiency, but no major design changes in the instruments were made over the next few decades.

In 1961, the ISO initiated standardization of the taper and geometry of the cutting tip of these instruments. Meanwhile, further modifications were focused on the geometry of their cross sections to improve flexibility and cutting efficiency. These modifications resulted in the introduction of different types of stainless steel instruments, such as improved hand instruments (conventional K-files, H-files, and K-reamers), medium-size instruments with greater flexibility (with or without a cutting tip), new hybrid-type instruments (Flex-R file, Moyco Union Broach, York, PA; Unifile,

Dentsply Maillefer, Ballaigues, Switzerland; and Helifile, Micro-Mega, Besancon, Cedex, France), and new designs (Canal Master Instruments, Brasseler, Savannah, GA).[12] The recent introduction of the nickel-titanium (Ni-Ti), nitinol-type, alloy as an alternative material for production of Ni-Ti endodontic files significantly increases their flexibility.[12,13] New engine-driven rotary cutting instruments with modified tapers, U-shaped cross sections, and flat outer edges known as "radial-land"[14] have been introduced.

The techniques for manufacturing these root canal instruments are of considerable importance. In the original fabrication process for K-files, tapered ground-wire blanks that have square, triangular, or rhomboid cross sections are prepared and then twisted counterclockwise.[12] This step of the manufacturing process accounts for the limited ductility of K-type instruments in counterclockwise torsion. In contrast, some newer K-type instruments and the Hedstrom files (H-files) are made by machine grinding from round-wire blanks.[12] Recently, a computer-assisted manufacturing (CAM) process has been used for the production of K-files.[15] This method facilitates the development of new instruments with a variable number of flutes per unit of length or a variable core thickness along the axis of the instrument, which can have considerable effect on the instrument's flexibility and cutting performance. Despite improvements in the design, manufacturing, and materials of endodontic files, even infrequent instrument fracture during clinical use endangers the success of endodontic therapy and remains the major problem in chemomechanical preparation of root canals.

Hedstrom Files

Fractured or extensively used Hedstrom files (H-files) of ISO sizes 20 to 40 were collected from different dental clinics and examined by means of optical microscopy and SEM. Figure 11-4 shows an optical microscope photograph of a polished cross section of a representative extensively used (but not fractured) H-file. Cracks are mostly located at the flute regions. While these cracks vary in size, they are oriented perpendicularly to the

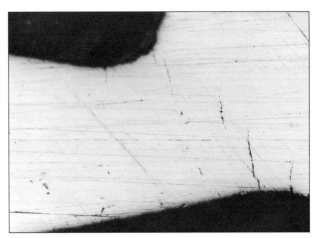

Fig 11-4 Optical microscope photograph of a representative region on the surface of an H-file where no abnormalities were observed after multiple uses in vivo. However, cracks are evident on the flutes of this file at the magnification of this figure (original magnification × 50).

long axis of the flutes. No evidence of such cracks or other manufacturing defects were found at the same magnification on the surfaces of the as-received H-files that were prepared for metallographic examination in the same manner (Fig 11-5).

The fracture surface of an H-file that failed during clinical use has a rough morphology when viewed at higher magnification with the SEM, and the machining grooves on the shaft of the instrument are also prominent (Fig 11-6). At the magnification of Fig 11-6, the dimpled-rupture morphology[16] characteristic of ductile fracture cannot be observed. The location, direction, and shape of the cracks within clinically fractured H-files were found to vary, depending on the observation level. This is clearly shown in the microcomputerized tomographic images of a fractured H-file (Fig 11-7), where two-dimensional reconstructed images taken at outer (Fig 11-7a) and middle longitudinal planes (Fig 11-7b) are presented.

Propagation of cracks must have occurred during extensive clinical use to cause failure of these H-files. There are two possible origins of the cracks in Figs 11-6 and 11-7. Machining grooves introduced during manufacture of these instruments and of rotary endodontic instruments[17-19] provide a myriad of sites for fracture initiation. Moreover, extension of the cracks into the depths

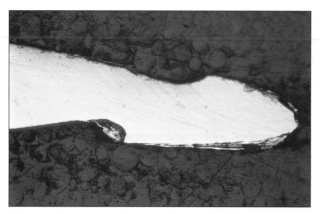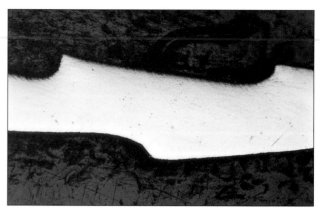

Fig 11-5 Two optical microscope photographs of the surface of an as-received H-file that does not exhibit structural defects, such as cracks or pores. These photographs should be compared with the photograph of the clinically used H-file in Fig 11-4 that was taken at the same original magnification (original magnification × 50).

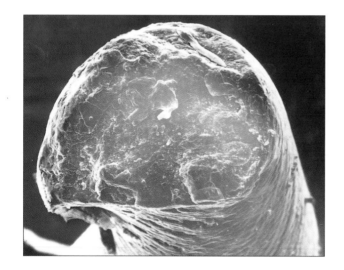

Fig 11-6 Scanning electron microscope photograph of the rough fracture surface of an H-file that failed after multiple clinical uses. A dimpled-rupture morphology characteristic of ductile fracture (see Fig 11-9) cannot be observed at this magnification. The array of surface grooves on the side of the instrument shaft arise from the machining process used to fabricate the instrument (original magnification × 390).

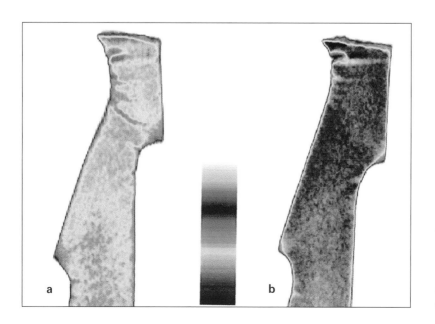

Fig 11-7 Two-dimensional x-ray microtomography images of an H-file that fractured after multiple clinical uses: *(a)* longitudinal plane at outer part (original magnification × 120); *(b)* longitudinal plane at middle part (original magnification × 120). *Bar* in center demonstrates the x-ray adsorption coefficient.

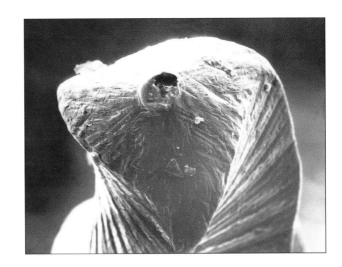

Fig 11-8 Scanning electron microscope photograph of the fracture surface of a stainless steel K-file with a triangular cross section after multiple uses in vivo. The surface is characterized by a symmetrical pattern of cracks that is oriented approximately perpendicular to the sides (cutting edges) of the triangular cross section and ends at a small circular feature at the center of the cross section. At this magnification, no dimpled-rupture morphology indicative of ductile fracture can be observed. This fracture pattern is produced by fatigue in torsion under low nominal stresses (original magnification × 420).

of the flutes may be attributed to the abrupt decrease in the cross-sectional diameter, which acts as a stress concentration factor, facilitating both crack initiation and propagation. In addition, there may be bulk microstructural features that serve as fracture initiation sites. Further fractographic analyses and detailed microstructural investigations will be required for unambiguous interpretation of the failure process in these instruments.

Although crack initiation and propagation may imply a fatigue failure mechanism for the H-files after extensive clinical use, the characteristic striations[16] associated with fatigue fracture under repeated loading were not observed. It is possible that these characteristic patterns may be eliminated by mutual attrition of the crack sides during instrumentation, or they may deteriorate by some corrosion process(es) during chemomechanical instrumentation, chemical disinfection, or sterilization. The presence of corrosion products is well-known in fractographic studies to hinder observation of certain details of the fracture surface, such as striations due to fatigue.[20]

Although no evidence of general corrosion, pitting, or other types of corrosion was found on the cutting surfaces of the fractured H-files, crevice corrosion might be activated after the introduction of cracks. While detailed mechanisms are presently conjectural, the mechanical stresses on the instruments during clinical use may interact with the biological environment, which could alter the fracture mechanism from conventional fatigue failure to corrosion fatigue (CF), SCC, or hydrogen embrittlement (HE). These mechanisms can be interrelated and may occur simultaneously during clinical use. Although classic CF cracking and SCC failures can be distinguished[21] by SEM examination, the characteristic surface patterns were not present on the observed fractured H-files. Fatigue or CF cracks have a more direct path of propagation, whereas cracks arising from SCC have a branched structure. Moreover, SCC and HE more often take place under static loading, whereas the cyclic loading conditions encountered in clinical use are more favorable for CF.[22] While fatigue or CF may be possible failure mechanisms for H-files during clinical use, further research is necessary to confirm this hypothesis.

Stainless Steel K-Files

Figure 11-8 shows the fracture surface of a representative clinically failed stainless steel K-file with a triangular cross section. Many cracks equally distributed over the fracture surface extend from the cutting edges to the circular feature in the center of the cross section. Because the greatest shear stresses during torsion are at the periphery of the cross section[23] and the likely locations of fracture initiation are at sites of machining damage along this periphery, it would be expected that crack propagation is directed toward the circular feature, which may have been caused by the spalling of material. At the SEM magnification used in Fig 11-8, the dimpled-rupture morphology characteristic[16–19] of ductile fracture cannot be seen, although the overall largely flat fracture surface suggests[16] a relatively ductile character for the failure. It is possible that residual stresses in the instrument arising from the manufacturing process were superimposed on the mechanical stresses applied during clinical use of the instrument to initiate the crack propagation. Comparison with published[20] fracture surfaces of metals suggests that the fracture pattern in Fig 11-8 was produced by torsional loading of the instrument under relatively low nominal stresses, ie, much less than the yield strength of the alloy. Further examination of the fracture surfaces of a variety of clinically failed K-files from several different manufacturers (including instruments fabricated by both twisting and grinding processes) is needed. These observations will provide insight into the different mechanisms for fracture initiation and propagation in these instruments (including a possible role for fatigue failure) that may occur in endodontic practice.

Ni-Ti Files

Quite different fracture mechanisms were observed for clinically failed files that were fabricated from Ni-Ti. A representative fracture surface for one of these instruments is shown in Fig 11-9. The center of the cross section is dominated by shallow dimples characteristic of ductile fracture[16] while a small area of the upper left corner of the cross section appears to contain some parallel planar features that may be indicative of cleavage fracture. These dimples on the fracture surface of Ni-Ti instruments are much shallower than the dimples that have been observed[17–19] on the fracture surfaces of rotary stainless steel instruments. This may be due to the much lower elastic modulus of Ni-Ti, resulting in less local permanent torsional deformation at the dimples for the stress at which fracture occurs (WA Brantley, personal communication, Nov 2000). At the relatively low magnification of Fig 11-9, it

is not possible to identify a fracture initiation site, such as might be expected at the periphery of the cross section where surface flaws are introduced by the grinding process used for instrument fabrication; the machining grooves are evident at the lower right corner of the cross section.

Figure 11-10a shows the overall complex fracture surface of a clinically failed Ni-Ti file with a U-shaped cross section. Figure 11-10b is a higher magnification photograph of the region near the edge at the left-center of the fracture surface in Fig 11-10a, showing in greater detail a series of striations that might be associated with the crack propagation process[16] occurring during cyclic fatigue failure. Neither Fig 11-10a nor Fig 11-10b shows areas of dimpled rupture, suggesting that this instrument experienced relatively brittle fracture during clinical use, a conclusion supported[16] by the overall nonplanar nature of the fracture surface. It is possible that fracture initiation and propagation were influenced[20] by stress concentrations associated with defects (cracks or microstructural flaws) in the Ni-Ti alloy. The quality of the parent metal and the manufacturing process are both critical factors associated with the clinical success of the Ni-Ti instruments.

The fracture mechanisms for endodontic files seem to be associated principally with the mechanical properties of the alloys (stainless steel and Ni-Ti) used for their fabrication, although there may be some differences for stainless steel files manufactured by twisting the tapered ground-wire blank compared to directly grinding the cross-section configuration and flutes. Examination of clinically fractured instruments by SEM has shown that files fabricated from the two different alloys, but having essentially the same cross sections (triangular stainless steel K-files and U-shaped Ni-Ti files), exhibited quite different fracture mechanisms. Therefore, the effect of cross-section geometry on the fracture mechanism seems to be much less important than the mechanical properties of the alloy used to fabricate the instrument. The much greater flexibility of the Ni-Ti files compared to stainless steel files of the same size and geometry is due to the considerably lower modulus of elasticity of Ni-Ti[13,24] (Table 11-1). Consequently, the Ni-Ti files can

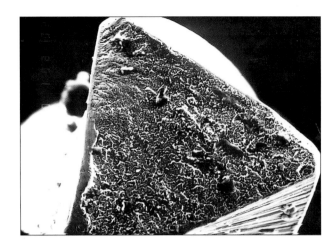

Fig 11-9 Scanning electron microscope photograph of a representative fracture surface for a clinically failed Ni-Ti file. Shallow dimples, particularly in the center of the cross section, are the characteristic surface pattern produced by ductile fracture, which yields a macroscopically flat fracture surface. Parallel fracture planes that appear to be present in the small area at the upper left corner of the cross section suggest that cleavage fracture may have occurred in this region (original magnification × 240).

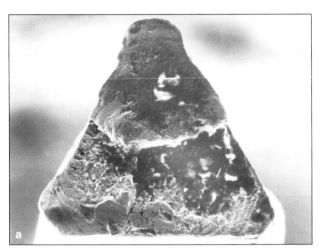
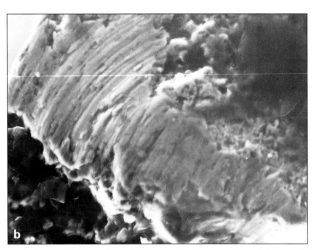

Fig 11-10 Scanning electron microscope photographs of a clinically failed Ni-Ti file with a U-shaped cross section. *(a)* Overall fracture surface morphology (original magnification × 240). *(b)* Higher magnification view of surface striations, assumed to arise from fatigue failure, that lie in the direction from the center to the periphery of the cross section. The failure process may be associated with structural defects in the bulk Ni-Ti alloy (original magnification × 1,250).

easily follow the curved root canals, avoiding severe stress concentrations that would result in clinical failure. Unfortunately, the yield strength of the Ni-Ti alloy also is much lower than that for stainless steel (see Table 11-1), so that the Ni-Ti file is more susceptible to catastrophic fracture when constrained in the root canal during clinical instrumentation.

From a clinical standpoint, knowledge of the fundamental fracture mechanisms for the stainless steel and Ni-Ti files can be of great practical importance. Although conclusive proof presently is not available for either the H-files or K-files, when stainless steel files undergo progressive mechanical degradation due to fatigue failure, instrument fracture is inevitable after some number of

Table 11-1 Approximate mechanical properties of materials used for the production of endodontic files*

Material	Modulus of Elasticity (GPa)	Yield strength (0.1%) (MPa)
Austenitic stainless steel	200	1,400
Ni-Ti	40	190

*Data from Mueller.[24]

chemomechanical root canal preparations. The occurrence of such failures would depend upon several instrument factors (eg, differences in file diameter, cross-section geometry, and manufacturing techniques), variations in root canal preparation techniques among clinicians, and other factors that cause stress development during instrumentation. Unfortunately, because fatigue cracks propagate without observable plastic deformation, there would be no macroscopic evidence to warn clinicians about the extent of mechanical degradation. This may explain the seemingly accidental fracture of stainless steel cutting instruments with no visual evidence of permanent shape deterioration.

In contrast, while additional studies are needed to establish the fundamental failure mechanism(s) for the Ni-Ti files, the present SEM observations of clinically failed instruments suggest that catastrophic failure occurs during instrumentation whenever the local stress in the root canal exceeds the fracture strength of the Ni-Ti alloy, rather than failure caused by some progressive fatigue process. The fracture strength of the Ni-Ti alloy would exceed its yield strength and depend upon the work-hardening characteristics of the particular alloy used to fabricate the instruments as well as upon details of the manufacturing process. Consequently, clinicians utilizing Ni-Ti files should carefully adjust their handling of these instruments to minimize the possibility of failure.

Solid-Core Filling Materials

Numerous materials, such as dental amalgams, gold foil, silver points, gutta-percha, and pharmaceutical pastes, have been used in endodontics to fill root canals. In recent decades, gutta-percha has been the most commonly selected solid-core filling material while the utilization of silver points has been progressively more limited. The gutta-percha formulation used in endodontic therapy is a partially crystalline viscoelastic material consisting of gutta-percha, ZnO, waxes, coloring and antioxidation agents, and opacifiers.[12] It is totally soluble in chloroform and halothane, but less so in other commonly used solvents.

Silver points have been used since 1920 because of their ease of handling, ready availability, and bacteriocidal effect, called their "oligodynamic property."[11] The silver points contain 98 to 99 wt % silver, with traces of nickel and copper. It is well known that silver points corrode in the root canal, and tissue fluids are considered the main corrosive factor. Experimental studies have shown that the corrosion products of silver points exhibit cytotoxicity in fibroblast cultures, and their involvement in the inflammation of periapical tissues has been hypothesized.[25,26] In vitro studies using curved root canals showed significantly less apical leakage in canals filled with silver points compared with those filled with gutta-

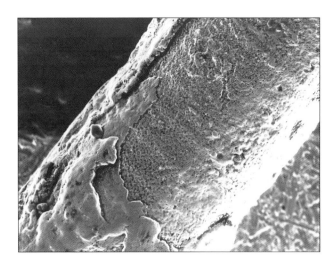

Fig 11-11 Corrosion pattern of a retrieved silver point after clinical use consists of surface pitting, limited notching, and small shallow craters (original magnification × 200).

percha,[27,28] and corroded silver points appear to be well tolerated in implantation studies.[29–32] However, in vitro studies are unable to answer questions about silver points that are pertinent to in vivo processes, such as:

- Is corrosion common for silver points after obturation?
- Which of the following is the main cause of the corrosion of silver points in vivo: tissue fluids, irrigating solution, eugenol, or sealers?
- Do the corrosion products of silver points cause failure of endodontic therapy?

Silver points were removed from teeth that had been treated endodontically 3 to 11 years previously and evaluated clinically and radiographically for success or failure using the clinical criteria of pain, swelling, sinus tract involvement, and radiographic evidence of a periapical lesion.[33] All silver points that were examined presented evidence of moderate to severe corrosion. The corrosion pattern was predominantly surface pitting, accompanied by limited notching and small shallow craters (Fig 11-11). The elements identified on the surfaces of silver-point tips (Fig 11-12a) using x-ray energy-dispersive spectroscopic analysis with the SEM were the following: sulfur (Fig 11-12b) from tissue fluids and sealer cements, as sulfur is also incorporated in endodontic cements as $BaSO_4$ for radiopacity; calcium and phosphorus (Figure 11-12c) originating from dentin and irri-

gating solutions; zinc and barium (Fig 11-12d), which are found in cements; and iron and vanadium (Fig 11-12e), which probably detached from root canal instruments. Electron spectroscopy for chemical analysis (ESCA), also known as XPS or x-ray photoelectron spectroscopy, of the silver points revealed the presence of carbon, nitrogen, and oxygen. An interesting finding was that the corrosion zone in silver points removed from failed cases was approximately 15 µm from the outer surface, contained numerous pits and fissures (Fig 11-13a), and was rich in sulfur, with an increasing concentration from the surface toward the bulk material. This pattern was not found in the silver points removed from successful cases (Fig 11-13b).

In addition, ESCA detected nitrogen in the form of N_2O_2 and NH/NH_2 binding phases on silver points in failed cases. An important difference between the successful and failed cases was the presence of these two nitrogen-containing phases. It is known that sulfate-reducing and nitrate-reducing bacteria affect considerably the corrosion of different alloys.[34,35] These anaerobic bacteria are aggressive and may induce inflammation. Thus, silver points are corroded in root canals due to handling factors, irrigant solutions, and sealers, whereas the presence of anaerobic bacteria is a potential factor not only for the induction of inflammation but also for the corrosion process.

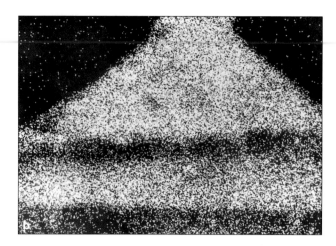

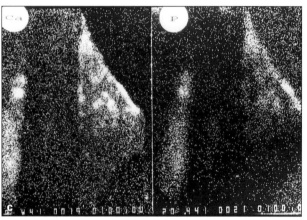

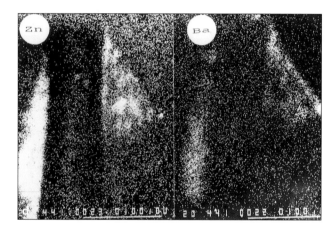

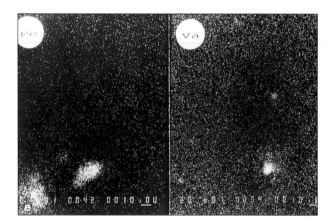

Fig 11-12 Scanning electron microscope photographs of a silver point removed after successful endodontic treatment. *(a)* Secondary electron image; *(b–e)* characteristic x-ray area scans for specific elements: sulfur *(b)*, calcium and phosphorus *(c)*, zinc and barium *(d)*, and iron and vanadium *(e)*.

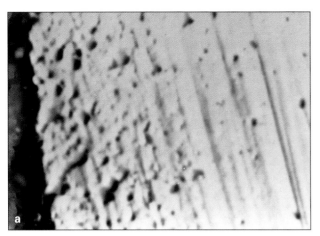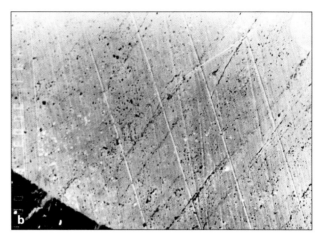

Fig 11-13 Scanning electron microscope photographs of the cross section of retrieved silver points. *(a)* From a failed endodontic case. A large number of fissures and pits can be seen (original magnification × 3,000). *(b)* From a successful endodontic case. The parallel grooves were created during the sectioning process to prepare the specimen (original magnification × 440).

Sealers

Sealer materials are routinely used to provide a hermetic seal in the obturating process for endodontically treated teeth. The function of these materials is to fill the voids between the dentin walls and the solid-core filling materials. They may be grouped on the basis of their mode of application and setting characteristics: Sealers are used in conjunction with a solid-core material (Grossman's sealer); cements are used to fill the entire canal, whether in setting form (Endo-methazone) or a nonsetting paste (calcium hydroxide).[36] Another classification is provided by ANSI/ADA specification 57, where type I cements are used with three different classes of core materials and type II filling materials are used with neither core materials nor the four classes of cements.

The most common endodontic sealers in current use are based upon zinc oxide–eugenol formulations. However, there are noneugenol sealers, such as Kloroperka N-O (Oriola, Espoo, Finland); Diaket (ESPE, Seefeld, Germany), an organic polyketone compound; AH-26 (Dentsply DeTrey, Zurich, Switzerland), an epoxy resin; and Ketac-Endo (ESPE), a glass-ionomer cement. Setting of these materials is achieved either by chemical reaction or polymerization within the root canal. The clinically relevant properties of the sealer materials are flow, film thickness, working time, setting time, dimensional alterations, radiopacity, solubility, and disintegration. Although clinical considerations dictate desirable levels of these properties, the available commercial products only partially meet these goals.

Many investigators have reported the cytoxicity of zinc oxide–eugenol cements and other sealers for periapical tissues, but no difference could be shown when the healing of apical periodontitis over a 3-year period was compared for different root canal sealers.[37] Uncured eugenol was released from zinc oxide–eugenol mixtures, which are subject to hydrolysis, and it is believed that eugenol is toxic to the periapical tissues. However, a recent study[38] reported that the level of eugenol released was very low and decreased over time. The immediate concentration was 10^{-4} to 10^{-5}, the one-day concentration was 10^{-5} to 10^{-6}, and after 1 month the concentration of eugenol was undetectable.

In closing, it is worthwhile to emphasize again that despite the usefulness of in vitro laboratory evaluations, only in vivo studies can provide evidence for the detrimental behavior of endodontic materials during clinical use. Nevertheless, information from laboratory tests can be used for the development of improved endodontic products and instruments, including new materials and geometric designs. It is particularly important to determine the basic failure mechanisms of these materials and instruments so that their clinical performance may be optimized by more efficient manipulation and clinical techniques.

References

1. Jedynakiewicz NM, Cunnigham J. Acid-etching and the fracture of rubber dam clamps. Br Dent J 1985;159:121–123.

2. Sutton J, Saunders WP. Effect of various irrigant and autoclaving regimes on the fracture resistance of rubber dam clamps. Int Endod J 1996;29:335–343.

3. Medical Procurement Item Description #2-27, January 1983. Cited in Svec TA, Powers JM, Ladd GD. Hardness and stress-corrosion of rubber dam clamps. J Endod 1997;23: 397–398.

4. Davis JR. Selection of wrought martensitic stainless steels. In: Olson DL, Siewert TA, Liu S, Edwards GL (eds). Welding, Brazing, and Soldering. ASM Handbook, vol 6. Materials Park, OH: ASM International, 1993:432–442.

5. Svec TA, Powers JM, Ladd GD. Hardness and stress-corrosion of rubber dam clamps. J Endod 1997;23:397–398.

6. Skoulikidis TN. Applied Electrochemistry. Athens, Greece: Symmetry Publications, 1991.

7. Mazia J, Lashmore DS. Electroplated coatings. In: Korb LJ, Olson DL (eds). Corrosion. ASM Handbook, vol 13. Materials Park, OH: ASM International, 1987:419–431.

8. Davidson RM, DeBold T, Johnson MJ. Corrosion of stainless steel. In: Korb LJ, Olson DL (eds). Corrosion. ASM Handbook, vol 13. Materials Park, OH: ASM International, 1987:547–565.

9. Woolson ST, Milbauer JP, Bobyn JD, Yue S, Maloney WJ. Fatigue fracture of a forged cobalt-chromium-molybdenum femoral component inserted with cement: A report of ten cases. J Bone Joint Surg Am 1997;79:1842–1848.

10. Masubuchi K. Residual stresses and distortion. In: Olson DL, Siewert TA, Liu S, Edwards GL (eds). Welding, Brazing, and Soldering. ASM Handbook, vol 6. Materials Park, OH: ASM International, 1993:1094–1102.

11. Guide to Dental Materials and Devices, ed 8. Chicago: American Dental Association, 1978:171, 184.

12. Miserendino LJ. Materials and devices. In: Cohen S, Burns RC (eds). Pathways of the Pulp, ed. 5. St. Louis: Mosby, 1991:388–399.

13. Walia H, Brantley WA, Gerstein H. An initial investigation of the bending and torsional properties of nitinol root canal files. J Endod 1988;14:346–351.

14. Thompson SA, Dummer PM. Shaping ability of ProFile .04 Taper Series 29 rotary nickel-titanium instruments in simulated root canals. Part 1. Int Endod J 1997;30:1–7.

15. Spangberg L. Endodontic treatment of teeth without apical periodontitis. In: Ørstravik D, Pitt Ferd TR (eds). Essential Endodontology. Oxford: Blackwell Science, 1998:217–221.

16. Dieter GE. Mechanical Metallurgy, ed. 3. New York: McGraw-Hill, 1986:394–398.

17. Luebke NH, Brantley WA. Torsional and metallurgical properties of rotary endodontic instruments. II. Stainless steel Gates Glidden drills. J Endod 1991;17:319–323.

18. Brantley WA, Luebke NH, Luebke FL, Mitchell JC. Performance of engine-driven rotary endodontic instruments with a superimposed bending deflection. V. Gates Glidden and Peeso drills. J Endod 1994;20:241–245.

19. Luebke NH, Brantley WA, Sabri ZI, Luebke FL, Lausten LL. Physical dimensions, torsional performance, bending properties and metallurgical characteristics of rotary endodontic instruments. VI. Canal Master drills. J Endod 1995;21: 259–263.

20. Vander Voort GF. Visual examination and light microscopy. In: Mills K (ed). Fractography. ASM Handbook, vol 12. Materials Park, OH: ASM International, 1987:91–165.

21. Sprowls DO. Evaluation of corrosion fatigue. In: Korb LJ, Olson DL (eds). Corrosion. ASM Handbook, vol 13. Materials Park, OH: ASM International, 1987:291.

22. Fraker AC. Corrosion of metallic implants and prosthetic devices. In: Korb LJ, Olson DL (eds). Corrosion. ASM Handbook, vol 13. Materials Park, OH: ASM International, 1987: 1324–1335.

23. Craig RG, McIlwain ED, Peyton FA. Comparison of theoretical and experimental bending and torsional moments of endodontic files and reamers. J Dent Res 1967;46:1058–1063.

24. Mueller HJ. Tarnish and corrosion of dental alloys. In: Korb LJ, Olson DL (eds). Corrosion. ASM Handbook, vol 13. Materials Park, OH: ASM International, 1987:1338.

25. Brady J, del Rio C. Corrosion of endodontic silver cones in humans: a scanning electron microscopy and x-ray microprobe study. J Endod 1975;1:205–210.

26. Seltzer S, Green DB, Weiner N, DeRenzis F. A scanning electron microscope examination of silver cones removed from endodontically treated teeth. Oral Surg 1972;33:589–605.

27. Vaughn DW. A Comparison of the Apical Seal of Silver Points to That of Gutta-percha in Finely Curved Root Canals [master's thesis]. Lexington: Univ of Kentucky, College of Dentistry, 1977.

28. Timpawat S, Jensen J, Feigal RJ, Messer HH. An in vitro study of the comparative effectiveness of obturating curved root canals with gutta-percha cones, silver cones and stainless steel files. Oral Surg Oral Med Oral Pathol 1983;55: 180–185.

29. Feldman NG, Nyborg H. Tissue reaction to root filling materials. II. A comparison of implants of silver and root filling materials AH-26 in rabbits' jaws. Odontol Revy 1964;15:33–40.

30. Zielke DR, Brady JM, del Rio CE. Corrosion of silver cones in bone: A scanning electron microscope and microprobe analysis. J Endod 1975;1:356–360.

31. Holland R, Souza V, Nery MJ, Mello W, Bernabe PFE, Otoboni FJA. Reaction of rat connective tissue to guttapercha and silver points: A long-term histological study. Aust Dent J 1982;27:224–226.

32. Zmener O, Dominguez FV. Corrosion of silver cones in the subcutaneous connective tissue of the rat: a preliminary scanning electron microscope, electron microprobe and histological study. J Endod 1985;11:55–61.

33. Margelos J, Eliades G, Palaghias G. Corrosion pattern of silver points in vivo. J Endod 1991;6:282–287.

34. Palaghias G, Soremark R, Nord C-E. Effect of Bacteroides corrodens on some dental alloys [abstract 105]. J Dent Res 1981;61:576.

35. Palaghias G, Soremark R. The electrochemical properties of three amalgam alloys in cultures of Streptococcus mutans [abstract 104]. J Dent Res 1984;63:583.

36. Ørstravik D. Properties of root canal sealers: measurements of flow, working time, and compressive strength. Int Endod J 1983;16:99–107.

37. Eriksen M, Ørstravik D, Kerekes K. Healing of apical periodontitis after endodontic treatment using three different root canal sealers. Endont Dent Traumatol 1988;4:114–117.

38. Hashieh IA, Pommel L, Camps J. Concentration of eugenol apically released from zinc oxide–eugenol-based sealers. J Endod 1999;25:713–715.

Section VI

ORAL AND MAXILLOFACIAL SURGERY

Aging of Stainless Steel Oral and Maxillofacial Surgical Implants

Elliott J. Sutow, PhD, MEd

Composition, Metallurgy, and Standards for Implants

Stainless steel is a term that represents a broad group of corrosion-resistant alloys of iron and chromium. These steels contain at least 11% chromium, with or without other elements.[1] Stainless steels may be divided into five families, four of which are based on the predominant phase constituent of their microstructure–martensite, ferrite, austenite, and austenite and ferrite (duplex). The fifth family consists of the precipitation-hardened stainless steels, which require heat treatment. The austenitic stainless steels generally have greater corrosion resistance than the other microstructures.[2] They may be supplied in the annealed, hot-forged, or cold-worked condition. Wrought stainless steels are identified by a three-digit code, established by the American Iron and Steel Institute (AISI). Stainless steel for surgical implantation is primarily used in the wrought form (eg, wires, miniplates, and screws). Austenitic steels that contain nickel as the primary austenite stabilizer are the AISI type 300 series,[3] which includes type 316L (Table 12-1), the most commonly used stainless steel for implantation applications.[4] The letter *L* denotes extra-low carbon content. The well-known wrought 18-8 stainless steels (18% chromium, 8% nickel) are exemplified by type 304.

Cast stainless steels are coded differently, according to the Steel Founders' Society of America.[1] In this code, the letter *C* indicates that the alloy is intended primarily for corrosion service, and the letter *H* denotes high-temperature service. Cast alloy compositions differ somewhat from their wrought counterparts in that they use higher silicon content to increase castability. The microstructures of these alloys may also differ. For example, CF-3M stainless steel nominally corresponds to AISI type 316L and contains ferrite in an austenite structure.[2]

Duplex stainless steels are some of the newest stainless steel alloys for biomedical application. The basic duplex alloy contains 28% chromium, 6% nickel,[2] and usually equal amounts of austenite and ferrite. (Weight percentages are used throughout this chapter for the elemental components.) Other elements (nitrogen, molybdenum, copper, silicon, or tungsten) may be added to control the balance of ferrite and austenite and to improve corrosion resistance. Some of these alloys have been tested and are reported to have better corrosion resistance and mechanical properties for orthopedic and osteosynthetic applications than type 316L stainless steel.[5,6] Additional ways of identifying stainless steels are the Unified Numbering System (UNS), compositional abbreviations, proprietary designations, and trademarks.[7]

Table 12-1 Wrought stainless steel chemical requirements for AISI type 316L, and for ASTM standards F 138-97 (bar and wire), F 139-96 (sheet and strip), and F 1350-96 (fixation wire)*

ELEMENT	COMPOSITION, %	
	Type 316L	F 138-97/F 139-96/F 1350-96
Carbon	0.030 max	0.030 max
Manganese	2.00 max	2.00 max
Phosphorus	0.045 max	0.025 max
Sulfur	0.030 max	0.010 max
Silicon	1.00 max	0.75 max
Chromium	16.00–18.00	17.00–19.00
Nickel	10.00–14.00	13.00–15.00
Molybdenum	2.00–3.00	2.25–3.00
Nitrogen	–	0.10 max
Copper	–	0.50 max
Iron	Balance	Balance

*Reproduced from American Society for Testing and Materials[15] with permission.

Although the addition of chromium has the greatest effect on corrosion resistance, other alloying elements are used to enhance corrosion behavior or to modify phase equilibria or metallurgical structure to meet specific application requirements. Among the most important alloying elements are carbon, nickel, molybdenum, and nitrogen. Various texts describe in depth the effects of alloying additions and the associated phase diagrams.[7,8] A brief overview of the corrosion behavior of stainless steel used for oral and maxillofacial surgical implantation will be presented in this chapter.

The pure elements iron (at room temperature) and chromium have a body-centered cubic (bcc) crystal structure.[3] The binary Fe-Cr phase diagram is dominated by alpha (α) ferrite, which has the bcc structure (Fig 12-1). A face-centered cubic (fcc) austenite (γ) phase region, which forms a so-called γ-loop, exists in the temperature range between 840° and 1,400°C and has a maximum chromium content of 10.7% at 1,075°C. The third region of major interest contains the sigma (σ) phase, which is a nonstoichiometric Fe-Cr compound. The σ region exists up to 821°C and at chromium percentages beyond those for the γ-loop. Restricting chromium in stainless steels to between 12% and 25% gives adequate corrosion resistance while avoiding the embrittling precipitation of the σ phase.

Carbon is a strong austenite stabilizer, and its addition to the Fe-Cr alloy system expands the size of the γ-loop to higher chromium percentages. Nickel, which in the pure element form has the fcc structure, is also a strong austenitizing element and expands the γ-loop toward both higher chromium contents and lower temperatures. The percentages of chromium and nickel in the Fe-Cr-Ni alloy system are balanced to help maintain a fully austenitic structure. The γ-loop does not extend to ambient temperatures, but the austenite structure is retained in practice because of its very slow rate of transformation at low temperatures.[3] Nitrogen is an austenite stabilizer and can be substituted for nickel. The addition of nitrogen reduces the possibility of precipitating the σ phase and improves the pitting and crevice corrosion resistance of molybdenum-containing austenitic stainless steels.[7] Molybdenum is second only to chromium in enhancing resistance to pitting and crevice corrosion, but the amount of molybdenum is normally restricted to < 3.5% to avoid σ-phase formation. In addition, molybdenum is a ferrite stabilizer that must be compensated for by decreasing the chromium content and increasing the nickel content. In austenitic stainless steel, manganese can be used to reduce the nickel content.

Certain austenitic stainless steels, such as type 316 (0.08% carbon), may be subject to intergranular corrosion due to precipitation of chromium or chromium-molybdenum carbides at grain boundaries when heated in or cooled through the temperature range of 480° to 815°C.[1] This temperature range may be achieved during hot-forging or welding operations. The area adjacent to the grain boundaries becomes depleted of chromium, which results in a smaller passive range and lower pitting potentials.[3] The affected material is said to be *sensitized*. Intergranular corrosion was reported sometimes for older stainless steel implants.[9] However, it should be virtually eliminated by modern metallurgic practices and fabrication techniques and by reducing the carbon content to a maximum of 0.03% (type 316L stainless steel; ASTM Standard F 138) or stabilizing the alloy with additions of carbon scavengers (titanium, niobium, or niobium plus tantalum).[1]

In the production of implant-quality stainless steel ingots, typical melting practice involves electric arc melting to produce an electrode, followed by argon-oxygen decarburization (AOD) and premium remelting (eg, vacuum arc remelting [VAR]) of the electrode.[10] Carbon is introduced naturally during the steel-making process. The AOD process, introduced in the 1970s, revolutionized steel making by allowing carbon to be reduced to very low levels while the percentage of other elements could be controlled within very narrow limits.[11] The use of remelted material improves alloy homogeneity and microcleanliness, which can enhance corrosion resistance.[12,13] Pitting corrosion is typically initiated at nonmetallic inclusions. Sulfide inclusions are particularly prone to attack,[14] but oxide inclusions are

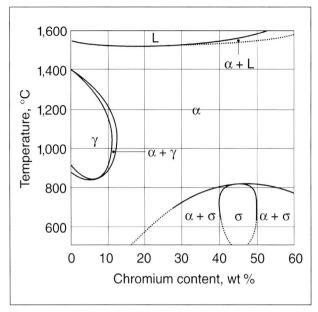

Fig 12-1 Binary Fe-Cr equilibrium phase diagram. (Reproduced from Davis[1] with permission from ASM International.)

also sites of original attack, though less active than sulfides.

The American Society for Testing and Materials (ASTM) is one of several organizations that set guidelines for standardization of medical and surgical implant alloys.[15] The ASTM stainless steel designations, which are designed in part to maximize corrosion resistance, are F 138-97, F 139-96, F 621-97, F 745-95, F 1314-95, F 1350-96, and F 1586-95. The last two digits of each designation indicate the standard's year of introduction. The specifications in standard F 138 for "Wrought 18 Chromium-14 Nickel-2.5 Molybdenum Stainless Steel Bar and Wire for Surgical Implants," for example, include producing an austenitic microstructure that is fine-grained, free of ferrite (at magnification × 100), and low in micro-inclusion content. The composition requirements for type 316L stainless steel, as well as for F 138 and other ASTM standards, are shown in Tables 12-1 to 12-3. The chemical composition requirements of ASTM F 138 include the pitting resistance equivalent (PRE), where %Cr + 3.3 × (%Mo) ≥ 26. The PRE is an empirical relationship whose use is intended to maximize resistance

Table 12-2 Cast and solution-annealed stainless steel chemical requirements in ASTM standard F 745-95*

ELEMENT	COMPOSITION, %	
	Minimum	Maximum
Carbon	–	0.06
Manganese	–	2.0
Phosphorous	–	0.045
Sulfur	–	0.030
Silicon	–	1.0
Chromium	17.00	19.00
Nickel	11.00	14.00
Molybdenum	2.00	3.00
Iron	Balance	Balance

*Reproduced from American Society for Testing and Materials[15] with permission.

Table 12-3 Wrought nitrogen-strengthened stainless steel chemical requirements in F 1314-95 (bar and wire) and F 1586-95 (bar)*

ELEMENT	COMPOSITION, %	
	F 1314-95	F 1586-95
Carbon	0.030 max	0.08 max
Manganese	4.00–6.00	2.00–4.25
Phosphorus	0.025 max	0.025 max
Sulfur	0.010 max	0.01 max
Silicon	0.75 max	0.75 max
Chromium	20.50–23.50	19.5–22.0
Nickel	11.50–13.50	9.0–11.0
Molybdenum	2.00–3.00	2.0–3.0
Nitrogen	0.20–0.40	0.25–0.5
Niobium	0.10–0.30	0.25–0.8
Vanadium	0.10–0.30	–
Copper	0.50 max	0.25 max
Iron	Balance	Balance

*Reproduced from American Society for Testing and Materials[15] with permission.

to pitting corrosion. An alloy meeting F 138 requirements must also pass an intergranular corrosion susceptibility test. The corrosion resistance of stainless steel may be enhanced by a final surface treatment, such as immersion in 20 to 40 volume percent nitric acid (ASTM F 86-91)[15] or electropolishing.[16–18] Other stainless steel standards for implant materials are Deutsches Institut für Normung (DIN) 1.4441 and Arbeitsgemeinschaft für Osteosynthesefragen [Association for the Study of Internal Fixation] (AO ASIF) 18% Cr–14% Ni–2.5% Mo. The relevant International Organization for Standardization document is ISO 5832-1.[19]

General Considerations for In Vivo and In Vitro Corrosion of Stainless Steel Implants

Various textbooks on corrosion science clearly introduce the subject and examine the corrosion of stainless steel in environments that pertain to implant applications.[2,7,20–23] Chromium is a highly reactive base metal whose corrosion resistance depends on its passive surface film, which spontaneously forms (passivation) and reforms (repassivation) in air and under most tissue fluid conditions. Oxygen is necessary for the formation and maintenance of the film, but acidic conditions and chloride ions can be particularly detrimental. Increasing the percentage of chromium tends to reduce the passive current density, raise the breakdown and pitting potentials, and lower the critical current density and potential necessary for passivation.[3] Nickel decreases the critical current density while molybdenum has a strong effect on lowering the critical current density and raising the pitting potential.

The passive film on stainless steel is composed mainly of chromium compounds, with smaller amounts of iron, nickel, and molybdenum. Studies have shown that the film formed in an aqueous environment consists of an inner oxide layer and an outer hydroxide layer. Olefjord and Wegrelius[24] examined the film formed on a 20Cr-18Ni-6Mo-0.2N stainless steel during anodic polarization in solution (0.1 M HCl + 0.4 M NaCl) at room temperature. The authors reported that the film consists of an inner Fe-Cr, Cr^{3+}-rich oxide layer and an outer monolayer of $Cr(OH)_3$. Chloride ions were found in both the inner and outer film layers. The film thickness was 12Å at –100 mV and 14.5Å at –500 mV (saturated calomel electrode). Lakatos-Varsányi, Wegrelius, and Olefjord[25] examined the passive film formed on type 304 stainless steel that was polarized in an oxygen-

free artificial saliva composed of NaCl, citric acid, and Na_2HPO_4 (pH = 6.4) at 38°C. This film also had a duplex structure, consisting of an inner layer of $(Cr_{0.5}Fe_{0.5})_2O_3$ and an outer layer of $Cr(OH)_3$ and $(Cr_xFe_y)PO_4 \cdot 2H_2O$. The $Cr(OH)_3$ transformed to Cr_2O_3 on exposure to air. The authors were unable to find chloride ions in the passive film and speculated that this was due to the cation-selective nature of the phosphate compound, which prevents penetration of chloride ions.

The nature of the oxide film on retrieved type 316L stainless steel wires used in maxillofacial surgery for skeletal fixation and pins used in hand surgery was examined by Sundgren et al.[26] The wires were removed after 20 to 136 days and the pins were removed after 20 to 49 days, then compared with unimplanted wires and pins. The oxides on both the unimplanted and implanted materials consisted mainly of chromium oxide. Iron and nickel were found in the outermost layers, but there was no evidence of molybdenum enrichment. The thickness of the oxide depended upon the surgical site, increasing three to four times in bone marrow compared with the 50Å thickness on unimplanted wires and pins. The differences were attributed to differences in oxygen pressure at the implant sites. The oxides on the implanted wires and pins contained calcium, phosphorus, and sulfur, and their presence was site dependent. Hazan, Brener, and Oron[27] heated type 316L stainless steel screws to 280°C for 200 minutes before implantation into the intramedullary canal of rats. They concluded that there was increased oxide thickness and augmented bony ingrowth compared with nonheat-treated controls, as indicated by higher shear stresses required for dislodgment. The dominant surface oxide on the heat-treated screws was iron oxide, compared with the dominant chromium oxide on the controls. Ungersböck, Pohler, and Perren[28] reported chromium oxide on electropolished type 316L stainless steel bone plates. Plates retrieved after 3 months implantation in the long bones of sheep showed x-ray energy-dispersive spectra with peaks for sodium, nitrogen, and calcium.

Surface and bulk chemical modifications of stainless steel for implant applications have been shown to improve corrosion resistance and other properties. Endo et al[29] demonstrated for an experimental high-nitrogen-containing austenitic stainless steel that CrN is formed in the outer region of the passive film, with nitrogen enrichment at the alloy surface under the passive film. The authors suggested that this may be the reason for the greater in vitro pitting corrosion resistance observed compared with type 316L stainless steel. In related studies, surface nitriding of stainless steel has been reported to be successful for increasing corrosion resistance. Veerabadran et al[30] showed a substantial increase in the pitting and crevice corrosion resistance of nitrogen-ion-implanted type 316L stainless steel in simulated body fluid compared with unimplanted material. Sundararajan et al[31] reported increased in vitro localized corrosion resistance for titanium-modified type 316L stainless steel and a further increase when the titanium-modified material received nitrogen-ion implantation. Bordji et al[32] showed that the surface treatments of nitrogen implantation and carbon-doped sputtering for type 316L stainless steel were biocompatible and that these surface-treated stainless steels displayed improved corrosion and wear resistance. Similarly, Rieu et al[33] demonstrated that nitrogen-ion implantation can reduce wear and crevice corrosion of type 316L stainless steel. Surface coatings with potentially bioactive glass also have been shown to increase corrosion resistance.[14,34] Nitrogen-stengthened, manganese-bearing austenitic stainless steel, such as 22Cr-12.5Ni-5Mn-2.5Mo (F 1314-95), has been introduced to provide greater localized corrosion resistance than type 316L. Rondelli, Vicentini, and Cigada[35] reported much better in vitro localized corrosion resistance for a high-nitrogen 20Cr-9Ni-2Mo-0.39N stainless steel than for type 316L and ASTM F 138. In vitro studies indicate that two "nitrogen-free" stainless steels also have improved localized corrosion resistance compared with type 316L.[36,37]

Identifying the possible effects of corrosion on the mechanical failure of implants has proved to be difficult. Morita et al[38] showed that the fatigue strength of type 316 stainless steel was lower in an animal model than in air. The authors sug-

gested that the observed effect was due to the corrosive action of body fluids. However, it is not known whether corrosion makes a significant contribution to the fatigue failure of orthopedic implants.[39] Stainless steel also is susceptible to stress-corrosion cracking in chloride-containing environments, but the likelihood of this form of breakdown occurring for orthopedic implants remains uncertain.[40–42]

Cold working austenitic stainless steel usually results in only a slight decrease in corrosion resistance.[20] However, there is little known about the effects of cold working on in vivo corrosion after performing procedures such as contouring miniplates. Following surgical handling and contouring of implants, it is recommended that stainless steel be repassivated,[43] for any mechanical damage to the passive film may adversely affect corrosion resistance. As-received implants with surface defects, especially on wires, may act as pitting or crevice corrosion initiation sites.[44]

Implant-quality stainless steels are less corrosion resistant than Co-Cr alloys or titanium and its alloys. It is generally recommended that stainless steel implants not be used in direct contact with these alloys because of the possibility of galvanic (or bimetallic) corrosion of the stainless steel.[45–47] Much of the research on metal-ion release from stainless steel deals with its susceptibility to pitting and crevice corrosion in chloride-ion-containing environments[48] and with the association between fretting and crevice corrosion.[49] Various methods measure localized corrosion susceptibility,[7] including polarization testing to determine the passive film breakdown potential of a noncrevice specimen[50] or the repassivation potential of a crevice specimen (ASTM F 746).[15] Fretting, pitting, and crevice corrosion may occur simultaneously on the same implant or at the same implant site, with fretting and crevice corrosion probably the main causes of significant in vivo corrosion of orthopedic stainless steel implants.[51]

Brown and Simpson[52] proposed that crevice corrosion at contact areas of stainless steel bone plates and screws is initiated by fretting rather than by electrochemical film breakdown. Recent evidence supports this hypothesis. Sutow et al[53] studied the long-term corrosion behavior of a modified type 302 endodontic obturator carrier. Specimens placed in a mechanically static, artificial crevice and tested in 0.9% NaCl solution at 37°C did not corrode at 174 weeks. Elemental analysis of the corrosive solution was done using inductively coupled plasma-mass spectroscopy. The maximum median mass loss rates (μg/cm^2/4 weeks) for iron, chromium, nickel, molybdenum, manganese, and copper were 3.67, 0.57, 0.75, 0.54, 0.53, and 0.47, respectively. Along with these low rates, there was no evidence of pitting or crevice corrosion as determined by scanning electron microscopy (SEM) examination of tested and untested specimens.

The extensive research literature on the corrosion of orthopedic implant stainless steels is relevant for oral and maxillofacial applications. Critical analysis is necessary, however, because various requirements, such as implant size and loading conditions, could affect the rate of metal-ion release.[54] For example, the reported frequency of crevice corrosion may be much higher for orthopedic fixation devices[13,48] than for mini-plates and screws.[55] Among the enormous number of surgical implantations being performed, implant-quality stainless steel continues to show highly successful clinical outcomes. The percentage of clinical failures attributed to corrosion is relatively small,[39] even though the frequency of corrosion is rather high,[12,56,57] with corrosion products reported in tissues adjacent to implants and in remote sites.[14,58] The amount of corrosion product typically shows little if any association with implant bulk composition or total time of implantation.[59] Nevertheless, stainless steel corrosion products remain a biocompatibility concern because they have been reported to induce tissue necrosis, pain, inflammation, and swelling and have been associated with implant loosening. Kohn and Ducheyne[60] reported that orthopedic stainless steel implants are now limited to temporary devices (about 6 to 12 months of service), such as intramedullary rods, bone plates, screws, and nails, because of corrosion.

Ions released from metallic implants may accumulate in significant levels in the surrounding tissues[61,62] and vital organs.[63–65] The major corrosion products of stainless steel are iron, chromium, and nickel, with nickel and chromium receiving the most attention because of their reported potential for producing allergic, toxic, or carcinogenic effects.[62,66–68] Caution should be used in interpreting these effects, however, because documented toxicities generally apply to the soluble forms of the elements, which may not be relevant to implant corrosion products.[69] For orthopedic implants in human patients, Jacobs, Gilbert, and Urban[69] concluded that any association between release of metal and any metabolic, bacteriologic, immunologic, or carcinogenic toxicity is conjectural insofar as cause and effect have not been demonstrated in vivo. Nevertheless, investigations continue to indicate concern for short- and long-term exposures to stainless steel corrosion products. For example, recent studies show histologic and ultrastructural changes in mice liver and spleen from the accumulation of stainless steel corrosion products.[64,65,70–72] Corrosion products may also play a role in bone loss.[73–78] Furthermore, in vitro studies suggest that while wear particles may become less toxic with age, they may induce more bone resorbing mediators over time.[79,80]

The most common metal sensitivity in the general population is to nickel, followed by cobalt, and chromium.[58] However, there are relatively few well-documented accounts of generalized allergic responses resulting from oral and maxillofacial surgical implantation of stainless steel.[81–83] For intraoral treatment using nickel-containing alloys, for example, even nickel-sensitized patients infrequently show intraoral lesions directly attributable to the alloys.[84] There is some evidence, using a guinea pig model, that oral contact with nickel and chromium may induce a state of partial tolerance to these metals in nonsensitized individuals.[85,86] The "nickel-free" stainless steels[36,37] were developed to avoid the potential problems associated with nickel-ion release from conventional nickel-containing stainless steels (see Tables 12-1 to 12-3).

Table 12-4 Typical applications of stainless steel in oral and maxillofacial surgery

APPLICATIONS	REFERENCE
Ramus blade and ramus frame implants	Lemons and Dietsh-Misch[43]
Suture wire for management of soft tissue injuries	Powers et al[90]
Wire fixation	Lew and Sinn[91]
Staple for skin grafts	Johnson et al[92]
Crib for mandibular reconstruction	Marx and Stevens[93]
Champy miniplates and screws	Scheerlinck et al[94]
Arch bars	Torgersen and Gjerdet[95]
Transmalar Steinmann pin	Panje and Hetherington[96]

Corrosion Behavior of Oral and Maxillofacial Surgical Implants

The research literature on the corrosion behavior of oral and maxillofacial stainless steel implants is much less extensive than comparable literature in the orthopedic area. Similarities have been reported in the forms of in vivo corrosion degradation, although there is some indication that there is less significant accumulation of corrosion products and less tissue reaction associated with oral and maxillofacial implants. Any evidence of corrosion degradation and adverse reaction must be interpreted along with clinical outcomes that show the many successful applications of stainless steel in oral and maxillofacial implantation.[54,55,87–89] Some applications[43,90–96] are listed in Table 12-4 and shown in Fig 12-2.

Millar, Frame, and Browne examined the tissue changes associated with stainless steel and titanium unthreaded screws that were inserted in the skull vault of beagle dogs.[97] The 5-mm screws were from a stainless steel Champy maxillofacial osteosynthesis set (KLS Martin, Jacksonville, FL) and a titanium Wurzburg miniplate set (Stryker Leibinger, Kalamazoo, MI). They were unloaded for the observation period, but the plates were not implanted. After 24 weeks, the histologic responses to the two materials were similar, with excellent long-term bone healing, and minimal con-

nective tissue had formed between the screws and bone. Earlier work by Linder and Lundskog[98] showed stable implant incorporation of unloaded type 316 stainless steel, titanium, and Vitallium (Austenal, Chicago, IL) cylinders in rabbit tibia. The stainless steel implants were in place for 7 months with no SEM evidence of surface degradation due to corrosion. No adverse tissue reaction was observed with light-microscopic histologic examination. More recently, Linder[99] and Linder, Obrant, and Boivin[100] reported evidence of osseointegration of stainless steel cylinders placed in the tibias of rabbits that was similar to the osseointegration observed with titanium, Ti-6Al-4V, and Vitallium specimens. The test periods were 4 and 11 months and showed identical healing conditions for the four materials.

Torgersen and Gjerdet[95] studied the in vitro corrosion of solid stainless steel arch bars with hooks that were made in one piece (Erich type) and arch bars in which the hooks were brazed with a silver solder (Dautrey type). Stainless steel ligatures were used to attach the arch bars to acrylic jaw models. The test electrolyte was 0.9% NaCl (pH 5.6 to 6.0) at 37°C. Elemental analysis of the electrolyte at 3, 10, and 28 days was conducted using atomic absorption spectrophotometry. Results showed that iron, chromium, and nickel were released from both types of arch bar, but the brazed arch bar released 140 to 660 times more metal, depending upon the element. Iron

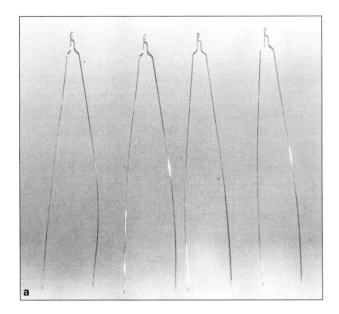

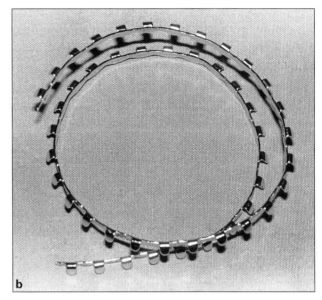

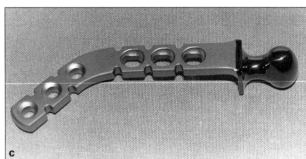

Fig 12-2 Applications of stainless steel in oral and maxillo-facial surgery: *(a)* Kobi-ashyi hooks, *(b)* arch bar, *(c)* condylar prosthesis. (Courtesy of DS Precious and S Giles.)

was found in the highest concentrations. There was no visible corrosion product on the solid arch bars, and SEM examination showed no corrosion defects. In contrast, the brazed arch bars showed major corrosion defects and gross corrosion deposits. Accumulation of corrosion products was observed adjacent to the junctions of the hooks and bars, which were easily separated at 28 days. The authors suggested that the observed corrosion of the brazed arch bars may be attributable to sensitization of the stainless steel caused by the high temperature of brazing plus a galvanic effect between the solder and stainless steel components.

The use of miniplates and screws for internal fixation of fractures and osteotomies in the maxillofacial region has greatly increased since its successful application was first documented in the 1970s.[101] Metal-ion release from the components occurs as the result of slow corrosion in the passive state, with greater rates occurring in the event of localized corrosion. Various studies show that particulate metal debris, which is found in the hard and soft tissues adjacent to the implants, is an additional source of metal ions. Although stainless steel initially was used for making miniplates, Baker, Dalrymple, and Betts[101] report that its selection has decreased considerably in favor of titanium or Vitallium.

Studies show that one source of particulate metal debris found in soft and hard tissue adjacent to miniplates results from fretting wear between the plates and screws.[54,102] Given that corrosion is a surface phenomenon, debris may significantly increase the total amount of metal ions released due to the high surface-volume ratio of these small wear particles. The work of Kovacs, Davidson, and Daigle[103] on orthopedic implant metals examined this hypothesis. These authors studied specimens of various materials, including hot-forged and cold-worked stainless steel, which were subjected to fretting wear in vitro. A good linear correlation was reported between the metal-ion concentration in the test solution and the calculated fretting wear volume. Additional metal-ion release may result from material-host interactions, such as enhanced corrosion due to a decreased local pH associated with phagocytosis of metallic wear particles by macrophages.[104] Ray, Matthew, and Frame[105] suggested that another source of metal particles found in tissue adjacent to miniplates and screws may be from surface defects consisting of rough edges and protuberances on as-received implants, which become detached and deposited in tissue during implantation. Over half of the stainless steel, titanium, and titanium alloy specimens examined by the authors had these defects. Torgersen and Gjerdet[55] reported that mechanical damage to retrieved miniplates and screws in handling and surgical procedures is common. Mechanical defects and corrosion together were reported in the countersink region, whereas tool marks on the free surface of the devices were free of corrosion.

Torgersen and Gjerdet[55] conducted a retrieval study of 43 stainless steel and 19 titanium miniplates and their matching screws for evidence of surface degradation. The authors reported that the majority of the implants were removed on a routine basis and that there was no history of adverse clinical reactions. Bone occasionally filled the microspace between the components of both the stainless steel and titanium implants, indicating that both materials are biocompatible. No corrosion was observed on the titanium devices. About one fifth of the stainless steel plates showed corrosion defects that were restricted to the countersink regions, and there were corrosion defects in the chamfer on the underside of the screw heads. No corrosion was detected on the free surface of the stainless steel implants, which is in contrast to orthopedic results that show pitting corrosion on the free surface of stainless steel bone plates.[56] Torgersen and Gjerdet also reported that there was no relationship between the frequency of corrosion and the implantation period.

Torgersen et al[54] studied retrieved stainless steel and titanium miniplates and screws (12 patients and 3 patients, respectively) used for jaw fracture healing to determine the nature of released metal particles and to evaluate the adjacent tissues histomorphologically. Removal of the stainless steel plates and screws occurred routinely between 15 and 47 weeks. The titanium plates and screws were removed at the patient's request between 39 and 41 weeks. Results showed tissue changes adjacent to both implant materials as well as evidence of fibrosis and areas of chronic inflammation in nonosseous tissues. For both implant materials, a connective tissue collar was observed between the bone tissue and the screws, with bone formation also evident adjacent to the screws. The authors concluded that both the stainless steel and titanium implants were well tolerated and that there were no local tissue changes, which suggest that asymptomatic patients with stainless steel or titanium implants should not be treated differently regarding removal of plates and screws following bone healing.

In a companion study, Torgersen, Moe, and Jonsson[106] examined subepithelial soft tissue and bone sections adjacent to 14 stainless steel and 5 titanium miniplates and screws to characterize the frequency and distribution of immunocompetent cells. The stainless steel implants were removed routinely between 15 and 47 weeks, and the titanium implants were removed at the patient's request between 39 and 41 weeks. The authors reported that the basis for an immune reaction existed for both the stainless steel and titanium implants because the cellular infiltrates in the examined tissues contained all of the cell types required for a delayed hypersensitivity reaction. However, the mild tissue reaction observed was thought to indicate that both materials were well tolerated by the body.

Matthew and Frame[107] studied the potential effect of additional friction between miniplates on corrosion and the fitting surface of screws that may be brought about by inadequate miniplate contouring. Experimental stainless steel miniplates were permanently deformed into a curved shape until the midpoint of the plate was raised 3 mm above the ends. The plates were inserted in the cranial vault of 12 beagle dogs and the screws tightened until enough stress was developed to make the plate conform to the skull curvature. Control plates were contoured properly before insertion. Comparison of atomic absorption spectrophotometry results at 24 weeks for the experimental and control implants showed no influence of stress due to poor contouring on the amount of iron, chromium, and nickel released into the surrounding soft and hard tissues. Also, there was no clear relationship between the results of the qualitative assessment of adjacent tissue pigmentation and the quantitatively determined concentration of metals.

The possibility of fretting and crevice corrosion and the production of corrodible debris are central to the issue of whether or not to remove nonfunctional stainless steel miniplates.[108] The in vivo corrosion research evidence and reports of associated long-term tissue response are very limited.[107] Brown et al[89] analyzed the surgical outcomes for 279 stainless steel Champy miniplates used routinely as permanent implants for management of maxillofacial trauma (62 patients) and orthognathic surgery (47 patients) over a 5-year period. Patients who had their plates removed were compared with patients who had retained their plates. Results showed that the morbidity associated with plate retention was within acceptable limits. No evidence of complications with long-term implantation was found, and there was no evidence of radiographic changes associated with orthognathic patients. The authors challenged the practice of routine removal of Champy miniplates three to four months postoperatively.

Rosenberg, Grätz, and Sailer[109] removed titanium and Champy stainless steel miniplates 3 months to 2 years and 8 months (mean: 8 months) after insertion in 32 patients and examined the surrounding soft tissue for evidence of corrosion. No visible pigmentation of the tissue was detected around stainless steel plates, whereas microscopic examination revealed pigmentation in 65.3% of the tissue. In comparison, 25.6% of the tissue surrounding the titanium miniplates had visible pigmentation, and 71.8% showed pigmentation on microscopic examination. X-ray energy-dispersive

analysis of one tissue specimen near a stainless steel implant showed the presence of chromium, nickel, iron, and molybdenum. Matthew et al[110] studied the surface of Champy stainless steel miniplates for evidence of surface degradation following fracture healing in the mandible of beagle dogs. The implants were retrieved after 24 weeks and compared, using SEM, with unused controls that had been stored in a solution of thymol and normal saline. The authors found no evidence that the risk of corrosion of stainless steel or titanium Champy miniplates warrants their routine removal up to 24 weeks postinsertion.

To determine risk factors contributing to symptomatic plate removal, Manor, Chaushu, and Taicher[111] studied the outcomes of stainless steel and titanium miniplates used in orthognathic surgery. Patient age was found to be the primary risk factor; implant material (15.5% stainless steel vs 6.7% titanium) was a secondary factor. Torgersen, Gilhuus-Moe, and Gjerdet[112] examined 15 patients for delayed hypersensitivity reaction to nickel before implantation and at removal (6 to 58 weeks, mean: 31 weeks) of stainless steel miniplates used for rigid fixation of mandibular fracture. Stainless steel arch bars were used for the first 2 weeks and then removed. The results of a lymphocyte transformation test with nickel showed stainless steel may increase lymphocyte activity, which has implications for removal or retention of nonfunctional implants. However, no adverse clinical complications were observed related to delayed hypersensitivity. The cited studies are important contributions to the issue of miniplate removal following bony healing in asymptomatic patients. Clearly, much additional research is needed to make an evidenced-based decision.

Stainless steels are used with a high degree of success in a wide variety of oral and maxillofacial implant applications because of their combination of corrosion resistance, hot and cold workability, and mechanical properties. The ongoing development of new stainless steel chemical formulations and new surface treatments reveals that there are many opportunities for continuing material advancement in the critical area of in vivo corrosion behavior.

References

1. Davis JR (ed). Stainless Steels, ASM Specialty Handbook. Materials Park, OH: ASM International,1994.

2. Bradford SA. Corrosion Control. New York: Van Nostrand Reinhold, 1993:193–194.

3. Talbot D, Talbot J. Corrosion Science and Technology. Boca Raton, Florida: CRC Press, 1998:253–277.

4. Tucker MR, Ochs MW. Basic concepts of rigid internal fixation: Mechanical considerations and instrumentation overview. In: Tucker MR, Terry BC, White RP, Van Sickels JE (eds). Rigid Fixation for Maxillofacial Surgery. Philadelphia: Lippincott, 1991:52.

5. Cigada A, Rondelli G, Vicentini B, Giacomazzi M, Roos A. Duplex stainless steel for osteosynthesis devices. J Biomed Mater Res 1989;23:1087–1095.

6. Cigada A, De Santis G, Gatti AM, Roos A, Zaffe D. In vivo behavior of a high performance duplex stainless steel. J Appl Biomater 1993;4:39–46.

7. Sedriks AJ. Corrosion of Stainless Steels, ed 2. New York: Wiley, 1996.

8. Peckner D, Bernstein IM. Handbook of Stainless Steels. New York: McGraw-Hill, 1977.

9. Sutow EJ, Pollack SR. The biocompatibility of certain stainless steels. In: Williams DF (ed). Biocompatibility of Clinical Implant Materials, vol 1. Boca Raton, FL: CRC Press, 1981: 45–98.

10. Disegi J. AO ASIF Wrought 18% Chromium-14% Nickel-2.5% Molybdenum Stainless Steel Implant Material. Davos, Switzerland:AO ASIF Materials Technical Committee, 1998.

11. Trethewey KR, Chamberlain J. Corrosion for Science and Engineering. Essex: Longman, 1995:341–347.

12. Harding AF, Cook SD, Thomas KA, Collins CL, Haddad Jr RJ, Milicic M. A clinical and metallurgical analysis of retrieved Jewett and Richards hip plate devices. Clin Orthop 1985; 195:261–269.

13. Cook SD, Thomas KA, Harding AF, et al. The in vivo performance of 250 internal fixation devices: A follow-up study. Biomaterials 1987;8:177–184.

14. Barbosa MA. Corrosion of metallic implants. Part II. In: Black J, Hastings G (eds). Handbook of Biomaterial Properties. London: Chapman & Hall, 1998:420–463.

15. American Society for Testing and Materials. Annual Book of ASTM Standards. Vol 13.01: Medical devices. Philadelphia: ASTM, 1998.

16. Sutow EJ. The influence of electropolishing on the corrosion resistance of 316L stainless steel. J Biomed Mater Res 1980;14:587–595.

17. Irving CC Jr. Electropolishing stainless steel implants. In: Fraker AC, Griffin CD (eds). Corrosion and Degradation of Implant Materials: Second Symposium, ASTM STP 859. Philadelphia: American Society for Testing and Materials, 1985:136–143.

18. Beddoes J, Bucci K. The influence of surface condition on the localized corrosion of 316L stainless steel orthopaedic implants. J Mater Sci Mater Med 1999;10:389–394.

19. Implants for Surgery—Metallic Materials—Part I: Wrought Stainless Steel. ISO 5832-1.Geneva, Switzerland: International Organization for Standardization; 1997.

20. Fontana MG. Corrosion Engineering, ed 3. New York: McGraw- Hill, 1986:236.

21. Trethewey KR, Chamberlain J. Corrosion for Science and Engineering. Essex: Longman, 1995.

22. Mattsson E. Basic Corrosion Technology for Scientists and Engineers. London: The Institute of Materials, 1996:135–156.

23. Talbot D, Talbot J. Corrosion Science and Technology. Boca Raton, FL: CRC Press, 1998.

24. Olefjord I, Wegrelius L. Surface analysis of passive state. Corros Sci 1990;31:89–98.

25. Lakatos-Varsányi M, Wegrelius L, Olefjord I. Dissolution of stainless steel in artificial saliva. Int J Oral Maxillofac Implants 1997;12:387–398.

26. Sundgren J-E, Bodö P, Lundström I, Berggren A, Hellem S. Auger electron spectroscopic studies of stainless-steel implants. J Biomed Mater Res 1985;19:663–671.

27. Hazan R, Brener R, Oron U. Bone growth to metal implants is regulated by their surface chemical properties. Biomaterials 1993;14:570–574.

28. Ungersböck A, Pohler OEM, Perren SM. Evaluation of soft tissue reactions at the interface of titanium limited contact dynamic compression plate implants with different surface treatments: An experimental sheep study. Biomaterials 1996;17:797–806.

29. Endo K, Abiko Y, Suzuki M, Ohno H, Kaku T. Corrosion resistance and biocompatibility of high nitrogen-bearing stainless steels. Corros Eng 1998;47:645–653.

30. Veerabadran KM, Kamachi Mudali U, Nair KGM, Subbaiyan M. Improvements in localized corrosion resistance of nitrogen ion implanted type 316L stainless steel orthopaedic implant devices. Mater Sci Forum 1999;318–320:561–568.

31. Sundararajan T, Kamachi Mudali U, Nair KGM, Rajeswari S, Subbaiyan M. Effects of nitrogen ion transplantation on the localized corrosion behavior of titanium modified type 316L stainless steel in simulated body fluid. J Mater Eng Perform 1999;8:252–260.

32. Bordji K, Jouzeau J-Y, Mainard D, Payan E, Delagoutte J-P, Netter P. Evaluation of the effect of three surface treatments on the biocompatibility of 316L stainless steel using human differentiated cells. Biomaterials 1996;17:491–500.

33. Rieu J, Pichat A, Rabbe L-M, Rambert A, Chabrol C, Robelet M. Ion implantation effects on friction and wear of joint prosthesis materials. Biomaterials 1991;12:139–143.

34. Galliano P, De Damborenea JJ, Pascual MJ, Durán A. Sol-gel coatings on 316L steel for clinical applications. J Sol-Gel Sci Tech 1998;13:723–727.

35. Rondelli G, Vicentini B, Cigada A. Localised corrosion tests on austenitic stainless steels for biomedical applications. Br Corros J 1997;32:193–196.

36. Xulin S, Ito A, Tateishi T, Hoshino A. Fretting corrosion resistance and fretting corrosion product cytocompatibility of ferritic stainless steel. J Biomed Mater Res 1997;34:9–14.

37. Brown RS, Gebeau R. Strength and corrosion resistance of BioDur® 108 alloy. In: Sixth World Biomaterials Congress Transactions [15–20 May 2000, Kamuela, Hawaii]. Minneapolis, MN, Society for Biomaterials, 2000:828.

38. Morita M, Sasada T, Hayashi H, Tsukamoto Y. The corrosion fatigue properties of surgical implants in a living body. J Biomed Mater Res 1988;22:529–540.

39. Sutow EJ. Iron-based alloys. In: Williams D (ed). Concise Encyclopedia of Medical and Dental Materials. Oxford: Pergamon Press, 1990:232–240.

40. Bundy KJ, Marek M, Hochman RF. In vivo and in vitro studies of the stress-corrosion cracking behavior of surgical implant alloys. J Biomed Mater Res 1983;17:467–487.

41. Sheehan JP, Morin CR, Packer KF. Study of stress corrosion cracking susceptibility of type 316L stainless steel in vitro. In: Fraker AC, Griffin CD (eds). Corrosion and Degradation of Implant Materials: Second Symposium, ASTM STP 859. Philadelphia: American Society for Testing and Materials, 1985:57–72.

42. Bundy KJ, Desai VH. Studies of stress-corrosion cracking behavior of surgical implant materials using a fracture mechanics approach. In: Fraker AC, Griffin CD (eds). Corrosion and Degradation of Implant Materials: Second Symposium, ASTM STP 859. Philadelphia: American Society for Testing and Materials, 1985:73–90.

43. Lemons JE, Dietsh-Misch F. Biomaterials for dental implants. In: Misch CE (ed). Contemporary Implant Dentistry, ed 2. St. Louis: Mosby, 1999:271–302.

44. Rentler RM, Greene ND. Corrosion of surface defects in fine wires. J Biomed Mater Res 1975;9:597–610.

45. Silva RA, Barbosa MA, Jenkins GM, Sutherland I. Electrochemistry of galvanic couples between carbon and common metallic biomaterials in the presence of crevices. Biomaterials 1990;11:336–340.

46. Lemons JE, Lucas LC, Johansson BI. Intraoral corrosion resulting from coupling dental implants and restorative metallic systems. Implant Dent 1992;1:107–112.

47. Reclaru L, Meyer J-M. Study of corrosion between a titanium implant and dental alloys. J Dent 1994;22:159–168.

48. Thomas KA, Cook SD, Harding AF, Haddad Jr RJ. Tissue reaction to implant corrosion in 38 internal fixation devices. Orthopedics 1988;11:441–451.

49. Brown SA, Merritt K. Fretting corrosion of plates and screws: an in vitro test method. In: Fraker AC, Griffin CD (eds). Corrosion and Degradation of Implant Materials: Second Symposium, ASTM STP 859. Philadelphia: American Society for Testing and Materials, 1985:105–116.

50. Semlitsch MF, Weber H, Streicher RM, Schön R. Joint replacement components made of hot-forged and surface-treated Ti-6Al-7Nb alloy. Biomaterials 1992;13:781–788.

51. Brown SA, Hughes PJ, Merritt K. In vitro studies of fretting corrosion of orthopaedic materials. J Orthop Res 1988; 6:572–579.

52. Brown SA, Simpson JP. Crevice and fretting corrosion of stainless-steel plates and screws. J Biomed Mater Res 1981;15:867–878.

53. Sutow EJ, Foong W-C, Zakariasen KL, Hall GC, Jones DW. Corrosion and cytotoxicity evaluation of Thermafil endodontic obturator carriers. J Endod 1999;25:562–566.

54. Torgersen S, Gjerdet NR, Erichsen ES, Bang G. Metal particles and tissue changes adjacent to miniplates: A retrieval study. Acta Odontol Scand 1995;53:65–71.

55. Torgersen S, Gjerdet NR. Retrieval study of stainless steel titanium miniplates and screws used in maxillofacial surgery. J Mater Sci Mater Med 1994;5:256–262.

56. Cook SD, Renz EA, Barrack RL, et al. Clinical and metallurgical analysis of retrieved internal fixation devices. Clin Orthop 1985;194:236–247.

57. Vieweg U, van Roost D, Wolf HK, Schyma CA, Schramm J. Corrosion on an internal spinal fixator system. Spine 1999; 24:946–951.

58. Black J. Biological Performance of Materials: Fundamentals of Biocompatibility, ed 3. New York: Marcel Dekker, 1999.

59. Walczak J, Shahgaldi F, Heatley F. In vivo corrosion of 316L stainless-steel hip implants: Morphology and elemental compositions of corrosion products. Biomaterials 1998;19: 229–237.

60. Kohn DH, Ducheyne P. Materials for bone and joint replacement. In: Cahn RW, Haasen P, Kramer EJ (eds). Materials Science and Technology: A Comprehensive Treatment, vol 14. Weinheim: VCH, 1991:29–109.

61. Merritt K, Brown SA. Biological effects of corrosion products from metals. In: Fraker AC, Griffin CD (eds). Corrosion and Degradation of Implant Materials: Second Symposium, ASTM STP 859. Philadelphia: American Society for Testing and Materials, 1985:195–207.

62. Merritt K, Brown SA. Release of hexavalent chromium from corrosion of stainless steel and cobalt-chromium alloys. J Biomed Mat Res 1995;29:627–633.

63. Abreu AM, Tracana RB, Carvalho GS, Sousa JP. Accumulation of metal ions in mouse organs following intraperitoneal injection of stainless steel corrosion products: Determination by atomic absorption spectroscopy and microelectrodes. Biomed Lett 1995; 52:133–148

64. Pereira MC, Pereira ML, Sousa JP. Histological effects of iron accumulation on mice liver and spleen after administration of a metallic solution. Biomaterials 1999;20:2193–2198.

65. Pereira MC, Pereira ML, Sousa JP. Individual study of chromium in the stainless steel implants degradation: An experimental study in mice. BioMetals 1999;12:275–280.

66. Granchi D, Cenni E, Ciapetti G, et al. Cell death induced by metal ions: Necrosis or apoptosis? J Mater Sci Mater Med 1998;9:31–37.

67. Shettlemore MG, Bundy KJ. Toxicity measurement of orthopedic implant alloy degradation products using a bioluminescent bacterial assay. J Biomed Mater Res 1999;45:395–403.

68. Savarino L, Stea S, Granchi D, et al. Sister chromatid exchanges and ion release in patients wearing fracture fixation devices. J Biomed Mater Res 2000;50:21–26.

69. Jacobs JJ, Gilbert JL, Urban RM. Current concepts review: Corrosion of metal orthopaedic implants. J Bone Joint Surg Am 1998;80A:268–282.

70. Pereira ML, Silva A, Tracana R, Carvalho GS. Toxic effects caused by stainless steel corrosion products on mouse seminiferous cells. Cytobios 1994;77:73–80.

71. Pereira ML, Abreu AM, Sousa JP, Carvalho GS. Chromium accumulation and ultrastructural changes in the mouse liver caused by stainless steel corrosion products. J Mater Sci Mater Med 1995;6:523–527.

72. Tracana RB, Pereira ML, Abreu AM, Sousa JP, Carvalho GS. Stainless steel corrosion products cause alterations on mouse spleen cellular populations. J Mater Sci Mater Med 1995;6:56–61.

73. Morais S, Sousa JP, Fernandes MH, Carvalho GS. In vitro biomineralization by osteoblast-like cells. I. Retardation of tissue mineralization by metal salts. Biomaterials 1998;19:13–21.

74. Morais S, Sousa JP, Fernandes MH, Carvalho GS, de Bruijn JD, van Blitterswijk CA. Decreased consumption of Ca and P during in vitro biomineralization and biologically induced deposition of Ni and Cr in presence of stainless steel corrosion products. J Biomed Mater Res 1998;42:199–212.

75. Morais S, Sousa JP, Fernandes MH, Carvalho GS, de Bruijn JD, van Blitterswijk CA. Effects of AISI 316L corrosion products in in vitro bone formation. Biomaterials 1998;19:999–1007.

76. Fernandes MH. Effect of stainless steel corrosion products on in vitro biomineralization. J Appl Biomater 1999;14:113–168.

77. Morais S, Dias N, Sousa JP, Fernandes MH, Carvalho GS. In vitro osteoblastic differentiation of human bone marrow cells in the presence of metal ions. J Biomed Mater Res 1999;44:176–190.

78. Costa MA, Fernandes MH. Proliferation/differentiation of osteoblastic human alveolar bone cell cultures in the presence of stainless steel corrosion products. J Mater Sci Mater Med 2000;11:141–153.

79. Haynes DR, Boyle SJ, Rogers SD, Howie DW, Vernon-Roberts B. Variation in cytokines induced by particles from different prosthetic materials. Clin Orthop 1998;352:223–230.

80. Haynes DR, Crotti TN, Haywood MR. Corrosion of and changes in biological effects of cobalt chrome alloy and 316L stainless steel prosthetic particles with age. J Biomed Mater Res 2000;49:167–175.

81. Schriver WR, Shereff RH, Domnitz JM, Swintak EF, Civjan S. Allergic response to stainless steel wire. Oral Surg Oral Med Oral Pathol 1976;42:578–581.

82. Roed-Petersen B, Roed-Petersen J, Dreyer Jørgensen KD. Nickel allergy and osteomyelitis in a patient with metal osteosynthesis of a jaw fracture. Contact Dermatitis 1979;5:108–112.

83. Guyuron B, Lasa CI. Reaction to stainless steel wire following orthognathic surgery. Plast Reconstr Surg 1992;89:540–542.

84. Hensten-Pettersen A. Nickel allergy and dental treatment procedures. In: Maibach HI, Menné T (eds). Nickel and the Skin: Immunology and Toxicology. Boca Raton, FL: CRC Press, 1989:195–205.

85. Vreeburg KJJ, de Groot K, von Blomberg BME, Scheper RJ. Induction of immunological tolerance by oral administration of nickel and chromium. J Dent Res 1984;63:124–128.

86. Vreeburg KJJ, van Hoogstraten IMW, von Blomberg M, de Groot K, Scheper RJ. Oral induction of immunological tolerance to chromium in the guinea pig. J Dent Res 1990;69:1634–1639.

87. Jackson IT, Adham MN. Metallic plate stabilisation of bone grafts in craniofacial surgery. Br J Plast Surg 1986;39:341–344.

88. Jackson IT, Somers PC, Kjar JG. The use of Champy miniplates for osteosynthesis in craniofacial deformities and trauma. Plast Reconstr Surg 1986;77:729–736.

89. Brown JS, Trotter M, Cliffe J, Ward-Booth RP, Williams ED. The fate of miniplates in facial trauma and orthognathic surgery: A retrospective study. Br J Oral Maxillofac Surg 1989;27:306–315.

90. Powers MP, Beck BW, Fonseca RJ. Management of soft tissue injuries. In: Fonseca RJ, Walker RV (eds). Oral and Maxillofacial Trauma, ed 2. Philadelphia: Saunders, 1997:792–854.

91. Lew D, Sinn DP. Diagnosis and treatment of midface fractures. In: Fonseca RJ, Walker RV (eds). Oral and Maxillofacial Trauma, ed 2. Philadelphia: Saunders, 1997:653–713.

92. Johnson PA, Fleming K, Avery CME. Latex foam and staple fixation of skin grafts. Br J Oral Maxillofac Surg 1998;36:141–142.

93. Marx RE, Stevens MR. Reconstruction of avulsion maxillofacial injuries. In: Fonseca RJ, Walker RV (eds). Oral and Maxillofacial Trauma, ed 2. Philadelphia: Saunders, 1997:1101–1203.

94. Scheerlinck JPO, Stoelinga PJW, Blijdorp PA, Brouns JJA, Nijs MLL. Sagittal split advancement osteotomies stabilized with miniplates. Int J Oral Maxillofac Surg 1994;23:127–131.

95. Torgersen S, Gjerdet NR. Metal release from arch bars used in maxillofacial surgery: An in vitro study. Acta Odontol Scand 1992;50:83–89.

96. Panje WR, Hetherington HE. Use of stainless steel implants in facial bone reconstruction. Otolaryngol Clin North Am 1995;28:341–349.

97. Millar BG, Frame JW, Browne RM. A histological study of stainless steel and titanium screws in bone. Br J Oral Maxillofac Surg 1990;28:92–95.

98. Linder L, Lundskog J. Incorporation of stainless steel, titanium and Vitallium in bone. Injury 1975;6:277–285.

99. Linder L. Osseointegration of metallic implants. I. Light microscopy in the rabbit. Acta Orthop Scand 1989;60: 129–134.

100. Linder L, Obrant K, Boivin G. Osseointegration of metallic implants. II. Transmission electron microscopy in the rabbit. Acta Orthop Scand 1989;60:235–239.

101. Baker S, Dalrymple D, Betts, NJ. Concepts and techniques of rigid fixation. In: Fonseca RJ, Walker RV (eds). Oral and Maxillofacial Trauma, ed 2. Philadelphia: Saunders, 1997: 1302.

102. Matthew IR, Frame JW. Ultrastructural analysis of metal particles released from stainless steel and titanium miniplate components in an animal model. J Oral Maxillofac Surg 1998;56:45–50.

103. Kovacs P, Davidson JA, Daigle K. Correlation between the metal ion concentration and the fretting wear volume of orthopaedic implant metals. In: St. John KR (ed). Particulate Debris from Medical Implants: Mechanisms of Formation and Biological Consequences, ASTM STP 1144. Philadelphia: American Society for Testing and Materials, 1992: 160–176.

104. Haynes DR, Rogers SD, Howie DW, Pearcy MJ, Vernon-Roberts B. Drug inhibition of the macrophage response to metal wear particles in vitro. Clin Orthop 1996;323: 316–326.

105. Ray MS, Matthew IR, Frame JW. Metallic fragments on the surface of miniplates and screws before insertion. Br J Oral Maxillofac Surg 1998;37:14–18.

106. Torgersen S, Moe G, Jonsson R. Immunocompetent cells adjacent to stainless steel and titanium miniplates and screws. Eur J Oral Sci 1995;103:46–54.

107. Matthew IR, Frame JW . Release of metal in vivo from stressed and non-stressed maxillofacial fracture and screws. Oral Surg Oral Med Oral Pathol Oral Radiol Endod 2000;90:33–38.

108. Matthew IR, Frame JW. Policy of consultant oral and maxillofacial surgeons towards removal of miniplate components after jaw fracture fixation: Pilot study. Br J Oral Maxillofac Surg 1999;37:110–112.

109. Rosenberg A, Grätz KW, Sailer HF. Should titanium miniplates be removed after bone healing is complete? Int J Oral Maxillofac Surg 1993;22:185–188.

110. Matthew IR, Frame JW, Browne RM, Millar BG. In vivo surface analysis of titanium and stainless steel miniplates and screws. Int J Oral Maxillofac Surg 1996;25:463–468.

111. Manor Y, Chaushu G, Taicher S. Risk factors contributing to symptomatic plate removal in orthognathic surgery patients. J Oral Maxillofac Surg 1999;57:679–682.

112. Torgersen S, Gilhuus-Moe OT, Gjerdet NR. Immune response to nickel and some clinical observations after stainless steel miniplate osteosynthesis. Int J Oral Maxillofac Surg 1993;22:246–250.

13

LEACHING OF METALLIC IONS FROM PLATES AND SCREWS USED IN JAW FRACTURE FIXATION

Ian R. Matthew, PhD, M Dent Sc, BDS, FDS, RCS (England and Edinburgh)

Plate and screw osteosynthesis is a method of internal fixation of jaw fractures using miniaturized metallic plates and screws (Fig 13-1).[1] Osteosynthesis is the functionally stable internal fixation of a fracture that allows the early recovery of function.[2] The goal of internal fracture fixation is early mobilization of the fractured bone.[3] Early mobilization is not feasible with conventional techniques such as open reduction and direct wiring because it is usually necessary to wire the jaws together to ensure adequate stability of the fracture (Fig 13-2). Rigid internal fixation plays an important role in maxillofacial trauma and orthognathic and reconstructive surgery.[4] Most jaw fractures now are treated with rigid internal fixation using plates and screws.[5] This technique represents the state of the art in the treatment of jaw fractures (Figs 13-3 and 13-4).[6,7]

The use of plates and screws to fix a jaw fracture has evolved from principles established in orthopedic practice, but it took years to develop suitable implants.[8] Plates and screws are typically manufactured from stainless steel, pure titanium, or titanium alloy. Vitallium also has been used in the manufacture of plates and screws. Vitallium is a trademark of Howmedica Osteonics (a subsidiary of Stryker Corporation, Kalamazoo, MI) for an alloy of cobalt (58.9% to 69.5%), chromium (27% to 30%), and molybdenum (5% to 7%), developed originally in 1929 by Austenal Laboratories in the United States.[9]

The surgeon may choose from a variety of implant materials and must then decide whether to remove the implants once bony union has occurred. These choices remain arbitrary because there is presently a shortage of published data that addresses the biologic performance of these materials in the treatment of jaw fractures.

There has been a trend toward the use of titanium and titanium alloy plates and screws rather than stainless steel because of the favorable response of bone to titanium during healing.[10] Furthermore, it is generally accepted that titanium is a suitable material for permanent implantation. Modern standards, eg, the American Society for Testing and Materials (ASTM) standard for the manufacture of surgical-implant alloys, ensure that leaching of metallic ions within the tissues from corrosion of a metallic implant in situ is minimized. However, is the biologic performance of titanium plates and screws superior to that of stainless steel components of similar design? A

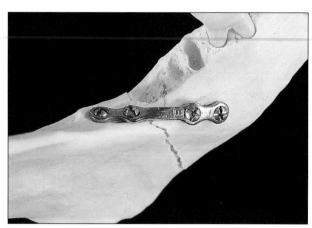

Fig 13-1 This view of a dried mandible shows a maxillofacial miniplate and four screws that have been used to fix a simulated fracture at the right angle of the mandible. Note that the miniplate has been bent to fit the contour of the jaw.

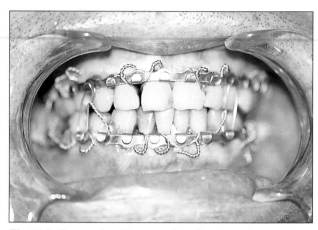

Fig 13-2 Conventional intermaxillary fixation using arch bars and interdental wires. The jaws may be wired together for 4 to 6 weeks to allow healing of a jaw fracture.

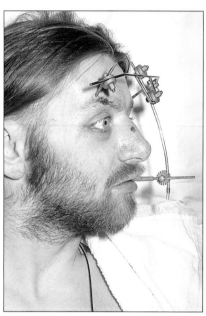

Fig 13-3 Skeletal fixation of a middle-facial-third fracture. Pins are screwed into the supraorbital bone to provide a rigid base for fixation of the maxillary fracture.

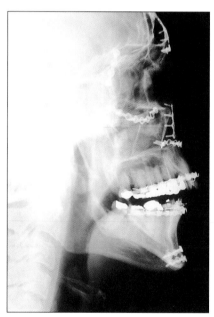

Fig 13-4 Internal fixation of maxillofacial fractures using plates and screws. The plates are placed via discrete (usually intraoral) incisions; therefore, there are no external scars, in contrast to the relatively severe external fixation visible in Fig 13-3.

fundamental aspect of the biologic performance of plates and screws is their resistance to degradation within the host tissues. Does degradation of the metallic implant have any effect on the host? If so, what is the nature of that effect?

If plates and screws may degrade within the harsh biologic environment of human tissues, should these devices routinely be removed after satisfactory healing of a jaw fracture (Figs 13-5 and 13-6)? Although most solid implant materi-

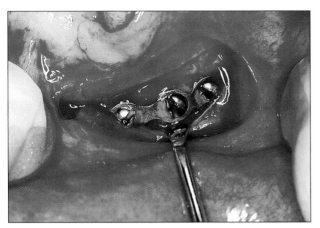

Fig 13-5 A miniplate and screws being removed prior to provision of an endosseous implant after treatment of a fractured mandible several years previously.

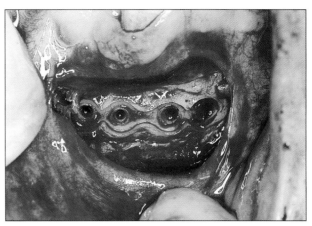

Fig 13-6 A view of the bone surface after removal of the miniplate and screws shown in Fig 13-5. Removal of the screws was difficult because of excellent adaptation of bone to their surfaces.

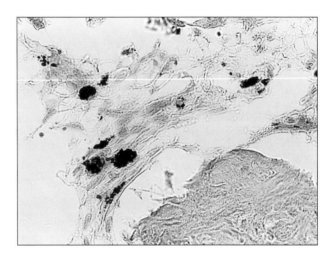

Fig 13-7 Metallic particles appear as dense, rounded clusters within the soft tissues next to a maxillofacial miniplate and screw. The soft tissues were biopsied at the time of plate removal because of metallosis (hematoxylin-eosin [h & e] stain, original magnification × 240).

als are inert and elicit little or no host response, events may occur after implantation that give rise to clinical symptoms.[11] Metal-ion release impairs the healing of bone in vitro and may cause hypersensitivity reactions in vivo.[7,12,13] Is the significance of metal-ion release from jaw plates and screws fully understood?

Metallic particles are present in soft and hard tissues adjacent to plates and screws (Fig 13-7).[3,7,14,15] What is the significance of such metallic debris? The particles will increase the surface area of a metallic implant, thus increasing the likelihood of ionic leaching. Macrophages play an active role in the phagocytosis of particulate debris and the assimilation of soluble metallic ions.[16] After the foreign material has been phago-

cytosed, immune function may be compromised through altered cellular responses.[11] Metallic implants or particulate debris may stimulate the production of cytokines, which subsequently influence interactions between macrophages and T cells.[11] Immune surveillance mechanisms may then fail. Ultimately, oncogenesis may arise within tissue adjacent to a metallic implant after chronic exposure to metallic ions.[11]

These are some of the principal concerns related to the use of metallic jaw fracture plates as permanent implants; such issues will be investigated during the course of this chapter. The orthopedic literature also is referenced throughout for comparison.

Evolution of Miniplating Methods for Jaw Fractures

Interest in plating of jaw fractures was stimulated in the late 1960s by reports of compression plates successfully used to fix long-bone fractures.[1] Compression plates were developed for jaw surgery but were difficult to adapt to the shape of the jaws. Extraoral incisions were necessary for surgical access. Meanwhile, monocortical plating of fractures gained further support after Michelet et al[17] described an original technique of maxillofacial osteosynthesis. Stellite (Vitallium) plates were fixed to the lateral cortical bone with 5- to 7-mm screws placed apical to the roots of the teeth. Access to the fracture was gained through an intraoral incision, a major advantage over compression osteosynthesis. Postoperative intermaxillary fixation (IMF) was not routinely employed.

Champy et al[18] modified the technique described by Michelet et al[17] to treat fractures of the mandible. Champy et al[18] defined the ideal anatomic location of plates by means of in vitro photoelastic studies of the mandible during simulated function. Modern principles of miniplate osteosynthesis are based upon the original work of Champy et al.[18,19]

The Roberts plating system, introduced in the early 1960s, was still used extensively in Great Britain two decades later.[20] The plates were effective for monocortical fixation of most jaw fractures, but IMF also was required for adequate stability of the fracture. Rowe[20] believed that the use of compression plating systems would become widespread in Great Britain. He argued that compression plating of a fracture of the mandible provided better stability than the use of monocortical fixation. This was possible because screws were inserted into both the buccal and lingual cortical bone, and an axial compression force brought the fracture into direct apposition. However, Rowe[20] conceded that compression plates were difficult to adapt to the shape of the jaws and that extraoral incisions were disadvantageous.

During the 1970s and early 1980s in Great Britain, plates were used to fix jaw fractures only when less invasive or simpler methods were un-suitable. For example, Frost et al[21] reported that bone plates (metacarpal plates) were used to fix only 75 fractures of the mandible out of 1,587 treated cases (4.7%) from 1973 to 1980. By the late 1980s, the use of internal fixation with plates and screws in treatment of fractures of the mandible was widespread across most of Europe, but not in the United States or in so-called Anglo-Saxon countries.[22]

Less than a third of oral and maxillofacial surgeons in the United States used miniplate fixation to treat jaw fractures in the late 1980s.[22] In a retrospective analysis of 200 fractures of the mandible treated in a Finnish oral surgery unit in the mid-1980s, only 6% underwent miniplate osteosynthesis[23]; 50% were treated with IMF, 17% with gunning splints, 16% with direct wiring, and 11% received no active treatment. Compression plating systems subsequently superseded the routine use of IMF in Finland.[24] Miniplate osteosynthesis by monocortical screw fixation subsequently has become the technique of choice in most European maxillofacial clinics, including those in the Anglo-Saxon countries.[5,25]

Biologic Performance of Metallic Plates and Screws

Biocompatibility has been defined as "the ability of a material to perform, with an appropriate response, in a specific application."[26] *Biologic performance* has been proposed as a more suitable term, however, because biocompatibility implies a harmonious interaction with the tissues and emphasizes the effect of the biomaterial on the host.[27] In contrast, biologic performance encompasses two aspects of the interaction: the host response (both local and systemic) to the implant and the response of the biomaterial to implantation.

Various types of corrosion in metallic implants have been described, and the mechanisms and implications of the process in the biologic performance of the materials have been emphasized. More evidence of the corrosion of plates has been provided in chapter 12.

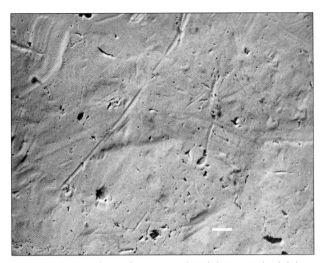

Fig 13-8 The surface of an unused stainless steel miniplate as received from the manufacturer (Martin GmbH, Solingen, Germany) and viewed by low-vacuum scanning electron microscopy (SEM) before autoclaving. Numerous surface pits and polishing and other abrasion marks are visible (original magnification × 750; bar = 10 μm).

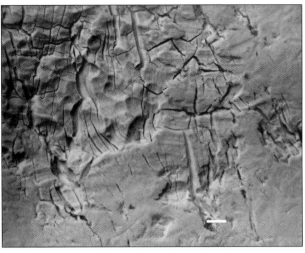

Fig 13-9 The surface of an unused titanium miniplate as received by the manufacturer (Martin GmbH) viewed by low-vacuum SEM before autoclaving. Numerous surface pits and polishing and other abrasion marks are visible (original magnification × 750; bar = 10 μm).

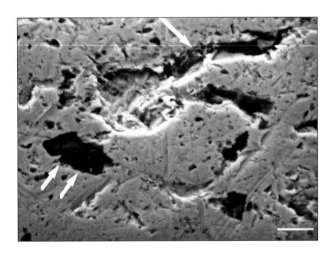

Fig 13-10 The surface of a stainless steel miniplate retrieved 4 weeks after surgery. The *single arrow* highlights a large surface irregularity, the base of which is partly obscured by soft tissue. Deposits of aluminum on the surface, one of which is highlighted by *twin arrows*, are also present (original magnification × 1,000; bar = 10 μm).

Evidence of Metallic Release from Implants into Tissues

Moberg et al[28] identified elevated levels of nickel (approximately 13 ppm wet weight) within tissues next to Champy stainless steel plates compared with controls. Aluminum levels also were higher (approximately 18 ppm wet weight) in soft tissues near titanium plates compared with controls. The normal level of aluminum within human tissues is typically 0.15 to 6.0 μg/g.[29] Moberg et al[28] did not discuss potential sources of the aluminum, nor did they explain why levels of aluminum within the tissues should be elevated.

Torgersen et al[15] also reported higher aluminum levels in tissues next to Champy titanium plates but offered no explanation. It is recognized that aluminum is ubiquitous and that dust is a major source.[30] Consequently, contamination was a possible explanation, but it subsequently has been shown that at least one brand of plates is marketed with aluminum and silicon deposits on their surfaces, probably due to the polishing process (Figs 13-8 to 13-10).[31]

In the study by Torgersen et al,[15] levels of chromium, cobalt, and molybdenum were not significantly elevated in the tissues with respect to controls. This may have been due to their high solubility or through binding to proteins. Although Moberg et al[28] reported increased levels of nickel, Pohler[32] observed that nickel was not usually present in the tissue next to implants in significant amounts. However, the results of Moberg et al[28] are equivocal because of the small study sample and the lack of valid controls. Furthermore, the plates were not inserted in a clinically analogous situation to fix an experimental fracture.

Agins et al[33] used atomic absorption spectroscopy (AAS) to quantify metal released into adjacent tissues from failed total hip replacement (THR) prostheses made of Ti-6Al-4V alloy. The average weight, in µg/g of dry tissue, was 1,047 for titanium (range, 56 to 3,700), 115 for aluminum (range, 2.1 to 396), and 67 for vanadium (range, 2.9 to 200). The normal weights (µg/g of dry tissue) for titanium, aluminum, and vanadium were reported as 0, 0, and 1.2, respectively.

Extensive pigmentation of tissues may occur next to metal-on-metal orthopedic prostheses because of fretting corrosion. Corrosion products may stain the tissues next to a metallic implant, giving rise to the term *metallosis*.[14,34] Huo et al[35] analyzed the tissues surrounding screw holes in mechanically stable cementless acetabular components of THR prostheses made of titanium alloy in three patients. The mean titanium level measured by AAS was 4,653 µg/g of dry tissue (range, 91 to 11,900 µg/g). The authors attributed the high levels of titanium in the tissues to fretting corrosion. Jorgenson et al[36] quantified titanium release from maxillofacial microplates into the adjacent soft tissues in four patients. The amount of titanium ranged from 7.92 to 31.8 µg/g of dry tissue. The microplates had been in situ from 84 to 116 weeks. There was no evidence of metallosis when the implants were removed.

Uniform attack releases approximately 12 to 32 µg/cm^2 of the exposed surface of a titanium implant each year.[37,38] Ferguson et al[39] reported normal titanium levels of 11.4 to 13.1 mg/g dry ash in rabbits. Steinemann et al[40] reported a figure of only 0.12 to 1.0 µg/g in humans. Smith[41] estimated the physiologic concentration of titanium in serum to be less than 10 µg/L, although Bianco et al[42] suggested that the actual figure was still

under debate. Maeusli et al[29] determined that the solubility of active titanium is approximately 0.15 µg/g at pH 7, according to the hydrolysis reaction:

$$TiO_2 + 2H_2O \longleftrightarrow Ti(OH)_4$$

When the solubility concentration of titanium (0.15 µg/g) is compared with the physiologic concentration of titanium within the tissues (0.12 to 1.0 µg/g), estimated conservatively by Steinemann et al,[40] titanium is at saturation point within the tissues. The corrosion products from a titanium implant may therefore precipitate in the tissues, as the titanium cannot be removed in solution from the site of implantation. When analysis of tissue yielded a significantly higher concentration of titanium than 0.15 µg/g, the excess is present in particulate form and will require phagocytosis for clearance. Maeusli et al[29] also stated that the formation of organometallic compounds was unlikely because dissolved neutral species such as $Ti(OH)^{3+}$ were likely to be inert. Bessho et al[43] suggested that titanium might enter the vascular system in solution. It is then disseminated from the implant site to distant organs.

Bianco et al[42] reported that titanium, released from an implant in the absence of wear, remains in the tissues near the implant. Local release of titanium was studied in the absence of wear from titanium-fiber felts that had been implanted into the tibia of rabbits for periods of up to 1 year. Titanium levels were greater within adjacent bone compared with controls at 4, 16, and 48 weeks after insertion of the implants (approximately 27 to 31 ng/g, limit of detection = 25.7 ng/g). The limit of detection of a trace element is the minimum concentration that may be detected with certainty by the given analytic method.[30] Titanium levels within muscle tissue also were raised (approximately 485 to 742 ng/g, limit of detection = 385 ng/g). Bianco et al[42] suggested that the rate of titanium release into bone increased up to 1 year after implantation.

Fatigue induced by fretting corrosion may be significant both in titanium and titanium alloys. Titanium alloys may be more susceptible to stress-corrosion cracking than commercially pure titanium,[44] but they do not exhibit galvanic corrosion under physiologic conditions.[45] The incorporation of molybdenum or tantalum in a titanium alloy enhances its resistance to corrosion and provides superior mechanical properties.

Before specifications for the manufacture of implant materials were introduced, corrosion of stainless steel implants was occasionally severe enough to form a so-called "rust-granuloma" containing iron oxides and other corrosion products within the tissues.[46] Cook et al[47] evaluated corrosion on 82 stainless steel orthopedic bone plates removed from patients between 4 and 676 weeks after insertion. Of the recovered implants, 89% displayed signs of surface (pitting) or plate-screw-interface (crevice and fretting) corrosion. All implants conformed to the ASTM F 138 standard for stainless steel. Cook et al[47] called for stricter manufacturing standards for stainless steel implants. Cook et al[48] subsequently examined 250 internal fixation plates after removal and reported a similar frequency of corrosion defects.

Influence of tissue proteins on corrosion of a metallic steel implant

Changes in the local environment affect the corrosion rate of stainless steel plates in vivo. Fretting corrosion in vitro of 316L stainless steel plates in a mixture of 10% fetal calf serum and normal saline solution is significantly greater than in the normal saline solution alone.[49] Merritt and Brown[50] immersed stainless steel AO (Davos, Switzerland) and Zimmer (Warsaw, IN) orthopedic plates in either sterile saline solution or in various sterile protein solutions in saline solution (at pH 6) for 16 hours per day over 14 days. There was significantly less corrosion in the protein solutions than in the saline solution. More nickel was released in the protein solutions than had been expected. Binding of metal ions from stainless steel to serum proteins such as β_2-macroglobulin and albumin occurs in serum next to the metal for chromium and nickel and in solution for cobalt from implant alloys.[51]

Sousa and Barbosa[52] studied the effect of proteins and calcium and phosphate ions on the resistance to corrosion of commercially pure (CP) titanium in vitro. The resistance to corrosion of titanium

decreased in the presence of calcium and phosphate ions, irrespective of whether the passive oxide film was intact or damaged. Resistance to corrosion of implants with an intact passive film was improved by immersion in 10% bovine serum. However, resistance to corrosion was compromised if the passive film was damaged.

Influence of Antibiotics on Corrosion of Metallic Implants

Antibiotics are usually administered prophylactically during open reduction of a jaw fracture. Soft tissue and bone adhere more easily to titanium than to other metallic implant materials, and thus the risk of infection is reduced.[40] Miniplate osteosynthesis of an infected fracture is usually satisfactory if the principles of adequate curettage of infection, rigid osteosynthesis, and appropriate antibiotic therapy are followed.[53,54] But infection may reduce the pH within the tissues and increase the rate of corrosion of an implant. Von Fraunhofer et al[55] studied the influence of antibiotics on corrosion of implants in vitro. Oxytetracycline inhibited corrosion at concentrations of 0.01 to 1.0 mg/mL. Von Fraunhofer et al[55] recommended preoperative administration of tetracycline for prophylaxis during the insertion of titanium, stainless steel, or Vitallium implants.

Von Fraunhofer and Stidham[56] studied the effect on metallic corrosion in vitro of doxycycline, oxytetracycline hydrochloride, and oxytetracycline dihydrate, other antibiotics that have the fused-ring structure of tetracycline. Oxytetracycline dihydrate inhibited corrosion of stainless steel. All three antibiotics inhibited corrosion of titanium. In contrast, all three antibiotics enhanced corrosion of Vitallium. Von Fraunhofer and Stidham[56] suggested that either topical or systemic administration of any of the three antibiotics would help to control infection and reduce corrosion whenever titanium components are implanted. Moura e Silva et al[57] studied the corrosion behavior in vitro of 316L stainless steel in diabetic serum, using isotonic saline solution alone and with two antibiotics as reference solutions. The addition of 4 g/L of ampicillin or cephradine to the saline solution did not influence the resistance of the stainless steel to pitting corrosion. Pooled samples of serum from diabetic patients with a total protein concentration of 68 g/L also had no significant effect on resistance to pitting corrosion.

Effect of Sterilization Techniques on Corrosion of Metallic Implants

Some sterilization techniques may adversely influence the surface properties of implants. Gamma-ray irradiation may alter the passive film on stainless steel, causing release of iron and the formation of a surface film enriched by chromium.[58] Sterilization by autoclave (one of the most common techniques for sterilizing maxillofacial plates and screws) may deposit a contaminating film on the surface of an implant. In contrast, pretreatment of an implant by radio-frequency glow discharge leaves the surface scrupulously clean, with a high surface energy. Chou et al[59] used radio-frequency glow discharge methods on titanium samples before tissue culture experiments. Vargas et al[60] used radio-frequency glow discharge on endosseous implants and found a statistically significant reduction of corrosion products after 2 and 12 weeks, compared with implants without pretreatment.

Fate of Corrosion Products

The fate of corrosion products from an implant is inadequately understood. Raised serum levels of metal from an implant may signal an increase in metallic content of some or all of the tissues in the body. Black et al[61] studied serum concentrations of chromium, cobalt, and nickel in patients with cobalt-chromium and polyethylene THR implants up to 24 weeks after surgery. Chromium levels reached a peak at 15 days after surgery and were still elevated by 50% after 24 more weeks. Cobalt levels remained the same or decreased. Nickel levels began to rise 2 to 6 weeks after surgery and gradually increased up to 24 weeks. Black et al[61] could not explain the significance of these changes. Autopsy was suggested as the most suitable method of studying long-term metal accumulation in the tissues from implants.

Pohler[32] discussed the fate of nickel, chromium, and iron after release from a stainless steel implant. Nickel is not usually present in significant amounts in the tissue adjacent to implants, suggesting that it is transported in solution. Chromium impregnates the tissue around the implant as a stable chromium oxide. Iron is partly dissolved and removed from the adjacent tissues and partly deposited both intra- and extracellularly.

Koegel and Black[62] studied the release of corrosion products from a cast cobalt-chromium alloy. The alloy was injected as a powder into the supraspinatus muscles of rats. Serum concentrations of chromium and cobalt rose in proportion to the amount of alloy present. The serum concentration of nickel reached a peak after 3 days and then diminished. Serum cobalt levels were elevated by a factor of 20, and chromium levels increased by a factor of 12. Koegel and Black[62] suggested that the serum concentrations of each element were short-term physiologic adaptations to the presence of biologically active organometallic complexes.

Brown et al[63] studied fretting corrosion of titanium and titanium alloy in vitro using a device that caused friction between a screw head and the countersink of a fracture plate. Accelerated fretting corrosion was simulated by anodic polarization during oscillation. The device was immersed in saline solution and 10% calf serum. After 1 hour, there were more metallic particles in saline solution than in calf serum. However, there was a greater loss of weight of titanium alloy and pure titanium components in calf serum than in saline solution. This was attributed to a greater percentage recovery of metallic ions by serum proteins. It was thought that the proteins formed complexes with metallic ions, preventing oxidation and precipitation of titanium oxide crystals.

Brown et al also undertook studies in vivo.[63] Titanium and titanium alloy implants were inserted subcutaneously in hamsters under anesthesia. The device that caused friction between a screw head and the countersink of a fracture plate was operated for 60 minutes. Fretting corrosion was simulated by applying electrodes to the skin during oscillation. Titanium levels were found to be elevated in serum and spleen samples but were not detected in urine. Vanadium was below detectable limits in serum, urine, liver, and spleen samples. The high solubility of vanadium was thought to account for the low levels detected, as vanadium is cleared rapidly from the body.

Bianco et al[64] studied the release of titanium from an implant in the absence of wear. Serum and urinary levels of titanium were assayed after insertion of titanium-fiber felts into rabbit tibiae. A sham group underwent surgery without the insertion of titanium felt, and a control group did not undergo surgery. Titanium in serum and urine for the implant group did not increase significantly compared to the control and sham groups up to 1 year after implantation. Bianco et al[64] also analyzed tissue from lymph nodes taken at autopsy. There was no difference in titanium content between the test group and controls. Bianco et al[64] suggested that titanium was excreted via feces and by incorporation into hair and nails.

Retrieval Studies

Retrieval studies are useful to evaluate the biologic performance of implants, both in patients and in animals. It is, however, unethical to insert implants in patients without reason or to withhold from a patient treatment that is known to be superior to other methods. Therefore, it is difficult to include valid controls in studies with patients. In contrast, retrieval studies in an animal model enable the use of controls and allow examination of tissues and even organs distant from the site of implantation.

Some early retrieval studies were unreliable because of doubtful methodology. For example, Brunski et al[65] found no corrosion or release of titanium into the tissues of dogs in a study of titanium endosseous blade-vent implants that had been removed after 8 to 48 weeks. However, the authors used only SEM and x-ray energy-dispersive spectroscopic (EDS) analysis, which was unsuitable to detect total amounts of metal released into the tissues. Moberg et al[28] fixed stainless steel, Vitallium, and titanium plates to the lateral surface of the mandible via a skin incision in seven monkeys. However, they did not create a fracture of the mandible before fixing the plates and therefore did not reproduce a clinically analogous situation.

Two studies by Bessho and coworkers[43,66] illustrate the use of retrieval studies in animals with the inclusion of control groups. The description below of the methods used in their study also highlights the dubious nature of their results. Bessho and Iizuka[66] conducted clinical and animal studies to determine the suitability of Champy titanium plates as permanent fixation devices. Titanium plates were removed 12 weeks following surgery in 50 patients after open reduction of a fracture of the mandible. Formation of new bone was reported in direct contact with the plate surface. Fibrous tissue was present around only 10 plates taken from six patients, and the fibrous capsules were described as thin. Light microscopy revealed titanium fragments in the fibrous capsule near the screws in 2 of the 10 plates where a capsule was present. Titanium levels of 0.1 ng/mg of wet tissue or less were determined within the fibrous tissue. The ability to detect such small amounts of titanium with accuracy is questionable, even with modern apparatus. The same authors, using the same equipment, reported a limit of detection for titanium of 0.5 ng/mg of wet tissue in a complementary animal study.[66]

Bessho and Iizuka[66] subjected each Champy miniplate surface to sandblasting, stone polishing, and natural passivation before insertion. This is not undertaken in clinical practice; most manufacturer's plates and screws are simply autoclaved before use. Bessho and Iizuka[66] reported surface depressions, identified by SEM examination, which the authors believed were caused by pitting corrosion. Stress-corrosion cracking also was identified, although the appearance of the plates was not described before implantation.

Bessho and Iizuka[66] also reported a study in rabbits in which a fracture of the mandible was created (the type of anesthesia was not stated). The fracture was reduced and fixed via an extraoral approach with a Champy continuous four-hole titanium miniplate and 5-mm screws. In a second group (nonfracture or control group), no fracture was created, but similar Champy titanium plates and screws were fixed to the mandible. Plates and screws remained in situ for 24 weeks. Plates were subsequently examined by SEM. Pitting corrosion was observed on the surfaces of all plates in both the fracture and nonfracture groups. The extent of pitting corrosion was not significantly different between the two groups. Furthermore, there was no distinct pattern of pitting on each plate. Stress-corrosion cracking, which the authors attributed to pitting corrosion, was observed more frequently on the miniplate surface next to the alveolar bone, between the two central screw holes. No stress-corrosion cracking was identified between the screw holes at either end of the plate. Stress-corrosion cracking is caused by a tensile stress within a corrosive environment and is virtually unheard of in CP titanium.[37] Bessho and Iizuka[66] also determined titanium levels in soft tissues next to the plates and in tissue from the left submandibular lymph node, lung, liver, spleen, and kidney. The titanium concentration in the tissues of the control group was less than 0.5 ng/mg of wet tissue. Titanium levels of this order of magnitude also were found in the submandibular lymph nodes and soft tissue surrounding the plates of the fracture group. More titanium was detected in lung, liver, spleen, and kidney tissue of both the fracture and nonfracture groups. The titanium concentration within the lungs was 14 times greater in the fracture group (248 ± 27.4 ng/mg) than in the nonfracture group (17.8 ± 2.4 ng/mg wet tissue). Titanium levels in the liver were three times greater in the fracture group (21.5 ± 6.9 ng/mg) than in the nonfracture group (7.8 ng/mg) and twice as great in the spleen and kidneys. Maximum titanium levels were detected after 12 weeks. Titanium levels were below the limit of detection in all of the submandibular lymph nodes of the test group.

Bessho et al[43] repeated the above study with titanium plates in situ for up to 2 years. As in the earlier study, plates and screws were conditioned before insertion, and the same operative procedure was adopted. Plates were removed 4, 12, 24, 52, and 104 weeks after surgery. The surfaces of the plates were examined by SEM before insertion and after retrieval. Corrosion pits were identified on the miniplate surface before insertion. However, the authors were probably describing natural features on the surface of the implants, for the plates had not been subjected to a corrosive physiologic environment before insertion.

Bessho et al[43] reported cracking of the miniplate surface caused by pitting corrosion. As in the previous study,[66] the cracks were more prevalent on the miniplate surface next to the bone between the central screw recesses. The extent of pitting was similar at each time interval. Bessho et al[43] described detachment of titanium oxide film from the surface of the plate, as shown by SEM. However, the surface of the implant would have undergone immediate passivation on exposure to air. In the usual secondary electron mode for observation, the SEM image detects topographical features but does not discriminate between different metallic elements or compounds on the surface of the miniplate. This distinction might be visible with the use of the backscattered electron imaging or EDS analysis, but the authors did not state whether these modes of SEM examination were used.

Bessho et al[43] did not identify titanium in any tissues of the control group. Furthermore, no titanium was found in the soft tissues surrounding the plates or in the submandibular lymph nodes of rabbits in either the fracture or nonfracture group at any time after implantation. However, titanium was present in lung and liver tissue of rabbits from the fracture and nonfracture groups. Titanium levels in the fracture group were 15 times greater in the liver and twice as high in the lungs than in the nonfracture group. Titanium levels were highest within organs of the fracture group 12 weeks after surgery but only 4 weeks after surgery in the nonfracture group. Titanium levels in both groups decreased gradually over the 2-year period of the study.

Surface analysis of retrieved plates and screws
Ionic leaching of metallic ions from plates and screws can occur in vivo through dissolution of the oxide layer on the surface,[67] but may be accelerated by damage to the surfaces of the implants during insertion and retrieval. Torgersen and Gjerdet[68] examined 43 stainless steel and 19 titanium plates and screws that were removed from the mandibles of patients after fracture healing. Titanium implants were in situ for 35 to 52 weeks, and stainless steel plates were in situ for 6 to 52 weeks. Two stainless steel plates and one titanium plate were removed because of wound dehiscence. The other plates were removed from asympt-

omatic patients. Handling defects were present on all plates on visual inspection, but more tool marks, appearing as sharp-edged scratches, were present on the stainless steel plates without corrosion.

There also was widespread damage to screw holes, attributed to drilling during their preparation. Tongues of metal and splinters also were present in the periphery of screw holes in both the titanium and stainless steel plates. Bone was identified within a screw countersink on three plates, one of titanium, and two of stainless steel. Scratches were present to a similar extent on all screw heads made of either material. A few small metallic splinters were present under the screw heads. Corrosion defects were localized to the countersink areas of stainless steel plates and were randomly distributed. Corrosion did not extend onto the flat surfaces of the plates. Corrosion defects also were observed on the fitting surface of the screw head, corresponding to similar defects at the contact point on the miniplate countersink. Titanium and stainless steel plates were rougher than unused plates of the same material, possibly because of degradation of the surface after implantation.

Matthew et al[31] investigated the surface features of titanium and stainless steel miniplates used to stabilize experimentally created fractures of the mandible in beagle dogs. Four animals were killed by rapid intravenous injection of sodium thiopentone after intervals of 4, 12, and 24 weeks. The soft tissues were elevated from the fracture sites, and the miniplates and screws were removed. Clinical healing was noted across all fracture sites. Bone growth had not occurred over the surface of the miniplates. EDS analysis was used to identify compositional variations at the miniplate surface. Low-vacuum SEM allowed examination of uncoated control (unused) and test miniplates from the same production batch and demonstrated typical features of both materials, with little difference in the surface characteristics of the miniplates at all time intervals. Screw heads made of both materials were damaged during use. Soft tissues had permeated surface defects of stainless steel plates over 4 mm wide and covered parts of the titanium surface from 4 weeks. Matthew et

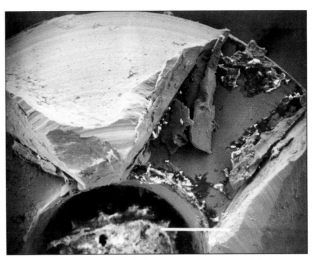

Fig 13-11 Low-vacuum SEM image of metallic debris present within the head of a titanium screw retrieved after healing of a jaw fracture (original magnification × 50; bar = 500 μm).

al[31] concluded that there was little evidence of surface corrosion damage by tissue fluids and cellular components up to 24 weeks following implantation, but the softness of titanium screws may render their removal difficult.

Formation of particles from the surface of a metallic implant Metallic protuberances have been shown to exist on miniplate and screw surfaces before insertion. Ray et al[69] identified metallic protuberances on the edges of the screw holes on the plates. These protuberances, if dislodged during plate and screw insertion, may increase the amount of particulate debris within the soft and hard tissues.

Metallic particles also may be created when a miniplate is bent to fit the contour of the jaw. Particles may be generated through friction between the bur and the countersink during preparation of the screw hole and through friction between the screw and the miniplate countersink during insertion or removal of screws. Damage to the head of a screw (or to the flat surface of the miniplate) during insertion or removal of the screw also may result in release of metallic particles (Fig 13-11). Damage to a screw head also may prevent proper engagement by the screwdriver, so that insertion or removal is difficult. Metallic particles may arise through fretting corrosion between the plate and screw. Aggregates of particles may represent the products of metallic degradation, originating from the interface between the miniplate and screw.[70] Levy et al[6] recommended copious irrigation of the wound after insertion of a miniplate to clear bony debris or metallic particles from the tissues. However, this may spread particles throughout the tissues.

Effect of a Metallic Biomaterial on the Host Tissues

Satisfactory integration of a biomaterial depends upon the direct attachment of host-matrix protein molecules or cell outer membrane molecules.[71] The tissue response is influenced by the surface energy, size, shape, and surface texture of the implant, as well as by movement at the interface between implant and tissue.[72–76] The solubility of the biomaterial, the rate of intercellular fluid turnover and macrophage activity, bacterial contamination, local pH, fretting corrosion in implants with two or more components, and electrochemical processes at the interface of metal and tissue are other important factors.

Impaired healing around an implanted material may be manifested as a failure of granulation tissue to organize the clot, failure of osteogenesis, granuloma formation, or the persistence of inflammatory cells.[77] Hypersensitivity also may occur, particularly in response to metallic ions released from stainless steel.[78] Corrosion products may cause chronic inflammation, abscess formation, delayed union or nonunion, osteomyelitis, aseptic inflammatory responses with associated swelling, or intractable pain.[70,79–82] Cells such as platelets, macrophages, lymphocytes, fibroblasts, and giant cells mediate the tissue reaction to a biomaterial. The clotting cascade, complement system, adhesion molecules, and cytokines are also important.[83–94]

Implants may cause resorption of bone or may interfere with tissue repair.[77] Release of metallic particles or other debris, eg, polymethyl methacrylate (PMMA) cement or polyethylene, may precipitate a foreign-body granuloma, necrosis, and/or resorption of bone.[95,96] Jacobs et al[97] and others have suggested that phagocytosis of metallic particles in the tissues by macrophages may stimulate bone loss around an implant. The process is mediated by cytokines that are released in response to macrophage activity.[98–100] The quantity of particulate material that precipitates resorption of bone is not known.[101]

Healing of Bone Next to a Metallic Implant

The host response to some biomaterials is similar to osteogenesis at the surface of bone.[102] Osseointegration is important for an endosseous implant, but it is of less importance in rigid internal fixation of jaw fractures. Miniplate fixation relies mainly on the stability of the self-tapping screws in cortical bone and on the maintenance or formation of healthy bone around the screws. Formation of bone over the surface of plates and screw heads can be disadvantageous if the plates and screws are subsequently removed (see Figs 13-5 and 13-6).

Southam and Selwyn[103] studied the structural changes in bone around Vitallium screws that had been used for fixation of jaw fractures but removed after the patients had died unexpectedly shortly after insertion (2 to 42 days). Bone fragments and hemorrhage were generated during preparation of the screw holes. The screws displaced the bone fragments into adjacent marrow spaces during insertion. By 8 days, the blood clot had undergone organization. However, acute and chronic inflammatory infiltrates were present next to multiple bone fragments around some screw holes. There was resorption of the cortical and cancellous bone trabeculae lining some screw holes. The rate and extent of resorption of bone were thought to depend on the mechanical forces applied to the screws and on their mechanical stability.

Linder and Lundskog[104] studied the reaction of bone to stainless steel, titanium, and Vitallium in rabbits. Copper implants acted as controls. They aimed to avoid operative trauma and implant instability in order to study the effect of corrosion only on the tissue response. The implants remained in situ up to 42 weeks. At autopsy, the tissues were analyzed by light microscopy. There was close apposition of bone to the implants, but with no adverse tissue reaction. Linder and Lundskog concluded that an atraumatic operative technique and implant rigidity were more important for stable incorporation of metallic implants in bone than the nature of the implant itself, yet the metal or alloy required high resistance to corrosion.

Using transmission electron microscopy, Albrektsson and Hansson[105] studied the ultrastructure of the interface between bone and magnetron sputter-coated titanium and stainless steel surfaces implanted in rabbits for 12 weeks. The titanium implants became directly anchored into bone with no cellular layers in the interface, but thick proteoglycan coatings and a cellular layer with inflammatory cells separated the surface of the stainless steel implant from bone. Sennerby et al[106] studied the ultrastructure of the interface between bone and titanium 48 weeks after inserting pure titanium endosseous implant screws in rabbit ulnas. Mineralized bone formed near the surface of the implant, but there was no direct contact.

Millar et al[4] found no difference in bone healing around titanium (Würzburg) and stainless steel (Champy) screws 4, 12, or 24 weeks after insertion into the skull bones of beagle dogs. However, the screws were not subjected to functional loads. Active bone formation was observed in conjunction with osteoclastic resorption of damaged bone. The damage to bone was attributed to thermal changes during preparation of the screw hole, although attempts were made during surgery to avoid overheating. Healing of bone was complete at 12 weeks. Cohen[107] commented that orthopedic screws were often difficult to remove at implant retrieval, a phenomenon more common with implants made of cobalt-chromium than of stainless steel.

Titanium ions may inhibit apatite crystal formation by binding to the surface of hydroxyapatite crystals and inactivating crystal growth sites in vitro.[108] Thompson and Puleo[109] studied the effect of Ti-6Al-4V alloy in solution on bone-marrow stromal cells harvested from juvenile rats. Cells were cultured in the presence of Ti-6Al-4V alloy in solution. After 4 weeks, total protein and alkaline phosphatase levels were similar for test and control solutions, but osteocalcin synthesis was inhibited by the Ti-6Al-4V alloy in solution. Calcium levels were reduced when the metallic ions were added before a critical stage of osteoblast differentiation, suggesting that Ti-6Al-4V alloy had inhibited the normal differentiation of bone-marrow stromal cells to mature osteoblasts in vitro. Formation of bone may also be impaired by corrosion products of cobalt-chromium alloys in vitro through the inhibition of enzymatic activity and protein production of osteoblasts.[13]

Titanium and stainless steel implants can become coated by a calcium phosphate substrate that is similar to apatite when the metal is immersed in a solution of similar pH to biologic fluids.[110] Leitão et al[111] immersed titanium alloy in Hank's solution at 37°C for 14 days. An apatite-like layer formed on the metal surface. Studies subsequently undertaken in vitro showed that the amorphous apatite structure improved the bonding characteristics of the titanium alloy to bone. However, the calcium phosphate layer must be at least 1 μm thick for induction of new bone on its surface.[111]

Larsson et al[112] showed that less bone formed around electropolished endosseous implants than machined implants with a similar oxide thickness in vivo. Könönen et al[113] studied the effect of electropolishing, etching, and sandblasting of commercially pure titanium surfaces on the adhesion, orientation, and proliferation of human gingival fibroblasts. Fibroblasts present on sandblasted titanium surfaces in vitro grew in clusters, suggesting that their ability to migrate in most directions was impaired. This feature would be desirable in metallic plates to minimize the possibility of fibrous tissue formation around the implant. Components of the Hall miniplate system (now obsolete) were electropolished after construction.

Formation of a Fibrous Connective-Tissue Capsule Around a Metallic Implant

The formation of fibrous connective tissue around an implant represents an attempt by the host tissue to sequester a foreign body.[77] Southam and Selwyn[103] stated that a layer of fibrous tissue always forms around a metallic implant after insertion into bone. Furthermore, the implant would subsequently never be as secure in the bone as it was immediately after insertion. However, capsule formation around an implant also has been regarded as a nonspecific response, regardless of the material implanted.[114] Formation of a fibrous capsule around a metallic implant in bone is also influenced by implant stability and corrosion.[104] Fibrous connective tissue present around an implant may itself compromise implant stability and precipitate loosening.[104] The concept of tissue tolerance to an implant previously has been evaluated by examining the amount of fibrous connective tissue that forms around an implant alloy.[115]

The extent of scarring or capsule formation around an implant depends on the severity of the surgical trauma, subsequent cell death, and the site of the implant.[27] After tissue injury, inflammatory, immune, and mesenchymal cells infiltrate the tissues.[116] Mesenchymal cells proliferate locally, and collagen is synthesized and deposited within the healing tissues. Laing et al[117] examined the tissue reaction to stainless steel, titanium, and titanium-alloy implants in rabbit muscle 24 weeks after implantation. Using light microscopy, two main zones were identified next to the implants: a pseudomembrane formed by the collection of cells next to the implant and a zone in which muscle had been replaced by fat and fibrous tissue. However, there was no effect on the muscle next to the pseudomembrane with 316L stainless steel. A thin pseudomembrane and mild fibrosis were identified next to Ti-6Al-4V alloy. The tissue reaction to titanium and titanium alloy implants was mild, explained by the wide exposure of animals and humans to titanium. Laing et al[117] attributed the mild tissue response to the titanium implants to the low toxicity of titanium.

The macrophage has an essential role in wound healing and in the physical removal of foreign material from the tissues. Macrophages are in contact with the surface of an implant within 24 hours, but their behavior is different at smooth and rough surfaces.[118] Macrophages and giant cells may coexist indefinitely next to the surface of an implant that is rough. Their presence

represents a chronic granulomatous reaction to the implant.[118] Macrophages activate the synthesis of collagen by fibroblasts.[118] The formation of fibrous tissue around an implant may therefore be mediated by cytokines released from macrophages.

Metallic particles within the tissues indirectly stimulate collagen synthesis in vitro.[119] At low (unspecified) concentrations, tumor necrosis factor alpha (TNF-α) stimulates fibroblast proliferation, and at higher concentrations, TNF-α inhibits the proliferation of fibroblasts.[116] TNF-α therefore may mediate the deposition of fibrous tissue around an implant. Tissue fluids degrade small metallic particles, producing even smaller particles, which are phagocytosed. Chronic inflammatory cells may remain within the fibrous capsule around an implant, and cellular immune responses may cause tissue damage mediated by cytokines,[71] which may increase the chances of infection or aseptic loosening of an implant. Hypersensitivity to the metal may cause loosening of an implant through a similar mechanism.[120]

Pigmentation in Soft Tissues Next to Plates and Screws

Corrosion may give rise to gray or black pigmentation of tissue next to the implant. Such pigmentation has been reported next to titanium and stainless steel plates and screws.[12,121–123] But pigmentation is not always present when plates and screws are removed. Torgersen et al[12] identified pigmentation in soft tissues next to stainless steel plates in 7 out of 15 patients. Nakamura et al[121] reported gray or black pigmentation next to Champy stainless steel plates in 7 out of 91 patients. On light-microscopy examination of biopsy samples, black or brown pigmented material was identified both within fibroblasts and in the extracellular tissues. Nakamura et al[121] attributed the pigmentation to release of metallic particles from the miniplate or bur during preparation of the screw hole. They found no evidence that retention of plates would cause complications but acknowledged that the cumulative effect of corrosion products was inadequately understood. Matthew and Frame[124] found no clear correlation between the extent of pigmentation of the soft tissues adja-

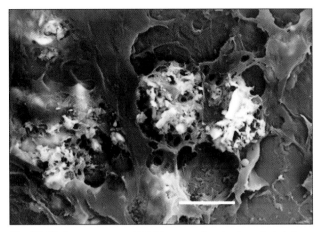

Fig 13-12 Low-vacuum SEM image of a cluster of stainless steel particles from the soft tissues immediately adjacent to the interface between a maxillofacial miniplate and screw. Some of the particles appear to be intracellular, and the void immediately above the bar suggests displacement of some debris during processing of the histologic sections (original magnification × 2,000; bar = 10 µm).

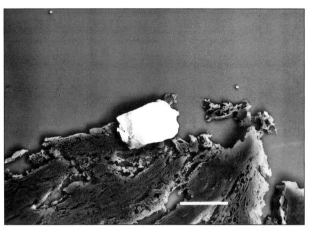

Fig 13-13 A solitary titanium particle within the soft tissues at the base of a screw hole. The particle shown is larger than those typically seen in histologic sections (normal range, 1 to 10 µm) (original magnification × 350; bar = 50 µm).

Characterization of Metallic Particles Within the Tissues

Rosenberg et al[14] analyzed black pigmentation in soft tissue covering titanium and stainless steel (Champy) plates in 32 patients treated for fracture of the mandible. The mean period between surgical repair and implant removal was 32 weeks (range, 12 to 128 weeks). The extent of pigmentation next to a fractured plate or loose screws was similar. On visual inspection, the tissues were pigmented next to 25% of the titanium plates but none of the stainless steel plates. Light microscopy revealed metallic particles in 72% of the soft tissues overlying the titanium plates and in 65% of the soft tissues overlying the stainless steel plates. Titanium dioxide was identified by EDS analysis in the soft tissue next to a titanium miniplate. Chromium, nickel, iron, and molybdenum were present in the tissues next to a stainless steel miniplate. Stainless steel particles up to 50 µm in diameter were identified within giant cells. No toxic systemic side effects occurred, although metallic

cent to Champy plates and screws and the amount of metal identified within soft tissue and bone samples immediately adjacent to the implants.

ions were present within the tissues next to the plates and screws.

Schliephake et al[7] used transmission electron microscopy to study particles liberated from titanium plates. Ten patients had undergone reduction and fixation of a fracture of the mandible with titanium plates. The tissues were biopsied when the implants were removed. Groups of opaque particles were identified within the connective tissue by light microscopy. There were no inflammatory cells next to the particles. Polygonal particles (0.5 to 5 µm in diameter) were present between collagen fibers. There was no cellular uptake or tissue degradation. Many smaller particles were grouped together and had a more diffuse outline than the larger particles.

Using low-vacuum SEM, Matthew and Frame[125] analyzed metallic particles identified in histologic sections of tissue retrieved after insertion of plates and screws under different conditions of loading. Most particles were 1 to 10 µm in diameter (Figs 13-12 and 13-13). The tissue response was variable; some particles were covered by fibrous connective tissue or surrounded by bone, and others appeared to be intracellular. The limitations of the SEM technique prevented analysis of the morphology of phagocytic cells.

Phagocytosis of Metallic Particles

Metallic particles (1 to 10 µm in diameter) are potent stimulators of macrophages in vitro.[119] Macrophages that are exposed to the surface of an implant or that phagocytose metallic particles may secrete inflammatory mediators. Over 100 secretory products have been isolated from macrophages.[126] Although titanium particles may act as a reservoir for collagenase, metallic particles released from implants may be responsible for stimulating collagen production from adjacent cells. Titanium, Ti-6Al-4V, and Co-Cr-Mo particles activate monocytes and macrophages to release Prostaglandin E_2 (PGE_2) in vitro and stimulate fibroblasts to increase collagen synthesis.[119] However, cell damage occurs in vitro after contact between fibroblasts and metallic particles.[127] The cell damage occurs regardless of the chemical nature of the particle, suggesting that the physical properties of the particles are responsible.

Toxic particulate material may affect the morphology of macrophages.[128] Pseudopodia retract, the cell-wall surface becomes smooth, and finally the cell is destroyed. The host response may depend on the number and size of particles. Goodman et al[129] studied the response to titanium alloy and polyethylene particles inserted via a bur hole in the proximal tibia of rabbits. The titanium alloy and polyethylene particles were small enough to stimulate phagocytosis. Up to 16 weeks after surgery, a histiocytic reaction was evoked, without extensive fibrosis, necrosis, or granuloma formation, in the presence of 10^6 to 10^9 particles per milliliter.

An implant that is not subjected to loading through functional stresses may generate wear particles at a rate that allows phagocytic cells to remove the particles from the tissues faster than they are generated.[130] This circumstance is analogous to the low-stress loading of maxillofacial plates, in contrast to orthopedic fracture plates, which might also explain differences in the cellular response within tissues next to maxillofacial plates compared with orthopedic prostheses.

Shanbhag et al[131] studied the effect of particle size of titanium and polystyrene samples on macrophage function in vitro. They analyzed bone-resorbing activity, fibroblast proliferation and secretion of interleukin-1 (IL-1) and PGE_2. Both IL-1 and PGE_2 stimulate resorption of bone.[119] Spherical particles of titanium dioxide (0.15 and 0.45 µm in diameter) and oxidized CP titanium (1.76 µm in diameter) were added to monocyte-macrophage cell cultures. Macrophages that were exposed to titanium particles released IL-1 but did not stimulate adjacent fibroblasts. Larger particles inhibited macrophage DNA synthesis, suggesting that cell damage or death occurred. Cells that were stimulated by the particles released small amounts of PGE_2 but increased resorption of bone by up to 125% compared with controls. Goldring et al[119] showed that the smaller particles were less injurious to macrophages than the larger ones.

Dissemination of Metallic Deposits from Implants via the Lymphatic System

Metallic deposits arising from implants have also been identified in regional lymph nodes, both in animals and in patients. Heath et al[132] showed that particulate cobalt-chromium alloy injected intramuscularly in rats is transported from the tissues to the regional lymph nodes, where the particles are present typically within macrophages. Meachim and Brooke[133] inserted particles of Vinertia (Vitallium) into the synovium of knee joints in guinea pigs. At autopsy, particles were identified in the ipsilateral inguinal lymph nodes. Biopsy of the knee joints revealed that particles (1 to 8 µm in diameter) had been phagocytosed by intimal cells, macrophages, multinucleate giant cells, and fibroblasts. Particles of 8 µm diameter or greater were typically present extracellularly, with adjacent multinucleate giant cells or macrophages. Clearance of the particles was slow, and fragments were present in the tissues after several months.

Inguinal lymphadenopathy has been reported in association with an orthopedic prosthesis that had been inserted after resection of an osteosarcoma from the lower femur and knee.[134] Metallic particles (0.5 to 5 µm in diameter) identified by light microscopy were present as irregular granules within histiocytes.

Onodera et al[135] reported titanium pigmentation in the submandibular tissues and an adjacent lymph node in a 41-year-old male treated for ameloblastoma of the mandible. There were no apparent local or systemic effects of titanium release. The mandible had been partially resected and then reconstructed with a titanium plate. Two years after surgery the plate was removed, along with the adjacent submandibular lymph node, because of loosening of screws. Microscopy revealed numerous black granules (1 to 20 µm in diameter) dispersed throughout the submandibular lymph node. Intracellular granules were identified within histiocytes by transmission electron microscopy. Dense particles (0.2 to 5 µm in diameter) were present and exhibited a well-defined outline with no jagged edges. EDS analysis showed that the particles were titanium. The authors attributed the generation of titanium particles to fretting corrosion between plate and screws.

Weingart et al[136] identified titanium within regional lymph nodes 36 weeks after insertion of endosseous implants in beagle dogs. Titanium levels were 0.16 to 9.0 µg/g in the regional lymph nodes of 12 of the 19 dogs in the test group and 0.01 to 0.21 µg/g in visceral organs. There was no relationship between the number of implants inserted and the presence of titanium in the regional lymph nodes.

Cytotoxicity of Corrosion Products

Corrosion products from an implant may be present in particulate form or in solution, and may be cytotoxic either within adjacent tissues or at distant sites. The intensity of the reaction diminishes in proportion to the distance from the implant.[137] Some cells are more vulnerable to metallic ions than others. Titanium, chromium and molybdenum in solution are well tolerated by macrophages in vitro.[138] Ions released from Co-Cr-Mo alloys and 316L stainless steel have been shown to be toxic in vitro to osteoblasts at concentrations similar to those measured in the fibrous capsule surrounding orthopedic implants.[139]

Rae[140] showed that nickel chloride (200 nmol/L) and cobalt chloride (50 nmol/L) solutions were toxic to cultured human synovial fibroblasts in vitro. Rae also showed that solutions of nickel (0.05 µmol/L) and cobalt (0.01 µmol/L) impaired the phagocytosis of bacteria by human polymorphonuclear leukocytes in vitro.[81] Tracana et al[141] injected a solution of iron (490 µg/mL), chromium (224 µg/mL), nickel (150 µg/mL), and molybdenum (26 µg/mL) from 316L stainless steel into the peritoneum of mice. White cell and macrophage counts in the peritoneal samples increased up to 1 week, suggesting that the metallic ions released caused only a transient and minor inflammatory response in the peritoneum. Lymphocytes were not stimulated by the presence of metals. However, this does not necessarily suggest a similar tissue response in other tissues around orthopedic or jaw implants made of 316L stainless steel.

Jacobs et al[97] examined the tissues next to THR implants after revision surgery. Chromium-phosphate particles (1 to 200 µm in diameter) were identified within the tissues, but there was no clinical evidence of metal toxicity. Carvalho et al[142] studied enzyme activity of human fibroblasts in response to corrosion products and metallic salts in vivo. Stainless steel corrosion products had no effect on cell morphology after 4 to 21 days. However, a solution of iron, chromium, and nickel stimulated cell proliferation and enzymatic activity. The effects of iron, chromium, and nickel together in solution were comparable with those of chromium alone. Chromium was therefore the metallic ion mainly responsible for the stimulatory effects.

Cytotoxicity may be influenced by the surface characteristics of an implant. Harmand et al[143] exposed rough-cast, microbead-blasted, specular-polished, and radio-frequency sputtered surfaces to human osteoblasts and gingival fibroblasts in vitro. Human osteoblasts were more sensitive than gingival fibroblasts to differences in the surface of the implant. Lysis occurred in cells next to rough-cast surfaces. Rapid corrosion, causing release of toxic chromium and cobalt compounds, was thought to be the cause. The best response was obtained with the microbead-blasted surface, followed by the specular-polished surface. However, specular polishing created a smooth surface finish that was unsuitable for cell adaptation, and the radio-frequency sputtered surface released toxic products.

Interference with Normal Cellular Function by Metallic Ions

Endogenous substances, eg, complement factor, leukotrienes, and denatured proteins, typically cause chemotaxis. Substances released from an implant may also cause chemotaxis. Nickel and copper ions affect chemotaxis of leukocytes, mediated by a change in shape.[144,145] Remes and Williams[146] studied the chemotactic response of human neutrophils to chromium, cobalt, and nickel ions at various concentrations in vitro in a protein-free environment. Cobalt and chromium ions did not stimulate chemotaxis of human neutrophils. Nickel ions inhibited chemotaxis at a concentration of 2.5 to 50 ppm. Hunt et al[144] incubated neutrophils in nickel and copper solutions and studied the kinetics of neutrophil locomotion by image analysis. Nickel and copper ions stimulated neutrophils to become aspherical and to move more slowly. Hunt et al[144] suggested that nickel ions might inhibit calcium-ion-dependent contractile activity by depolarizing the neutrophil cell membrane.

Stainless steel corrosion products may interfere with hepatocyte function in vivo. Pereira et al[145] obtained corrosion products from stainless steel by electrochemical dissolution. At intervals of 3 days they injected 0.5 mL of the solution (6.8 μg/mL iron, 138.6 μg/mL chromium, and 114.7 μg/mL nickel) subcutaneously into mice for 10 or 14 days. AAS analysis of dry livers from treated mice showed that chromium levels increased significantly compared with controls. Light microscopy revealed extensive hepatic degeneration in mice from both test groups compared with controls. Hepatocytes were swollen and had clear cytoplasm; the nuclei were hyperchromatic.

Puleo and Huh[139] showed that chromium, cobalt, iron, molybdenum, and nickel ions in solution were toxic in vitro to cells in bone marrow that were capable of producing bone. In contrast, aluminum, manganese, titanium, and vanadium ions were not toxic at concentrations below

25 ppm. Other cells have a different susceptibility to metallic ions. Human neutrophils are not activated or damaged in vitro by solutions containing up to 10 ppm Co^{2+}, 50 ppm Ni^{2+}, or 10 ppm Cr^{3+}.[82,144] Daniel et al[147] showed that cell death occurred in fibroblast cultures exposed to 5 ppm of cobalt in solution. However, growth of fibroblasts in vitro was only inhibited by a 7.5-ppm solution of cobalt in another study.[148] Sublethal doses of certain metallic ions may also inhibit the function of bone cells.[139]

Oncogenesis

No amount of experimental study can guarantee absolute safety for any substance.[149] However, toxicologic investigations provide results from which reasonable assumptions may be made about the conditions under which a product can be safely used. Heath et al[132] showed that metallic particles, produced by the movement of an artificial cobalt-chromium alloy joint in Ringer's solution, were oncogenic in rat muscle. Titanium dioxide, administered orally in doses ranging from 6,250 to 100,000 ppm, was not oncogenic in rats and mice.[150] Nickel is a known occupational carcinogen, predisposing nickel-refinery workers to lung and nasal cancer.[151] Trace amounts of trivalent chromium are essential for carbohydrate metabolism in mammals, but hexavalent chromium is oncogenic.[151] Deposits of iron in the tissues suppress function of the immune system in vivo, and prolonged exposure may predispose subjects to opportunistic infection or neoplasia.[152]

Implant materials have specific electrostatic, hydrophilic, ionic, and other surface properties that may influence the onset of neoplastic change. Any biomaterial may cause neoplasia in animals if the material has a smooth continuous surface and is not degradable in vivo.[153] The frequency of oncogenesis may be reduced and latency prolonged when materials with roughened surfaces are used.[153] Latency is the time from insertion of an implant to confirmation of neoplastic change.

Bessho et al[154] reported the induction of a neoplasm by a metallic implant used in jaw reconstruction, but the authors gave no details. There have been no other published reports of oncogenesis in association with maxillofacial plates and screws. Friedman and Vernon[155] reported an intraoral squamous cell carcinoma arising next to a gold mandibular staple implant 36 weeks after implantation. However, the onset of the neoplasm was regarded as coincidental because of the short latent period.

Malignant lesions have been reported in relation to orthopedic implants, eg, malignant fibrous histiocytoma,[156] osteosarcoma,[157] and epithelioid carcinoma.[158] The average period for development of a neoplasm is 20 years after insertion of an implant, although the minimum period of exposure may be as little as 5 to 10 years.[34]

McDougall[159] reported the case of a patient who fractured an arm, which was subsequently plated. The arm was fractured again 25 years after the initial injury. This time the fracture was treated conservatively. Five years later the patient presented with a history of painless swelling at the site of the original fracture for 10 weeks. The lesion was a Ewing sarcoma. The stainless steel plate and screws were dissimilar on metallurgic examination; a potential difference of 80 mV existed between plate and screws. The patient underwent radiotherapy but died from metastases a year later.

Dube and Fisher[160] reported a hemangioendothelioma in an 84-year-old man arising 30 years after insertion of a metallic plate used to treat nonunion of a fracture of the tibia. The plate was type 316 stainless steel and displayed moderate surface corrosion. Dense sheets of macrophages were present in the fibrous tissue surrounding the plate. Nickel and chromium deposits were identified within the malignant tissue.

Sunderman[161] reviewed the incidence of malignancy arising at the site of metallic orthopedic implants in 13 patients from 1956 to 1987. The latent period averaged 11 years (range, 2 to 30 years). The case histories suggested that most neoplasms were induced by the implanted prostheses, and most implants were of Fe-Cr-Ni (stainless steel, AISI type 316) or Co-Cr-Mo (Vitallium, ASTM type F 75) alloys. In two of the reported cases, orthopedic plates and screws made of different stainless steel alloys were used. Galvanic corrosion appeared to contribute to development of the neoplasms.

The latent period for development of a malignant lesion varies among species. Sinibaldi et al[162] reported eight malignant lesions that originated near metallic implants used in the treatment of common fractures in cats and dogs. In 6 years, 2,600 fractures were treated by open reduction and fixation. Five osteosarcomas, one fibrosarcoma, and two undifferentiated sarcomas with the characteristics of malignant histiocytomas were diagnosed. All eight neoplasms occurred in the midshaft of the femur. None were infected. All of the implants showed signs of corrosion. The latent period varied from 24 weeks to 6 years.

Epidemiologic studies suggest that the incidence of malignancy related to implants may remain low in the future.[163] However, as more implants are used and the duration of implantation increases, the incidence may rise.[164] Hamblen and Carter[165] reviewed the literature on cases of sarcoma arising after hip arthroplasty. They argued that the number of reported cases was so small compared with the number of hip replacements undertaken that neither patients nor surgeons should be concerned. However, clinicians are not obliged to report adverse reactions to prostheses, and the true incidence of malignancy associated with metallic implants therefore cannot be estimated reliably.[161]

Titanium has been available as an implant material over a shorter period than stainless steel, but its use has increased considerably over the past decade. The long-term biologic effect of titanium as an implant material in humans, both on adjacent tissues and on distant organs, therefore is not established. Infants who have undergone craniofacial surgery might have metallic plates within the tissues for 40 to 60 years or longer if the components remain in situ. The same is true of some adolescents who have had orthognathic surgery or other patients in their late teens and early 20s who have sustained facial fractures.

It is reassuring that there are few reports in the literature of oncogenesis arising either next to an implant or at remote sites. However, the incidence of oncogenesis may increase in the future through the increasing use of metallic implants as permanent fixtures.[34] Although titanium is considered to be a safe biomaterial, our knowledge of the long-term tissue response to titanium remains incomplete, suggesting the need to maintain a cautious approach to its use as a permanent implant.[166] Long-term follow-up of patients with metallic implants is important in order to identify any link between release of metallic ions and development of a malignant neoplasm.[162,164]

A metallic implant, or wear particles that are released from it, may influence interactions between macrophages and T lymphocytes by stimulating the production of cytokines.[11] Prolonged exposure may cause failure of antineoplastic surveillance mechanisms, and a neoplasm may develop. Tracana et al[167] studied the effect of stainless steel corrosion products on spleen tissue in mice. Iron, chromium, and nickel ions in physiologic solution were injected subcutaneously, and the spleens were removed after 4, 10, and 14 days. The levels of iron, chromium, and nickel in the spleens were assayed, and the tissues were examined by light microscopy. The metallic ions, especially iron, had accumulated in the spleen and induced changes in cell populations. There were more multinucleate giant cells and fewer lymphocytes. Tracana et al[167] concluded that stainless steel corrosion products induced cellular changes in the spleen and may impair immune function, possibly offering a clue to the mechanism of impaired immune surveillance and oncogenesis in association with metallic implants.

Suitability of Metallic Plates and Screws As Permanent Implants

There has been uncertainty in the past over the need to remove asymptomatic plates and screws after healing of a jaw fracture. Plates and screws also may have to be removed for specific indications. These include infection, wound dehiscence, the subsequent provision of a dental or maxillofacial prosthesis, or pain from thermal conductivity. Plates and screws also may have to be removed when the device is visible or palpable through the skin or oral mucosa or for psychological reasons. The plate or screw may fracture

or elicit local radiographic changes, or operator error may have resulted in poor placement of the plates and screws.[168] However, is it safe to leave metallic plates and screws in situ after a jaw fracture has healed? Scales et al[169] recommended the removal of all stainless steel orthopedic appliances after healing because the extent of corrosion that might be harmful to the host was impossible to determine. At that time of Scales and coworkers' study[169] there was no standard for the production of implant-grade stainless steel. It is difficult to study the long-term physiologic effects of metallic implants in animal models because of the high cost of animal maintenance, the animals' short life expectancy, and uncertainty over the relevance of such studies to humans. These difficulties have essentially made the patient the laboratory for long-term testing of biomaterials.[137]

Should Jaw Plates and Screws Be Removed Routinely After Osteosynthesis?

Cawood[1] suggested that plates should be removed after 12 weeks to avoid interference of the plate with jaw function. Moberg et al[28] advised removal of nickel-chromium and cobalt-chromium alloy implants after satisfactory healing because metallic elements released from the surface could induce allergic sensitization. Nakamura et al[121] commented that plates in the tooth-bearing region might be involved in dental infections in later life.

Nakamura et al[121] recommended removal of all plates and screws but did not specify a minimum time after surgery for their removal. Iizuka and Lindqvist[170] removed stainless steel plates about one year after surgery because there were no grounds for leaving a foreign metallic object in situ after bone healing had occurred. In contrast, it has been suggested that titanium and titanium alloys are suitable for use as permanent maxillofacial implants because of their superior biocompatibility over stainless steel.[171,172]

Moberg et al[28] used titanium plates and screws if they decided that the implants were to remain in situ. Rosenberg et al[14] removed titanium plates only if the patient experienced symptoms or in the presence of infection or wound dehiscence.

The authors believed that the black deposits occasionally found within the adjacent soft tissues did not necessitate removal of the plates. Williams[173] stated that titanium had gained its position within the hierarchy of biocompatibility despite the observed gross discoloration of adjacent tissue.

Titanium vs Stainless Steel Plates and Screws As Permanent Implants

It is uncertain whether titanium plates and screws are superior to those of stainless steel when used as permanent implants. Breme et al[171] examined the tissue reaction to titanium and stainless steel plates and screws 8 to 20 weeks after insertion into the tibias of guinea pigs with no experimental fractures. New bone formed next to the titanium fixtures, and it was difficult to identify the location of the titanium plates at autopsy. Granulation tissue was present between the surface of the stainless steel plates and surrounding bone, but not between titanium plates and adjacent bone. The authors recommended removal of all stainless steel plates because of the risk of metallosis and allergy to nickel and chromium. However, they concluded that it was not necessary to remove titanium plates after healing of bone because titanium was well tolerated by the surrounding tissues. The experimental method of Breme et al[171] did not take into account the clinical situation of a fracture of the jaws.

Brown et al[174] studied the fate of 279 stainless steel Champy plates used in maxillofacial trauma and orthognathic surgery. Plates were removed only if there was swelling, discharge, or dehiscence, or if pain was experienced that was not caused by infection. The symptoms resolved once the implants were removed. Of the 30 plates removed, 24 (80%) were removed within the first year. Plates were removed because of infection within the trauma group in 8 of 12 patients, in contrast to 5 of 7 patients within the orthognathic group. Plate survival was not influenced by the time interval between injury and surgery, the cause of the trauma, the severity of the trauma, or the use of IMF. The authors challenged the practice of removing all Champy stainless steel plates 12 to 16 weeks after insertion.

In a review paper, Haug[172] commented that stainless steel should not be used as a permanent implant material to treat a jaw fracture because of corrosion toxicity, hypersensitivity, and stress protection. There is no evidence that stainless steel plates and screws adversely affect the healing of a jaw fracture through stress protection. Haug[172] also stated that titanium and Ti-6Al-4V alloy implants may be retained as permanent implants because of their superior resistance to corrosion, non-oncogenicity, hyposensitivity, nontoxicity, and excellent tissue compatibility. Furthermore, he argued that the possible complications associated with the removal of plates and screws and the costs incurred in removal did not justify the benefits derived.

It is misleading for Haug[172] to state that titanium implants are not oncogenic in humans because there is a lack of evidence to support this statement. Conversely, it is generally assumed that titanium is not an oncogenic biomaterial simply because of a lack of reports. It is only after sufficient individuals have had titanium implants in situ, both subperiosteally (plates) and endosteally (miniplate screws and endosseous implants), for two or more decades that the evidence will become available.

Removal of orthopedic implants may be unjustifiable because of the severity of complications. Brown et al[175] studied the outcome of 297 orthopedic procedures involving metallic implants in 284 patients. Forty-two percent of the implants were removed, and the postoperative complication rate was unacceptably high. The risk of complications associated with the removal of orthopedic implants outweighed the theoretical disadvantages of leaving the implants in situ. Brown et al[175] stressed that removal of an implant is technically difficult and should not be undertaken by inexperienced surgeons without supervision. French et al[70] studied the tissue reaction in patients undergoing orthopedic implant removal and concluded that tissue reaction decreases with time. Furthermore, they suggested that internal fixation devices do not need to be removed routinely.

Llewelyn and Sugar[176] argued that removal of stainless steel lag screws used in oral and maxillofacial surgery procedures was unnecessary. They examined 26 stainless steel lag screws removed after a mean of 42 weeks. The implants, all of which complied with the ASTM specification, showed no signs of corrosion on visual inspection, and none was loose or infected at the time of removal. However, visual inspection is a crude and inadequate measure of corrosion. Lag screws are single-component implants and not prone to crevice or fretting corrosion. The authors concluded that stainless steel lag screws inserted for sagittal split osteotomy do not cause significant morbidity and should not require removal.

In 1991, the Strasbourg Osteosynthesis Research Group (SORG) issued a statement recommending the removal of plates and screws once the fracture had healed:

> A (titanium) plate, which is intended to assist the healing of bone, becomes a non-functional implant once this role is complete. It may then be regarded as a foreign body. While there is no clear evidence to date that a (titanium) plate causes any actual harm, our knowledge remains incomplete. It is therefore not possible to state with certainty that an otherwise symptomless (titanium) plate left in situ in the long term is harmless. The removal of a non-functioning (titanium) plate is desirable provided that the procedure to remove the plate does not cause any undue risk to the patient.[177]

The SORG statement was published in the technical brochures of Martin Medizin-Technik (Tuttlingen, Germany) and in a textbook on maxillofacial trauma.[177] However, the statement was not published in contemporary journals for the benefit of a wider audience.

The Arbeitgemeinschaft für Osteosynthesefragen (AO) study group (Davos, Switzerland; http://www.ao-asif.ch/) for internal fixation held a similar view of the permanent retention of plates and screws.[3] The AO study group commented that plates do not appear to have a deleterious effect on health in the long term, but internal fixation devices should be removed after healing, especially in patients with a long life expectancy.

Orthopedic bone plates typically are used in mature patients, some of whom may have coexisting disease. It may be inappropriate to remove implants in these patients because of the risks associated with general anesthesia.[178] In contrast, most patients who sustain fractures of the mandible are in their 20s or 30s.[179] If surgical access is satisfactory, it may be desirable to remove nonfunctional plates in younger patients because it is not proven that the permanent retention of metallic maxillofacial implants over four or five decades is safe. However, the arguments in favor of removal of plates after bone healing, either by experienced surgeons or by junior surgeons under direct supervision, remain valid in order to avoid complications.

Conclusions

It is recognized that metallic ions leach from the surface of a metallic implant. Metallic debris is also present within the tissues adjacent to metallic jaw plates and screws. The tissue reaction to metallic ions and particulate debris is inadequately understood. The current practice of leaving metallic miniplates and screws in situ after healing of a jaw fracture is undesirable in view of our lack of knowledge of the long-term tissue response to these implants.[180–182]

References

1. Cawood JI. Small plate osteosynthesis of mandibular fractures. Br J Oral Maxillofac Surg 1985;3:77–91.
2. Hayter JP, Cawood JI. The functional case for plates in maxillofacial surgery. Int J Oral Maxillofac Surg 1993;2:91–96.
3. Spiessl B. Internal Fixation of the Mandible: A Manual of AO/ASIF Principles. Berlin: Springer Verlag, 1989.
4. Millar BG, Frame JW, Browne RM. A histological study of stainless steel and titanium screws in bone. Br J Oral Maxillofac Surg 1990;28:92–95.
5. Stoelinga P. Oral surgery [editorial]. Int J Oral Maxillofac Surg 1996;25:413.
6. Levy FE, Smith RW, Odland RM, Marentette LJ. Monocortical miniplate fixation of mandibular angle fractures. Arch Otolaryngol Head Neck Surg 1991;117:149–154.
7. Schliephake H, Lehmann H, Kunz U, Schmelzeisen R. Ultrastructural findings in soft tissues adjacent to titanium plates used in jaw fracture treatment. Int J Oral Maxillofac Surg 1993;22:20–25.

8. Ellis E III. Rigid skeletal fixation of fractures. J Oral Maxillofac Surg 1993;51:163–173.

9. Herschfus L. Histopathologic findings on Vitallium implants in dogs. J Prosthet Dent 1954;4:413–419.

10. Matthew IR, Frame JW. Policy of consultant oral and maxillofacial surgeons towards removal of miniplate components after jaw fracture fixation: Pilot study. Br J Oral Maxillofac Surg 1999;37:110–112.

11. Tomazic VJ, Withrow TJ, Hitchins VM. Adverse reactions associated with medical device implants. Period Biol 1991; 93:547–554.

12. Torgersen S, Gilhuus-Moe OT, Gjerdet NR. Immune response to nickel and some clinical observations after stainless steel miniplate osteosynthesis. Int J Oral Maxillofac Surg 1993; 22:246–250.

13. Tomás H, Carvalho GS, Fernandes MH, Freire AP, Abrantes LM. Effects of Co-Cr corrosion products and corresponding separate metal-ions on human osteoblast-like cell-cultures. J Mater Sci Mater Med 1996;7:291–296.

14. Rosenberg A, Grätz KW, Sailer HF. Should titanium plates be removed after bone healing is complete? Int J Oral Maxillofac Surg 1993;22:185–188.

15. Torgersen S, Gjerdet NR, Erichsen ES, Bang G. Metallic particles and tissue changes adjacent to plates: A retrieval study. Acta Odontol Scand 1995;53:65–71.

16. Lee FD, Anderson JR. Lympho-reticular tissues. In: Anderson JR (ed). Muir's Textbook of Pathology. London: Edward Arnold, 1988:18.8–18.19.

17. Michelet FZ, Deymes J, Dessus B. Osteosynthesis with miniaturized screwed plates in maxillo-facial surgery. J Maxillofac Surg 1973;1:79–84.

18. Champy M, Loddé JP, Jaeger JH, Wilk A. Mandibular osteosynthesis according to the Michelet technique. I. Biomechanical bases [in French]. Rev Stomatol Chir Maxillofac (Paris) 1976;77:569–577.

19. Champy M, Loddé JP, Schmitt R, Jaeger JH, Muster D. Mandibular osteosynthesis by miniature screwed plates via a buccal approach. J Maxillofac Surg 1978;6:14–21.

20. Rowe NL. Maxillofacial injuries: Current trends. Injury 1985; 16:513–525.

21. Frost DE, El-Attar A, Moos KF. Evaluation of metacarpal bone plates in the mandibular fracture. Br J Oral Maxillofac Surg 1983;21:214–221.

22. Hardman FG, Boering G. Comparisons in the treatment of facial trauma. Int J Oral Maxillofac Surg 1989;18:324–332.

23. Oikarinen K, Altonen M, Kauppi H, Laitakari K. Treatment of mandibular fractures: Need for rigid internal fixation. J Craniomaxillofac Surg 1989;17:24–30.

24. Oikarinen K, Ignatius E, Silvennoinen U. Treatment of mandibular fractures in the 1980s. J Craniomaxillofac Surg 1993; 21:245–250.

25. Lindqvist C. Future of biodegradable osteosynthesis in maxillofacial fracture surgery. Br J Oral Maxillofac Surg 1995;33: 69–70.

26. Williams DF (ed). Definitions in Biomaterials. Amsterdam: Elsevier, 1987:38.

27. Black J. Biological Performance of Materials, ed. 2. New York: Dekker, 1992.

28. Moberg L-E, Nordenram Å, Kjellman O. Metal release from plates used in jaw fracture treatment: A pilot study. Int J Oral Maxillofac Surg 1989,18:311–314.

29. Maeusli P-A, Bloch PR, Geret V, Steinemann SG. Surface characterisation of titanium and Ti-alloys. In: Christel P, Meunier A, Lee AJC (eds). Biological and Biomechanical Performance of Biomaterials. Amsterdam: Elsevier, 1986: 57–62.

30. Dean JR. Atomic absorption and plasma spectroscopy. In: Ando DJ (ed). Analytical Chemistry by Open Learning, ed. 2. London: Wiley, 1997:1–71.

31. Matthew IR, Frame JW, Browne RM, Millar BG. In vivo surface analysis of titanium and stainless steel plates and screws. Int J Oral Maxillofac Surg 1996;25:463–468.

32. Pohler G. Interaction between the implant and tissue. In: Spiessl B (ed). Internal Fixation of the Mandible: A Manual of AO/ASIF Principles. Berlin: Springer, 1989:133–135.

33. Agins HJ, Alcock NW, Bansal M, et al. Metallic wear in failed titanium-alloy total hip replacements: A histological and quantitative analysis. J Bone Joint Surg Am 1988;70:347–356.

34. Black J. Does corrosion matter? J Bone Joint Surg Br 1988; 70:517–520.

35. Huo MH, Salvati EA, Buly RL. Wear debris in cemented total hip arthroplasty. Orthopedics 1991;14:335–340.

36. Jorgenson D, Mayer MH, Ellenbogen RG, et al. Detection of titanium in human tissues after craniofacial surgery. Plast Reconstr Surg 1997;4:976–979.

37. Williams DF. Titanium and titanium alloys. In: Williams DF (ed). Biocompatibility of Clinical Implant Materials, vol 1. Boca Raton, FL: CRC Press, 1981:9–44.

38. Brune D, Evje D, Melsom S. Corrosion of gold alloys and titanium in artificial saliva. Scand J Dent Res 1982;90: 168–171.

39. Ferguson AB Jr, Laing PG, Hodge ES. The ionization of metal implants in living tissue. J Bone Joint Surg Am 1960; 42:77–89.

40. Steinemann SG, Eulenberger J, Maeusli P-A, Schroeder A. Adhesion of bone to titanium. In: Christel P, Meunier A, Lee AJC (eds). Biological and Biomechanical Performance of Biomaterials. Amsterdam: Elsevier, 1986:409–414.

41. Smith DC. Surface characterization of implant materials: Biological implications. In: Davies JE (ed). The Bone-Biomaterial Interface. Toronto: Univ of Toronto Press, 1991:3–18.

42. Bianco PD, Ducheyne P, Cuckler JM. Local accumulation of titanium released from a titanium implant in the absence of wear. J Biomed Mater Res 1996;31:227–234.

43. Bessho K, Fujimura K, Iizuka T. Experimental long-term study of titanium ions eluted from pure titanium plates. J Biomed Mater Res 1995;29:901–904.

44. Williams DF. The deterioration of materials in use. In: Williams DF, Roaf R (eds). Implants in Surgery. London: Saunders, 1973:137–201.

45. Brown D. All you wanted to know about titanium, but were afraid to ask. Br Dent J 1997;182:393–394.

46. Cohen J, Lindenbaum B. Fretting corrosion in orthopedic implants. Clin Orthop 1968;61:167–175.

47. Cook SD, Renz EA, Barrack RL, et al. Clinical and metallurgical analysis of retrieved internal fixation devices. Clin Orthop 1985;194:236–247.

48. Cook SD, Thomas KA, Harding AF, et al. The in vivo performance of 250 internal fixation devices: A follow-up study. Biomaterials 1987;8:177–184.

49. Brown SA, Merritt K. Fretting corrosion in saline and serum. J Biomed Mater Res 1981;15:479–488.

50. Merritt K, Brown SA. Effect of proteins and pH on fretting corrosion and metal ion release. J Biomed Mater Res 1988; 22:111–120.

51. Woodman JL, Black J, Jiminez SA. Isolation of serum protein organometallic corrosion products from 316LSS and HS-21 in vitro and in vivo. J Biomed Mater Res 1984;18:99–114.

52. Sousa SR, Barbosa MA. Corrosion resistance of titanium CP in saline physiological solutions with calcium phosphate and proteins. Clin Mater 1993;14:287–294.

53. Johansson B, Krekmanov L, Thomsson M. Miniplate osteosynthesis of infected mandibular fractures. J Craniomaxillofac Surg 1988;16:22–27.

54. Rix L, Stevenson ARL, Punnia-Moorthy A. An analysis of 80 cases of mandibular fractures treated with miniplate osteosynthesis. Int J Oral Maxillofac Surg 1991;20:337–341.

55. von Fraunhofer JA, Berberich N, Seligson D. Antibiotic-metal interactions in saline medium. Biomaterials 1989;10:136–138.

56. von Fraunhofer JA, Stidham SH. Effects of fused-ring antibiotics on metallic corrosion. J Biomed Eng 1991;13:424–428.

57. Moura e Silva T, Monteiro JM, Ferreira MGS, Vieira JM. Corrosion behaviour of AISI 316L stainless-steel alloys in diabetic serum. Clin Mater 1993;12:103–106.

58. Capobianco G, Palma G, Granozzi G, Glisenti A. Electrochemical and XPS studies of the effects of gamma-ray irradiation on the passive film on 446 stainless steel. Corros Sci 1992;33:729–734.

59. Chou L, Firth JD, Nathanson D, Uitto VJ, Brunette DM. Effects of titanium on transcriptional and post-transcriptional regulation of fibronectin in human fibroblasts. J Biomed Mater Res 1996;31:209–217.

60. Vargas E, Baier RE, Meyer AE. Reduced corrosion of CP Ti and Ti-6Al-4V alloy endosseous dental implants after glow-discharge treatment: A preliminary report. Int J Oral Maxillofac Implants 1992;7:338–344.

61. Black J, Maitin EC, Gelman H, Morris DM. Serum concentrations of chromium, cobalt and nickel after total hip replacement: A six month study. Biomaterials 1983;4:160–164.

62. Koegel A, Black J. Release of corrosion products by F-75 cobalt base alloy in the rat. I. Acute serum elevations. J Biomed Mater Res 1984;18:513–522.

63. Brown SA, Margevicius RW, Merritt K. Fretting and accelerated corrosion of titanium in vitro and in vivo. In: Heimke G, Soltész U, Lee AJC (eds). Clinical Implant Materials (Advances in Biomaterials), vol. 9. Amsterdam: Elsevier, 1990:37–42.

64. Bianco PD, Ducheyne P, Cuckler JM. Titanium serum and urine levels in rabbits with a titanium implant in the absence of wear. Biomaterials 1996;17:1937–1942.

65. Brunski JB, Moccia AF Jr, Pollack SR, Korostoff E, Trachtenberg D. Investigation of surfaces of retrieved endosseous dental implants of commercially pure titanium. In: Luckey HA, Kubli F (eds). Titanium Alloys in Surgical Implants ASTM STP 796. Baltimore: American Society for Testing and Materials, 1983:189–205.

66. Bessho K, Iizuka T. Clinical and animal experiments on stress corrosion of titanium plates. Clin Mater 1993;14:223–227.

67. Solar RJ, Pollack SR, Korostoff E. In vitro corrosion testing of titanium surgical implant alloys: An approach to understanding titanium release from implants. J Biomed Mater Res 1979;13:217–250.

68. Torgersen S, Gjerdet NR. Retrieval study of stainless steel and titanium plates and screws used in maxillofacial surgery. J Mater Sci Mater Med 1994;5:256–262.

69. Ray MS, Matthew IR, Frame JW. Metallic fragments on the surface of plates and screws prior to insertion. Br J Oral Maxillofac Surg 1999;37:14–18.

70. French HG, Cook SD, Haddad RJ Jr. Correlation of tissue reaction to corrosion in osteosynthetic devices. J Biomed Mater Res 1984;18:817–828.

71. Gristina AG. Implant failure and the immuno-incompetent fibro-inflammatory zone. Clin Orthop 1994;298:106–118.

72. Michel R. Trace element analysis in biocompatibility testing. CRC Crit Rev Biocomp 1987;3:235–317.

73. Ratner BD. Biomaterial surfaces. J Biomed Mater Res 1987; 21:59–90.

74. Finnegan M. Tissue response to internal fixation devices. Crit Rev Biocompat 1989;5:1–11.

75. Aspenberg P, Goodman S, Toksvig-Larsen S, Ryd L, Albrektsson T. Intermittent micromotion inhibits bone ingrowth: Titanium implants in rabbits. Acta Odontol Scand 1992;63: 141–145.

76. Ungersböck A, Hunt JA. Comparison of visually controlled and automatic histomorphometric evaluation of soft tissue. J Mater Sci Mater Med 1994;5:702–704.

77. Collins DH. Structural changes around nails and screws in human bones. J Pathol Bacteriol 1953;65:109–121.

78. Merritt K, Brown SA. Tissue reaction and metal sensitivity: An animal study. Acta Orthop Scand 1980;51:403–411.

79. Byrne JE, Lovasko JH, Laskin DM. Corrosion of metal fracture fixation appliances. J Oral Surg 1973;31:639–645.

80. Hierholzer S, Hierholzer G, Sauer KH, Paterson RS. Increased corrosion of stainless steel implants in infected plated fractures. Arch Orthop Trauma Surg 1984;102:198–200.

81. Rae T. The action of cobalt, nickel, and chromium on phagocytosis and bacterial killing by human mononuclear and polymorphonuclear leukocytes: Its relevance to infection after total joint arthroplasty. Biomaterials 1983;4:175–180.

82. Black J. Biological Performance of Materials, ed 2. New York: Dekker, 1992.

83. Atkinson PJ, Farries T. Separation of self from non-self in the complement-system. Immunol Today 1987;8:212–215.

84. Albelda SM, Buck CA. Integrins and other cell-adhesion molecules. FASEB (Federation of American Societies for Experimental Biology) J 1990;4:2868–2880.

85. Damas J, Bourdon V, Remacle-Volon G, Adam A. Proteinase-inhibitors, kinins and the inflammatory reaction induced by sponge implantation in rats. Eur J Pharmacol 1990;175: 341–346.

86. van Wachem PB, van Luyn MJA, Olde Damink L, Feijen J, Nieuwenhuis P. Tissue interactions with dermal sheep collagen implants: A transmission electron microscopical evaluation. Cells Mater 1991;1:251–263.

87. Zaoui P, Green W, Hakim RM. Hemodialysis with cuprophane membrane modulates interleukin-2 receptor expression. Kidney Int 1991;39:1020–1026.

88. Putz D, Barnas U, Luger A, Mayer G, Woloszczuk W, Graf H. Biocompatibility of high-flux membranes. Int J Artif Organs 1992;15:456–460.

89. Cardona MA, Simmons RL, Kaplan SS. TNF and IL-1 generation by human monocytes in response to biomaterials. J Biomed Mater Res 1992;26:851–859.

90. De Mol Van Otterloo JC, Van Bockel JH, Ponfoort ED, Brommer EJ, Hermans J, Daha MR. The effects of aortic reconstruction and collagen impregnation of Dacron prostheses on the complement-system. J Vasc Surg 1992;16: 774–783.

91. Remes A, Williams DF. Immune-response in biocompatibility. Biomaterials 1992;13:731–743.

92. Rozema FR, de Bruijn WC, Bos RRM, Boering G, Nijenhuis AJ, Pennings AJ. Late tissue response to bone-plates and screws of poly(l-lactide) used for fracture fixation of the zygomatic arch. In: Doherty PJ, Williams RL, Williams DF (eds). Biomaterial-Tissue Interfaces (Advances in Biomaterials), vol 10. Amsterdam: Elsevier, 1992:349–355.

93. Klein CL, Nieder P, Wagner M, et al. The role of metal corrosion in inflammatory processes: Induction of adhesion molecules by heavy metal ions. J Mater Sci Mater Med 1994;5:798–807.

94. Wälivaara B, Aronsson B-O, Rodahl M, Lausmaa J, Tengvall P. Titanium with different oxides: In vitro studies of protein adsorption and contact activation. Biomaterials 1994;15: 827–834.

95. Buchhorn GH, Willert H-G, Semlitsch M, Schon R, Steinemann S, Schmidt M. Preparation, characterization, and animal testing for biocompatibility of metallic particles of iron-, cobalt-, and titanium-based implant alloys. In: St. John KR. (ed). Particulate Debris from Medical Implants: Mechanisms of Formation and Biological Consequences. ASTM STP 1144. Philadelphia: American Society for Testing and Materials, 1992:177–188.

96. Chiba JC, Schwendeman LJ, Booth RE Jr, Crossett LS, Rubash HE. A biochemical, histologic, and immunohistologic analysis of membranes obtained from failed cemented and cementless total knee arthroplasty. Clin Orthop 1994;299:114–124.

97. Jacobs JJ, Urban RM, Gilbert JL, et al. Local and distant products from modularity. Clin Orthop 1995;319:94–105.

98. Santavirta S, Konttinen YT, Hoikka V, Eskola A. Immuno-pathological response to loose cementless acetabular components. J Bone Joint Surg Br 1991;73:38–42.

99. Lalor PA, Revell PA. T-lymphocytes and titanium aluminium vanadium (TiAlV) alloy: Evidence for immunological events associated with debris deposition. Clin Mater 1993;12:57–62.

100. Al Saffar N, Kadoya Y, Revell P. The role of newly formed vessels and cell adhesion molecules in the tissue response to wear products from orthopaedic implants. J Mater Sci Mater Med 1994;5:813–818.

101. Bobyn JD, Tanzer M, Krygier JJ, Dujovne AR, Brooks CE. Concerns with modularity in total hip arthroplasty. Clin Orthop 1994;298:27–36

102. Nanci A, McCarthy GF, Zalzal S, Clokie CML, Warshawsky H, McKee MD. Tissue response to titanium implants in the rat tibia: Ultrastructural, immunocytochemical and lectin-cytochemical characterization of the bone-titanium interface. Cells Mater 1994;4:1–30.

103. Southam JC, Selwyn P. Structural changes around screws used in the treatment of fractured human mandibles. Br J Oral Surg 1971;8:211–221.

104. Linder L, Lundskog J. Incorporation of stainless steel, titanium, and Vitallium in bone. Injury 1974;6:277–285.

105. Albrektsson T, Hansson H-A. An ultrastructural characterization of the interface between bone and sputtered titanium or stainless steel surfaces. Biomaterials 1986;7:201–205.

106. Sennerby L, Thomsen P, Ericson LE. Ultrastructure of the bone-titanium interface in rabbits. J Mater Sci Mater Med 1992;3:262–271.

107. Cohen J. Tissue reactions to metals: The influence of surface finish. J Bone Joint Surg Am 1961;43:687–699.

108. Blumenthal NC, Posner AS. In vitro model of aluminium-induced osteomalacia: Inhibition of hydroxyapatite formation and growth. Calcif Tissue Int 1984;36:439–441.

109. Thompson GJ, Puleo DA. Ti-6Al-4V ion solution inhibition of osteogenic cell phenotype as a function of differentiation time course in vitro. Biomaterials 1996;17:1949–1954.

110. Hanawa T. Titanium and its oxide film: A substrate for formation of apatite. In: Davies JE (ed). The Bone-Biomaterial Interface. Toronto: Univ of Toronto Press, 1991:49–67.

111. Leitão E, Barbosa MA, De Groot K. In vitro calcification of orthopaedic implant materials. J Mater Sci Mater Med 1995;6:849–852.

112. Larsson C, Thomsen P, Lausmaa J, Rodahl M, Kasemo B, Ericson LE. Bone response to surface-modified titanium implants: Studies on electropolished implants with different oxide thicknesses and morphology. Biomaterials 1994;15:1062–1074.

113. Könönen M, Hormia M, Kivilahti J, Hautaniemi J, Thesleff I. Effect of surface processing on the attachment, orientation, and proliferation of human gingival fibroblasts on titanium. J Biomed Mater Res 1992;26:1325–1341.

114. Meachim G, Pedley B. The tissue response at implant sites. In: Williams DF (ed). Fundamental Aspects of Biocompatibility, vol 1. Boca Raton, FL: CRC Press, 1981:107–144.

115. Cohen J. Metal implants: Historical background and biological response to implantation. In: Rubin LR. (ed). Biomaterials in Reconstructive Surgery. St. Louis: Mosby, 1983: 46–61.

116. Kovacs EJ. Fibrogenic cytokines: The role of immune mediators in the development of scar tissue. Immunol Today 1991;12:17–23.

117. Laing PG, Ferguson, AB, Hodge ES. Tissue reaction in rabbit muscle exposed to metallic implants. J Biomed Mater Res 1967;1:135–149.

118. Salthouse TN. Some aspects of macrophage behavior at the implant interface. J Biomed Mater Res 1984;18:395–401.

119. Goldring SR, Bennett NE, Jasty MJ, Wang J-T. In vitro activation of monocyte macrophages and fibroblasts by metallic particles. In: St. John KR (ed). Particulate Debris from Medical Implants: Mechanisms of Formation and Biological Consequences. ASTM STP 1144. Philadelphia: American Society for Testing and Materials, 1992:136–142.

120. Evans EM. Metal sensitivity as a cause of bone necrosis and loosening of the prosthesis in total joint replacement. J Bone Joint Surg Br 1974;56:626–642.

121. Nakamura S, Takenoshita Y, Oka M. Complications of miniplate osteosynthesis for mandibular fractures. J Oral Maxillofac Surg 1994;52:233–238.

122. Katou F, Andoh N, Motegi K, Nagura H. Immuno-inflammatory responses in the tissue adjacent to titanium plates used in the treatment of mandibular fractures. J Craniomaxillofac Surg 1996;24:155–162.

123. Meachim G, Williams DF. Changes in non-osseous tissue adjacent to titanium implants. J Biomed Mater Res 1973; 7:555–572.

124. Matthew IR, Frame JW. Release of metal in vivo from stressed and non-stressed maxillofacial fracture plates and screws. Oral Surg Oral Med Oral Pathol Oral Radiol Endod 2000;90:33–38.

125. Matthew IR, Frame JW. Ultrastructural analysis of metal particles released from stainless steel and titanium miniplate components in an animal model. J Oral Maxillofac Surg 1998;56:45–50.

126. Nathan CF. Secretory products of macrophages. J Clin Invest 1987;79:319–326.

127. Evans EJ. Cell damage in vitro following direct contact with fine particles of titanium, titanium alloy, and cobalt-chrome-molybdenum alloy. Biomaterials 1994;15:713–717.

128. Waters MD, Gardner DE, Aranyi C, Coffin DL. Metal toxicity for rabbit alveolar macrophages in vitro. Environ Res 1975;9:32–47.

129. Goodman SB, Davidson JA, Song Y, Martial N, Fornasier VL. Histomorphological reaction of bone to different concentrations of phagocytosable particles of high-density polyethylene and Ti-6Al-4V alloy in vitro. Biomaterials 1996;17:1943–1947.

130. Trumpy IG, Lyberg T. In vivo deterioration of Proplast-Teflon temporomandibular joint interpositional implants: A scanning electron microscope and energy-dispersive x-ray analysis. J Oral Maxillofac Surg 1993;51:624–629.

131. Shanbhag AS, Jacobs JJ, Black J, Galante JO, Glant TT. Macrophage/particle interactions: Effect of size, composition, and surface area. J Biomed Mater Res 1994;28:81–90.

132. Heath JC, Freeman MA, Swanson SAV. Carcinogenic properties of wear particles from prostheses made in cobalt-chromium alloy. Lancet 1971;1:564–566.

133. Meachim G, Brooke G. The synovial response to intra-articular Co-Cr-Mo particles in guinea pigs. Biomaterials 1983;4:153–159.

134. Shinto Y, Uchida A, Yoshikawa H, Araki N, Kato T, Ono K. Inguinal lymphadenopathy due to metal release from a prosthesis: A case report. J Bone Joint Surg Br 1993;75: 266–269.

135. Onodera K, Ooya KO, Kawamura H. Titanium lymph node pigmentation in the reconstruction plate system of a mandibular defect. Oral Surg Oral Med Oral Pathol 1993; 75:495–497.

136. Weingart D, Steinemann S, Schilli W, et al. Titanium deposition in regional lymph nodes after insertion of titanium screw implants in maxillofacial region. Int J Oral Maxillofac Surg 1994;23:450–452.

137. Dumbleton JH, Black J. An Introduction to Orthopaedic Materials. Springfield, IL: Thomas, 1975.

138. Rae T. A study of the effects of particulate metals of orthopaedic interest on murine macrophages in vitro. J Bone Joint Surg Br 1975;57:444–450.

139. Puleo DA, Huh WW. Acute toxicity of metal ions in cultures of osteogenic cells derived from bone marrow stromal cells. J Appl Biomater 1995;6:109–116.

140. Rae T. The toxicity of metals used in orthopaedic prostheses: An experimental study using cultured human synovial fibroblasts. J Bone Joint Surg Br 1981;63:435–440.

141. Tracana RB, Sousa JP, Carvalho GS Mouse inflammatory response to stainless-steel corrosion products. J Mater Sci Mater Med 1994;5:596–600.

142. Carvalho GS, Castanheira M, Diog I, et al. Inhibition and stimulation of enzymatic-activities of human fibroblasts by corrosion products and metal-salts J Mater Sci Mater Med 1996;7:77–83.

143. Harmand M-F, Naji A, Jeandot R, Ducassou D. Cytocompatibility study of cobalt-chromium alloys using human cell cultures. In: Heimke G, Soltész U, Lee AJC (eds). Clinical Implant Materials (Advances in Biomaterials), vol 9. Amsterdam: Elsevier, 1990:19–24.

144. Hunt JA, Remes A, Williams DF. Stimulation of neutrophil movement by metal ions. J Biomed Mater Res 1992;26:819–828.

145. Pereira ML, Abreu AM, Sousa JP, Carvalho GS. Chromium accumulation and ultrastructural changes in the mouse liver caused by stainless steel corrosion products. J Mater Sci Mater Med 1995;6:523–527.

146. Remes A, Williams DF. Chemotaxis and the inhibition of chemotaxis of human neutrophils in response to metal ions. J Mater Sci Mater Med 1990;1:26–32.

147. Daniel M, Dingle JT, Webb M, Heath JC. The biological action of cobalt and other metals. I. The effect of cobalt on the morphology and metabolism of rat fibroblasts in vitro. Br J Exp Pathol 1963;44:163–176.

148. Bearden LJ, Cooke FW. Growth inhibition of cultured fibroblasts by cobalt and nickel. J Biomed Mater Res 1980;14:289–309.

149. Stanley HR. Biological evaluation of dental materials. Int Dent J 1992;42:37–46.

150. US National Cancer Institute. NCI: Bioassay of Titanium Dioxide for Possible Carcinogenicity. National Cancer Institute Carcinogenesis Technical Report Series No. 97-1347. Washington, DC: US Dept of Health, Education & Welfare, 1979.

151. Goyer RA. Toxic effects of metals. In: Klaassen CD, Amdur MO, Doull J (eds). Casarett and Doull's Toxicology: The Basic Science of Poisons, ed 5. New York: MacMillan, 1995:691–737.

152. Carvalho GS, Bravo I. In vitro immuno-cytotoxicity of iron evaluated by DNA synthesis of human T lymphocytes stimulated via CD2 and CD3. J Mater Sci Mater Med 1993;4:366–371.

153. Brand KG. Exploration of implant-associated carcinogenesis in animals. In: Rubin LR (ed). Biomaterials in Reconstructive Surgery. St. Louis: Mosby, 1983:27–35.

154. Bessho K, Hirano Y, Ishihama N, Furuta M, Murata M. A study on metallic implant for jaw reconstruction: Changes and damaging action of Champy miniature screwed plate in the body. Jpn J Oral Maxillofac Surg 1988;34:1406–1413.

155. Friedman KE, Vernon SE. Squamous cell carcinoma developing in conjunction with a mandibular staple bone plate. J Oral Maxillofac Surg 1983;41:265–266.

156. Bagó-Granell J, Aguirre-Canyadell M, Nardi J, Tallada N. Malignant fibrous histiocytoma of bone at the site of a total hip arthroplasty. J Bone Joint Surg Br 1984;66:38–40.

157. Penman HG, Ring PA. Osteosarcoma in association with total hip replacement. J Bone Joint Surg Br 1984;66:632–634.

158. Weber PC. Epithelioid carcinoma in association with total knee replacement: A case report. J Bone Joint Surg Br 1986;68:824–826.

159. McDougall A. Malignant tumour at site of bone plating. J Bone Joint Surg Br 1956;38:709–713.

160. Dube VE, Fisher DE. Hemangioendothelioma of the leg following metallic fixation of the tibia. Cancer 1972;30:1260–1266.

161. Sunderman FW. Carcinogenicity of metal alloys in orthopaedic prostheses: Clinical and experimental studies. Fundam Appl Toxicol 1989;13:205–216.

162. Sinibaldi K, Rosen H, Liu S-K, et al. Tumours associated with metal implants in animals. Clin Orthop 1976;118:257–266.

163. Brand KG. Human foreign-body carcinogenesis in animal experiments and assessment of cancer risk at implant sites. In: Rubin LR (ed). Biomaterials in Reconstructive Surgery. St. Louis: Mosby, 1983:36–39.

164. Cutright DE. Dental implants. In: Rubin LR (ed). Biomaterials in Reconstructive Surgery. St. Louis: Mosby, 1983:647–661.

165. Hamblen DL, Carter RL. Sarcoma and joint replacement [editorial]. J Bone Joint Surg Am 1984;66:625–627.

166. Alpert B, Seligson D. Removal of asymptomatic bone plates used for orthognathic surgery and facial fractures. J Oral Maxillofac Surg 1996;54:618–621.

167. Tracana RB, Pereira ML, Abreu AM, Sousa JP, Carvalho GS. Stainless-steel corrosion products cause alterations on mouse spleen cellular-populations. J Mater Sci Mater Med 1995;6:56–61.

168. Kline SN, Stevens MR. The case for conventional versus rigid internal fixation in maxillofacial trauma. In: Worthington P, Evans JR (eds). Controversies in Oral and Maxillofacial Surgery. Philadelphia: Saunders, 1994:201–208.

169. Scales JT, Winter GD, Shirley HT. Corrosion of orthopaedic implants, screws, plates, and femoral nail-plates. J Bone Joint Surg Br 1959;41:810–820.

170. Iizuka T, Lindqvist C. Rigid internal fixation of mandibular fractures: An analysis of 270 fractures treated using the AO/ASIF method. Int J Oral Maxillofac Surg 1992;21:65–69.

171. Breme J, Steinhäuser E, Paulus G. Commercially pure titanium Steinhäuser plate-screw system for maxillofacial surgery. Biomaterials 1988;9:310–313.

172. Haug, RH. Retention of asymptomatic bone plates used for orthognathic surgery and facial fractures. J Oral Maxillofac Surg 1996;54:611–617.

173. Williams DF. Titanium: Epitome of biocompatibility or cause for concern. J Bone Joint Surg Br 1994;76:348–349.

174. Brown JS, Trotter M, Cliffe J, Ward-Booth RP, Williams ED. The fate of plates in facial trauma and orthognathic surgery: A retrospective study. Br J Oral Maxillofac Surg 1989;27:306–315.

175. Brown RM, Wheelwright EF, Chalmers J. Removal of metal implants after fracture surgery: Indications and complications. J R Coll Surg Edinb 1993;38:96–100.

176. Llewelyn J, Sugar A. Lag screws in sagittal split osteotomies: Should they be removed? Br J Oral Maxillofac Surg 1992;30:83–86.

177. Heslop IH, Cawood JI, Stoelinga PJW, et al. Mandibular fractures: Treatment by closed reduction and direct skeletal fixation. In: Williams JLI (ed). Rowe and Williams' Maxillofacial Injuries, ed 2. Edinburgh: Churchill Livingstone, 1994:341–386.

178. Williams DF. The selection of implant materials. In: Williams DF, Roaf R (eds). Implants in Surgery. London: Saunders, 1973:299–358.

179. Zachariades N, Mezitis M, Rallis G. An audit of mandibular fractures treated by intermaxillary fixation, intraosseous wiring and compression plating. Br J Oral Maxillofac Surg 1996;34:293–297.

180. Matthew IR, Frame JW. The debate about debris. J Oral Maxillofac Surg 1997;55:1504.

181. Matthew IR, Frame JW. Detection of titanium in human tissues after craniofacial surgery. Plast Reconstr Surg 1998;101:1148–1149.

182. Matthew IR, Frame JW. Allergic responses to titanium. J Oral Maxillofac Surg 1998;56:1466–1467.

Section VII

PERIODONTOLOGY

14

SUTURES IN THE ORAL CAVITY

J. Anthony von Fraunhofer, PhD

Successful wound closure is essential in any invasive surgical procedure, and the most common approach is tissue approximation with sutures. The healing of a sutured wound is profoundly affected by the approximating force exerted by the suture loop, which in turn is determined by several physicomechanical factors. These suture-related factors include the suture's tensile properties; the knotting method; the tautness of the suture loop; the in vivo environment; and particularly, the stress relaxation characteristics of the suture, which affect the postplacement approximating force applied by the suture loop.

Sutures may be defined as filamentous materials used to approximate wound edges after surgery or trauma, or as filamentary biomedical devices used to hold tissues in place following surgical transposition of soft tissues. Sutures are manufactured from a wide variety of natural and synthetic materials and, accordingly, differ markedly in their properties and characteristics. The selection criteria for a suture include the clinical function and required in vivo longevity, the anatomic location of the suture site, and the nature and characteristics of the tissues being sutured. A variety of other factors are also important in suture selection and use, notably local and systemic pathology, physiology, and often esthetic considerations of the sutured wound.

The clinical success of surgical procedures depends on good wound healing, and this healing is profoundly affected by the type and properties of the suture used for wound closure, the surgical technique, and the behavior of the suture during placement and throughout the wound-healing process. Thus, a stainless steel suture used to "wire" a fractured jaw together has markedly different physical and mechanical characteristics than a suture material used following mucoperiosteal flap surgery. Sutures that are required to perform a long-term biomechanical function, such as permanent anastomosis of blood vessels, must retain their structural integrity and strength over extended periods. Completely different characteristics are required of sutures that have a short-term or temporary function. Thus, absorbable sutures may be used for the short-term approximation of wound edges or apposition of repositioned soft tissues, because they will dissolve in the body within a specified, usually limited, time.

Sutures are used routinely in only two dental specialties: *(1)* periodontology and *(2)* oral and maxillofacial surgery. Although most surgeons recognize that proper suture selection and use are central to the successful outcome of clinical procedures, there is a paucity of literature on sutures and suturing techniques for these two fields. Consequently, this chapter provides an overview of surgical suture materials and discusses the factors that contribute to the successful clinical use of sutures.

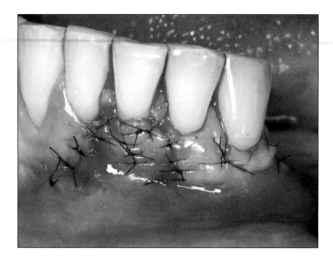

Fig 14-1 Interrupted sutures following periodontal surgery. Sutures were placed to support but not compromise the wound. (Courtesy of K Zeren, Lutherville, MD.)

Wounds and Wound Healing

There are various classifications of wounds. Wounds that are heavily contaminated prior to surgery are usually caused by trauma—eg, open fractures, lacerations, and penetrating wounds. Clean wounds are acquired in elective surgery performed under aseptic conditions. Because of the flora and saliva that occur naturally within the oral cavity, the type of wound most often found in periodontal surgery is the clean contaminated wound. A further, and distinct, difference between periodontal surgery and other surgical disciplines is that in the latter, wound healing involves approximation of the edges of vascularized soft tissues, whereas in periodontal surgery, one surface of the wound can be approximated over tooth structure, and the avascular tooth surface tends to be contaminated through exposure to the oral environment (Fig 14-1).

Despite the distinction between wounds in general and wounds in periodontal surgery, a review of the basic processes of wound healing can help clarify suture selection criteria.[1,2] Wound healing is a multiphase, dynamic process involving the integrated actions of different cells. When there is no infection, minimal edema, and negligible fluid discharge, and the wound edges are well approximated, the healing process is commonly referred to as *healing by primary intention* or *healing by primary union,* and it occurs in three phases. In phase 1, which lasts 1 to 5 days, an inflammatory response induces a flow of tissue fluids (comprising plasma proteins, fibrin, blood cells, and antibodies) into the wound. During phase 1 there is increased blood supply to the wound, together with cellular and fibroblast proliferation. Leukocytes and macrophages release proteolytic enzymes that remove damaged tissue and debris, and a protective scab forms on the surface and is accompanied by the initiation of collagen fiber production. In phase 2, occurring from about the 5th to the 14th day, there is increased formation and deposition of collagen within the wound, and fibroblasts form fibrin and fibronectin. At this stage, closure and contraction of the wound begin, together with formation of granulation tissue. From the 14th day onward, phase 2 gradually merges into phase 3, during which there is reorganization and maturation of the collagen fibers, together with deposition of fibrous connective tissue. The third phase also involves increased wound contraction and revascularization. In the absence of pathology, wound healing by primary intention occurs in a rapid and straightforward manner.

Healing by primary union may not occur if a wound is infected or there has been trauma, tissue loss, or poor tissue approximation. In such cases, healing is more complex and requires more time. The wound is often left open, and *healing by secondary intention* occurs from within the wound toward the outermost surface. Granulation tissue forms within the wound, and the wound edges come together through contraction,

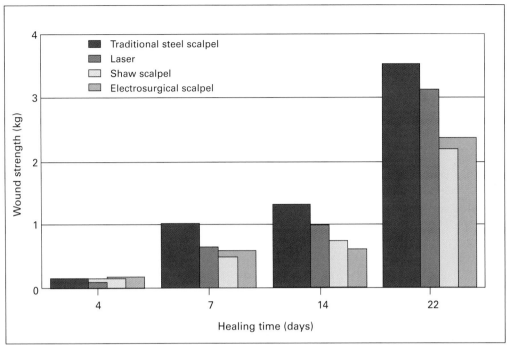

Fig 14-2 Effect of surgical incision method on wound tear strength. (Data from Sowa et al.[5])

which is secondary to epithelial growth over the connective tissue. The healed wound is usually characterized by granulation and scar tissue. Secondary intention healing occurs after periodontal flap surgery when the flaps have been slightly displaced or improperly scalloped.

Finally, with deep, contaminated, and/or infected wounds, or where tissue loss is extensive, the healing process is categorized as *delayed primary closure* or *healing by third intention*. As in second intention healing, the wound is left open after cleaning and debridement of dead or damaged tissue, but third intention healing involves the approximation of two surfaces or the edges of granulation tissue. Myofibroblasts deep within the wound form granulation tissue, and although there is subsequent approximation of the skin edges and deeper tissues, the wound is usually characterized by granulation and scar tissue. Third intention healing is found in extraction sockets and after periodontal surgery when bone is left exposed and healing follows resorption of the cortical layer.

The rate of wound healing varies with the type of tissue and depends on a number of factors. In the absence of pathology, a graph of wound strength versus time during wound healing follows a sigmoidal curve, with the healing tissue asymptotically approaching the strength of uninjured tissue.[3,4] Significant wound tear strength is normally achieved within 28 days, although this time scale is affected by many factors, including local and systemic pathology, surgical and suturing techniques, and the properties of the suture. Abnormal wound healing can occur because of malnutrition; vitamin deficiencies; diseases such as diabetes and uremia; and therapy with systemic drugs, especially cytotoxic drugs and certain steroids.

The method of surgical incision has been shown to affect wound strength (Fig 14-2). The use of the traditional steel scalpel and the carbon dioxide laser achieves higher wound strengths than the use of the self-cauterizing electrosurgical or hemostatic Shaw scalpel.[5]

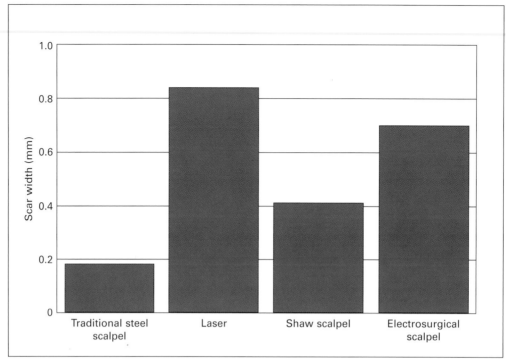

Fig 14-3 Residual scar width at 22 days. (Data from Sowa et al.[5])

The width of the residual scar also varies with the surgical tool (Fig 14-3). The traditional steel scalpel creates the most narrow scar, whereas thermal injury induced by thermal knives delays wound healing.[5] Thus, it would appear that although the steel scalpel has the disadvantages of mechanically dividing tissue, not coagulating small vessels, and requiring good manual dexterity, its convenience, economy, ready availability, and superior wound healing effects may offset the faster cutting and concomitant tissue and vessel coagulation achievable with thermal knives.

The tautness of the suture used to approximate the edges of a wound can have a marked effect on wound healing.[6] This subject, together with stress relaxation of sutures, will be discussed in a later section. A comprehensive treatise on sutures and wound closure devices also has been published.[7]

Suture Types, Sizes, and Configurations

Surgeons may choose among a wide variety of sutures that differ in diameter, physical configuration, and chemical composition. All these factors affect the properties and in vivo behavior of sutures.

Suture Sizes

Sutures are categorized according to their diameters in two coding systems: the US Pharmacopeia (USP) and the European Pharmacopeia (EP) size codes. The EP size codes are the same for absorbable and nonabsorbable sutures, whereas the USP system differentiates between natural

Table 14-1 Suture size classifications

Natural absorbable materials	Synthetic nonabsorbable and synthetic absorbable materials	Absorbable and nonabsorbable materials	Range (mm)
–	11-0	0.1	0.010–0.019
–	10-0	0.2	0.020–0.029
–	9-0	0.3	0.030–0.039
8-0	8-0	0.4	0.040–0.049
7-0	7-0	0.5	0.050–0.069
6-0	6-0	0.7	0.070–0.099
5-0	5-0	1	0.10–0.14
4-0	4-0	1.5	0.15–0.19
3-0	3-0	2	0.20–0.24
2-0	2-0	2.5	0.25–0.29
0	0	3	0.30–0.39
1	1	4	0.40–0.49
2	2	5	0.50–0.59
3	3	6	0.60–0.69
4	4	7	0.70–0.79
5	5	8	0.80–0.89
6	6	9	0.90–0.99
–	7	10	1.00–1.09

Columns: USP size codes (Natural absorbable materials; Synthetic nonabsorbable and synthetic absorbable materials), EP size codes (Absorbable and nonabsorbable materials), Suture diameter (Range mm).

absorbable materials on the one hand and synthetic nonabsorbable and absorbable sutures on the other hand. Table 14-1 indicates the sizes of suture materials under the two classification codes. Oral and maxillofacial surgeons use predominantly 3-0 sutures, and sometimes 4-0 sutures, particularly at implant sites. Periodontal surgeons commonly use 4-0 sutures for conventional flap surgery but use the finer-gauge 5-0 and 6-0 sutures for microsurgical procedures (eg, soft tissue grafting). Thus, for wound approximation in oral and maxillofacial surgery, suture diameters commonly range from 0.15 to 0.24 mm. Periodontal surgeons use sutures 0.15 to 0.19 mm in diameter for flap surgery and much finer sutures (0.07 to 0.14 mm in diameter) for soft tissue

grafts. The type of sutures used, however, differs between the two specialties for many procedures.

Both the USP and EP size codes encompass a range of diameters for each nominal suture size. The range is approximately 0.10 mm for larger sutures (sizes 7 to 0 USP) but drops to 0.04 mm for sizes 2-0 to 5-0 and is even narrower for the smallest-diameter sutures. This variability in diameter affects the tensile strength of the suture. Sutures that are of nominally the same code size but that differ in diameter show marked differences in tensile breaking load and tensile strength, as shown by a study of six sutures of sizes 1 to 3-0.[8] The permissible size range for sutures commonly used in oral surgery is 0.20 to 0.24 mm for 3-0 sutures, 0.15 to 0.19 mm for 4-0 sutures,

0.10 to 0.14 mm for 5-0 sutures, and 0.070 to 0.099 mm for 6-0 sutures. Thus, the actual diameters of sutures that are nominally the same size can vary by as much as 20% to 40%. However, although the attendant strength differences are measurable in the laboratory, they are very unlikely to be significant during surgery.

Suture Classifications

Sutures are classified in various ways, but the most common designations are absorbable (ie, bioabsorbable) and nonabsorbable (ie, biostable). Absorbable sutures dissolve in the body at a rate determined by such factors as composition, size, and morphology. These sutures generally do not require removal after surgery and are composed of materials that degrade in vivo; complete loss of suture tensile strength and mass occurs within 2 to 3 months. A variety of monofilament (single-strand) and both braided and twisted multifilament sutures manufactured from bioabsorbable materials are used in general and oral surgery. The trade (commercial) and generic names of available absorbable sutures are given in Table 14-2.

Nonabsorbable sutures do not dissolve in situ, and they may or may not require later removal, depending on the application and surgeon's preference. These sutures retain their structural integrity and tensile strength for longer periods—ie, longer than 2 to 3 months. Commercially available nonabsorbable sutures are listed in Table 14-3. Table 14-4 lists, by manufacturer, both the brand and generic names of a wide variety of both absorbable and nonabsorbable sutures.

Suture Surface Coatings

Frictional resistance to the passage of sutures through tissue is an important factor in surgery, and the surfaces of many sutures are coated to improve frictional behavior and handling properties, as noted in Tables 14-2 and 14-3. Traditionally, such coatings were nonabsorbable—eg, beeswax, paraffin wax, silicone, and polytetrafluoroethylene (Teflon [duPont, Wilmington, DE])—but the modern trend is to use absorbable coatings, particularly for bioabsorbable sutures.[9] Some

of these coatings are water soluble (typically surfactants), whereas others are poorly soluble and have a chemical formulation similar to that of the suture (eg, polyglactin 910, which is used for Vicryl sutures [Ethicon, Somerville, NJ]). Such surface coatings have no effect on the host defense mechanisms against microorganisms and do not increase the risk of wound infection.[10]

The often-observed "stick-slip" behavior of sutures, particularly with finer-gauge materials, can cause tensile failure of a suture or traumatize the tissue through which the suture is being drawn. Surgeons using polybutester cardiovascular sutures have a novel approach to this problem; they subject the sutures to radiofrequency glow discharge in hexamethyldisiloxane or hexamethyldisilazane vapor, which deposits a thin, stable, very hydrophobic surface coating.[11] The coating does not affect the tensile strength of the suture but effectively eliminates stick-slip behavior during suturing; such coatings have obvious appeal for suturing the thin, friable oral mucosa in periodontal surgery. Although these surface coatings improve handling and reduce frictional effects during suture passage through tissue, they may reduce knot security and necessitate a greater number of throws to achieve a secure knot.

Surface coatings may affect the rate of bioabsorption of absorbable sutures. The classic example was Lister's stabilization of the biologic properties of catgut through chromate treatment in 1860. Since then, a variety of surface treatments have been developed to improve the properties of sutures, as noted above. Such coatings can modify in vivo absorption, as shown by the large difference in biodegradation rates of the two polyglycolide-L-lactide sutures, Polysorb (USS DG Sutures, Norwalk, CT) and Vicryl, which have different surface treatments.[12]

Suture Configurations

Suture configurations fall into two broad categories: monofilament (single-strand) and multifilament (multistrand), the latter being subdivided into twisted and braided sutures, as noted in Tables 14-2 and 14-3. Nylon, polyester, and stainless steel sutures are available in both multifilament and

Table 14-2 Absorbable sutures

TRADE NAME	GENERIC NAME	CONFIGURATION	SURFACE
Natural absorbable sutures			
Catgut/surgical gut (Ethicon)	Catgut	Twisted multifilament	Plain and chromic
Chromic gut/plain gut (USS DG Sutures)	Catgut	Twisted multifilament	Plain and chromic
Collagen (Ethicon)	Reconstituted collagen	Twisted multifilament	Plain and chromic
Stericat (Stericat Gutstrings PVT, New Delhi, India)	Catgut	Twisted multifilament	Plain and chromic
Synthetic absorbable sutures			
Biosyn (USS DG Sutures)	Glycomer 631	Monofilament	None
Caprosyn (USS DG Sutures)	Polyglytone 6211 (glycolide, caprolactone, trimethylene carbonate, lactide)	Monofilament	None
Dexon II (USS DG Sutures)	Polyglycolide	Braided multifilament	None
Dexon "S" (USS DG Sutures)	Polyglycolide	Braided multifilament	None
I-COL (Stericat Gutstrings PVT)	Polyglycolide	Braided multifilament	None
Maxon (USS DG Sutures)	Polyglycolide-co-trimethylene carbonate	Monofilament	None
Medifit (JMS, Hiroshima, Japan)	Polyglycolide	Braided multifilament	None
Monocol (Stericat Gutstrings PVT)	Poly-p-dioxanone	Monofilament	None
Monocryl (Ethicon)	Polyglycolide co-ϵ-caprolactone	Monofilament	None
PDS II (Ethicon)	Poly-p-dioxanone	Monofilament	None
Polysorb (USS DG Sutures)	Polyglycolide-L-lactide	Braided multifilament	Coated
Vicryl (Ethicon)	Polyglycolide-L-lactide	Braided multifilament	Polyglactin 370 and Ca stearate
Vicryl Rapide (Ethicon)	Polyglycolide-L-lactide	Braided multifilament	Irradiated

monofilament forms. Twisted multifilament sutures may be made of catgut, reconstituted collagen, or cotton; braided multifilament sutures may be of polyglycolic acid, polyglycolide-L-lactide, polyester, polyamide (nylon), or silk. One polyamide (nylon 6) suture, Supramid (S. Jackson Inc, Alexandria, VA), is unique in having a twisted core covered by an outer sheath or jacket of the same material. Some sutures are available only as monofilaments—notably Maxon, Monocryl, PDS, and polypropylene and polytetrafluoroethylene sutures.

Table 14-3 Nonabsorbable sutures

TRADE NAME	GENERIC NAME	CONFIGURATION	SURFACE TREATMENT
Cotton (Ethicon)	Cotton	Twisted multifilament	—
Dacron (USS DG Sutures)	Polyester	Braided multifilament	None
Dermal (Ethicon)	Silk	Twisted multifilament	Tanned gelatin
Dermalon (USS DG Sutures)	Polyamide (nylon 6 and 66)	Monofilament	None
Ethibond (Ethicon)	Polyester	Braided multifilament	Polybutylate
Ethiflex (Ethicon)	Polyester	Braided multifilament	PTFE (Teflon) coated
Ethilon (Ethicon)	Polyamide (nylon 6 and 66)	Monofilament	—
Flexon (USS DG Sutures)	Stainless steel	Twisted multifilament	—
Gore-Tex (WL Gore)	Polytetrafluoroethylene	Monofilament	None
Linen (Ethicon, USS DG Sutures)	Linen	Twisted multifilament	—
Mersilene (Ethicon)	Polyester	Braided multifilament	—
Mirafil (B. Braun, Bethlehem, PA)	Polyester	Monofilament	—
Novafil (USS DG Sutures)	Polyester	Monofilament	None
Nurolon (Ethicon)	Polyamide (nylon 6 and 66)	Braided multifilament	Coated
Prolene (Ethicon)	Polypropylene	Monofilament	—
Silk (Ethicon, USS DG Sutures)	Silk	Braided multifilament	Tanned gelatin
Silky Polydek (USS DG Sutures)	Polyester	Braided multifilament	PTFE (Teflon) coated
Sofsilk (USS DG Sutures)	Silk	Braided multifilament	Coated
Stainless steel (USS DG Sutures)	Stainless steel	Monofilament or twisted multifilament	—
Steel (USS DG Sutures)	Stainless steel	Monofilament or twisted multifilament	—
Sterilene (Stericat Gutstrings PVT)	Polyester	Braided multifilament	PTFE (Teflon) coated
Supramid (S. Jackson Inc)	Polyamide (nylon 6)	Core-sheath	—
Surgical cotton (Ethicon)	Cotton	Twisted multifilament	—
Surgical silk (Ethicon)	Silk	Braided multifilament	Tru-permanizing
Surgidac (USS DG Sutures)	Polyester	Braided multifilament and monofilament	Coated with braid
Surgilene (USS DG Sutures)	Polypropylene	Monofilament	None
Surgilon (USS DG Sutures)	Polyamide (nylon 66)	Braided multifilament	Silicone
Surgipro (USS DG Sutures)	Polypropylene	Monofilament	None
Ti-Cron (USS DG Sutures)	Polyester	Braided multifilament	Silicone
Vascufil (USS DG Sutures)	Polybutester	Monofilament	Coated
Virgin silk	Silk	Twisted multifilament	—

*PTFE, polytetrafluoroethylene.

Table 14-4 Suture manufacturers and sutures (partial listing)

MANUFACTURER	TRADE NAME	GENERIC NAME
Ethicon	**Absorbable sutures:**	
	Monocryl	Poliglecaprone 25
	PDS II	Polydioxanone
	Vicryl	Polyglactin 910
	Surgical gut	Chromic gut
	Nonabsorbable sutures:	
	Ethibond	Polyester
	Ethilon	Nylon
	Mersilene	Polyester
	Nurolon	Braided nylon
	Perma-Hand	Silk
	Prolene	Polypropylene
	Pronova	Polyhexafluoropropylene-VDF
USS DG Sutures	**Absorbable sutures:**	
	Biosyn	Glycomer 631
	Caprosyn	Polyglytone 6211
	Dexon	Polyglycolic acid
	Maxon	Polyglycolide-co-trimethylene carbonate
	Polysorb	Polyglycolide-L-lactide
	Nonabsorbable sutures:	
	Dermalon	Nylon
	Novafil	Poly(tetramethylene ether)terephthalate-co-tetramethylene terephthalate
	Surgilene	Polypropylene
	Surgilon	Nylon
	Ti-Cron	Polyethylene terephthalate
WL Gore	**Nonabsorbable sutures:**	
	Gore-Tex	Polytetrafluoroethylene

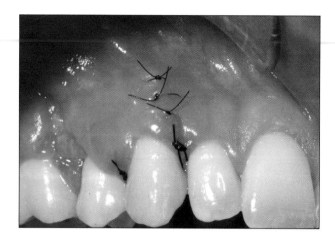

Fig 14-4 Interrupted sutures at a periodontal surgical site where there is postsurgical edema. The sutures stabilize the transposed flap and resist displacement by the edema. (Courtesy of K Zeren, Lutherville, MD.)

Properties of Sutures

Sutures are essentially fibrous materials that are evaluated in terms of interrelated, clinically relevant characteristics—namely, physical and mechanical properties, handling characteristics, and biologic properties.

Physical and Mechanical Properties

The physical and mechanical properties of a suture are central to its biomechanical function in periodontal surgery—specifically, wound closure and withstanding physiologic loads during healing (Fig 14-4). Most important are the tensile properties (strength, elongation at break, and elastic modulus), viscoelasticity, bending stiffness, fluid sorption/capillarity, and coefficient of friction. The tensile strengths of unknotted (straight pull) and knotted sutures differ, with strength being markedly decreased by the presence of a knot. Likewise, strength varies according to whether a suture is tested dry or wet (soaked).

The strengths of commercial suture materials vary markedly, and the tensile properties of sutures used in periodontal surgery are summarized in Table 14-5.[8,9,13] It should be noted that by convention, strength is expressed in terms of the cross-sectional area of the material, so sutures of different sizes and composition can be compared. This normalization of strength often causes confusion, because the surgeon in the clinical setting is concerned with how much force a suture of a given gauge or nominal size can resist before breaking. Thus, a 4-0 suture with a larger diameter will exhibit a greater resistance to breakage (ie, a larger knotted and unknotted breaking force) than a smaller-diameter suture of the same nominal size, even though the larger suture will have a lower tensile strength due to its larger diameter. Consequently, surgeons should evaluate sutures on the basis of breaking force rather than tensile strength per se.

Another important tensile property is compliance or ease of elongation under tensile loading. Ideally, the compliance of a suture and the tissue being sutured should be comparable, and it has been suggested that compliance mismatch contributes to clinical failure of grafts. It should be noted, however, that if the tensile force applied during knotting is too high, a compliant suture may lose its compliance and be stiffer. Suture compliance is of major importance in vascular anastomoses.[14]

An additional important property that has received little attention in the literature is the bending or flexural stiffness of sutures, a complex parameter that affects their handling characteristics, particularly knot security. Most reported suture stiffness data were derived from the moduli of elasticity calculated from tensile strength testing. These values, however, poorly quantify knot strength, knot security, and tie-down,

Table 14-5 Mechanical properties of sutures

SUTURE	BREAKING STRENGTH (MPA)	KNOTTED STRENGTH (MPA)	ELONGATION AT BREAK (%)
Catgut	310–380	110–220	15–35
Nylon 6 and 66	460–710	300–330	17–65
Polydioxanone (PDS)	450–560	240–340	
Polyglactin 910 (Vicryl)	570–910	300–400	18–25
Polyglycolide-co-ε-caprolactone (Monocryl)	760–920	310–590	18–25
Polyglycolic acid (Dexon)	410–460	280–320	24–62
Polypropylene (Prolene)	1,859	1,437	33
Polytetrafluoroethylene (Gore-Tex)	480–550	290–370	29–38
Poly(tetramethylene ether)-terephthalate-co-tetramethylene terephthalate (Novafil)	370–570	240–290	9–31

because knotting of a suture involves bending its strands, behavior that is not addressed in tensile testing. There are few reported studies of bending stiffness of sutures, but one important study[15] defined *suture flexural stiffness* as the force required to bend a suture to a predetermined angle. The study showed that braided sutures were generally more flexible than monofilaments, regardless of chemical composition. It also noted that the flexural stiffness of coated materials was significantly higher than that of the corresponding uncoated sutures, particularly when the sutures were coated with a polymer other than wax or silicone. The greater bending stiffness was attributed to the reduced mobility of the suture strands during bending. Flexural stiffness also increases with suture size, although the actual increase depends on the composition and structure of the suture; an example is Gore-Tex, which has low flexural stiffness because of its large pore volume (Fig 14-5). Suture flexural stiffness also depends on the duration of loading in stiffness testing. Monofilament sutures show a greater time-dependent stiffness than braided sutures, although nylon sutures, regardless of physical form, apparently do not exhibit this time dependence.

Two interrelated suture properties that are significant in periodontal surgery are capillarity and fluid sorption. Suture capillarity is the ease with which fluid can be transported along the suture strand. High capillarity is an inherent characteristic of multifilament sutures because of the large amount of interstitial space, whereas monofilament materials generally have low capillarity. Suture capillarity is important because it regulates the ability to transport microorganisms. In fact, microorganism uptake by braided nylon suture is three times that of monofilament nylon.[16] One qualitative study demonstrated capillarity in twisted polyamide with cover, braided polyester, and twisted linen but did not find this property in monofilament polypropylene or either monofilament or braided, waxed polyamide sutures.[17] It is interesting to note that the same study did not detect capillarity in plain or chromic catgut or with wax-coated braided silk; presumably, in the latter case the wax coating inhibited capillarity. The three sutures with demonstrated capillarity showed a marked (more than 10-fold) difference in their rates of fluid transport, and their respective rate constants were 0.24, 0.04, and 0.01 cm^2/s.[17]

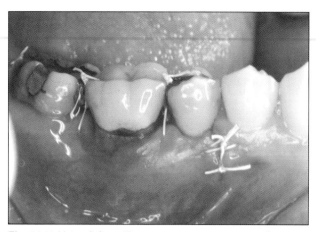

Fig 14-5 Use of Gore-Tex sutures as suspensory ligatures following periodontal surgery. The low-stiffness sutures permit tissue movement while retaining coaptation. (Courtesy of M Reynolds, Baltimore, MD.)

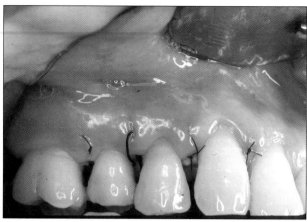

Fig 14-6 Loosening of silk sutures following subsidence of postsurgical edema. (Courtesy of M Reynolds, Baltimore, MD.)

Fluid sorption by a suture also may be responsible for the spread of microorganisms within tissues, and although both the chemical composition and the physical structure of the suture determine sorption behavior, chemical nature appears to be the more important property.[17] In general, synthetic sutures exhibit less sorption than natural fibers because of their greater hydrophobicity. Multifilament sutures show greater fluid sorption than monofilaments because of their associated capillarity. Natural sutures (gut, silk, and linen) show markedly higher sorption rates of saline and blood plasma than do synthetic materials, apparently because natural fibers have higher bulk fluid absorption and surface fluid absorption rates.[17] The higher sorption of catgut arises from its proteinaceous nature, which provides numerous bonding sites for fluid molecules, with such attachments not limited to the surface. In contrast, most of the sorbed fluid in synthetic sutures is retained on the surface.

Viscoelasticity and stress relaxation

The *viscoelasticity* of a material indicates its ability to change dimensions with time under static loading (ie, creep) or to change strength during time-dependent dimensional changes (ie, stress

relaxation). For sutures, this property determines whether tissue approximation is maintained. Suture loops often loosen after edema subsides (Fig 14-6). With sutures subject to high creep, the relaxation following recession of wound edema may result in suture loops becoming too loose to properly appose the wound edges. Not much information is available on the viscoelastic behavior of suture materials, however.

Semicrystalline synthetic polymeric and natural fibers show a decrease in applied load with time under constant strain (the viscoelastic phenomenon of stress relaxation). Thus, when these fibers are elongated to a fixed strain at a constant temperature and humidity, the stress within the fiber will decay with time. Depending on the chemical structure of the fiber, the strain level, the relative humidity, and the temperature, the stress may decay to a limiting value or decrease to zero. The usual pattern is a rapid initial decay of the stress, followed by a much slower decay rate later. Stress relaxation can occur under other modes of stress application, such as torsion[18]; this is an important consideration, because the knotting of sutures must account for torsional loading. Research has shown that relaxation of torque stress is a function of the number of turns and twists; there is a linear relationship between log (torque stress) and log (time in minutes),[19] similar to the stress relaxation under tensile loading.

Stress relaxation occurs because the mobility of the segments of the constituent polymer chains allows them to achieve a new equilibrium position under applied loads. Consequently, any factor that affects segmental mobility will influence stress relaxation. Generally, stress decay increases with increasing temperature and humidity, the effect of the latter being due to the plasticizing effect of the absorbed water through disruption of secondary bonding between polymeric chain segments. The disruption of the secondary linkages increases the structural mobility and leads to faster stress decay under a fixed strain. Fiber pretreatments that stabilize or disrupt the secondary bonds affect stress relaxation behavior.

The solution pH should have little effect on the rate of stress decay of nonabsorbable sutures (which are hydrophobic materials) immersed in liquid media. The stress decay of nylon 66 fibers is independent of pH over a range of pH 2.95 to 10.02.[13,20] The solution pH may significantly affect the stress decay behavior of hydrophilic absorbable sutures, however, particularly because their degradation has been shown to be pH dependent.[21,22]

The composition, structure, and stereoregularity of the polymer can affect stress relaxation. The isotactic form of polypropylene, for example, exhibits a lower rate of stress relaxation than the atactic form.[23] Under dynamic mechanical analysis (DMA), atactic polypropylene exhibits a relationship of log (relaxation modulus) and log (time) characteristic of amorphous polymers—ie, an initial glassy region is followed by a rapid reduction in Young's modulus with time (the viscoelastic region in which there is breakdown of secondary bonds) and then by a rubbery region in which the molecular chains, now free of the secondary linkages, can react to thermal vibrations of the solid. In contrast, isotactic polypropylene is semicrystalline, and the stress relaxation master curve does not show as pronounced a viscoelastic region as that of amorphous polymers. Likewise, the orientation of fibers and the extent of fiber drawing affect stress relaxation. In general, it

appears that the rate of stress decay decreases with increases in the degree of drawing.[13,20,22]

Handling Characteristics

Surgeons refer to the *hand* of a suture, and experienced surgeons rate the hand of sutures quite similarly. However, the handling characteristics of sutures are difficult to evaluate quantitatively because they are so subjective. Handling characteristics actually encompass various properties, and the many qualities that are determined by the physical and mechanical properties of the sutures are quantifiable. A pliable suture is one that a surgeon can bend easily and tie in a knot without the knot quickly reopening. Pliability, therefore, is determined by both the modulus of elasticity and the frictional behavior of the suture. However, suture knotting also is affected by the packaging memory, ie, the tendency of the suture to remain kinked after being taken from the package. A kinked suture typically is more difficult to manipulate after being straightened and then tied into a knot. Sutures with high packaging memories—eg, nylon, PDS, and polypropylene—tend to untie themselves as they try to resume the kinking from packaging. Generally, monofilament sutures have greater packaging memories than braided ones, but two monofilament sutures, Monocryl and Gore-Tex, appear to have exceptionally low packaging memory.[13,24]

The nature of the suture surface and its coefficient of friction determine two clinically important properties, knot tie-down and knot security.[25] *Knot tie-down* is the ease with which a surgeon can slide a knot down to the wound edge; *knot security* is how well a knot stays in position without untying or slipping after it is tied. Generally, sutures with smooth surfaces (eg, monofilaments or coated braided sutures) have better knot tie-down than sutures with rougher surfaces, such as uncoated braided sutures. Thus, although a high coefficient of friction may make knot tie-down difficult, it generally leads to a more secure knot, because frictional forces help hold the knot together. One method of quantifying the knot tie-down properties of sutures has generated data on knot tie-down resistance and roughness for two

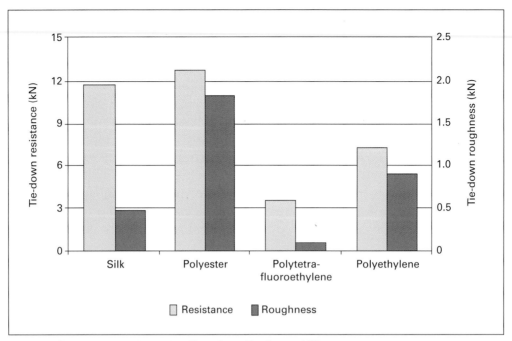

Fig 14-7 Suture knotting behavior. (Data from Tomita et al.[26])

monofilament sutures (polytetrafluoroethylene and polyethylene) and two braided sutures (silk and polyester).[26] As expected, the braided sutures had higher values of resistance to knot sliding, and these materials required fewer throws to ensure good knot security than did the monofilaments (Fig 14-7). Silk suture, which is generally recognized as having excellent handling characteristics, had the largest difference between knot tie-down resistance and tie-down roughness. The high knot security of these braided sutures was thought to be due to both surface friction and additional resistance to knot opening arising from deformation (bending and flattening) of the suture within the knot.

Another clinically important characteristic of a suture is the ease with which it can be drawn through tissue, during both wound closure and suture removal. This characteristic, known as *tissue drag*, clearly should be as low as possible to avoid tearing soft tissue as the suture is drawn through it. The tissue drag of a suture is determined by both its surface roughness and the coefficient of friction. In general, monofilaments and coated sutures have less tissue drag than uncoated and braided sutures because of their smoother surfaces. The few reported studies on tissue drag evaluated the ease of suture removal; the data indicated that less force was required to withdraw monofilament sutures than braided sutures, and surface coatings reduced tissue drag for even braided sutures.[27] Tissue drag for braided (multifilament) sutures may also be increased by the ingrowth of connective tissue within the suture during wound healing. This consideration is important because of the rapid healing in periodontal surgery.

Biologic Properties

The biologic properties of sutures encompass both biocompatibility and biodegradability. Because sutures are foreign materials to the body, they can affect the surrounding tissues, and the surrounding tissues may affect the properties of sutures. In other words, the biocompatibility between suture and soft tissue is a two-way relationship. The type and extent of tissue reactions to a suture are

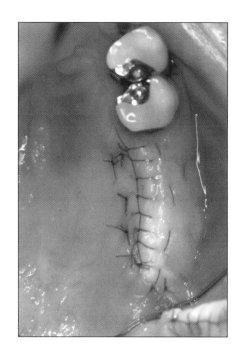

Fig 14-8 Continuous mattress suturing of a healing periodontal surgical site in the palate. Internal mattress sutures maintain tissue approximation while external sutures maintain the integrity of the wound margins. (Courtesy of K Zeren, Lutherville, MD.)

determined by the chemical formulation and, to a degree, the physical form of the suture, as well as the degradation products if the suture is biodegradable. Sutures fabricated from natural materials, such as catgut and silk, usually provoke more intense tissue reactions than synthetic ones because of the availability of enzymes that can react with them. Consequently, surgeons generally try to use as little suture material as possible when closing wounds, eg, by tying smaller knots or using a smaller-gauge material (Fig 14-8).

In general, smaller-diameter sutures are preferred, provided that they adequately support the healing wound and add no risk of cutting through wound tissue. The use of smaller-diameter sutures reduces the volume (V) of material in tissue; $V = \pi D^2 L/4$, where D is the suture diameter, and L is its length. Clearly, even a small change in suture diameter will have a large effect on the tissue volume.

The pliability of a suture is another important characteristic. A suture with poor pliability when knotted may leave stiff ears projecting from the knot, which can mechanically irritate the surrounding tissues. Certain monofilaments have this problem, but it is less common with braided multifilament sutures.

The biocompatibility of suture materials is clearly important, and this property may be evaluated by cellular response, enzyme histochemistry, or both.[20,24,28–30] Cellular response is used more frequently and provides information about the type and density of inflammatory cells at a suture site. The enzyme histochemistry approach is based on the fact that any cellular response to a suture is always associated with the presence of enzymes that degrade absorbable sutures. Many biocompatibility studies of suture materials have been performed in rat gluteal muscle. Although this site provides a consistent and reproducible cellular response that permits comparison of the responses to implanted sutures, it is not a common surgical site, and its usefulness has been questioned.[31] Suture biocompatibility studies also have been performed using the dorsum of New Zealand White rabbits and the mucosa of beagles.[29,32] However, the cellular responses are rated through subjective histologic evaluation of tissue sections, which requires a skilled and experienced evaluator.

Evaluating suture biocompatibility through enzyme histochemistry is an objective, reproducible, consistent, and quantifiable approach, but it is time-consuming and requires more sophisticated facilities. However, because of the role of enzy-

Table 14-6 Stages in tissue reactions to sutures

STAGE	TIME (DAYS)	REACTION
Phase 1	0–4	Acute response: infiltration of polymorpho-nuclear leukocytes, lymphocytes, and monocytes
Phase 2	4–7	Macrophagic and fibroblastic activity
Phase 3	7–10	Chronic inflammation and start of fibrous connective tissue maturation

matic activity in suture degradation and metabolization of the degradation products, enzyme histochemistry is useful for studying the biodegradation of absorbable sutures.

The normal tissue reaction to sutures proceeds through three stages, which are differentiated according to the appearance and activity of various inflammatory cells, as outlined in Table 14-6. Generally, there are virtually no differences in the tissue and cellular responses to synthetic absorbable and nonabsorbable sutures over the first 7 days after implantation. Synthetic absorbable sutures may elicit a slightly greater inflammatory reaction that persists until the suture is completely absorbed and metabolized. In contrast, nonabsorbable sutures elicit minimal chronic inflammatory reactions, and by 28 days they are often surrounded by a thin, fibrous connective tissue capsule. A consequence of the normal tissue reaction is the ingrowth of fibrous tissue into multifilament sutures, and there may also be ingrowth of epidermis with sutures that pass through the cutaneous surface. Such tissue ingrowth may hamper easy removal of sutures from the healing wound, as noted above.

Various adverse tissue reactions may arise because of the nature of the surgical suture site or the characteristics of the suture itself. In general, monofilament sutures are preferred for closing contaminated wounds, because multifilament sutures elicit more tissue reactions due to penetration of inflammatory cells into the interstitial spaces within the sutures. This process may adversely affect the healing of infected wounds. Further-

more, where multifilament materials exhibit capillarity, microorganisms may migrate throughout the wound area.

Absorbable sutures must biodegrade and be absorbed when placed in the body, characteristics that nonabsorbable sutures do not have. As a result, absorbable sutures do not elicit the long-term inflammatory reactions found with nonabsorbable sutures. Furthermore, unlike nonabsorbable sutures, absorbable materials progressively lose both strength and mass from the time of implantation, with the rate of strength loss always exceeding the rate of mass loss. Consequently, as wound healing progresses, the suture may no longer maintain wound closure, although significant amounts of material may remain in the wound area. This consideration is clearly important in treating infected and/or contaminated wounds, particularly for braided materials.

A number of factors determine the rate of absorbable suture biodegradation, including the suture type, the tissues involved, temperature, pH, electrolytes, the applied stress, and any microorganisms within the wound area.[20,30] The biocompatibility of degradation products from absorbable sutures generally is not a problem, because these sutures are manufactured from well-established biocompatible polymers. Nevertheless, both the accumulation rate and the metabolization of the degradation products in the surrounding tissues are important factors. In general, degradation products are rapidly metabolized in well-vascularized tissue, which tends to minimize tissue reactions.

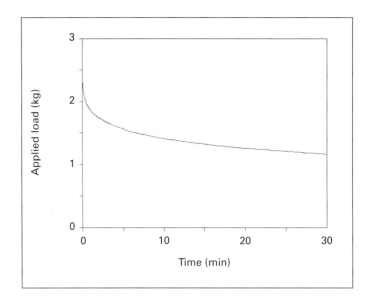

Stress Relaxation and Wound Healing

Tensile studies of suture materials indicate differences in their strength, elongation at failure, and failure energy; the shapes of their force-elongation curves also differ.[8,13,33] Although the elastic moduli of the suture materials vary, most display a virtually linear stress-strain curve almost to failure; ie, the elastic modulus does not change significantly with the applied stress, although the polypropylene (Prolene) suture had an elastic modulus that decreased with increasing stress until the suture failed. Nevertheless, most sutures exhibited the load-elongation behavior characteristic of semicrystalline materials and therefore should show some degree of viscoelasticity. In fact, most sutures, when held under tension at a fixed strain, have a similar relationship of applied load to time; the applied load decreases rapidly over the first few minutes, with a slower rate of stress decay thereafter.[34,35] Figure 14-9 shows this behavior for Prolene.

The load-vs-time behavior of three sutures—Prolene (polypropylene), PDS (polydioxanone), and Dexon (polyglycolic acid) was characterized by an initial rate of stress relaxation that was dependent on the rate of elongation, but the final or steady-state residual load fraction was independent of the strain rate, except at very low loading rates. Furthermore, the bulk of stress relaxation occurred within the first 2 minutes, and the subsequent rate of relaxation was much slower. The degree of stress relaxation varied with the suture material, and the percentage residual load for the three suture materials was approximately 70% for polydioxanone, 62% for polyglycolic acid, and 40% for polypropylene (Fig 14-10).

The stress relaxation modulus can be determined by calculating the ratio P_t/ϵ, where P_t is the applied load at time t, and ϵ is the applied strain; a plot of log (relaxation modulus) vs log (time) yields a characteristic curve. Such curves often indicate that the relaxation modulus (E_r) has different regions of behavior, typically a constant value for the first few seconds followed by a transition region and then a region where there is a constant decrease with time. Stress relaxation studies indicate that there is a change in E_r of sutures at 1 to 2 minutes, ie, the period when the greatest stress relaxation occurred.

The viscoelastic properties of materials may be characterized by DMA, and this technique has been applied to sutures.[13,36] In DMA, a sinusoidal time-varying tensile force is applied to the specimen, which elongates, and the resulting strain also is a sine wave. If the specimen is viscoelastic,

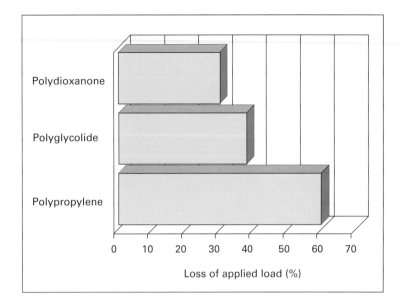

Fig 14-10 Load decrease (percentage) for sutures under constant strain. (Data from Metz et al.[34])

the strain is out of phase with the applied stress such that there is a phase shift or lag between them. This lag is defined as the phase angle (δ), which is used to calculate the loss tangent (tan δ), an index of material viscoelasticity because it is the ratio of the viscous and elastic moduli. Dynamic mechanical analysis also permits determination of both the tensile storage modulus, or E′ (the ratio of the in-phase strain to the applied stress), and the loss modulus, or E″ (the ratio of the out-of-phase strain to the applied stress). E″ reflects the ability of the material to dissipate mechanical energy by conversion to heat through molecular motion.

In practice, a tensile force is applied to the test specimen at a temperature below the glass transition event, which is normally characterized by the temperature T_g at which the material transforms from being rigid to rubberlike. This applied force is maintained as the temperature is raised. The values of elastic moduli (E′ and E″) and of tan δ are determined at temperatures above and below those at which the material is used, and they indicate the α and β transitions for the material. The α transition, also known as the *glass transition* or T_g *event*, is the main amorphous phase change for a polymer and is characterized as the transition from a rigid, glasslike state to a rubbery condi-

tion. The β relaxation event is associated with molecular rearrangements arising from motion occurring within the amorphous regions of the material, and it affects viscoelastic or stress relaxation behavior. Clearly, the temperatures at which the α and β transitions occur markedly affect polymer behavior.

Long-term polymer behavior can be evaluated by shifting the modulus data with respect to frequency to determine the properties at short times (high frequencies) or long times (low frequencies). This procedure generates master curves that characterize the long-term mechanical properties.[13,23,36–38]

In DMA studies of the viscoelastic properties of suture materials, marked differences were found; these viscoelastic data are summarized in Table 14-7.[13,36] The polydioxanone suture (PDS) did not show a β relaxation event, and the α transition occurred at 1°C; it had the lowest elastic modulus of the materials tested. Consequently, at room temperature, PDS is above its T_g and might be expected to exhibit "soft" characteristics. In contrast, silk had a relatively high elastic modulus and showed a change in elastic modulus and glass transition temperature (T_g) only at temperatures higher than 200°C; ie, changes in properties occurred only at temperatures close to the decomposition temperature.

Table 14-7 Dynamic mechanical analysis data for 4-0 sutures at 30°C

SUTURE MATERIAL	TRADE NAME	STORAGE MODULUS E′ (GPA)	LOSS MODULUS E″ (GPA)	TAN δ* (°C)	TAN δ† (°C)
Polydioxanone	PDS	2.2	1.2	—	1
Polyglactin 910	Vicryl	19.5	2.1	−65	68
Polyglycolide	Dexon	39.0	3.8	−55	72
Polyglycolide-co-trimethylene carbonate	Maxon	2.8	3.8	−78	30
Polypropylene	Prolene	4.4	1.1	2	106
Silk	Silk	41.2	3.2	—	226

*β transition.
†α transition.

Vicryl and Dexon have a similar chemistry and showed comparable thermomechanical behavior. Both materials exhibited subambient β relaxation events, and their main amorphous phase relaxation events (the α or glass transitions) occurred well above room temperature, as shown in Table 14-7. As would be expected, changes in the elastic modulus for these materials occurred only well above room temperature.

The polypropylene suture Prolene exhibited its β relaxation event at 2°C and its α transition at approximately 100°C. Because the β relaxation transition occurred slightly below room temperature, the transition should have a major impact on the properties—notably stress relaxation—exhibited by the suture at room or body temperature. Furthermore, Prolene had a low loss modulus and a low storage modulus, and it was found to undergo pronounced changes in both elastic moduli close to room temperature. The polyglyconate suture Maxon had storage and loss moduli comparable to those of Prolene, and although its β relaxation transition occurred at approximately −78°C, its T_g was close to room temperature (see Table 14-7).

Master curves, generated through frequency multiplexing data, show that both Prolene and Maxon undergo changes in the storage modulus and tan δ at room temperature with respect to time.[13,36] PDS shows similar behavior. In contrast, the frequency multiplexing data for silk and Vicryl show very flat responses in E′ and tan δ in the vicinity of 25°C, indicating that the elastic moduli of both suture materials are very stable with respect to time at this temperature. Dexon presumably has a similarly stable elastic modulus.

These preliminary DMA data suggest that silk and the "artificial silk" sutures (Dexon and Vicryl) may be best suited for ligation, because these materials retain a high degree of stiffness over a long period and thus in this application should minimize the risks of delayed hemorrhage. Prolene, Maxon, and PDS, in contrast, exhibit elastic moduli that change (relax) with time, so these sutures may give better results during normal healing.

Effect of Suturing on Wound Healing

It is a clinical maxim that sutures should not be tied tightly across a wound, and junior residents in all surgical specialties are admonished not to snug sutures down too tightly to avoid wound

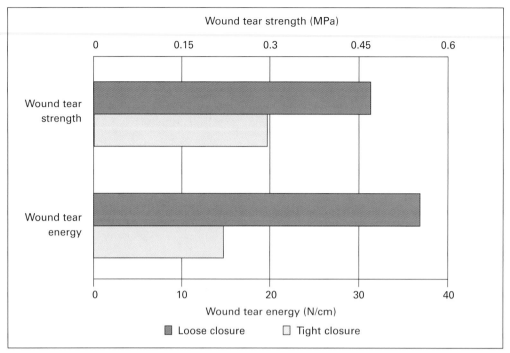

Fig 14-11 Effect of suture tautness on wound healing. (Data from Stone et al.[6])

dehiscence, tissue strangulation, and poor healing. This advice is particularly pertinent for periodontal surgical procedures involving highly vascularized tissues. Despite wide acceptance of the time-honored principle that wound healing is affected by the tension applied by sutures across the approximating tissue edges, until recently the literature had sparse quantitative data to support this contention. However, recent work has demonstrated that the tautness of the suture across a healing wound can significantly affect the healing process. In particular, it was shown that healing wounds exhibit greater tear strengths and tear energies when tied with loose sutures than tight sutures.[6]

In a wound-healing study,[6] wound edges approximated under the force routinely used by an experienced surgeon for suturing were designated as being closed with "tight" sutures. The edges of another series of wounds were approximated by normal suturing technique, but the sutures were tied over a rod 3 mm in diameter laid adjacent to

the wound. After the wound was closed, the rod was removed and the wound allowed to heal in the normal manner. These wounds were designated as being closed with "loose" sutures. Wounds that were approximated with loosely tied sutures achieved a statistically significantly greater wound tear strength and wound tear energy than tightly sutured wounds, as shown in Fig 14-11. This in vivo study clearly demonstrated that the apposition force applied across a healing wound by a suture may profoundly affect the normal course of wound healing, in that a small reduction in the approximating force across the wound edges achieved greater wound tear strength and tear energy. The effects on wound tear strength arising from suture tautness were far greater than the effects due to the mode of surgical incision.[5]

Improved wound healing through reduction of the approximating force across a wound is clearly beneficial, but the use of an external aid, such as a rod placed beside a healing wound, is impractical during most surgical procedures. However, reducing the approximating force by stress relaxation within the suture will facilitate wound healing.

The research data summarized here suggests that wound closure with stress-relaxing sutures may be beneficial in wound healing, and this idea has important implications for periodontal surgery. Insufficient data exist to accurately predict surgical outcomes, but careful suture selection and surgical technique may markedly improve the prognosis for wound healing in many periodontal and oral surgical procedures.

References

1. Cohen IK, Diegelmann RF, Lindblad WJ (eds). Wound Healing: Biochemical and Clinical Aspects. Philadelphia: Saunders, 1992.

2. Lin PH, Hirko MK, von Fraunhofer JA, Greisler HP. Wound healing and inflammatory response to biomaterials. In: Chu CC, von Fraunhofer JA, Greisler HP (eds). Wound Closure Biomaterials. Boca Raton, FL: CRC Press, 1996.

3. Capperauld I, Bucknall, TE. Wound Healing for Surgeons. London: Bailliere Tindall, 1984.

4. Peacock EE, Van Winkle HW. Surgery and Biology of Wound Repair. Philadelphia: Saunders, 1970.

5. Sowa DE, Masterson BJ, Nealon N, von Fraunhofer JA. Effects of thermal knives on wound healing. Obstet Gynecol 1985;66:436–439.

6. Stone IK, von Fraunhofer JA, Masterson BJ. The biomechanical effects of tight suture closure on fascia. Surg Gynecol Obstet 1986;163:448–452.

7. Chu CC, von Fraunhofer JA, Greisler HP (eds). Wound Closure Biomaterials. Boca Raton, FL: CRC Press, 1996.

8. von Fraunhofer JA, Storey RJ, Stone IK, Masterson BJ. The tensile strength of suture materials. J Biomed Mater Res 1985;19:595–600.

9. Casey DJ, Lewis OG. Absorbable and nonabsorbable sutures. In: von Recum AF (ed). Handbook of Biomaterials Evaluation: Scientific, Technical and Clinical Testing of Implant Materials. New York: MacMillan, 1986:chap 7.

10. Rodeheaver GT, Foresman PA, Brazda MT, Edlich RF. A temporary nontoxic lubricant for a synthetic absorbable suture. Surg Gynecol Obstet 1987;164:17–20.

11. Griesser HJ, Chatelier RC, Martin C, Vasic ZR, Gengenbach TR, Jessup G. Elimination of stick-slip of elastomeric sutures by radiofrequency glow discharge deposited coatings. J Biomed Mater Res 2000;53:235–243.

12. Debus ES, Geiger D, Sailer M, Ederer J, Thiede A. Physical, biological and handling characteristics of surgical suture material: A comparison of four different multifilament absorbable sutures. Eur Surg Res 1997;29:52–61.

13. von Fraunhofer JA, Chu CC. Mechanical properties. In: Chu CC, von Fraunhofer JA, Greisler HP (eds). Wound Closure Biomaterials. Boca Raton, FL: CRC Press, 1996:chap 6.

14. Megerman J, Hamilton G, Schmitz-Rixen T, Abbott WM. Compliance of vascular anastomoses with polybutester and polypropylene sutures. J Vasc Surg 1993;18:827–834.

15. Chu CC, Kizil Z. Quantitative evaluation of stiffness of commercial suture materials. Surg Gynecol Obstet 1989;168: 233–237.

16. Bucknall TE. Factors influencing wound complications: A clinical and experimental study. Ann R Coll Surg Engl 1983; 65:71–77.

17. Blomstedt B, Osterberg B. Fluid absorption and capillarity of suture materials. Acta Chir Scand 1977;143:67–70.

18. Hammerle WG, Montgomery DJ Mechanical behavior of nylon filaments in torsion. Textile Res J 1953;23:595–604.

19. Permanyer F. [PhD thesis]. Manchester, England: University of Manchester, 1947.

20. Chu CC. Biodegradation properties. In: Chu CC, von Fraunhofer JA, Greisler HP (eds). Wound Closure Biomaterials. Boca Raton, FL: CRC Press, 1996:chap 7.

21. Chu CC. In-vitro degradation of polyglycolic acid sutures: Effect of pH. J Biomed Mater Res 1981;15:795–804.

22. Chu CC. The biodegradation of polyglycolic acid suture, I. Effect of buffer. J Biomed Mater Res 1981;15:19–27.

23. Tobolsky AV. Properties and Structure of Polymers. New York: Wiley, 1960.

24. Pinheiro AL, de Castro JF, Thiers FA, et al. Using Novafil: Would it make suturing easier? Braz Dent J 1997;8:21–25.

25. Herrmann JB. Tensile strength and knot security of surgical suture materials. Am Surg 1971;37:209–217.

26. Tomita N, Tamai S, Morihara T, et al. Handling characteristics of braided suture materials for tight tying. J Appl Biomater 1993;4:61–65.

27. Homsy CA, McDonald KE, Akers WW, Short C, Freeman BS. Surgical suture-canine tissue interaction for six common suture types. J Biomed Mater Res 1968;2:215–230.

28. Outlaw KK, Vela AR, O'Leary JP. Breaking strength and diameter of absorbable sutures after in vivo exposure in the rat. Am Surg 1998;64:348–354.

29. Setzen G, Williams EF III. Tissue response to suture materials implanted subcutaneously in a rabbit model. Plas Reconstr Surg 1997;100:1788–1795.

30. Hirko MK, Lin PH, Greisler HP, Chu CC. In: Chu CC, von Fraunhofer JA, Greisler HP (eds). Wound Closure Biomaterials. Boca Raton, FL: CRC Press, 1996:chap 8.

31. Walton M. Strength retention of chromic gut and monofilament synthetic absorbable suture materials in joint tissues. Clin Orthop 1989;242:303–310.

32. Selvig KA, Biagiotti GR, Leknes KN, Wikesjo UM. Oral tissue reactions to suture materials. Int J Periodontics Restor J Dent 1998;18:474–487.

33. von Fraunhofer JA, Storey RJ, Stone IK, Masterson BJ. Tensile properties of suture materials. Biomaterials 1988;9: 324–327.

34. Metz SA, von Fraunhofer JA, Masterson BJ. Stress relaxation of organic suture materials. Biomaterials 1990;11:197–199.

35. Chu CC. Stress relaxation of synthetic sutures. In: Winter GD, Gibbons DF, Plenk H (eds). Advances in Biomaterials, vol 3. Chichester, England: Wiley, 1982:655–660.

36. von Fraunhofer JA, Sichina WJ. Characterization of surgical suture materials using dynamic mechanical analysis. Biomaterials 1992;13:715–720.

37. Leaderman H. Elastic and creep properties of filamentous materials and other high polymers. Washington, DC: Textile Foundation, 1943.

38. Sichina WJ. A practical technique for predicting mechanical performance and useful lifetime of polymeric materials. Am Lab 1988;20(January):4–7.

15

Aging of Bioactive Glass Bone-Grafting Materials

John C. Mitchell, PhD

Bone tissue is frequently lost through trauma, disease, developmental deformity, or tumor removal. Repairing such bone defect sites currently involves various surgical techniques, including the use of bone-grafting materials. In the treatment of many diseases today, surgical resection of large regions of bone is the only viable option. In these cases, the gap left by tissue removal must be filled immediately. In addition, the loss of bone and gingival tissue following the traumatic removal or surgical extraction of a tooth often leads to both functional and cosmetic deficiencies. Such tissue loss often results in a nonesthetic appearance, especially in the anterior portion of the mouth, where proper maintenance of bone crestal height is critical to normal esthetics.

Functionality is severely compromised because loading of the jaw bones occurs through the teeth. Wolff's law[1] has long held that bones grow in response to applied loading. Thus, when loading does not occur (because of the absence of teeth), the existing bone will continue to undergo resorption,[2] potentially leading to complete edentulism. Additionally, loss of adequate bone width often compromises a dental practitioner's ability to adequately replace the missing tooth or teeth with either conventional prosthodontic appliances or implant-supported restorations. Many times, the lack of bone within the region of tooth loss is so severe that surgical procedures to augment the existing bone are required prior to replacing missing teeth.

The search for an ideal bone substitute has spanned hundreds of years and continues today. A variety of materials have been, and continue to be, used to graft bone tissues. Conservative estimates suggest that in 1998, practitioners performed more than 500,000 bone-grafting procedures in the United State alone, with an even greater number performed in subsequent years.[3] The use of grafting is widespread in dental practices for such purposes as filling osseous defects, maintaining the alveolar ridge width and height following tooth loss, and sinus lift grafting to support dental implants.[4–7]

Categories of Bone-Grafting Materials

Categorization of the various types of bone augmentation materials available is complicated, and its terminology merits a quick review. Briefly, grafting materials are classified according to origin. *Autografts* are bone fragments or blocks harvested from an alternative location—commonly, the mandibular symphysis or the iliac crest—in the patient. Although they have long been considered the gold standard for grafting, autografts subject the patient to additional surgical procedures (with associated discomfort and potential morbidity of the donor site) and additional operative time and expense, and their supply is relatively limited.[8–11]

Allografts are composed of bone obtained from other human individuals. Currently, these materials are by far the most commonly used extenders and substitutes for autogenous bone. Fresh allogenous grafts are never used, as they initiate an unacceptable immune response in the recipient. Bone banks therefore provide this material as a gamma-sterilized, lyophilized powder. Although freezing and gamma sterilizing greatly reduce the immunogenic response, they may also reduce the mechanical properties of the graft.[12–15] The compromised strength and possibility of disease and viral transmission have led researchers to continue the search for superior alternative materials.

The final two categories of materials, *xenografts* and *alloplasts*, have only relatively recently been developed for use in bone replacement surgery. Xenografts are natural materials obtained from nonhuman sources. Cross-species materials used in bone grafting include bovine bone, porcine bone, and coral. Although considered less risky than allografts, these materials still hold the potential for viral transmission and invoke an immune reaction. Alloplasts, in contrast, are completely nonbiologic synthetic materials. Bioactive glasses, ceramics, polymers, and even metals have been investigated as alloplastic materials for bone replacement therapy.[8–10,16]

The broad categories of graft materials are also commonly subclassified according to their biologic potential. All grafting substances must possess one or more of three essential capabilities to be accepted as a successful graft material: *(1) osteoconduction*, which implies that a material provides a physical scaffold on which cells might migrate into a defect site and begin the repair process; *(2) osteoinduction*, in which various factors initiate the cascade of reactions that ultimately lead to the formation of new bone; and *(3) osteogenesis*, in which resident mesenchymal stem cells differentiate to osteoblasts to form new bone. Numerous articles describe the capabilities of materials that have been used in an attempt to accomplish these goals. This chapter focuses on what happens when one alloplastic material type, the bioactive glasses, is placed in vivo and allowed to react

with the physiologic system. Determining the chemical and physical exchanges (or aging processes) that take place is of critical importance in understanding bone growth in these grafts and their vicinity.

Bioactive Glasses

Bioactive glasses are a unique class of synthetic metal oxide materials that react in the presence of body fluids to enhance and augment the body's self-healing capability. They not only assist the normal physiologic regeneration of tissues but also are ultimately resorbed in the process. These glasses have the singular ability to form a chemical bond with living tissues, thereby helping stabilize a filled defect site and maintaining a rigid scaffold upon which cells can migrate and grow. In contrast, materials considered to be nearly inert elicit the production of a fibrous capsule at the tissue-material interface.

In addition to chemical bonding to natural tissues (both soft and hard tissues), the glasses stimulate and attract essential physiologic components produced by the body for healing and help bind them at the defect site during healing and repair. Although many different physical conformations of these glassy solids have been proposed and tested for use as a defect filler, bioactive glasses are almost always produced as size-sorted granules or a very fine powder. They are commonly used either as a stand-alone product or combined with other materials at the time of placement in the body, and they almost always are combined with autogenous blood as a minimum adjuvant.

Introduced as Bioglass (US Biomaterials, Alachua, FL) in 1971 by Hench et al,[17] bioactive glasses are an amorphous mixture of one or more oxides. Typically, they have a silica-rich composition with minor, yet very important, secondary constituents, such as Na_2O, P_2O_5, and CaO. The minor constituents play important roles in determining the bioactive behavior and resorbability of these materials. These glasses are extremely surface-active in physiologic solution; ie, they undergo a rapid, spontaneous ion exchange with the body fluids. It is because of this bioactive behavior, along with the high silica content and amorphous nature of the material, that Hench coined the name *Bioglass*. The bioactive glass materials have proven to be both hemostatic and easy to manipulate.[18] Their use provides full-strength restoration of bone in 6 weeks, in comparison with the 12 weeks necessary for particulate hydroxylapatite to produce a comparable response.[19] Also, unlike hydroxylapatite particles, bioactive glass is completely resorbed in the restoration process, so potential problems associated with production of a bone-biomaterial composite interface are avoided in the fully restored bone.[20,21]

A key characteristic of these glasses is that their spontaneous ion exchange with the surrounding solution leads to the chemical deposition of a layer of biologic apatite on their surfaces when immersed in a physiologic fluid. During its formation, this layer incorporates organic molecules, such as fibrin and collagen fibers, from the surrounding solution into its structure, enabling easier cell migration over the surface of the particles.[22–28] This deposit is initially an amorphous carbonate apatite layer that over time matures, reorganizes, and mineralizes to become physically and chemically equivalent to the apatitic phase found in natural bone. This layer becomes extremely well bonded to both the underlying glass particles and the surrounding bone. In fact, the interface becomes indistinct over time as epitaxial growth of the bone cell–produced hydroxylapatite crystals occurs and the interface is incorporated into the deposited layer.[29]

Because of a growing body of evidence that this reaction of the glass (or of its dissolution products) stimulates a response at the cellular level to engender bone synthesis, the term *osteoproduction* was coined by Wilson and Low.[30] This term contrasts with the more familiar term *osteoconduction*, used to refer to what occurs with materials that merely provide a framework along which bone might grow, as discussed previously. As such, the bioactive glasses are now designated as Class A bioactive materials, as opposed to Class B bioactive materials such as hydroxylapatite.[31]

The bioactive glass originally developed by Hench had only a single amorphous phase and three crucial compositional requirements to maintain bioactivity: *(1)* less than 60 mol% SiO_2, *(2)* high contents of both Na_2O and CaO, and *(3)* a relatively high ratio of CaO to P_2O_5 (5:1 in Hench's original formulation). The most famous of these melt-derived bioactive glasses was designated 45S5, indicating 45 weight % SiO_2, silicon (S) as the glass network–forming cation, and a CaO-to-P_2O_5 molar ratio of 5.[31,32]

Recent advances in sol-gel chemistry, however, have enabled the production of bioactive sol-gel glasses with fewer compositional restrictions. These improvements include a much greater surface area (which results in a higher number of chemically reactive silanol groups on the surface), a much greater concentration of silicon dioxide in the glass, and the complete removal of Na_2O from the structure. Compositions with as much as 85% SiO_2 have been shown to exhibit bioactivity when prepared by the sol-gel method. These glasses generally contain only SiO_2, CaO, and P_2O_5 (and sometimes even the P_2O_5 is omitted).[33–44]

The concentration of silica in the glass network has a major effect on the survivability of the glass particles, with higher concentrations having longer in vivo lifetimes.[34–37,40,44] Additionally, the lack of Na_2O in the composition eliminates the uncontrollable rapid pH change associated with its release and allows greater control over the pH rise. These next-generation bioactive glass materials hold the promise of enabling precise control over the structure, composition, and surface texture of the resulting glass materials to an extent never before possible. They ultimately may allow surgeons to custom design the composition and texture of graft material for each recipient and thereby match the glass degradation (or resorption) rate with the new bone growth rate for each patient. These new designs may not only alleviate the development of short-term interfacial gaps but also permit the delivery of therapeutic compounds, adsorbed to the glass surface, which would enhance the speed of new tissue growth and repair.[45–51]

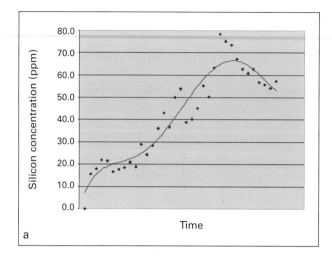

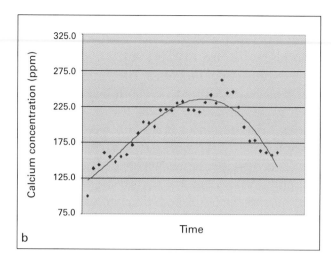

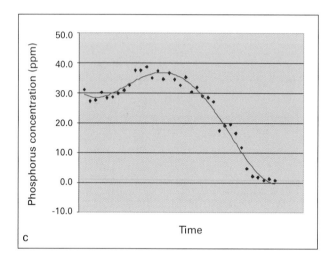

Fig 15-1 Inductively coupled plasma–optical emission spectroscopy data from simulated body fluid solution in which sol-gel–derived bioactive glass particles have been immersed for 7 days, the period of time represented on the horizontal axis. *(a)* The initial, very rapid release of silicon from the glass, which slows as the solution begins to saturate, increases again to a maximum and ultimately declines in concentration. *(b)* The elemental release of calcium ions into solution. Note that this element has a rapid initial release but quickly starts decreasing in concentration as the layer of carbonate apatite begins forming on the glass particles. *(c)* Phosphorus ion release into solution. This behavior is markedly different from that of the other two elements, as there is an initial reduction in solution phosphate content, followed by a small increase and a rather precipitous decline as the apatite layer is formed.

Ionic Exchange Sequence and Biologic Processes

The sequence of ionic exchange reactions that occur when a bioactive glass is immersed in physiologic fluid has been studied extensively. These reactions reproducibly result in the initial formation of a silica gel layer on the surface of the glass particles.[22–44,46–52] This gel layer is the result of condensation and polymerization of silanol groups on the surface of the glass. To observe and predict the elemental compositional changes that occur within and on bioactive glass materials, the author[44] soaked bioactive glass particles in a simulated body fluid (SBF), as originally described by Kokubo et al.[53] This liquid is an acellular, chemically defined solution that mimics the ionic composition of human blood plasma. As such, it allows direct observation of the step-by-step chemical processes that occur when bioactive glasses are immersed in physiologic solutions.

Figures 15-1a to 15-1c are graphs of data obtained by soaking sol-gel–prepared bioactive glass particles in SBF for various time periods up to 7 days. The graphs plot the actual concentration values obtained by inductively coupled plasma–optical emission spectroscopy (ICP-OES) on the SBF fluids, along with a superimposed regression line indicating the general trends of the ion concentration changes moving into, or precipitating out of, the SBF solutions.

As can be seen in Figs 15-1a and 15-1b, upon exposure of the glass particles to the SBF, there is a very rapid initial increase in the concentration of the soluble silicon and calcium ions in the solution. These ions are released from the glass surfaces and are carried nearly instantaneously out into the solution. However, as the solution becomes saturated with these ions, they begin to precipitate back onto the surface of the glass. These initial steps occurring on the surface of the glass particles are extensively reviewed in the literature[21,53-62] and summarized below. Although the steps are described here in sequence, they actually occur in an overlapping and continuous manner, with no definitive conclusion of any step prior to the commencement of the next.

Initial Steps Occurring on Surfaces of Glass Particles

Step 1a

When either K^+ or Na^+ network modifiers exist in the glass composition, the initial reaction is the diffusion of these ions from the glass, in exchange for H^+ or H_3O^+ from the solutions:

$$-Si-O-Si-O-Na^+ + H_3O^+ \rightarrow$$
$$-Si-O-Si-OH^+ + H_2O + Na^+$$

The Na^+ (or K^+) ion enters into the solution and is responsible for a rapid pH rise.

Step 1b

In the case of sol-gel–derived bioactive glasses, in which these alkali ions are absent, the initial step is the loss of soluble silicon in the form of $Si(OH)_4$ to the solution. This reaction also occurs in the melt-derived glasses, along with the ionic exchange shown in step 1a. This reaction results from the breaking of the Si–O–Si bonds at the glass-solution interface and the formation of silanol groups on the surface of the particles. This step similarly may result in an alkalinization of the surrounding microenvironment, albeit a greatly reduced one:

$$-Si-O-Si-O-Si-O-Si + H_2O \rightarrow$$
$$-Si-O-Si-OH + HO-Si-O-Si$$

There is evidence that this very minor shift in pH has potential beneficial effects, as it has substantial influence on cellular metabolism and function.[63] This alkaline shift plays a particularly important role in bone formation, because the cross-linking of collagen fiber chains, the intracellular release of calcium (which stimulates osteoblast adenosine triphosphate production), and the subsequent precipitation of hydroxylapatite depend on the attainment and maintenance of an optimal, slightly alkaline pH. Evidence for the loss of soluble silicon to the solution is shown in Fig 15-1a, where there is an initial rapid release of silicon into the solution.

Step 2

Next, as the silicon levels begin to reach saturation near the surface of the particles, they undergo a condensation and repolymerization reaction, which results in the formation of a silica gel layer on the surface of the glass particles:

$$-Si-O-Si-OH + HO-Si-O-Si \rightarrow$$
$$Si-O-Si-O-Si-O-Si + H_2O$$

This reaction step is highly exothermic and accounts for the slowing of the silicon release from the glass shown in Fig 15-1a. It is worth noting, however, that this reaction stage occurs simultaneously and continuously with step 1b, resulting in the formation of a relatively thin silica gel layer.

Step 3

The gel layer formed in step 2 is completely interpenetrated with pore liquid, enabling the subsequent migration of other species through this layer. The next sequence of reactions involves the migration of Ca^{2+} ions through this layer and into solution. After a slight lag, this process is followed by migration of the bulkier PO_4^{3-} ions. As these groups reach the surface of the silica gel layer, they are released into solution; they quickly reach the saturation concentration, however, and are precipitated back onto the glass surface as a new layer rich in $CaO-P_2O_5$. This amorphous layer continues to grow in thickness by the incorporation of soluble Ca^{2+} and PO_4^{3-} ions from the solution (see Figs 15-1b and 15-1c).

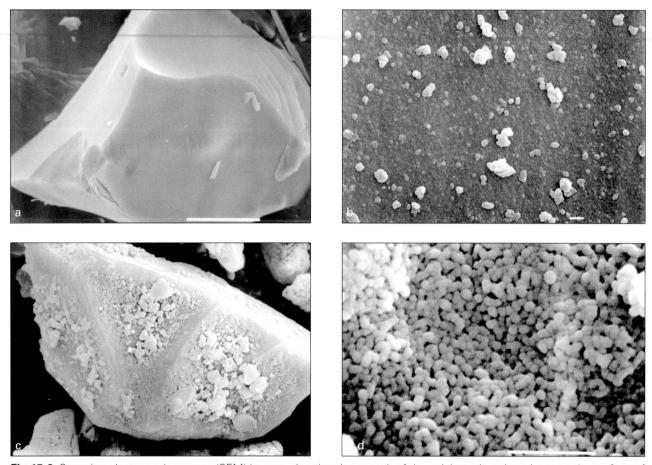

Fig 15-2 Scanning electron microscope (SEM) images showing the growth of the calcium phosphate layer on the surface of sol-gel–derived bioactive glass particles and the corrosion degradation of the particle surface: *(a)* soaking time (t) = 0 minutes; *(b)* the same particle as in *(a)* at a higher magnification; *(c)* a particle after t = 168 hours; and *(d)* the same particle as in *(c)* on a "clean" region at higher magnification (bar = 100 μm in *[a]* and *[c]* and 1 μm in *[b]* and *[d]*).

Notice that the initial solution calcium level slowly increases as the Ca^{2+} ions migrate through the glass and then drops dramatically as the precipitation occurs. The phosphate level, however, undergoes an initial drop, as the PO_4^{3-} ions cannot migrate as quickly through the glass and are depleted from the solution before reaching the surface, following a trend similar to that of the calcium level.

Formation of the Carbonate Apatite Layer

The initial series of steps are purely chemical, with each reaction occurring at its own time- and concentration-dependent rate. The ultimate for-

mation of the carbonate apatite layer has been confirmed by the author using several analytical techniques: direct observation with the SEM, Fourier transform infrared (FTIR) spectroscopy, and x-ray diffraction (XRD).[44] Typical results of these observations are shown in Figs 15-2 to 15-4.

The SEM images, shown in Figs 15-2a to 15-2d, are from a sol-gel–derived glass that has undergone aging in SBF. Figure 15-2a shows an original starting glass particle. It displays a conchoidal fracture pattern and a generally glassy appearance. However, the higher-magnification micrograph in Fig 15-2b shows that the surface is actually composed of nanometer-sized spherical particles of glass formed as a result of the sol-gel process. Even though these spherical glass particles pack together with spatial efficiency, this particulate nature greatly increases the surface area of the resulting bulk glass particles. Laboratory results obtained by the author[44] show that glasses prepared via the sol-gel route have a surface area four orders of magnitude greater than conventionally prepared glass materials.

Images of the glass after soaking for 168 hours in SBF are shown in Figs 15-2c and 15-2d. The obvious chemical corrosion of the glass surface results in the "opening up" of the porous structure. Microscale and nanoscale pores now seen between the particles increase the surface area for chemical reaction even further. Note also a new deposition of spherical particles of calcium phosphate laid down on the surface of the original glass particles. The composition of these new micrometer-sized particles has been confirmed[44] by x-ray energy-dispersive spectroscopy as being rich in both calcium and phosphorus.

The FTIR analysis of the newly synthesized (unsoaked) sol-gel bioactive glass shown in Fig 15-3a[44] reveals several peaks that have been previously interpreted.[64,65] The peak at 450 cm^{-1} corresponds to Si–O–Si bending and Si–O rotation modes. The peak near 785 cm^{-1} corresponds to Si–O bending, along with its associated cation movement. The small peak between 850 and 900 cm^{-1} corresponds to an Si–O–Ca structural unit. The peak at 1,060 cm^{-1} corresponds to P–O stretching. The peak at 1,190 cm^{-1} corresponds to Si–O–Si stretching, and the peak at 1,410 cm^{-1} is a result of a small amount of CO_3^{2-} in the structure. It is significant that the initial bioactive glass material prepared by the author had no characteristic peaks for the presence of apatite, a finding in agreement with the lack of peaks seen in the XRD results discussed below.

Compared with XRD, the FTIR technique is more sensitive to the initial stages of deposition and growth of the apatitic phases on the glass surface. When the bioactive glass materials are soaked in physiologic solution for as little as 30 minutes, two new broad peaks appear, at 550 cm^{-1} and approximately 960 cm^{-1} in the FTIR spectrum, as shown in Fig 15-3b. The first of these locations corresponds to the presence of a small amount of amorphous phosphate (P–O

bending), and the latter is characteristic of Si–O stretching where there are two nonbridging oxygen atoms in the structure (confirming the initial dissolution of the silicate network). Note also the diminished size of the former peak for the Si–O–Ca structure. This result again is probably due to disruption of the glass network and migration of calcium into solution.

Figure 15-3c shows that with increasing time in solution, the initially broad peak for amorphous phosphate (indicating the presence of the newly forming amorphous calcium phosphate layer) evolves into two discrete peaks located at 560 cm^{-1} and 590 cm^{-1}. These locations represent the P–O stretching and bending modes in the PO_4 tetrahedrons, and as such, these two peaks are each considered characteristic for the presence of crystalline hydroxylapatite.[66,67] Additionally, a new peak for carbonate is found in this spectrum at approximately 880 cm^{-1} (indicating the formation of hydroxyl carbonate apatite as the predominant species in the calcium phosphate layer).

Thus, within minutes of immersion in SBF, a detectable layer of amorphous carbonate apatite forms on the surface of the bioactive glass particles. This layer not only continues to grow in thickness but also undergoes chemical and physical rearrangement, resulting ultimately in the formation of a new integrated crystalline layer of hydroxyl carbonate apatite. The crystallinity of this growing layer has been confirmed[44] using XRD, as shown in Figs 15-4a and 15-4b. Figure 15-4a displays the XRD pattern produced by newly synthesized (unsoaked) glass particles. The only broad peak extends between diffraction angles (2θ) of approximately 15 and 40 degrees. This XRD pattern is characteristic of an amorphous material, in which there is no long-range atomic arrangement into a crystal structure with well-defined lattice parameters; only short-range order exists for the basic structural unit.[68,69] Figure 15-4b shows that after soaking in SBF, the area of the broad amorphous peak diminishes, and a new peak close to 31.8 degrees appears, which corresponds to the most intense diffraction peak (the 211 plane) of crystalline hydroxyl carbonate apatite.[70,71]

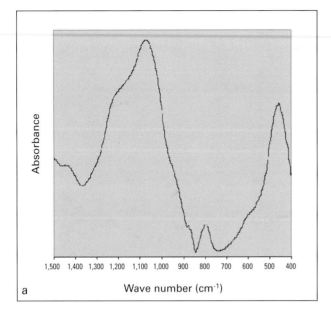

a

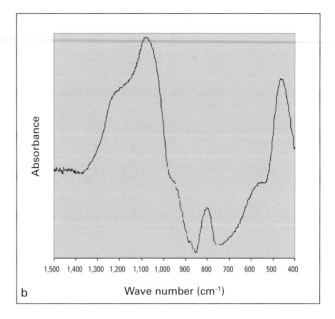

b

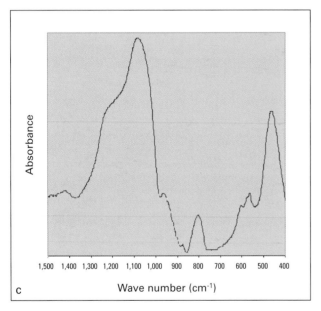

c

Fig 15-3 Fourier transform infrared spectra of a sol-gel–derived bioactive glass after exposure for *(a)* 0 hours, *(b)* a half hour, and *(c)* 72 hours in simulated body fluid solution.

It is during this stage of the in vivo reaction, which is ongoing for several days after implantation, that this growing layer of apatite entraps and incorporates glycosaminoglycans, fibronectin, bone proteoglycans, collagen fibers, and bone growth factors into its evolving structure. Fibronectin, which is known to facilitate osteogenic cell adhesion to surfaces, appears to have an affinity for this newly forming layer. These proteins appear to get trapped within the fluid inside pores as the slow increase in apatite gel layer thickness begins to envelop them. It is significant that while they are thus entrapped, partially inside the gel layer and partly free, these proteins are able to maintain their conformation and biologic activity. This protein-studded surface interaction layer continues to grow, ultimately becoming as much as 30 μm thick. The end result is a smooth transition from a protein-rich composition on the outer surface to a relatively inorganic calcium phosphate layer that overlies the silica-rich gel layer initially formed on the surface of the glass particles.[54,56,63,72,73]

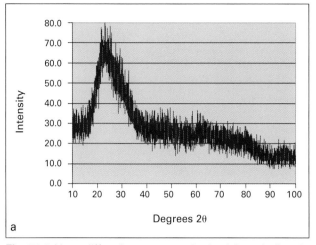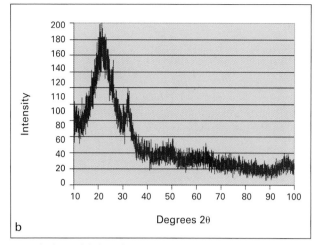

Fig 15-4 X-ray diffraction patterns obtained from bulk sol-gel–prepared glass: *(a)* the glass as synthesized and *(b)* the same glass particles after soaking in simulated body fluid for 168 hours at 37°C.

These bound proteins play crucial roles in the biointegration of the glass particles, as they form a chemical interconnection with the fibrin network of the surrounding blood clot. This blood clot fills the surgically created gap between the edge of the defect site and the glass particles, as well as between the glass particles. It is along this protein network that circulating stem cells, macrophages, fibroblasts, and other cells begin to migrate to reach the glass particle surfaces.[73,74] As the cell population increases, a stabilizing chemical bond develops between the proteins within the glass surface and the surrounding cells and resulting tissues. This helps to initially anchor the glass particles and prevent any micromotion at the particle surface. (Micromotion has been implicated as contributing to fibroblast proliferation and the formation of a fibrous capsule.[75]) This stability at the interface allows the osteoblast population to proliferate on the particle surfaces because of a series of cell membrane attachments and specific protein adsorptions, which are currently under investigation.[76] Soon after this migration and proliferation, cellular differentiation of circulating mesenchymal cells occurs, and new bone trabeculae can be seen forming between and among the particles. In Figs 15-5a and 15-5b, which are typical SEM photographs at a slightly later stage, the bioactive glass particles have been enveloped by this newly forming bone tissue. Note the direct contact between the surface of the glass and the bone tissue.

Once these cells reach the surface, the glass begins to biodegrade. The glass is now undergoing both chemical resorption and gel layer synthesis, while cells are developing and maturing on its surface. The formation process has been described above; the resorption process involves both the native chemical dissolution of the surface, enhanced by a reduction in pH caused by cellular and phagocytic activities, and the normal physiologic degradation action of osteoclasts.[77–79] Additionally, macrophages can engulf smaller particles and enzymatically eliminate them from the implantation site. Lai et al[80] describe the results of this degradation of the glass and report that by 28 weeks after implantation, the removal of silicon from the body is complete. They additionally report that the excretion of silicon in a soluble form through the urine has no significant adverse effect on any tissues or organs involved in its removal.

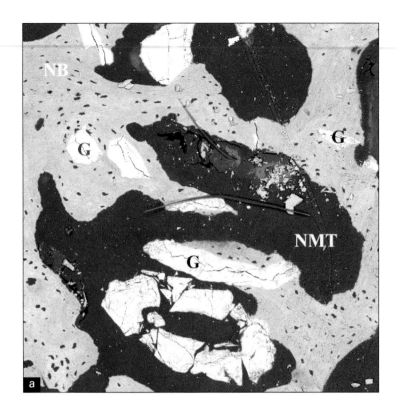

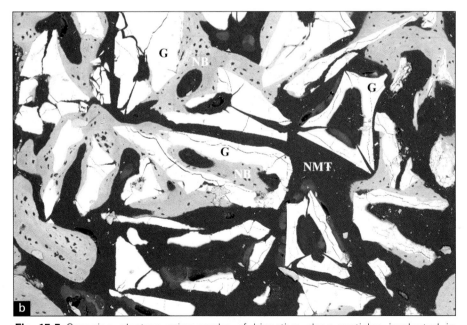

Fig 15-5 Scanning electron micrographs of bioactive glass particles implanted in human maxillary sinus for 3 months. NMT indicates nonmineralized tissue; NB, newly formed bone; and G, residual glass particles. Note the bone growth directly on and surrounding the glass particle surfaces in *(a)*, as well as in pores created by dissolution of the interior structure of the glass particles *(b)*. Also note the complete lack of intervening fibrous capsule formation (original magnification × 75).

Perspective on Future Biologic Studies

The molecular biologic and genetic details of the subsequent cellular differentiation events are beyond the scope of this chapter. Although the type of new tissue growth initiated is determined by the location of the wound site, the specific proteins present, and myriad other factors, one particular point merits mention. The formation of a crystalline hydroxyl carbonate apatite (such as the layer formed on the glass particle surfaces) intermediary has been implicated as being necessary in the formation of mineralized bone.[81,82] Subsequent growth of the mineralized apatitic phase in bone appears to use this layer as a template in the epitaxial growth of new crystals. Even in the "normal" nonaugmented physiologic growth and repair of bone, the growth of bone crystals requires an initial ionic adsorption of calcium and phosphorus onto some organic substrate and the formation of nanoparticles that ultimately serve as a stable transition state prior to true crystal formation. So the importance of the initial events, which occur within seconds to minutes of implantation, cannot be overstated.

Considerable research is currently investigating the underlying mechanisms and modes of action for the unexpected finding that certain compositions of glass particles are biocompatible and osteoproductive.[83–86] This chapter has touched upon the reactions that have been observed in vivo and in vitro, but the contribution of specific biologic molecules and genetic effects in general to the cell–bioactive glass interaction is relatively unknown. Because of the inexplicable beneficial effects of bioactive glasses, among other substrates, Hench has even gone so far as to advance a bioactive substrate theory of the origin of life; he suggests that inorganic glass-crystal assemblages (associated with volcanic activity) played a significant role in the creation of life by providing a substrate capable of achieving selective adsorption and ordering of macromolecules into replicative structures.[87] However, regardless of the origin of these phenomena, these glasses can effect an ion exchange with their surrounding solution in vivo and ultimately form an extremely biocompatible layer of material on their surfaces, thereby enhancing the ability of the body to regenerate damaged tissue and heal itself.

References

1. Wolff J. The Law of Bone Remodeling. Maquet PGJ, Furlong R (trans). Berlin: Springer-Verlag, 1986.
2. Cowin SC, Hegedus DH. Bone remodeling, I. Theory of adaptive elasticity. J Elasticity 1976;6:313–325.
3. Shors EC. Coralline bone graft substitutes. Orthop Clin North Am 1999;30:599–613.
4. Garg AK. Preservation, augmentation, and reconstruction of the alveolar ridge. Dent Implantol Update 2001;12:81–85.
5. Block MS, Kent JN. Maxillary sinus bone grafting. Atlas Oral Maxillofac Surg Clin North Am 1994;2:63–76.
6. Kent JN, Craig MA. Secondary autogenous and alloplastic reshaping procedures for facial asymmetry. Atlas Oral Maxillofac Surg Clin North Am 1996;4:83–105.
7. Rosen PS, Reynolds MA, Bowers GM. The treatment of intrabony defects with bone grafts. Periodontol 2000 2000;22:88–103.
8. Schallhorn RG. Present status of osseous grafting procedures. J Periodontol 1977;48:570–576.
9. Misch CE, Dietsh F. Bone-grafting materials in implant dentistry. Implant Dent 1993;2:158–167.
10. Stevenson S. Biology of bone grafts. Orthop Clin North Am 1999;30:543–552.
11. Raghoebar GM, Louwerse C, Kalk WW, Vissink A. Morbidity of chin bone harvesting. Clin Oral Implants Res 2001;12:503–507.
12. Boyce T, Edwards J, Scarborough N. Allograft bone: The influence of processing on safety and performance. Orthop Clin North Am 1999;30:571–581.
13. Pelker RR, Friedlaender GE. Biomechanical aspects of bone autografts and allografts. Orthop Clin 1987;18:235–239.
14. Simonian PT, Conrad EU, Chapman JR, et al. Effect of sterilization and storage treatments on screw strength in human allograft bone. Clin Orthop 1994;302:290–296.
15. Hamer AJ, Strachan JR, Black MM, et al. Biomechanical properties of cortical allograft bone using a new method of bone strength measurement: A comparison of fresh, fresh-frozen and irradiated bone. J Bone Joint Surg Br 1996;78:363–386.
16. Damien CJ, Parsons JR. Bone graft and bone graft substitutes: A review of current technology and applications J Appl Biomater 1991;2:187–208.
17. Hench LL, Splinter RJ, Greenlee TK, Allen WC. Bonding mechanisms at the interface of ceramic prosthetic materials. J Biomed Mater Res 1971;2:117–141.

18. Schepers E, de Clercq M, Ducheyne P, Kempeneers R. Bioactive glass particulate material as a filler for bone lesions. J Oral Rehabil 1991;18:439–452.

19. Oonishi H, Kushitani S, Yasukawa E, et al. Particulate Bioglass compared with hydroxyapatite as a bone graft substitute. Clin Orthop 1997;334:316–325.

20. Kokubo T. Bioactive glass ceramics: Properties and applications. Biomaterials 1991;12:155–163.

21. Rawlings RD. Bioactive glasses and glass-ceramics. Clin Mater 1993;14:155–179.

22. Neo M, Nakamura T, Ohtsuki C, Kokubo T, Yamamuro T. Apatite formation on three kinds of bioactive material at an early stage in vivo: A comparative study by transmission electron microscopy. J Biomed Mater Res 1993;27:999–1006.

23. Kitsugi T, Nakamura T, Oka M, Cho SB, Miyaji F, Kokubo T. Bone-bonding behavior of three heat-treated silica gels implanted in mature rabbit bone. Calcif Tissue Int 1995;57:155–160.

24. Thomsen P, Gretzer C. Macrophage interactions with modified material surfaces. Curr Opin Solid State Mater Sci 2001;5:163–176.

25. Rehman I, Knowles JC, Bonfield W. Analysis of in vitro reaction layers formed on Bioglass using thin-film X-ray diffraction and ATR-FTIR microspectroscopy. J Biomed Mater Res 1998;41:162–166.

26. Gatti AM, Valdre G, Andersson OH. Analysis of the in vivo reactions of a bioactive glass in soft and hard tissue. Biomaterials 1994;15:208–212.

27. Li J, Liao H, Sjostrom M. Characterization of calcium phosphates precipitated from simulated body fluid of different buffering capacities. Biomaterials 1997;18:743–747.

28. El-Ghannam A, Ducheyne P, Shapiro IM. Effect of serum proteins on osteoblast adhesion to surface-modified bioactive glass and hydroxyapatite. J Orthop Res 1999;17:340–345.

29. El-Ghannam A, Ducheyne P, Shapiro IM.. Formation of surface reaction products on bioactive glass and their effects on the expression of the osteoblastic phenotype and the deposition of mineralized extracellular matrix. Biomaterials 1997;18:295–303.

30. Wilson J, Low SJ. Bioactive ceramics for periodontal treatment: Comparative studies in the Patus monkey. J Appl Biomater 1992;3:123–129.

31. Hench LL, West JK. Biological applications of bioactive glasses. Life Chem Rep 1996;13:187–241.

32. Hench LL, Paschall HA. Direct chemical bond of bioactive glass-ceramic materials to bone and muscle. J Biomed Mater Res 1973;7:25–42.

33. Brinker CJ, Scherer GW. Sol-Gel Science: The Physics and Chemistry of Sol-Gel Processing. Boston: Harcourt Brace Jovanovich, 1990.

34. Qiu Q, Vincent P, Lowenberg B, Sayer M, Davies JE. Bone growth on sol-gel calcium phosphate thin films in vitro. Cells Mater 1993;3:351–360.

35. Hench LL, West JK. The sol-gel process. Chem Rev 1989;90:33–72.

36. Li P, Clark AE, Hench LL. Effects of structure and surface area on bioactive powders by sol-gel process. In: Hench LL, West JK (eds). Chemical Processing of Advanced Materials. New York: Wiley, 1992:627–633.

37. Hench LL. Biomaterials: A forecast for the future. Biomaterials 1998;19:1419–1423.

38. Li P, Clark AE, Hench LL. An investigation of bioactive glass powders by sol-gel processing. J Appl Biomater 1991;2:231–239.

39. Kamiya K, Yoko T, Sakka S. Preparation of oxide glasses from metal alkoxides by sol-gel method. NASA Technical Translation 20124. Washington, DC: National Aeronautics and Space Administration, 1987.

40. Li P, Ye X, Kangasniemi I, de Blieck-Hogervorst JMA, Klein CPAT, deGroot K. In vivo calcium phosphate formation induced by sol-gel prepared silica. J Biomed Mater Res 1995;29:325–328.

41. Pereira MM, Clark AE, Hench LL. Homogeneity of bioactive sol-gel-derived glasses in the system CaO-P2O5-SiO2. J Mater Synth Process 1994;2:189–196.

42. Pereira MM, Clark AE, Hench LL. Calcium phosphate formation on sol-gel derived bioactive glasses in vitro. J Biomed Mater Res 1994;28:693–698.

43. Zhong J, Greenspan DC. Processing and properties of sol-gel bioactive glasses. J Biomed Mater Res 2000;53:694–701.

44. Mitchell JC. A Bioactive Glass Material for the Delivery of Bone Morphogenetic Proteins: Synthesis by the Solution Sol-Gel Method, Physical and Chemical Analyses, and In Vitro Testing [doctoral dissertation]. Columbus: The Ohio State University, 1999. [Available from University Microfilms, Inc, Ann Arbor, MI; no. 9941388].

45. Varshneya AK. Fundamentals of Inorganic Glasses. San Diego: Academic Press, 1994.

46. Radin S, Falaize S, Lee MH, Ducheyne P. In vitro bioactivity and degradation behavior of silica xerogels intended as controlled release materials. Biomaterials 2002;23:3113–3122.

47. Santos EM, Radin S, Ducheyne P. Sol-gel derived carrier for the controlled release of proteins. Biomaterials 1999;20:1695–700.

48. Nicoll SB, Radin S, Santos EM, Tuan RS, Ducheyne P. In vitro release kinetics of biologically active transforming growth factor β1 from a novel porous glass carrier. Biomaterials 1997;18:853–859.

49. Gao T, Aro HT, Ylanen H, Vuorio E. Silica-based bioactive glasses modulate expression of bone morphogenetic protein-2 mRNA in Saos-2 osteoblasts in vitro. Biomaterials 2001;22:1475–1483.

50. Radin S, Ducheyne P, Kamplain T, Tan BH. Silica sol-gel for the controlled release of antibiotics, I. Synthesis, characterization, and in vitro release. J Biomed Mater Res 2001;57:313–320.

51. Radin S, El-Bassyouni G, Vreslovic EJ, Schepers E, Ducheyne P. Tissue reactions to controlled release silica xerogel carriers. In: LeGeros RZ, LeGeros JP (eds). Bioceramics, vol 11. New York: World Scientific, 1998:529–532.

52. Kangasniemi IMO, Vedel E, deBlick-Hogerworst J, Yli-Urpo AU, deGroot K. Dissolution and scanning electron microscopic studies of Ca,P particle-containing bioactive glasses. J Biomed Mater Res 1993;27:1225–1233.

53. Kokubo T, Kushitani H, Sakka S, Kitsugi T, Yamamuro T. Solutions able to reproduce in vivo surface-structure changes in bioactive glass-ceramic A-W. J Biomed Mater Res 1990;24:721–734.

54. Effah Kaufmann EAB, Ducheyne P, Radin S, Bonnell DA, Composto R. Initial events at the bioactive glass surface in contact with protein-containing solutions. J Biomed Mater Res 2000;52:825–830.

55. Gross UM, Strunz V. The anchoring of glass ceramics of different solubility in the femur of the rat. J Biomed Mater Res 1980;14:607–618.

56. Jallot E, Benhayoune H, Kilian L, et al. STEM and EDXS characterization of physiochemical reactions at the interface between a Bioglass coating and bone. Surf Interface Anal 2000;29:314–320.

57. Jallot E, Benhayoune H, Kilian L, Irigaray JL, Balossier G, Bonhomme P. Growth and dissolution of apatite precipitates formed in vivo on the surface of a bioactive glass coating film and its relevance to bioactivity. J Phys D: Appl Phys 2000;33:2775–2780.

58. Gatti AM, Valdre G, Andersson OH. Analysis of the in vivo reactions of a bioactive glass in soft and hard tissue. Biomaterials 1994;15:208–212.

59. Li P, Ohtsuki C, Kokubo T, Nakanishi K, Soga N. Apatite formation induced by silica gel in a simulated body fluid. J Am Ceram Soc 1992;75:2094–2097.

60. Hench LL. Bioactive glasses and glass-ceramics: A perspective. In: Yammamuro T, Hench LL, Wilson J (eds). CRC Handbook of Bioactive Ceramics. Vol 1: Bioactive glasses and glass ceramics. Boca Raton, FL: CRC Press, 1990:7–23.

61. Kokubo T. Bonding Mechanism of Bioactive Glass-Ceramic A-W to Living Bone. In: Yammamuro T, Hench LL, Wilson J (eds). CRC Handbook of Bioactive Ceramics. Vol 1: Bioactive glasses and glass ceramics. Boca Raton, FL: CRC Press, 1990:41–49.

62. Radin S, Ducheyne P, Falaize S, Hammond A. In vitro transformation of bioactive glass granules into Ca-P shells. J Biomed Mater Res 2000;49:264–272.

63. Silver IA, Deas J, Erecinska M. Interactions of bioactive glasses with osteoblasts in vitro: Effects of 45S5 Bioglass, and 58S and 77S bioactive glasses on metabolism, intracellular ion concentrations and cell viability. Biomaterials 2001; 22:175–185.

64. Bell RJ, Dean P. Atomic vibrations in vitreous silica. Discuss Faraday Soc 1970;50:82–93.

65. Jones JR, Sepulveda P, Hench LL. Dose-dependent behavior of bioactive glass dissolution. J Biomed Mater Res 2001; 58:720–726.

66. Fowler BO. Infrared studies of apatites, I. Vibrational assignments for calcium, strontium, and barium hydroxyapatites utilizing isotopic substitution. Inorg Chem 1974;13:194–207.

67. Ruyter IE. IR-spectroscopy and chemical analysis of four commercial "hydroxyapatites" intended for implantation. Adv Biomater 1992;10:495–501.

68. Kingery WD, Bowen HK, Uhlmann DR. Introduction to Ceramics, ed 2. New York: Wiley, 1976.

69. Doremus RH. Glass Science, ed 2. New York: Wiley, 1994.

70. Okazaki M, Taira M, Takahashi J. Rietveld analysis and Fourier maps of hydroxyapatite. Biomaterials 1997;18: 795–799.

71. McConnell D. Apatite: Its Crystal Chemistry, Mineralogy, Utilization, and Geologic and Biologic Occurrences. Vienna: Springer-Verlag, 1973.

72. Nimni ME. Polypeptide growth factors: Targeted delivery systems. Biomaterials 1997;18:1201–1225.

73. Kubo M, Van de Water L, Plantefaber LC, et al. Fibrinogen and fibrin are anti-adhesive for keratinocytes: A mechanism for fibrin eschar slough during wound repair. J Invest Dermatol 2001;117:1369–1381.

74. Drew AF, Liu H, Davidson JM, Daugherty CC, Degen JL. Wound-healing defects in mice lacking fibrinogen. Blood 2001;97:3691–3698.

75. Viceconti M, Monti L, Muccini R, Bernakiewicz M, Toni A. Even a thin layer of soft tissue may compromise the primary stability of cementless hip stems. Clin Biomech 2001;16: 765–775.

76. Cao W, Hench LL. Bioactive materials. Ceram Int 1996;22: 493–507.

77. Li P, Ohtsuki C, Kokubo T, Nakanishi K, Nakamura T, Yamamuro T. Effects of ions in aqueous media on hydroxyapatite induction by silica gel and its relevance to bioactivity of bioactive glasses and glass-ceramics. J Appl Biomater 1993;4:221–229.

78. Gough JE, Christian P, Scotchford CAA, Rudd CD, Jones IA. Synthesis, degradation, and in vitro cell responses of sodium phosphate glasses for craniofacial bone repair. J Biomed Mater Res 2002;59:481–489.

79. Roman J, Salinas AJ, Vallet-Regi M, Oliveira JM, Correia RN, Fernandes MH. Role of acid attack in the in vitro bioactivity of a glass-ceramic of the 3CaO·P2O5-CaO·SiO2-CaO·MgO· 2SiO2 system. Biomaterials 2001;22:2013–2019.

80. Lai W, Garino J, Ducheyne P. Silicon excretion from bioactive glass implanted in rabbit bone. Biomaterials 2002;23: 213–217.

81. Cuisinier FGC. Bone mineralization. Curr Opin Solid State and Mater Sci 1996;1:436–439.

82. Wen HB, Moradian-Oldak J, Fincham AG. Modulation of apatite crystal growth on Bioglass by recombinant amelogenin. Biomaterials 1999;20:1717–1725.

83. Hench LL, Wheeler DL, Greenspan DC. Molecular control of bioactivity in sol-gel glasses. J Sol-Gel Sci Tech 1998;13: 245–250.

84. Xynos ID, Edgar AJ, Buttery LDK, Hench LL, Polak JM. Ionic products of bioactive glass dissolution increase proliferation of human osteoblasts and induce insulin-like growth factor II mRNA expression and protein synthesis. Biochem Biophys Res Comm 2001;276:461–465.

85. Dieudonne SC, van den Dolder J, de Ruijter JE, et al. Osteoblast differentiation of bone marrow stromal cells cultured on silica gel and sol-gel-derived titania. Biomaterials 2002;23:3041–3051.

86. Kamitakahara M, Kawashita M, Kokubo T, Nakamura T. Effect of polyacrylic acid on the apatite formation of a bioactive ceramic in a simulated body fluid: Fundamental examination of the possibility of obtaining bioactive glass-ionomer cements for orthopaedic use. Biomaterials 2001;22: 3191–3196.

87. Hench LL. Bioceramics and the origin of life. J Biomed Mater Res 1989;23:685–703.

INDEX

Deutschland, Deutschland über alles

A Picture-book by Kurt Tucholsky

Deutschland, Deutschland über alles

Photographs assembled by John Heartfield

Translated from the German by Anne Halley

Afterword and Notes by Harry Zohn

The University of Massachusetts Press Amherst 1972

Contents

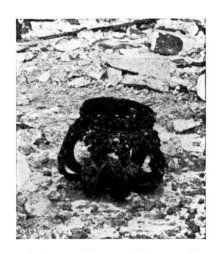

So I came to live among the Germans. I expected little and was prepared to accept even less. I came humbly, the way homeless blind Oedipus came to the gate of Athens. But beautiful spirits received Oedipus in the mystic grove, while those who received me were of another kind.

Dear friend, the people who received me were known as barbarians in the old days. Today, with the help of hard work, science, all learning, and even religion, they have made themselves even more barbarous. They are incapable of noble emotions, spoiled to the marrow, unable to feel any joy or spirit. Their distortion by every kind of excess and impoverishment is an insult to any well-formed soul. They are tuneless, as inharmonious as a slag-heap.

These are hard words, but true. I can think of no people more torn apart and separated from themselves than the Germans. You find workers, thinkers, priests, rich and poor, young and old, but no human beings. Germany looks like a battlefield on which dismembered hands, legs, arms, and other parts lie scattered, while the blood of life runs forgotten into the sand.

You may say that each man must follow his own calling. I agree. But let him follow it completely, with his whole being. Let him not smother those energies and impulses that don't happen to fit his job. Let him not limit himself fearfully and deceitfully to the letter of his official title, but let him be whole, seriously and lovingly. Then his actions might after all be informed by spirit: if he finds that his work kills his spirit, let him throw off the work contemptuously, and learn to plow. But your friends, the Germans, like to justify all their actions by utility—that is why they do so much idiotic busy-work, and so little that is really free and pleasureable. This by itself might not matter, but in the process they lose all joy in life; their unnatural denial of spirit curses them everywhere.

These barbarians, who invent and calculate, carry on even those customs which among other tribes retain their original purity, like mechanical assigned tasks. They can do no other. Whenever human beings are trained only for use, they will learn to serve their purpose and look to their own advantage, but love and warmth cannot survive the training. I tell you, there is nothing holy that these people have not perverted and desecrated to serve a poverty-stricken opportunism. Let them try to celebrate or love or pray—while spring seems to renew the innocence of nature and magically to drive away guilt, when even a slave might be able to forget his chains in the warm sunshine and the enemies of mankind seem momentarily as peaceful as children in the divinely inspired air, when caterpillars grow wings and bees hum—the Germans will be sticking to business, paying no attention to the weather.

Hölderlin°

I

Foreword

**or, it is impossible to write
captions for photographs**

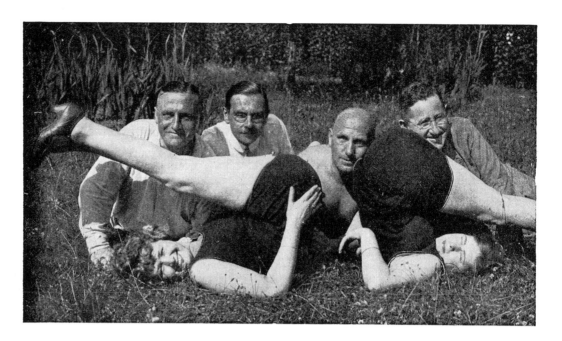

Well, this is the picture.

We've looked at hundreds and thousands of them: all of ordinary German life, all more or less typical of a class or group, a district, or a region. We've looked at them all. A single image was supposed to materialize:

GERMANY

It's easy, and then again, difficult.

Easy, because once you've studied the pictures a while, they begin to speak. The people in the pictures hold still—so patiently, that you can study them at your leisure. And when you're wholly inside the picture, the people speak.

They tell you their life-stories. Their political opinions. They confess. They accuse. They laugh. They sigh because they're tired. They open their hearts to you. This is how we love, they say, and this is how we hate, and this is why we didn't get anywhere, and this is our youth, and these our dreams of glory, and this is what our parents looked like, and here is my weak point, and here my strength, and, they say, I'm a good guy, but I don't want to admit it, and I'm a bastard at the office—more and more crowd around, and the pictures have no ending: faces and backsides and the well-to-do and the rich and the millions who work, and the places where they work, and the houses they live in, the fields around the house, the meadows, the little lakes, the oceans, the towers of the city, the forest, the workshops, foundries, plowland, the factories, the offices, movie-houses—an unending picture book:

Germany

They are all speaking pictures. But captions can be written for only a very few. Because:

Photographs always have a double import. These are all typical of something in Germany, but they are also private. In the first picture, for example, some members of the upper middle-class are having their fun. But at the same time, it is Mr. *A*, and Mr. *B* and *C* and *D* with their ladies. If I were to let these people speak as types, as representatives of a group, as examples—it would certainly end badly. Even if the Messrs. *A, B, C,* and *D* didn't object—and they might not, since they look as if they had a sense of humor. They have something else—they have enemies.

You're in trouble the moment you take a photograph of a middle-class citizen, or a worker, or anybody not in public life, and write a caption which lets that person express sentiments typical of his group. First there's the copyright problem. One might just ignore that. But all these men and women have enemies who will take delighted advantage of a joke and say, "Look! Here's the foreman, Mr. Pomuchelskopp, to the life! And there! So that's what our representative thinks!" And then the private soul which inhabits these collective-beings is enraged. Then the subjected peoples arise, the oppressed claim their freedom, flex their muscles, and hire a lawyer. And this book cannot be published.

It can't be published because the bright illumination of the flashbulb, which was meant for the whole group, has fallen on only one member—the individual pays the whole group's debt. You can do it in complete freedom with drawings. The case is quite clear—a drawing of a judge shows only the type. The particular judge doesn't exist. But in our pictures the judge has a double presence. He is typical, because the photographer saw him that way, and because he really is. But he is also the circuit judge, His Honor, Mr. Puschke. The Germans are not

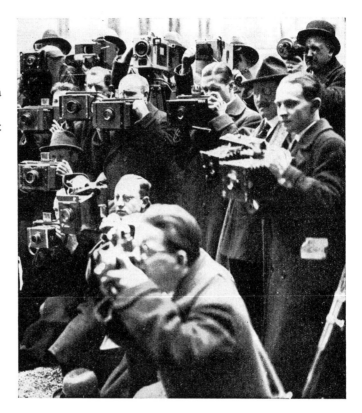

free enough to understand what an attack on Puschke means. If I hit Mr. Puschke where it hurts, this book could not be published.

But we want the book published. We want—as much as possible—to extract the typical from snapshots, posed photographs, all kinds of pictures. And all the pictures together will add up to Germany—a cross-section of Germany.

Official cross-sections always cut the cheese without hitting the maggots. We wanted to do it differently. Whatever you see moving as you cut, is a maggot. And part of Germany.

To return to the first picture—I'll have to ask you to write your own caption. Look at

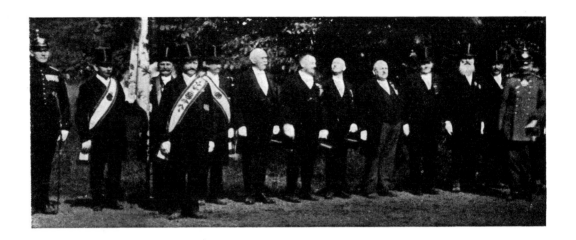

it closely. Look into the people's eyes and let
them speak. They will tell you about their
lives: they will tell you about part of
Germany.

All our pictures tell about Germany. But
why did we pick the resounding title for our
book? This line from a really bad poem,
which a really demented Republic chose for
its national anthem—and, unhappily, chose
with a good deal of reason? Well, we'll tell
each other that story when we meet again
at the end.

On the Rhine in 1918

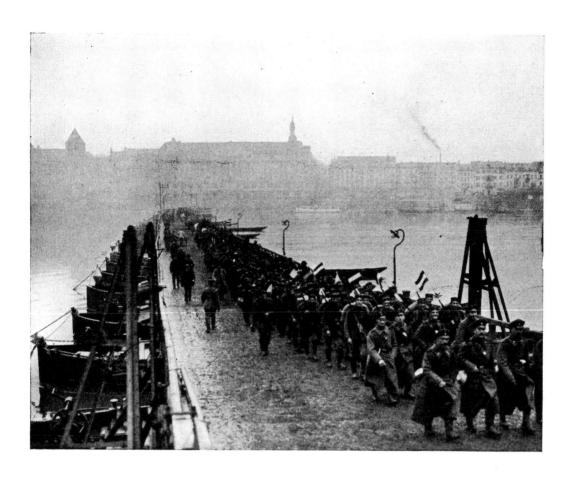

They're coming home. What did they go for? For whom?

Miners, laborers, pipe-fitters, business employees, in disguise—they're coming home. The enemy, who was not their real enemy, is behind them. The enemy behind them was just a partner in war, and only the class-conscious ones among them have yet recognized the enemy ahead. They don't know yet what awaits them or how the Fatherland will thank them at home. Inflation—the deceitful bankruptcy of the state, hunger, unemployment, and 1.67 Mark a week disability payments. Why?

And for whom? For the croupiers who work your wars and your peace.

The Country of Orderlies

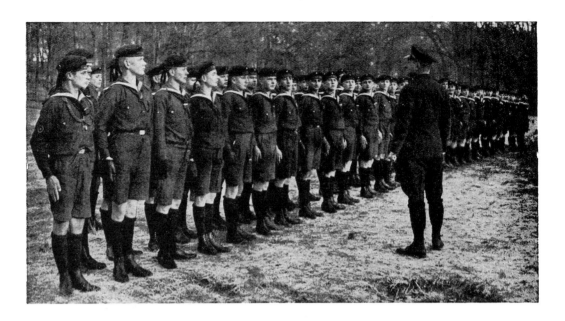

Under this picture, we read:

The club "Marine-youth Fatherland" takes as its objective to provide without consideration of political or social differences further physical and intellectual training, supplementing that provided in the schools, for German youth. Our effort is to harden the youth for the life-struggle, to form a new generation of able men to serve the community.

It's all clear in the picture. Intellectual training, preparation for life, encouraging ability. The German people can achieve these goals by standing at attention.°

And what exactly is the new generation up there doing? We read that too. They're preparing to march on the Potsdam Observatory. To observe. If Mars-people could see them—those arms tightly pressed into position, those eyes thirsting for astronomy, that general reviewing the battle-line—then surely the Mars-people would call their Earth-expert to the telescope. And he could say, with absolute certainty: "There may be life on earth. But human beings—no, there are no human beings."

The Harmfulness of Civilian Dress

Erich Lindström, born Ludendorff° . . . after all, there must be more important things on earth than one scrapped general. But it may be proper to reflect a little on this one. He's no longer successful.

Why isn't he successful any longer?

Actually all the prerequisites for popularity in Germany seem to be given. The man brought nothing but disaster to his country —but he brought it with pomp and circumstance; he was a general; he had power, and there was the possibility that he would have power again some day; he got fat enough to display that degree of tough solidity that seems to be required of those who want their picture on the beer-mugs of fame in this country. Nevertheless, it's not working. I want to let him in on the secret of his unsuccess.

Especially in the spring, a young man's fancy sometimes turns to the household-help.° He feels attracted to the kitchen maid, or to the nice waitress in her cap, to the housemaid in her flirtatious little apron, or maybe to a nurse, looking delicious, totally wrapped in aseptic white. But the affair does not always run smoothly enough for courtship, passionate declaration, and fulfillment, to take place during working hours. So the impassioned lover requests a rendezvous. The provocatively costumed beloved blushes and agrees, but already the door is opening: enter Madame or inn-keeper or head-physician. In a flash, the beloved is gone. That evening she appears— "dressy" as for Sunday, freshly washed and in street clothes or evening dress. A faint disappointment takes hold of the lover. Can this be she? The sweet little beribboned

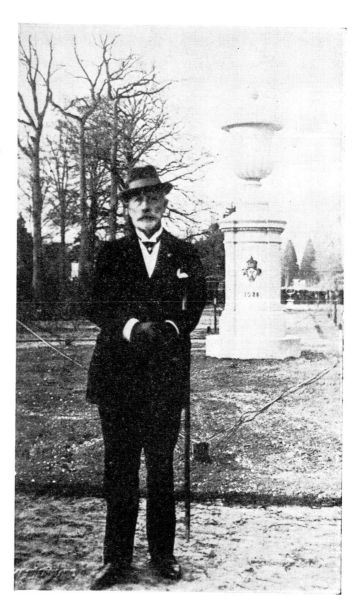

H.R.H. in Civilian Dress

one, the aproned, white-uniformed? It is.
But herself no longer. Civilian dress has
killed both attraction and love. Civilian
dress kills. And Lindström feels it. He gets
himself up in his unreal, fantasy uniform, a
costume for masked balls, to attend festivi-
ties, regimental holidays, flag-dedications,
and parades. But it doesn't help. He knows
civilian dress doesn't suit him. It really
doesn't suit him. I saw him stammering his
piece before the investigating committee.
Like a stern teacher caught in the Turkish
bath. All authority gone. It's the same first
principle for housemaids and generals: To
be loved, stay in uniform. Civilian dress is
always harmful. Poor general!

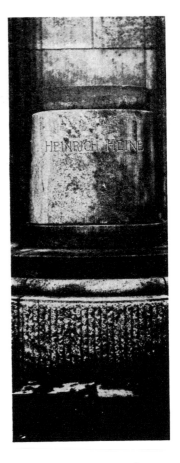

*In Germany the ratio of war-memorials to
Heine-memorials is the same as the ratio of
force to spirit.*

The People

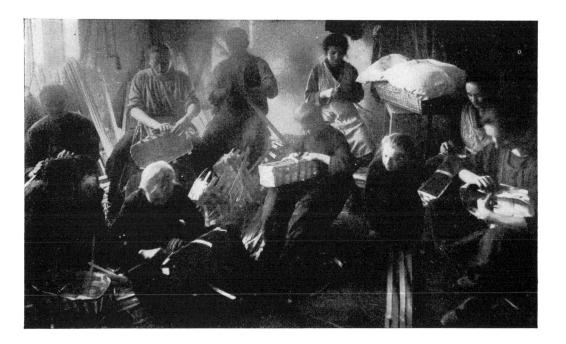

"Religion must be preserved for the people."—"You have to understand—the people have a different sense of . . ."—"The people are simply . . ." The speakers? Middle-class citizens with delusions of grandeur. Let's give our subject its proper name, say what we mean: the workers. And no more nonsense about the workers' need for Culture. They need other things. For me to write this picture-book, I need:

Enough to eat. A roof over my head. Leisure and time to look at the pictures the publishers send me. A father who gave me enough money in my youth so that I could learn a little more than the ABC and the multiplication tables . . . I need all those conditions. Occasionally a heroic proletarian may overcome his limitations: in epic struggles and in spite of hunger, cold, and inadequate education, working at night,

with enormous strength of will, the worker may achieve what the businessman's son accomplishes with ease. But to expect the worker to accomplish all this as a matter of course, shows an insulting lack of sensitivity; to despise him for not accomplishing it is shameless.

Perhaps the basket-weavers pictured here should read the French mystic Paul Claudel? Or think about the concept of immortality in Lao-tse? Should we criticize them for not doing so? And should we deny them the opportunity to do so forever? Which is not to suggest that environment is all important; of course heredity, and possibly some inexplicable "X," also matter in human development. But why not grant these workers three things:

The wages that they really deserve but don't get under the present system.

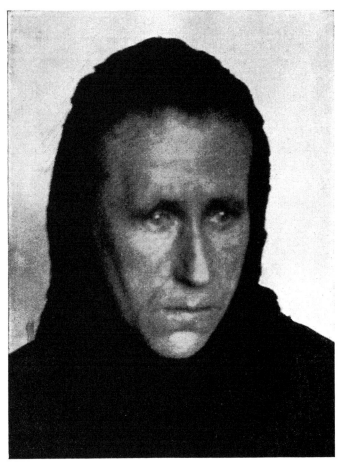

Healthy working conditions. People ought not to have to work herded together, eight to a single room.

The chance to share in humanity's goods—and not just to wonder at them once in their lives, on a Sunday afternoon museum visit. Why shouldn't they have these things?

We are told that there isn't enough for everybody, but that's a lie. Capitalists will only work for an income that exceeds the workers' by thousands and thousands. But surely we don't believe that even the shrewdest and best investor or manager really earns what he earns—that is, as much as five hundred of his workers? Five hundred people. And actually there are at least seven hundred more who have to survive on the earnings of the five hundred. At the very least. A single man is allowed to take in so much, because—as he says—he risks so much. (The worker risks his health.) And because he has such great ideas? Still, he only does his job as the worker does his—and believe me, there are deeper, more creative ideas than those of a stock-market speculator.

Well, there they sit—weaving baskets. Does labor have to be a curse—?

German Judges of 1940

We meet here united
in padded leather rigs,
our sacred honor plighted
and bleeding like stuck pigs.
    In duel stout and steady
    butchering ourselves bloody!
    En garde!
           Ready!

German spirit takes its stand
on a precise low quarte!
We make chopped meat by hand
and let red juice squirt!
    The Aryan's finest flower,
    we despise the low
    crude and common worker—
    En garde!
           Ready!
                  Go!

Just twenty years, and then
high on the bench in court,
we scar-faced blackrobed men
pass judgment on your sort!
    In chambers and office hours
    you'll learn what you need to know:
    keep still! eyes down! show some respect!
    En garde!
           Ready!
               Set!
                  Go!

How long will you, men and women,
let it stay the same?
Today they wallop each other—
tomorrow you're fair game!
    You are the people, the masses
    from Adige to Rhine are you:
    Are these our ruling classes?
    Shall these be our leaders?
           Go!

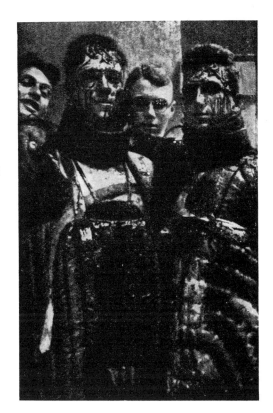

Three Glasses

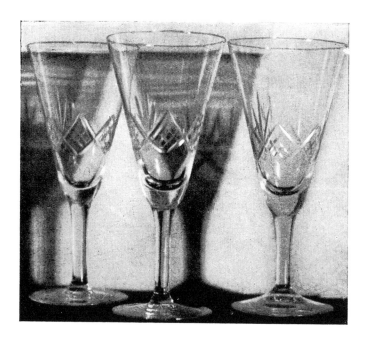

Look, wine glasses like these have been the cause of much evil in Germany. You wouldn't believe what men and women will do—or fail to do—just to drink from these glasses.

In our country the word, champagne, still has remarkable resonance. As if it were something special. As if champagne meant high-society. The idea, no doubt, comes from the novels and movies in which upper-class gentlemen—Yippee!—lead the high life with "wine, women, and song." Is it really all that high?

Anyone who knows wine would pass up the best champagne for a good, old Rhine-wine or 1911 Burgundy. But the fact is, people don't have champagne. Champagne has them. It gives them that lift. It makes them believe they're more than they are. Little middle-class housewives suddenly get a teasing glow in their eyes, as if they were capable of anything. We all witnessed what

happens when Social-Democratic function-aries get at the champagne. They fall on their faces. They drown in it. They aren't even drinkers—that wouldn't be so bad. But it's much worse. They're overcome by the idea. That he—plain Gustav Kunze him-self—should be drinking real champagne that he's always read about! And the stuff's pretty good too! Cheers!

Maybe you have to be really wise to escape. Or, it may be better just to pass through the champagne-experience early. If one drank champagne in one's youth, and then grew up with some sense, one might not need to chase after the stuff—or after the things traditionally associated with it. You could smile knowingly and be on your way.

There's so much boredom inside these glasses. Hell-raising is no great pleasure, in spite of popular belief. Besides, no drink can change a man's social position. The word "wine-section" is one of the most disgusting in the language. German elegance too often looks like the "wine-section" of the local beer-hall: artificially heightened, forced upward, separated by a barrier from the common people. Nothing there, without the fence. You can't even call the customers "the dissipated bourgeoisie." That's slogan-eering. They complain, while they manage to lead a nice life, but they're not dissipated. They're noisy and puffed-up with self-importance, and they don't know how to enjoy life. Possibly *their* life, but not life itself. You have to see it: the way they enjoy themselves.

Crammed hotels with sloppy kitchens, but beautiful "presentations" at the table.

German cooking is only for the eyes. And the cut and sugared, adulterated wines, insanely expensive—"Germans, drink German wine!" The little red lamp that means "wine-section" glows above the scene. The people are really convinced that they're something special because they don't have a beer in front of them. Of course, most of this silliness goes on in the parts of Germany that have no open wine; the wine lands are simpler, more sensible and democratic, by nature. If the plain man-in-the-street can order his measure of wine at breakfast, then wine loses some of its upward-mobility-inducing powers.

But many people have betrayed their cause for these three glasses.

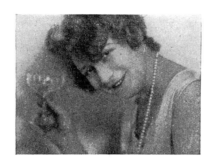

The Prison School

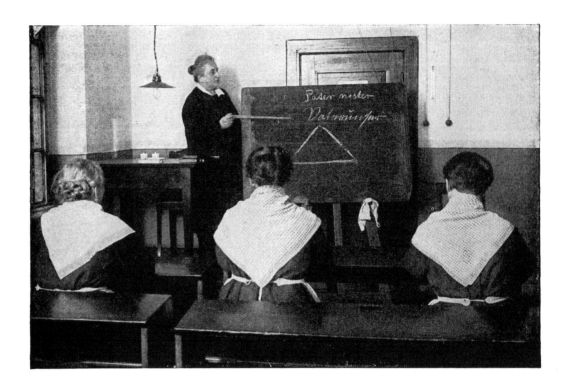

When an African falls, he falls on his back-side. When a European falls, he falls back on his religion.

Religion must be preserved for the people. When prison administrators get their hands on a law-breaker, then not even God—I almost said—can help him. He gets religion. These female prisoners, who had no voice in the establishment of law, broke the law out of poverty, hereditary inclina-tion, and social discontent. Now they are being taught that there is a final court in heaven, to which possible appeals may be submitted orally—though, of course, with-out guarantee of hearing. I'm sure it's a comfort to them. Amen.

I am a Murderer

"I, Ignaz Wrobel,° like to cheat the bus conductor and ride free. I have a terrible temper: twice I've ripped my bathrobe to punish it; I have cut up neckties; I've smashed glasses on purpose. I can't stand the sight of blood. No—I can stand blood. Animal blood. It's an odd feeling—unpleasant. But maybe it's pleasant after all—I'm sort of afraid to say. Yes, it's pleasant. I have often had love affairs with two women at the same time. They didn't know about each other. I knew. Once, at one in the morning, I had a strange sensation. I was lying on the sofa next to Conrad and we were talking about women. I began to tremble and I wanted to touch him. I didn't do it, because I was afraid of making myself ridiculous. I wasn't afraid of anything else. Sometimes I dream about bloody things. I eat irregularly—nothing for days at a time, and then much too much. I'm not respectable. If I weren't afraid of infections, I'd pick up a girl on the corner every few days. I'm a sneaky coward. I poured ink in my cousin's new hat and ripped Mother's lace handkerchief. Afterwards, I look innocent. 'I have no idea. Good Heavens—it's all torn! It's finished!' I like to listen to people making love. And to people fighting. I lie for the sake of lying and my heart races, wondering if I'll be found out. I'm a pretty good liar. I hate my father. As a boy I did something with my brother; afterwards I wanted to beat him up. But he was stronger. I have irregular habits—but I've already said that. What does it all mean?"

"Nothing special. Look around—everyone carries a larger or a smaller bundle like yours. Everyone carries his bundle. We're all spiritual hunchbacks and we're all ashamed of our humps. People may strip down, but not far enough to reveal their humps. Usually not even to themselves. It's nothing special."

"Nothing special? Then I don't have to be afraid?"

"Nothing special. You don't have to be afraid. Unless . . ."

"Unless?"

"Unless you're brought to trial in a court of law. As long as you're not suspected of a crime—Should that happen—"

"—?"

"Well, in that case the facts you've just told me change. What were only anomalies —things that every judge, district attorney, and juror could find, at least potentially, in himself if he were going to be honest—are transformed. Suddenly different."

"What . . . what happens? If everyone's the same?"

"Facts like these don't get in to the front parlors of the law. There, everyone pretends that he lives a different kind of life, conforms to a nonexistent morality, has a purity of which no human being is capable. Children in their Sunday clothes suddenly can't understand that there are mud-stains on earth. And these little characteristics of yours—"

"Are what?"

"Suspicious circumstances, Mr. Wrobel."

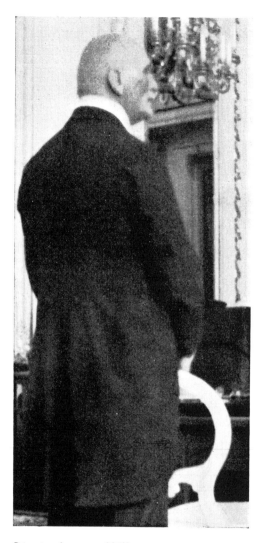

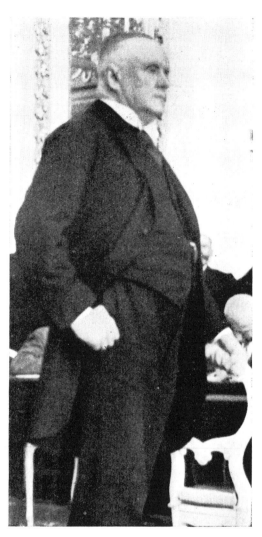

District Attorney Müller

Minister Hustaedt

"—and therefore your verdict can only
be: The accused is guilty as charged and
must suffer the death penalty."

Prayer for Prisoners

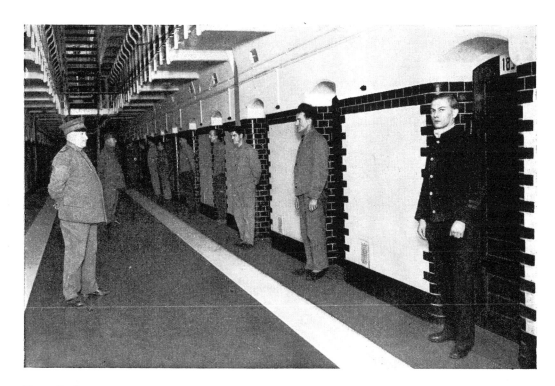

Dear God:

If you happen to have time, do you think you could spare
a minute for the poor? Could you possibly care
that, between stockmarket crises, the fighting in Morocco,
and other important details,
there are seven-thousand Communists locked-up and miserable
in German jails?

$\qquad\qquad\qquad$ Kyrie eleison!

Unlucky boys, who went along for the ride,
and the judges got hold of them. So now they're inside.
They got their skulls cracked, and down they went
under the policeman's club that hangs above us all
world without end.

$\qquad\qquad\qquad$ Kyrie eleison!

And there are old guys, who had conviction
and the courage to fight well.
Our judges don't think much of that—
they put them in jail.

$\qquad\qquad\qquad$ Kyrie eleison!

Some believed they were protecting
a republic that turned their help down cold.
Fritz Ebert found his friends more frightening
than his enemies—in this sense: black, red, and gold!°
Kyrie eleison!

Dear God: it's years in a little cell,
getting sick and pale, and missing your wife,
getting pushed around by warders who always yell,
and sometimes beat you up, and put you in the hole.
Kyrie eleison!

A lot of guys get mean, and they've all lost hope,
but some may have a spider to be their friend.
Sometimes, God, it takes a thousand years before one day will end—
Kyrie

Do you think that maybe, you could take another look
at the New Testament?
Preachers read it on Sundays, but during the week
it's the criminal-code and the High Court's judgment!
eleison!

Dear God: do you know why these seven-thousand men
are locked-up in Germany, in jail?
I know, but I won't tell. You can imagine!
Amen.

Penance

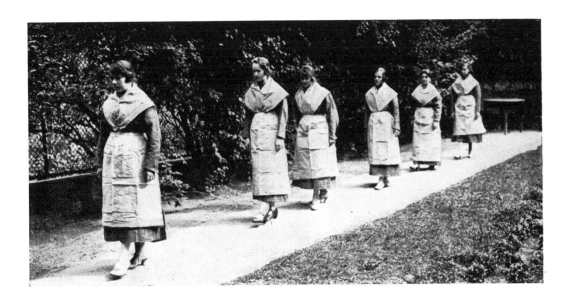

Prison administrators are especially proud of this way of executing a sentence. What about it? Most noticeable is the will of someone whom we might call the obedience-trainer. These girls and women don't belong to themselves; they belong to someone not in the picture: the prison administrator. He is possessed by the same organizing madness as the staff-officers in the field, who—with raised batons—organize barracks and people and cannon and the whole theater of war, right up to the well-known end.

These prisoners are "good"; they represent ideal sentence-servers. What heavy humiliation and mortification of the will they have to suffer! Any psychologist understands the effects of such psychic flagellation. Now they walk, like geese in single file, and no doubt some male or female guard, out of the camera's range, calls: "Keep your distance." And this is penance

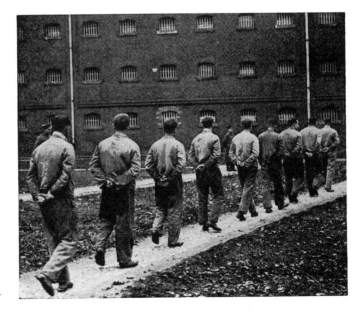

for infanticide, embezzlement, thievery, or libel.

To take away freedom from those who have committed criminal acts against society is enough. Enough to protect society against them. But no one has the right to assign penance. No one has the right to punish.

This discipline, set against those inhumanities to man that are not pictured, may be a small step forward. It is worthless.

Democracy°

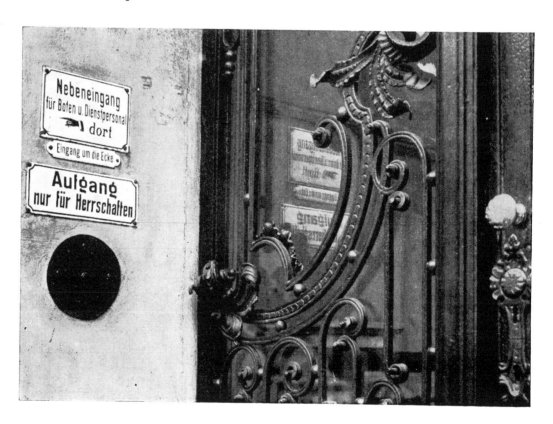

The Member of the Reichstag

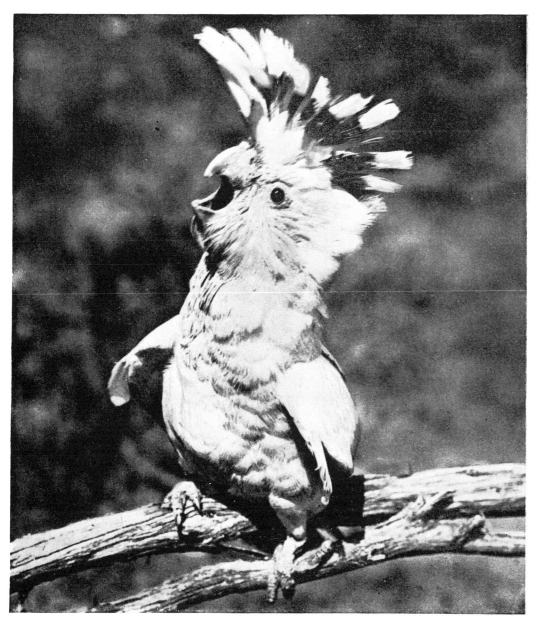

"We will force the government to . . ."

Experienced Jackasses

Nowadays everyone's a "specialist with experience." We have tried and true glider fliers (three years' experience) and truly tried radio technicians (two years). When they get together to talk shop they foam at the mouth with nonsense. They get happier —absolutely glowing—the more they can manage to sound like an official report: superior, objectively distanced, elegantly impersonal.

Like this:

"Yesterday evening Fridolin, the eight-year-old son-on-duty in the household of the professional dwarf, Nietzke, reported the incumbent drainpipe as in a state of blockage. The report was delivered to Mrs. Nietzke at ten minutes after nine P.M. Mrs. Nietzke immediately referred the report to her household employee, Miss Anna Koschmann. Miss Koschmann, however, had already gone off duty, and was consequently unable to take further action. At half past eleven P.M. immediately upon his return from the Scala, his place of employment, Mr. Nietzke was apprised of these circumstances. In accord with his instructions, all action was postponed until the following day.

"On the following day—that is, the next morning—a commission visited the drainpipe in question. The members of the commission were: Professional Dwarf Nietzke, Mrs. Nietzke, in an advisory capacity, and their eleven-year-old son Hadubrand. Mr. Dwarf Nietzke undertook leadership of the commission. Mr. Nietzke inferred immediately that the drainpipe was unable to function because it was in a state of blockage. He thereupon personally called on the building superintendent, Schippanofsky,

although the latter had not yet begun his tour of duty. As a result, Schippanofsky issued a challenge to Nietzke, but the latter refused. A defamation suit has been filed.

"After further negotiations, Mrs. Schippanofsky appeared during the afternoon. The drainpipe cleaning team was composed of the following members: Technical-Direction: Mrs. Building Superintendent Schippanofsky. Personnel-Supervision: Mrs. Dwarf Nietzke. Management of Subsidiary-Assistance-Brigade Membership, composed of son, Hadubrand Nietzke: Hadubrand Nietzke. General Manager: Mr. Nietzke. Surrounded by his staff, Manager Nietzke himself undertook the specialized technical functions.

"The conference resulted in the following conclusions: Although from the viewpoint of the individual household economy, the installation of a new drainpipe might be considered desirable, over-all economic considerations, as well as certain technical problems, make such a step questionable. There was no objection, on aesthetic grounds, to the insertion of a mop-handle, so-called, into the drainpipe, but this act could not be undertaken since, as the Personnel-Supervisor pointed out, from the standpoint of the household economy, such an implement was not available. The Technical-Direction asserted that it could not contribute to the acquisition of such an implement, but this was hotly contested by both Personnel and Subsidiary-Assistance Management. Finally, the Management decided that for both hygienic and nutritional-scientific reasons, the immediate acquisition of the drainpipe-cleansing implement should be considered, since the Management, in view of its longtime specialized experience, was eminently fit to advise in this matter. As a longtime professional, the Manager denied that the appellation 'Old Bullhead' applied to him by the Technical-Direction was acceptable.''

Pretty funny?

But it's not funny if three officials, about to drive in a nail, indulge in the same business, just to inflate their sense of significance, necessity, and importance. We know the Germans are a thorough people: every child its potty, every adult his specialized university education, his title, and his swollen head.

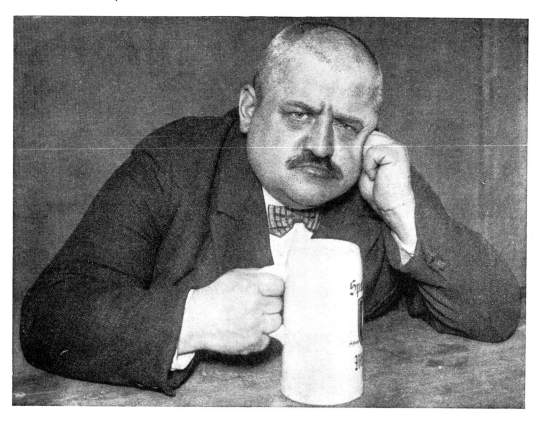

Rebellion in Central Germany

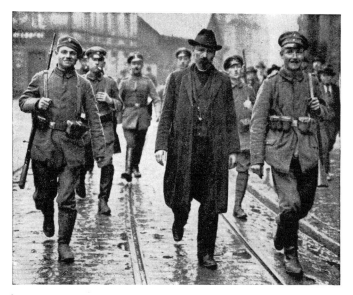

The horrible thing about pictures like this one is that the arrested man in the middle, and the guards who walk beside him, are the same people. But the victors in their uniforms, especially, are unaware of it. If these sons of building-superintendents and farmers had happened into different neighborhood bars with different companions and a few different conversations, they might now be marching behind the man who wanted to free the workers. Their eyes are shining with pleasure, like boys playing cowboys and Indians. They won, and life is beautiful. Try to tell me, they're interested in the "Re-establishment of Law and Order." They don't even know what that means. One of them will tell about it later, in the guard-room. "This noon," he'll say, "one of the brothers gave me a funny look. I smashed him right across the skull. Hey look—the butt's splintered . . ."

Civil war is brothers' war? Worse. Members of the same class fight each other, and their rulers benefit.

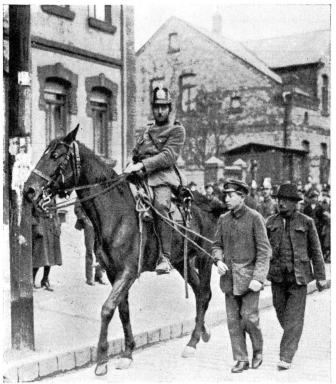

Good Times

Those were the good times . . . here's our dear Philipp Sh.° standing up to address the people on the government's good window-sill. Wouldn't you think he'd put down a newspaper first? He's addressing the people. Listen to the picture. "The German Republic is a people's republic. The system of masters and servants is past—we are establishing the most libertarian government in the world! We will . . . you will . . . they will . . . Hail the new free German Republic!" The people yelled "hurray!" and took off their hats. Those were good times.

No they weren't. Today we understand what happened then. Today we know that there was treachery on one side, and overconfidence, muddle, and muck on the other. We've learned something. We know how Fritz Ebert° telephoned Groener° on the secret line, to save the system that should have been destroyed—today we know. But not even ten people in the crowd knew it then. The people standing there were mainly *tired*; they had had their fill of war and were sick of the whole business; they didn't want to stand in rationing lines anymore; they were tired and they wanted to go home and they had had enough. Had you asked them what they really wanted, you would have gotten some very strange, vague answers. But political battles cannot be fought vaguely—they need clarity and a dogmatically strict program. Although the program also has to be as pliable and elastic as the best steel. Revolutions cannot be made with emotion alone.

But not without feelings either.

Someone like Fritz Ebert, who worked up his documents coolly from the beginning, isn't—as they say—a *Real*-politician. Not at

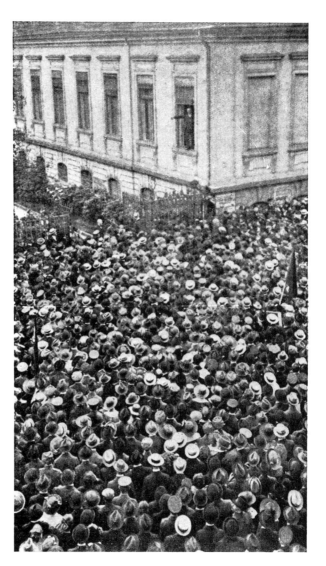

all. He's just a clerk. Nothing can be accomplished without the vital spark; nothing on earth has ever been overthrown or changed or rebuilt without heroism. That it might be, is a German fairy tale.

Good times . . . But those who lived through them at least know one thing—as I know it, and as we all do:

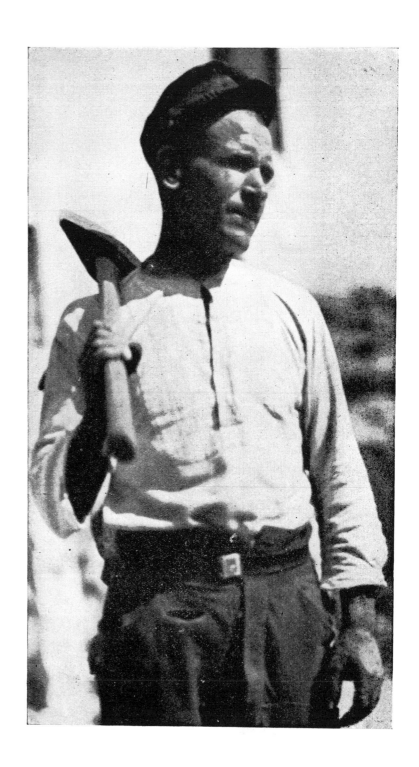

Once, just once, in Prussia in 1918, the earth shook. Just once a new wind, foreign to us, blew down the streets and the ground heaved under our feet; once a breath of freedom and an intimation of what it means to say, the People, passed this way. We should not compare these unforgettable hours and days to the drunken street spirit of 1914—that was just German champagne. And that's how it affected us. But what moved us in 1918 was different, entirely different. It was not a good time, certainly not a magnificent time—but Germany was moving. This frozen, overdisciplined, tight country was spinning like a top. The workers accomplished it, and the returning soldiers and the vanguard of sailors. Let us keep the tune in our hearts. It passed: choked in blood, betrayed and beaten to the ground, driven back inside the limits of "order." Liebknecht, Luxemburg° . . . gone. In the memoirs of certain Social Democrats the "good times" live on in counterfeit, fictionalized, lying versions. Those who unmade a Revolution, can still get a modest income by writing their dreary life-stories. The blood of those who died in the war was shed in vain. They died for nothing. The revolutionaries' blood must not be shed in vain. They died for a cause. Let it grow.

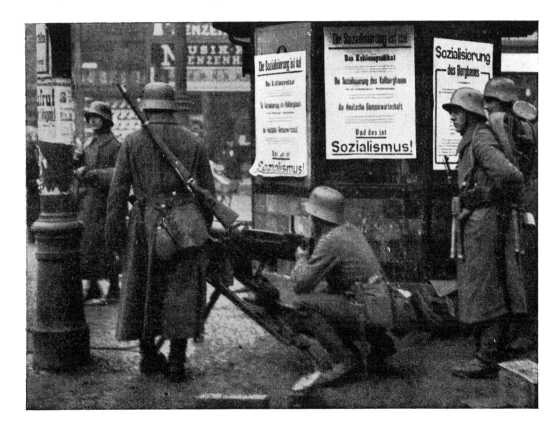

Such Terrible Scenes

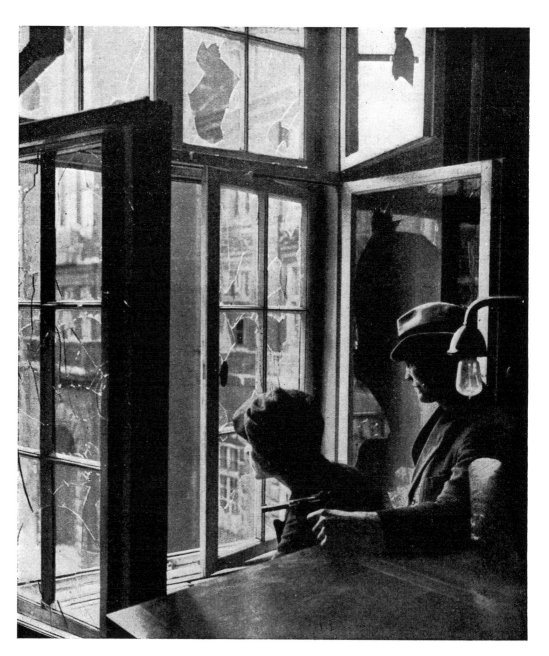

Are Part of our Daily Life—When

the workers take over a city hall—for instance the one in Mülheim on the Ruhr.
Broken windows and bare desks—the
property damage must be enormous.

And just look at these peoples' faces! They
have brutality and crudity written all over
them. No one could deny that these two
people are the image of brute irrational
violence. They will show no mercy. The
solid citizen's blood will have to flow. Probably their pockets are full of stolen gold
fillings and jewelry. The practiced physiog-
nomist can tell at a glance, and the judge
can tell without even looking, that here the
revolution has brought the lowest elements
to the top. As a matter of fact, the two
gentlemen in the picture are police agents
in disguise.

This Performance

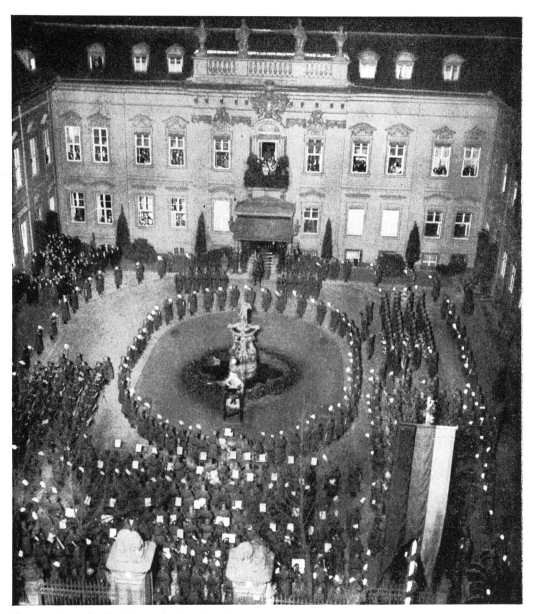

Tattoo before the Reich President's palace.

was put on for the former ruler of Afghanistan by the Republic now in residence, which lacks a king of its own. The cost of receptions and gifts just about equaled the monetary value of a year's German exports to Afghanistan.

Those Who Live by Dying!

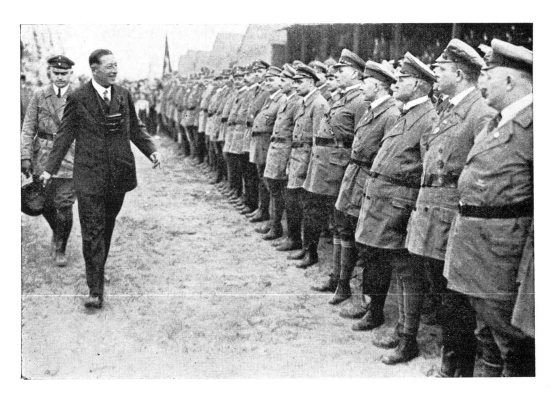

What if the German earth decline,
God's poorhouse in the world?
We'll put our last boy on the line,
We'll offer our last herd.
We gave bright gold for iron gray,
When we had that to give,
And, if our last gifts pass away,
We'll die, that we may live!

*Dr. von Eickstädt, Regional Leader of
the* Stahlhelm° *in Kyritz*

Arithmetic Problems

A peasant owns a field of 18 hectares. His 54-year-old neighbor disputes his ownership. How high will the court costs be, if the prosecuting attorney's name is Cohn XVII ?

A High-President's mouth measures 4×2 meters. How long can he remain an SPD member, if he has the murder of 1100 workers on his conscience?

An investigating judge lets a businessman, suspected of being a Jew, remain in custody for 11 weeks. In how much time will the judge be promoted to the district court?

Problem using imaginary quantities: A social-democratic party has 0 successes in 8 years. In how many years will the party notice that its tactics are mistaken?

A people's state, Saxony, always gets its own shit together. How many Augusts of Saxony can get all the Reimann° stories together?

A Kaiser costs 50,000 Mark° unemployment benefits a month. How much do two Kaisers on the throne of an eight-year-old Republic cost? (Solve the same problem using the German Republic—equation with one unknown.)

A German judge jails one communist a day. How many German judges can jail every German communist in how many days?

A crown-prince has an illegitimate child. (A theoretical problem.) How many crown-princes are needed to populate Mongolia, if the Mongolian morality co-efficient is taken as 218?

(Solutions are intended only for teachers.)

Anniversary Celebration

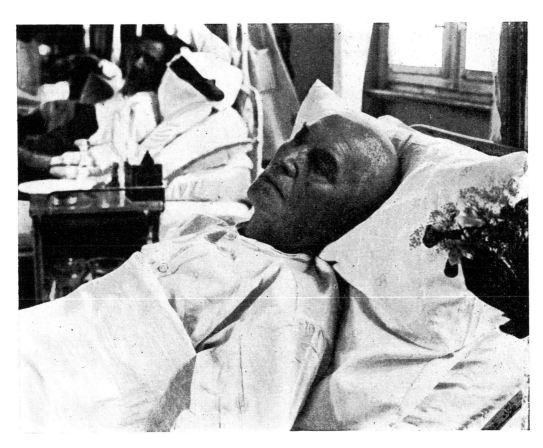

Are you watching from the other beds?
Yes, that's him, lying there.
He worked for fifty years, at Stelzner's, on
Great Frankfurt Street in Berlin. Well, and
so he was over seventy and they fired him,
told him to go collect Social Security. And
so he tried to get rid of what little life they'd
left him. But it didn't work. So here he is in
bed. Oh, of course, somebody sent him
flowers, and one of the ministries got interested in his case: when he gets out of the
hospital he's going to be allowed to go back
to work. That's a firm promise. Oh, you
think that after all those years of pasting in
Social Security stamps, he ought to be able

to . . . in his old age . . . ? You must be out of
your mind! He's got to work until he drops!

You want to know about the company?
Nothing—what do you expect? First of all,
they're not responsible; second, it was an
administrative error on a lower level; and
third, the man just couldn't do his job anymore. What should happen to the company?
Since when is a corporation responsible for
its actions? Railroad engineers and chauf-
feurs are responsible for their actions. But
groups?

After all, this isn't the United States.
There they fire anybody, any day they
please. No one ever expects to have a job by

33

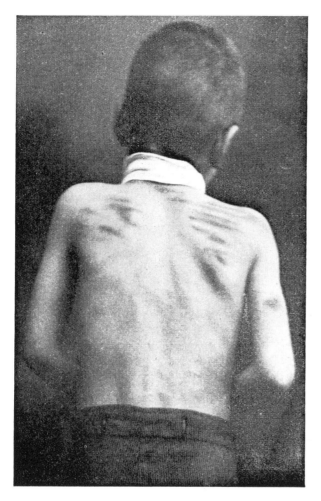

rights. It's an honest system, at least. But to use a man, until he's seventy-two and then throw him out! Surely that's . . .

Don't despair. Take it up with the SPD and its unions. They'll show those people what's what. Inexorably. Even if they have to pass a resolution! And in any case, we've learned the exchange value of a working life: one bunch of flowers.

Camouflage

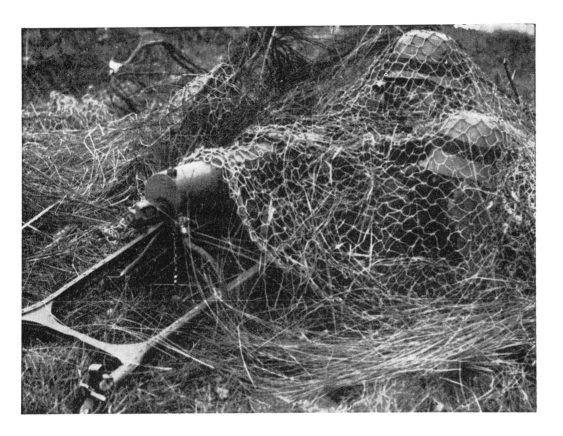

The German army's newest protective
device makes machine-gun divisions almost
invisible.

    This net is not a net. It's an allegory.

Idols of the
Maigoto-Blacks

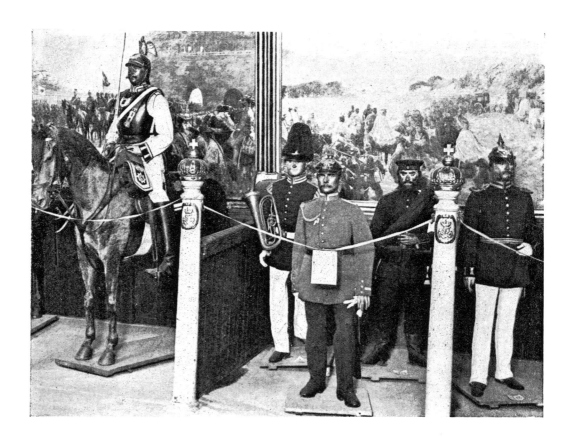

"... a curious practice. The tribe erects costumed idols of wood, or even wax, in special halls and dances around them on ceremonial occasions. The writer has had opportunity to enter these rooms: he saw truly terrifying figures, wild masks expressing insensitive, brute primitivism. One idol, enthroned on a totem-animal, held a spear in its hand ... the Maigoto-Blacks are exceedingly proud of these works of art ..."

The Ancestral Ruling
Family

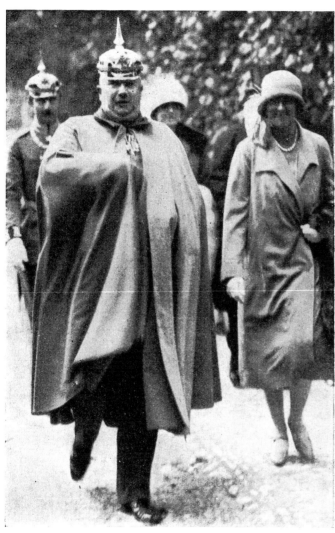

Prince Eitel Friedrich°

I'm a fat man.
I don't give a damn
for the Republic.
Let 'em kick.
Let 'em be hollerin'—
we Hohenzollern
have to live.
You'll give.
Until Doomsday,
you'll pay.
We'll stay.

How's that again? Did you say stay
            until Doomsday?

Study in Statistics

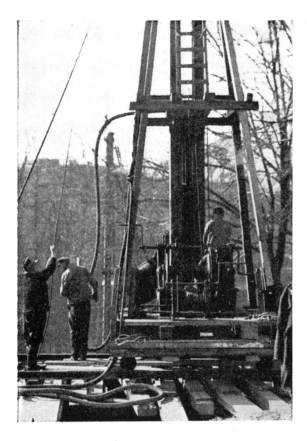

This is a poor country. I am a worker, with a trade, and I have a wife and three children. Fifty days out of the year, I work not for myself.

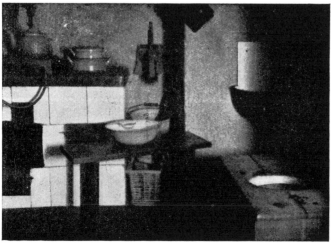

I work a little more than two days for the army. Two other days in the year I work so that we can have a nice police station.

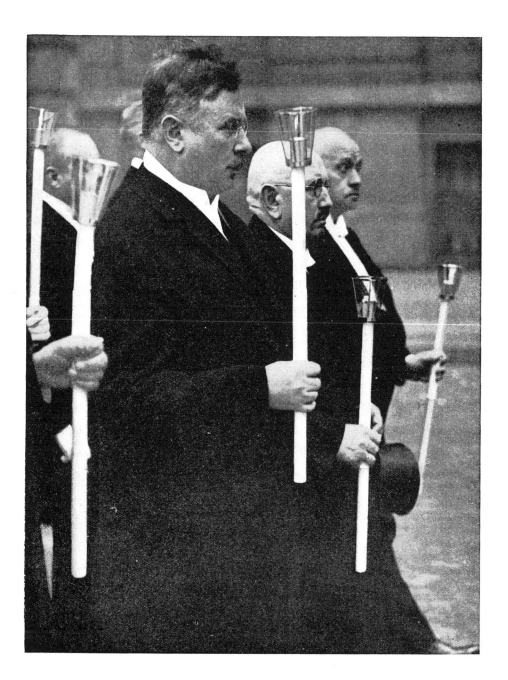

I have to work half a day for the church to which I don't
belong anymore, and

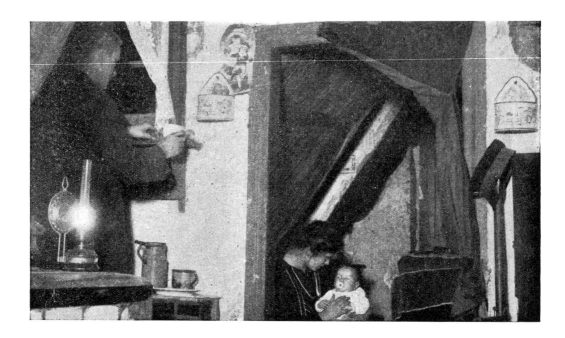

a whole week for the civil servants—for the many, unnecessary civil servants. Science and the arts are easier; they only take three hours.

This is a poor country!

In Prussia we have 28,807,988 Mark just for horse-breeding and

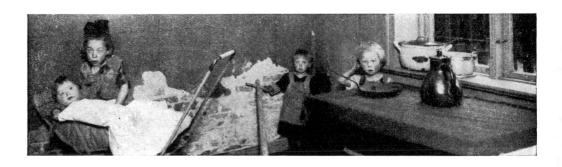

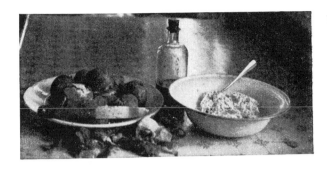

very little to eat.

But we have 230,990 Mark to pay for religion in the army, and 2,164,000 Mark for ambassadors' and diplomats' moving expenses. What would they have to do, if they didn't move. And

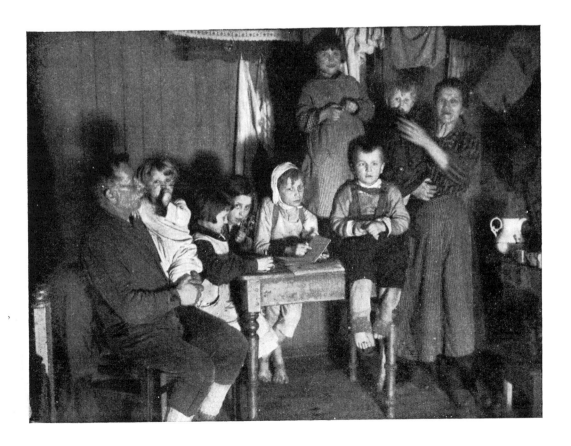

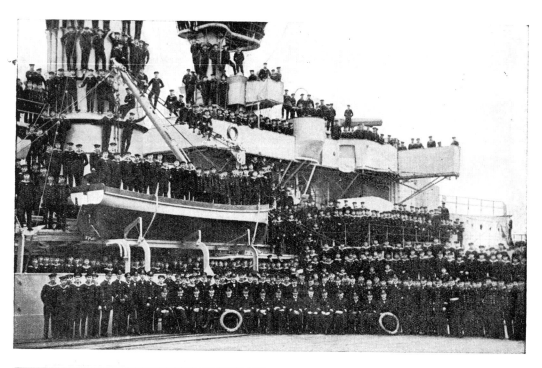

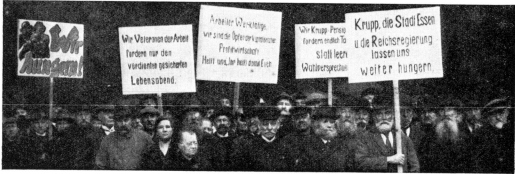

I am a book-keeper with a yearly salary of 3,600 Mark. My wife spends 40 Mark a week. I would have to work 433 weeks, to earn what Mr. Tirpitz,° who mismanaged the German fleet, gets on pension. Mr. Loser-of-battles Ludendorff gets 17,000 Mark.

We pay the old monarchists 206,931,960 Mark a year in pensions. After all, we've got the money. Well, actually, we haven't, but what are you going to do if you need a new battleship that costs 80 million Mark? And if the officers have to take morning rides, you can't expect beautiful eye clinics. We need our money for other things.

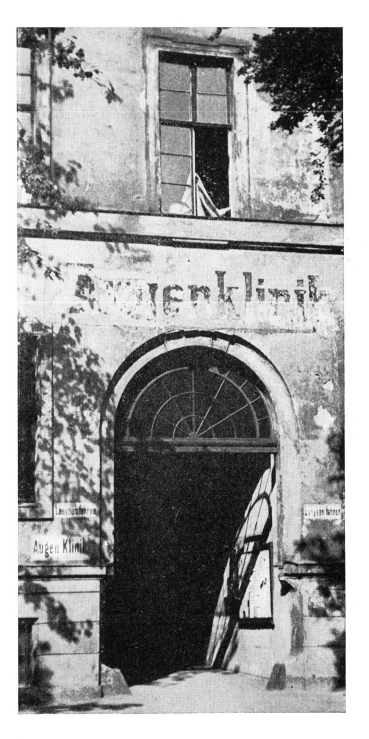

Where is Germany's money?

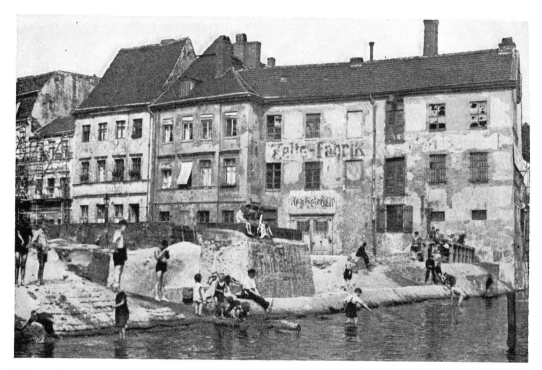

Here?

or maybe here?

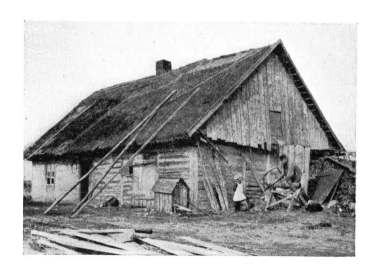

No, it's here.

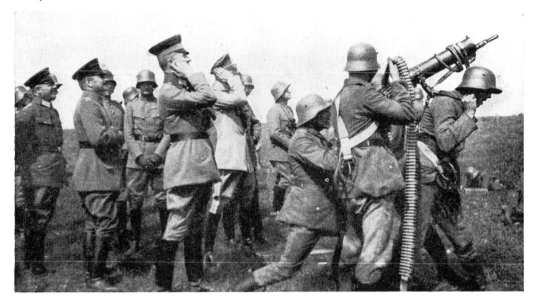

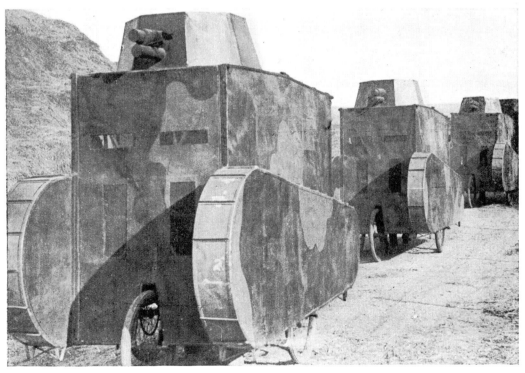

And here—

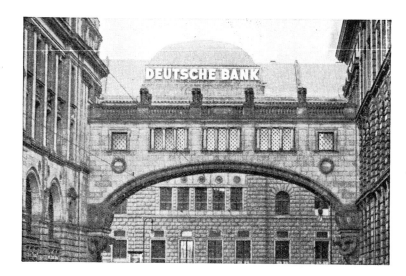

And here—

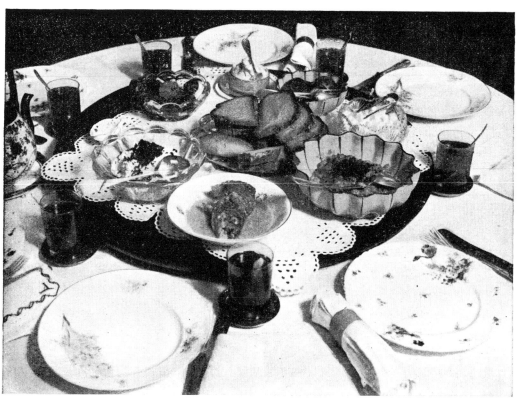

because

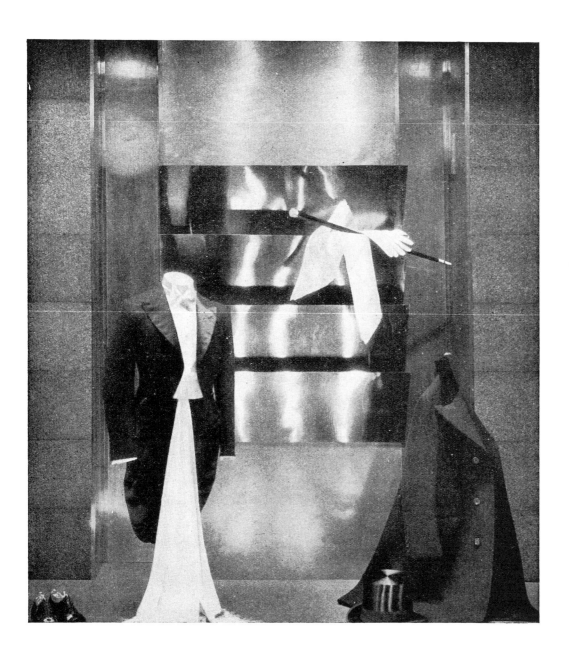

this is a very poor country.

The Cup

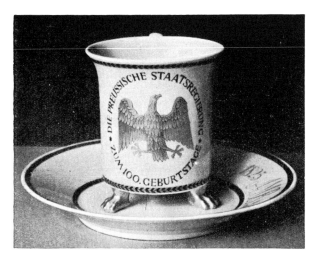

The State of Prussia presents this cup to everyone of its citizens who lives to be a hundred years old. Isn't that nice? Maybe to give the citizen courage for his next hundred years; maybe to say: "You made it to a hundred, in spite of being a Prussian—in spite of war, tuberculosis, and taxes, you survived! Good boy! Here have a cup on me." You can't say it's not a nice gesture, though the cup looks like a chamber pot with lion's feet.

But what's funny about this gesture?

The little external details express the true nature of a state better than anything else. This cup represents the patriarchal state's last gasp. The state, wanting to play Daddy, gives the good child who has reached a hundred a pat on the back, and we feel the emptiness of the gesture. It is done in vain— an anachronism. None of that is true anymore.

The state isn't a Daddy anymore—if it ever was—and the children are damnably grown up. All that has been drowned in faceless anonymity. The gesture isn't even hypocritical. It's nothing.

A village might congratulate an old inhabitant on his hundredth birthday. It makes sense when people know each other. But a modern state cannot congratulate private individuals . . . the gesture has an air of kindly belittling charity extended to little people. Unthinkable, that a well-to-do businessman with official titles and functions would be satisfied with a coffee cup—but successful businessmen, anyway, live too strenuously to get to be a hundred. The cup is whole—the idea shattered. Whom can they mean by "The Prussian State Government"? The ministers who change every month?—Marie, the fifteenth is the first, you can start stopping by that date—? The "Eternal Idea of the State"—Just park it over there, for now, Sir!—? Or do they mean the bureaucrats who stay, after the poor minister leaves? Who chose those particular representatives of the will of the people? No, it won't work.

People aren't subjects anymore, but they can't be citizens until they have a voice. Well, what are they then?

They are subscribers without choice.

They have to join, whether they want to or not. They are united by no common birth, race, or political opinion. Their language? It means less than we think—there are hundreds of different kinds of German and I cannot believe that a good writer and a bad judge speak the same language. The people are forced subscribers—where else could they get gas, mail delivery, a railroad? Surrounded by monopolies, they play at being citizens. And aren't by a long shot. Only the smallest of the small still believe. The clever ones let them. But the State exists in a queer mixture—half in the interest of its own self-serving bureaucracy which asks no one's permission to perpetuate itself, half controlled by the real lords of the land—the defense industry, the coal-barons, the steel-lords, the large landowners, and the manufacturers. The state doesn't have much to say.

But the state, poor thing, does get itself together on the occasion of an old railway guard's birthday—to present him with a coffee cup.

With kindest regards
from the Prussian state.

"Right," the old man will say. "There is a state too." He'll nod his old white head, remembering all the lovely times that his state gave him.

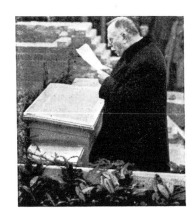

Lockout

We stand and wait
At the company gate.
Krause's are closing shop.
Father's with the comrades,
Father won't show up.
    Father's locked-out

The *I.G. Farben*° bloom
But there's no milk at home.
And down the Rhine, a shout:
Two hundred thousand men
Done out of work by force:
    Father's locked-out

We exist
To take our father's place
And be caught in the same vise.
Grandmother, teach them younger,
They mustn't cry with hunger,
But stand up for their right!
With father and his brothers,
Everyone together,
Towards freedom! Towards the light!

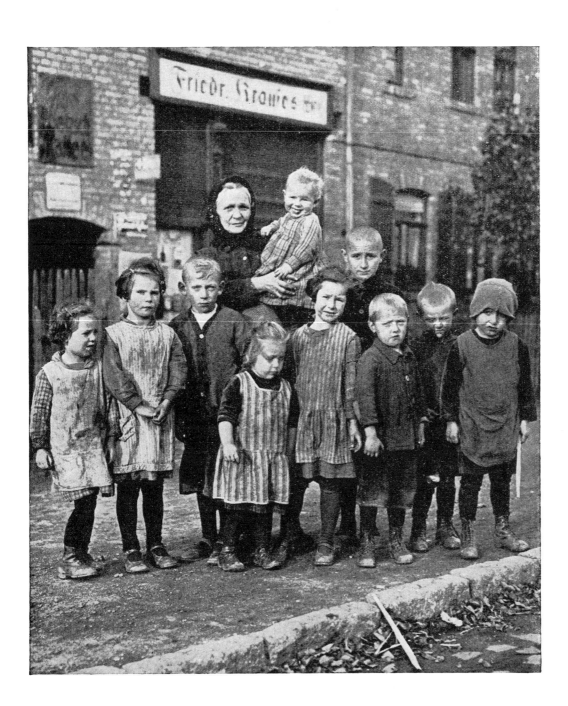

The Ecologist

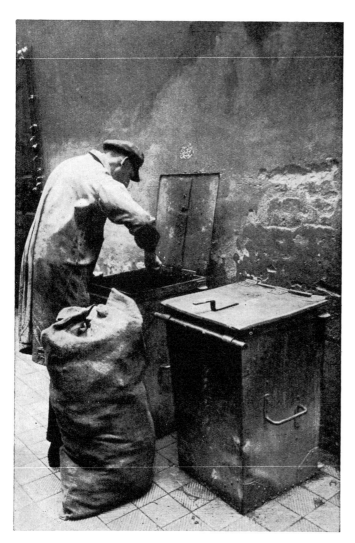

"Aw, you find quite a lot. The other day, I'm poking around in here, I feel something hard. Hey, what's this? I say—grab it. It's an old army helmet. I think, yep, still useful. Little Willie's always yelling for a potty. In the sack.

"Well sure, you're careful, you come into quite a lot of stuff. Other day, I'm poking around in there, all of a sudden, there's something soft. Hey, what's that? I think. Take a look. It's old Kahl's° long beard. You know, guy who made that new criminal law. Must have two—one for work, one for Sundays. In the sack.

"Yeah, well the best was yesterday. In the morning in a yard on Kloster Street, I'm going through a can. What do you think? Some joke. The Socialist Program of 1870. Read it to the guys—best laugh we've had in years.

"What'd I do with it? That nice paper?

"Show you in a minute."

The National Economy

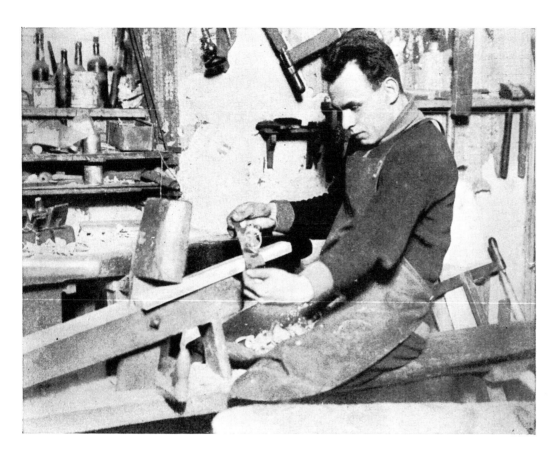

A railroad engineer's wages aren't high. For consolation the state grants him a pension to sweeten his declining years. The pension tends to be very small.

Well-to-do men, however, who make guest-appearances in political life, not only profit from their visits to cabinets and ministries, but take home pensions like the following:

Dr. Georg Michaelis,° the same chancellor who demonstrated his absolute lack of ability in 1917: 27,600 Mark a year.

Dr. Wilhelm Cuno,° whose job it was to conduct reparation proceedings with the large shipping concerns, and who subse-quently became—as chance would have it—director of such a concern. As chancellor, he was not responsible for the inflation because he cannot be held responsible for anything: about 19,000 Mark.

Gottlieb von Jagow°—that's right, the one who warned off investigators and later tried to overthrow the government: about 24,000 Mark.

Dr. Lewald,° a former government official of great, but so far undisclosed, merit: about 17,000 Mark.

Von Tirpitz, the old man with the beard. Having deceived the Reichstag for years, he forced through the building of a fleet. The

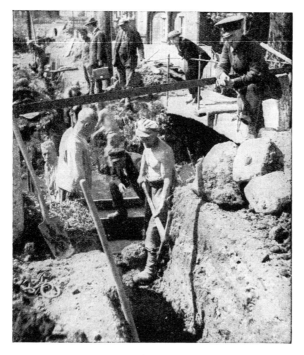

fleet accomplished nothing and was of no use during the war—in other words, it was unnecessary. To our beloved Tirpitz, from his grateful country: about 25,000 Mark. While we contemplate these figures, we should remember that the country spending these insane sums—more than 23 million —every year, is deeply in debt. That we have already touched bottom once. That while we fatten these others, our working taxpayers carry the heavy burden.

Of course, these pensioneers work hard. Many of them are still active enough to hold well-paid positions in industry. They get their positions because of their former titles—their service to the state is thus already well rewarded. But the country keeps on paying. We still pay each and every one of the former German ministers of war for their destructive and harmful activities: 25,000 Mark on the nose.

We pay Mr. Gustav Bauer°: 11,000 Mark.

We pay Mr. Hermes (Mosel)°: 11,000 Mark.

We pay the Mr. Emminger° who destroyed the German jury system: 19,000 Mark. We pay and pay, and will continue to do so, because the beneficiaries themselves make the laws. The workers and wage-earners have no idea what is being done to them.

In the lives of our contemporaries the state has come to represent what religion was to their great-grandparents: a dark, mysterious something that must, at all costs, be worshipped.

Animals looking at you°

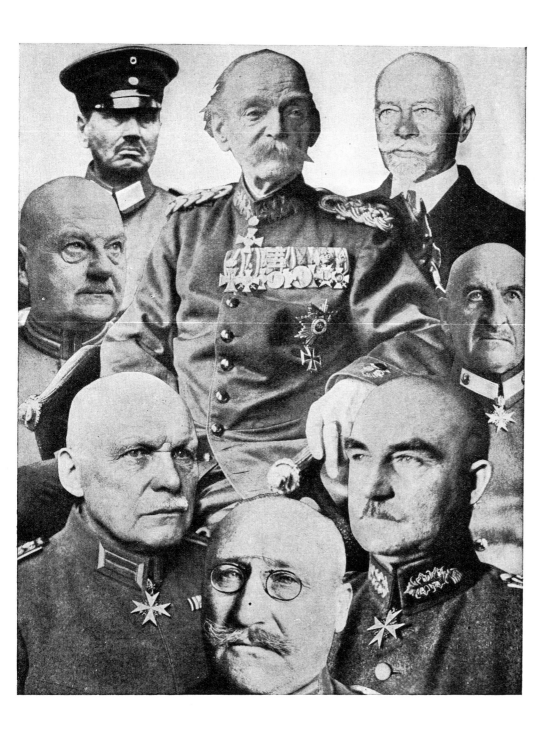

The Theater of War

"Hauser°—Man—long time no see, huh? How's it going, boy? Me? Just great! Well sure, I've been away! Most of the year— let's see, ten, well ten and a half months exactly. Yeah, took off last December—you didn't even know? Man, don't you read the papers? Siberia! At the TW! Hauser, you must be kidding! The Theater of War! You never heard of it? Come on, let's have a drink in this joint—you've got to hear this! Never even heard of it! Well, listen to this:

"You know who General Wrobel is don't you? Little fat guy, right? Well, two years ago at the Military Preparedness Conference in Dortmund he—I'll have a Curaçao—no, just a minute, a brandy, a double. One for this gentleman, too—O.K. by you, or—? Well, in Dortmund he said we ought to set up a Theater of War for National Defense Preparedness Training. To keep the youth physically fit . . . How'd he get that idea? Simple. Like the radical papers always said: 'If the gentlemen want to wage war, let them establish and open their own Theater.' So we did it! Yeah—here's looking at you! Wow—that's real stuff! Remember the one about the old farmer in the ditch. He's just had a good swig, enough to give him the shakes. And the preacher passing by, says: 'Well, Zeke, I can tell you're drunk, but you're shaken! That's the first step to re-formation.' And Zeke says: 'No Siree— I'm a-shakin' to spread the whiskey out even!' Yeah, I was going to tell you . . . a Theater of War to encourage Strength and Fitness in the Youth, Preparedness and Patriotism and National Power—well, you know the line. O.K. So Wrobel gets going: to the Ministry of Defense, to the Russians, Geneva, Paris—he had himself a time!— but he did it! All under wraps, sure, but they got us this great Theater of War in Siberia. Told the French it was against the Bolshies—Grumbach° believes Breitscheid° —they keep each other in the picture you know—told the English it was against the French, the Russians that we'd organize their army. And our boys, well, they'd be there anyway. Bon.

"A few hundred miles past Krasnoyarsk, you know where that is? Alright, here's the Yenisey—let the matchbox be the Upper Tunguska, your cigarette case the Sayan mountains. Right here's our TW. Well, the thing's got to have a snappy abbreviation, so that was it. Here's to you! I tell you, that's good stuff. Really great! Now listen. It's all fenced in with barbed wire—nobody gets in or out. And they've got everything: trenches, front lines, artillery positions, observation posts, field telephones, the whole business complete. And Rest and Recreation! Hauser, you wouldn't imagine! Huge staff headquarters, two really first rate casinos. You couldn't ask for better chow. Terrific wine—contributed by the Red Cross, you know how international those people are—and liquor—why this stuff here is plain rotgut by comparison. Oh waiter, another double—yes, two—and we had chaplains and orderlies and communication officers and antiaircraft artillery and field radio—everything. We had a fleet too—kept coursing up and down the Yenisey. Ludendorff and Brüninghaus° and Killinger,° the bigshots—all there too. I'm not kidding! Cheers!

"I got to be lieutenant—made sergeant first, then lieutenant in the field. Oh yeah— we had an enemy too. The first general meeting, they all fought so much that we got two sides—the red and the green—enemies. Even one battle, though most of the time it was just organizing. But that once—we had a body count of four hundred. The officer in charge—some big butter-and-egg man from Leverküsen—got drunk and didn't know what he was doing, so his gas-gun discharged. That's how it happened. Locals? No, we didn't have any of them. I mean, the men did have to have something for requisitions and women and stuff. So we put in two-hundred girls with their pimps to be native population, like they say. Yeah, and the men went to them, and we did too—I mean, we got them to headquarters mostly. And let me tell you, we had some great old times! Fantastic! Here's to you!

"How come I'm back? You won't believe this, Hauser, you'll laugh—and it is sort of funny. But I'll try to explain. Listen. After a while it just wasn't any fun.

"Here we had everything, right? War correspondents—I even kicked one guy in the pants—and rabbis—those were the only Jews on the place. We really had everything. But you know, I had this feeling there was something missing. At night, checking the posts—alone with my bottle and God—I'd keep thinking about it. Why I wasn't having fun. What was missing? I really felt that, Hauser. Cheers! You know what it turned out to be? These people were all volunteers, right? They all *wanted* to do it, understand?

"It wasn't fun. Look, I was in the service, put in my fourteen years before the war, I know what it's like. It's when they first come in—the recruits. They've always looked right through you before, walked by without seeing you even—but now, all of a

sudden, they're nothing. It cuts them down to size. Well anyway, they'd come, and the waiters would want to wait on you, and the actors dying to be clerks in the office, and the hotshot lawyers . . . boy, they'd all do their act—Sergeant this and Sergeant, Sir, that and up and back and all around. Because we had them! They'd perform like trained puppy dogs! They'd have to stand there, stockstill, and you go up real close: they couldn't move—couldn't do anything except just look back. And no expression. You think I didn't know what they were thinking! But there's no thinking in the army. Go ahead, think all you want, I'd say to myself. Discipline! Well, that's what was missing. All of it. Even complaints from the locals, even when we yelled and broke up their stuff. Everything paid for in advance. And the men got good pay too. What was missing was the guy who didn't want to play. Do you get me? Dissent, resistance, the insubordinate elements—that's what was missing. The Socialists—well no, not them, they're willing—but the Commies and Pacifists and the women who cry for real, you know—when it means something. The girls who worship you because they believe in you; the kids that run away and hide when they see you coming; the Belgians that you could sock —all them. It just wasn't real—you get it? It was phony. So I got out. They're still fighting . . . but its not the real front-line spirit anymore. Most of them went into some little business—Ludendorff is a bricklayer—he has a shop; Tirpitz sells hair-oil; Noske° breeds bloodhounds—they're all doing pretty well. But the real thing—*that* it wasn't . . . With swastikas on our helmets°. . . Oh they were good times, all right. But it

57

just wasn't right. I'm going to look around in Berlin now, see what's doing in cars and industry—they always need somebody to do organizing. And things have to get organized. You know, against the workers. Well yes, so I'm back.

"And how about you—what've you been doing all this time?"

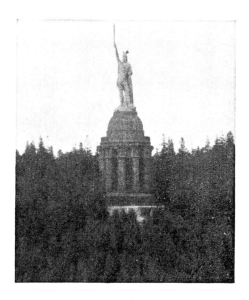

Rudolf Herzog°—a German Man

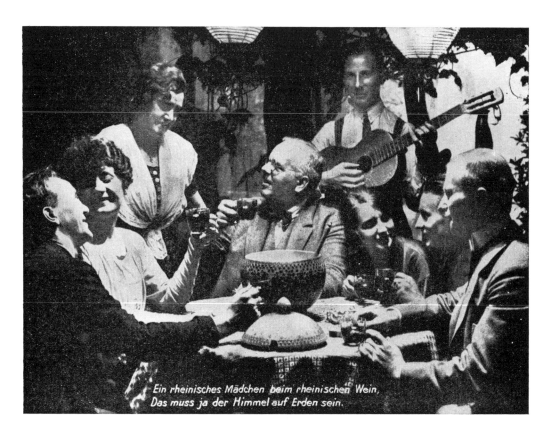

Ein rheinisches Mädchen beim rheinischen Wein,
Das muss ja der Himmel auf Erden sein.

*The local girls and the native wine
Make Heaven on Earth along the Rhine.*

Subordination is an inferior's continued and successful attempt to seem less intelligent than his superior.

German Article of War

We've all experienced a first journey. We watch every tree along an unfamiliar section of track. By the third time, however, our interest dies. Difficulties with customs, passport inspection, the endless jolting of the wheels, the little low houses to right and left—we know it all too well. What to do? We read. The latest Conan-Doyle isn't available. We need suspense and amusement in our compartment—what could be better than *Kameraden*, a novel by Rudolf Herzog. First printing, 150 thousand (Stuttgart and Berlin: J. G. Cotta, 1922). Cotta, who published Goethe and Schiller. But that's already long ago.

Now, I'm not quite as ignorant as most generals look. I've read two other novels by Herzog: *Die Wiskotten* and another, whose title I've forgotten. But I know it by heart, could recite it page by page. I could make it up as I go along. I snickered my way very carefully through *Kameraden*. It's a classic of German sensibility.

Bad novels have always existed. That Mrs. Courts-Mahler° can't write German and that Mr. Herzog can't write novels, isn't the point. Popular literature has always ex-expressed character—not the author's, of course, but the consuming public's. In the past the theme of popular novels in most countries has been that of the conquering hero: knights, bandits, pirates, detectives, famous criminals—they are all braver, stronger, less law-abiding than their readers. The heroes behave as the readers would like, if it were allowed. We read Clauren°, and the romances of that period, to learn what small, nineteenth-century business-men dreamed about; to find today's ideal, read Arnolt Bronnen°—a second Herzog. Philistines are really Napoleons without opportunity: during the war we learned the disastrous effects of—for once—allowing them their heroics. But let's see what the educated, north-German middle-class ideal looks like.

Like a reserve officer.

One of Mr. Herzog's favorite words is "tight." All his heroes are unspeakably rigid: ". . . he answered tight-lipped"; "no, she said stiffly"; "deep seriousness tightened his features." Tight and stiff, they march through his volumes. Since that's what his heroes look like, it must be—to judge by the publication figures—how his public wants them. They are rigid, abrupt and cold officials or merchants of a certain social standing. They are on the best terms with the existing social order, which they affirm, but do not understand. They are brave, as long as they stay inside their group. Alone they're nothing. They show courage mainly by treating all outsiders with an infinite boorishness. "With a stiff gesture, he made room for himself and his companion." Other people don't exist. There's no one as aristocratic as a Mr. Schulze, member of the Board of Governors, striding through the common crowd. These are the aristocrats of the "wine-section." If everyone drank wine, shield and coat-of-arms would fade away.

The terminology and slang in the book are taken from the casino, the riding-stables, and the hunt. The fine distinctions between "the man fell to, heartily" and "the gentle-men sat down to dine" are scrupulously upheld. The formal contortions of army-post social structure appear in the wildest situations. A drowning man might call, "Private Klopp obediently requests per-mission to be pulled out, Sir!" Or something like it. Herzog is good at that.

The kind of sugary, stupid love story that a large part of womanhood seems to demand, also runs through the book. To each his own: Ewers° does it for hysterical Jewish readers, Bonsels° for Christians, and Mr. Herzog satisfies the normal German woman. And besides loving, there's beating.

"But surely, first, you gave them some-thing to remember you by? I mean, these contemporaries had backsides to be kicked, didn't they?" The contemporaries are fellow-Germans. "Niklas, let's have an immediate lesson in good manners." " 'Right away,' the hunter growled. He bent far back and laid his long strap across the abus-ive fellow's pelt." The owner of the pelt is German. The novel also contains a second— or maybe a thousandth—case of Corporal Lyck (the character in Heinrich Mann's *Der*

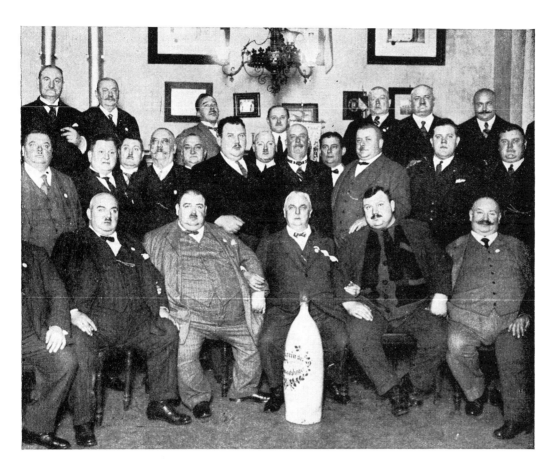

Untertan [The Underling] who shot at the workers and earned the Kaiser's praise). Here's a soldier in the same situation. "Give the bandit both barrels. And if the rotten rabble doesn't run away, you won't have to take the long trip alone." " 'Yes, Sir,' the man murmured, his eyes staring fixedly into the distance." "You conducted yourself like a hero. I congratulate the Fatherland on its brave son. Come. We'll go together." In short, the slap in the face, the kick, the saber-blow, are seen as the basic necessities for our country's reconstruction. You find the same stuff in Bronnen.

Herzog is political. And such politics! The kind his readers practice and see, understand and accept. This what his politics look like: "And what—what would you have done?" (The reference is to November 1918.) "The Rhine, Dülkingen! I would have held firm and fought all along the Rhine! Every day of hard-bitten resistance would have softened the enemy—would have won us better peace terms. Only a whimpering coward is kicked in the teeth, humiliated. Not the man who trades blood for blood." "Right, Volker, right. And if the Rhine-front had broken?" "Behind the Weser! Behind the Elbe!—

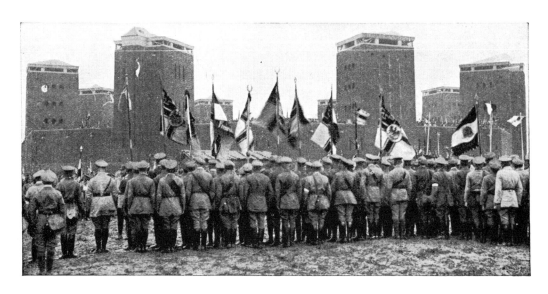

Slow and tough and step by step."

There was a telegram from Baron von Lersner,° the representative of the Foreign Office at Main Headquarters, on October 1, 1918, at one in the afternoon. "General Ludendorff has just requested Baron von Grünau° and me, in the presence of Colonel Heye,° to convey to Your Excellency his urgent request to begin peace negotiations at once. Today the troops hold the line; what may happen tomorrow cannot be predicted." A further telegram from the Acting Embassy Counselor, von Grünau, was sent the same day at two. "General Ludendorff, in the presence of Colonel Heye and Lersner, has just requested me to forward to Your Excellency his urgent plea to begin peace negotiations at once. To wait until the formation of a new government would be unwise. Today the lines are holding and our situation is still dignified, but a breakthrough might occur at any moment. Our offer would then come at the least favorable time. He is gambling against time; a division could col-

lapse suddenly at any point. My own impression is that there has been a complete loss of nerve; I believe that, at worst, we could publicly justify this step with reference to Bulgaria's position. Grünau."

Now what are we to call Mr. Herzog's treatment of events? We call it poetic license. Although no one could accuse me of a too great tenderness for this Republic, Mr. Herzog's nonsense is too much! And one of his *raisonneur*-heroes, himself, openly admits the foolishness, the incompetence and mistakes, of pre-war attitudes and policies: "All those decades, while we struggled and labored and suffered through our development abroad, the whole Berlin crew was sound asleep. The Fatherland ignored our physical and spiritual suffering, and our need. Until—the Fatherland needed us." True enough. Neither the Kaiser nor his country were much concerned about Germans in the colonies and abroad. But who was asleep? Why, Mr. Herzog's own readers. And who had all—but literally all— the

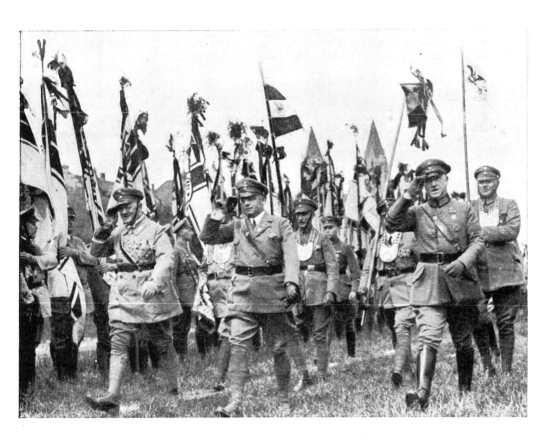

positions of power and influence? The noble souls he writes about—members of fraternal orders, sons of large landowners, officers: those who still collect large dowries in "good matches" (with a stiff gesture). They certainly didn't want the war. They never wanted anything that extended beyond Outer-Pomerania or the Weser country. With your kind permission: Idiots. The middle-class aristocrats (especially the women) who read Mr. Herzog shudder with delight when the lending-library-laureate proves to them that, thank God, we belong to the better class of people. "And do you have neighborly relations with the common folk?" asked Volker. "My God, you go to the zoo on Sundays, sometimes, if there's one in the neighborhood." The zoo-dwellers spilled their dirty blood at Verdun and carried their skins—at world-market prices —into the trenches. Volker got the *Pour le Mérite*.

Herzog rises to the same heights in his treatment of the Polish uprising in Upper-Silesia. What patently false nonsense, as "Berlin" comes under attack! Even the readers whose views are circumscribed by their neighborhood bar's horizons must know who paid off the *Freikorps°* whose deeds are glorified in these pages. Once, the truth appears here too. "The men who, with Volker, belonged to the inner circle."

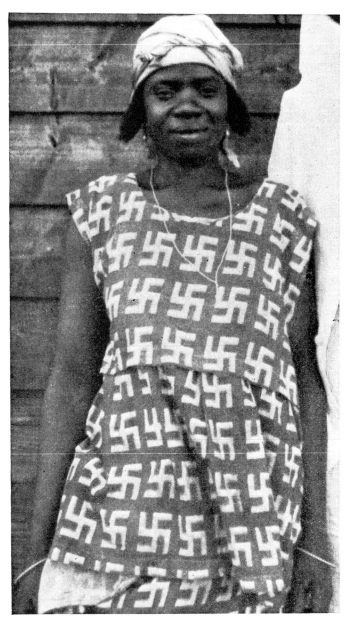

White Shame in Africa

(Herzog's heroes, incidentally, always belong to the inner circle; his books tell little about the life and death of ordinary men.) "They had eyes and ears and hands everywhere . . . their hands were on the Rifle-Corps in the Bavarian mountains, and on the universities in the German provinces." You may well say so. And I have heard it said, that (when they withdrew them) their hands were red up to the wrists. Details can be found under Gustav Landauer.°

They're not very refined, the fine gentlemen. But apparently that's what life in these circles is like, otherwise the books would not be so popular. For instance, a country is in deep trouble. "Didn't I tell you, all my money is in dollars. If the Mark falls to zero, I'll pay a dollar to buy an ox." An uncircumcised one, of course. And once, after the main hero has done the subhero a service: "I got my comrade out, he thought as he walked, well-content with his day's work, towards Dülkingen's estate. And since giving my dollar doesn't cost me a cent, the deal is tolerable, and the loss only imaginary." This way of being a good German is intolerable; its value only imaginary.

But I got good value for my money: love and moonlight, wine-shop owners who come "from up and down the Rhine" to attend the funeral of a sentimental balladeer, even a criminal rape with the guaranteed black shame and—ha!—powerful fisticuffs won by the blond saviour. Everything is there. Foreign soldiers always stare "insolently"; traveling North-Germans get slapped in a Bavarian train station; "the noise of French deportment and French speech everywhere." You'd have to hear what an old French soldier—say, Gaston

Moch—says about Germany, to understand the ugliness of these false observations. An excellent student of the French, Arthur Eloesser,° once told me that at first he felt strange in French society; something seemed to be missing. Finally he realized that he missed our rather loud and animated conversations. French socializing is quieter.

Herzog's characters are refined gentlemen. And clever! When the cattle-trading Jew goes past the stable with the "Master," he says, "What beautiful oxen you have! What beautiful oxen the Baron has!" Dülkingen misheard. " 'Yes, yes. It's beer from the brewery in Dortmund.' And they quickly joined the others." That's real wit for the readers. What a clever man! He simply doesn't hear! And with such admirable cleverness men like him afterwards ruled the world. Admirable, refined, but they can be jolly into the bargain. Dülkingen —would you like to be named Dülkingen? —complains that his housekeeper always folds her hands under her breasts. But what does he call the breasts? The rascal! "Whatsis" and "the pudding"—it's riotous! The gentlemen are historically-minded too: only the old Kaiser interests them. "My feeling for the grandson is only one of honest sympathy." That's telling them! And lyricism? There's lyricism too. The Prussian kind, naturally. In one sentence, we have all of Prussian lyric poetry. "The trained male voices carried their cry of yearning through the room." I still hear the sound of those male voices! "Attention!" Finally, a pearl which brings the innermost lives of the whole group which reads this junk into focus:

"Superiority—?" Volker repeated. "Can one

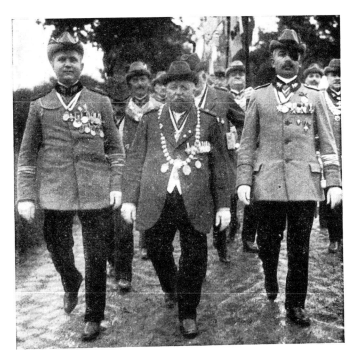

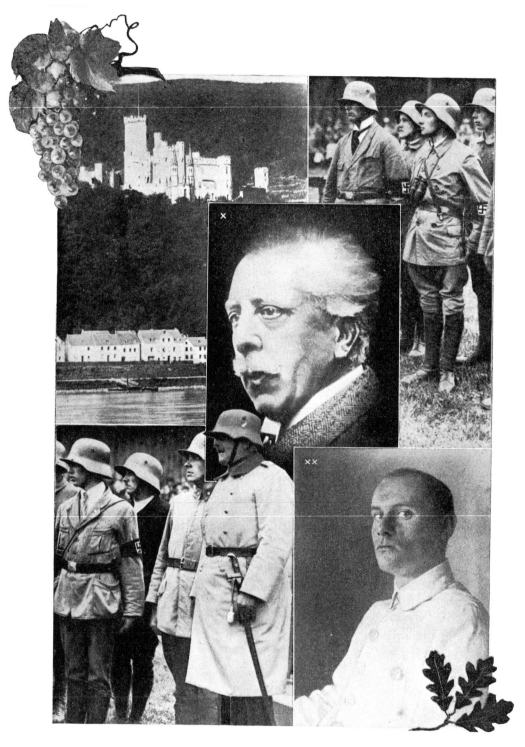

x Rudolf Herzog   xx Arnolt Bronnen

be superior, and careless? To be careless? To be careless is to be unprincipled.''

Can superiority be careless?—Certainly, real superiority is relaxed and loose; these people's strict and tight character is like the excessively tight, high, and stiff collar worn by a noncommissioned officer on Sunday leave. He needs the collar. It's his moral principle. If he were to open it—but that's a question for animal-husbandry. Millions and millions read this stuff. Tight-muscled heroes let fly with their fists so that the sound of the blows is deafening; count-less loving couples walk across the moonlit fields at chapter's end; everyone looks down his nose—with a tight and controlled ex-pression—at the messy crowd below. Who are the readers?

The wage-earner who imagines himself

lord of the castle, the library official on salary-step IV in a helmet with movable visor, the chairman of a policedog-breeding association being August the Strong.° These books read so pleasantly, so smoothly; they are our times' never-never-land. A whole broad stratum enjoys these delicacies. At the back of the book an edition of 2,485,000 copies is listed. That means ten million readers, generously calculated: this Herzog is the Duke° of the rental libraries. Ten million people want the world in this book.

And there's another little thing.

Where was the bard during the war? It would be senseless to ask this question of a pacifist whom one could, at most, criticize for not having refused service. Where was Mr. Herzog? He probably has all the excuses ready. Walter Bloem,° whose novels aren't

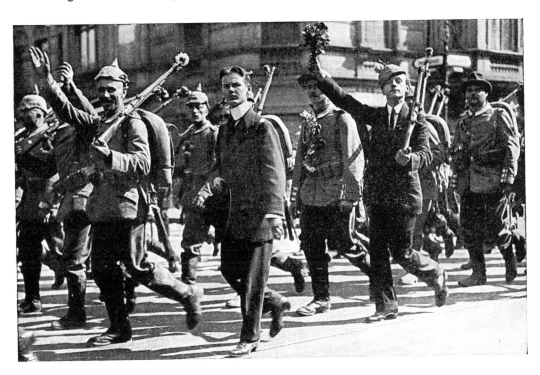

very delightful either, had no excuses. I shall
never say a word against the man who
sealed his patriotism with his blood. He
believed in the thing, and, as soon as he recovered from his wounds, he always went
back. Mr. Höcker° was making money in
Lille. Mr. Herzog wrote novels. God bless
his name, inscribed among the founders.

A horrible face looks back at us from his
books: a little mustache brushed stiffly up-
wards, sparse hair short on top, cold horn-
rimmed glasses. The face stands out from a
background of white tiles: it must be the
"Gentlemen's" in an inn on the Rhine.
White-tiled, with church-windows of
colored glass, and the windows show the
German Rhine and the German girl doing
something-or-other, clean, correct, up-
standing, and German. I've already forgotten
Mr. Herzog. But his millions of readers—
business men, civil servants, students, land-
surveyors, priests, doctors, fathers of families, and their wives—have erected a worthy
memorial for themselves and their times in
the works of this universally honored poet.

Bock Beer Festival

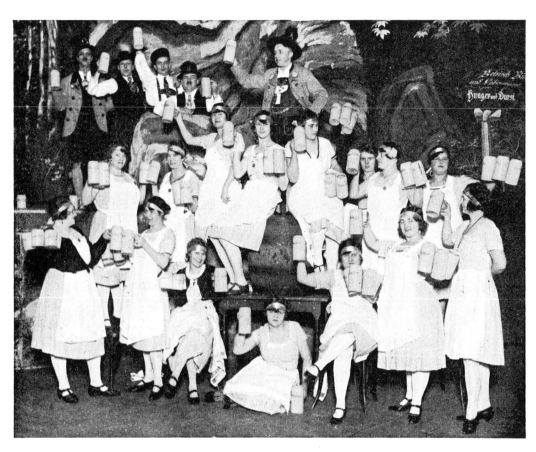

We're the Bavarian
dirndls—Yoohoo!
With a glad-eye, a come-on,
a—good health!—to you!
    Yodelayeeoo!

We're the Bavarian
fellows—Yoohoo!
We work on commission
and we're thirsty too!
    Yodelayeeoo!

We're the Bavarians
having a drop!
    For business the Prussians
      golldurned
      danged
      cussed Prussians
are just good enough!
Yodelayeeoo!
    Lalalahui!

Frozen Blood

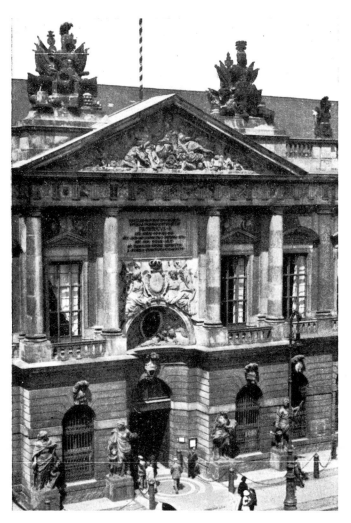

This bombastic trumpet blast is the façade of the Armory in Berlin.

It's even worse inside.

Inside they kept their trophies. Old generals' overcoats and cannon and tin soldiers and—that's right—bits of tattered cloth.

A lot of poor jerks marched to their deaths behind the bits of cloth. Some got paid, others went for honor—gratis. Flags . . .

You will not find a single word expressing regret or disapproval, or humanity, anywhere inside this advertisement for war. The whole building is single-minded propaganda for a blissfully slavish obedience. "The State has never bothered itself about your troubles, but should the State demand your life, you must give it." We'll play them a new tune. Maybe an East Pomeranian non-com, bleeding to death on barbed wire, really does feel comforted by the fact that his name will be engraved on a stone tablet somewhere; it may be a comfort that—at least in other days—people could die so picturesquely. But it's no comfort to us. We think, what's all the dying for? It's for nothing. It's in someone else's interest.

But the Republic loves tradition (only, not its own). So they've left this building-block playhouse nicely standing, just the way it was. Because we have to keep the people in touch with their glorious history. And so this shaming building is also the first thing they show foreign visitors. This building is what they show the English employee, Fuad,° when he comes from Egypt to visit Berlin. And any king understands immediately. It's like touring the advertising department of a friendly business concern.

Everything stays just the way it was.

These are "honorably earned rights and privileges." Nothing moves. It's as eternal as people's stupidity. Because the church and their own, beaten-in preconceptions about "the dignity of family life" tell people to want things the way they are, they can't decide to change the criminal law that prohibits abortion. But the way the salvaged fruit-of-the-womb finally croaks—that's another story. There will be no peace on earth, while people still believe that the wax-work junk, displayed in armories like this one, has anything to do with a people's real worth. Until they learn that these are the memorabilia of degradation. Although all war is economically caused, some of its aspects can only be explained biologically.

Primitive power-worship, for instance— especially when power happens to appear in a colorful costume. Women get excited— even though, as Ludwig Thoma° pointed out, soldiers take off their bright uniforms for the act in question. But men, too, are stirred strongly by the intoxicating memories of spilled blood, and fall into unusual moods better served in another kind of public "house" than an armory.

If you should pass this building, remember that hundreds and thousands of tortured human bodies cry out to the heavens, behind the colored cloth, the uniforms, the coats of arms. Cry out to heaven, and to earth: to you, fellow sufferer. To you.

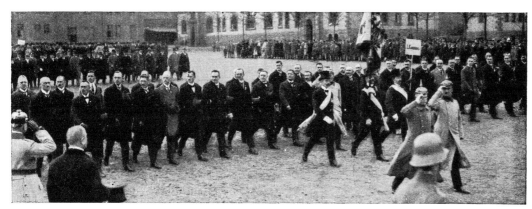

An Empty Cell

As soon as they've taken him away, the guard opens the window. It always smells bad in prison cells—but the air in this cell is especially foul. It's a sour air; the sweatiness of last fears sticks to the walls; and final prayers, wishes, vague images, escape through the little, barred window, while outside the passing bell tolls. The door is open—you can look inside from the passage.

There isn't much inside: the chair, the bed that still shows the outline of a human being who won't be back, the table at which they let him write a last letter, the water jug from which he drank—why did he still bother?—the pail into which he emptied his last terror. Now he's gone. The room is completely still. Although door and window are open, it doesn't get better—something sticks to the walls and the air seems clotted. You feel so tight in here. He still pretended to be a human being; he breathed, as if it still mattered; he cried; he retreated into himself—in this moment he could not have fathered a child; all his glands shrank in an extremity of tension, defensively cramped, as if they had been injected with alum. His pores exuded bitter fear.

Yes, he did deserve it—didn't he? He mutilated my child, my sweet blond baby. It looked just like her, had her round nose, and we wanted a boy so much, and then it was a boy—and that pig attacked him . . . in the park—the little one lost his way in the bushes. I can't even say what that monster— oh the damned dog! Is my child alive? Is his mother's pain gone? She'll have another child, but not that one. Maybe even a boy, but not that boy. Bending over the new cradle, she will cry. But what has happened?

They haven't even avenged my wrong. What good does it do to satisfy my lowest instincts, and to satisfy them senselessly— perhaps even by offering me a front seat to watch his head roll in the sack? I don't want to watch. Something unalterable happened through him—a part of myself is gone. And nothing has been accomplished except another murder, with all the terrors of the first. To make us secure? Yes. To make us parents secure, so that no other little boy will be found like . . . oh, the dog! No: God's failed handiwork. The cell is empty now; the sweated smell of death is almost gone; the jug that he touched with his lips is empty; the bed is made and the pail clean. The cell waits. For the next one.

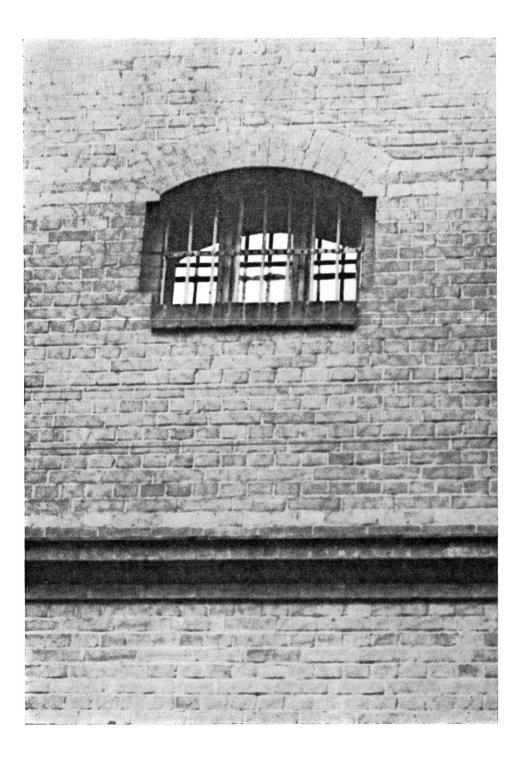

73

The Fire Brigade

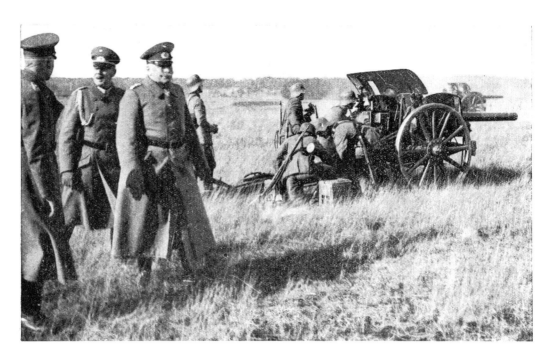

The repair works of the Dnieper steamship line are located on the Island of Truchany, across from Kiev. For years the voluntary fire brigade there had nothing to do. Last year six firemen, worried about the future of their voluntary organization, set fire to one of the company's buildings. The voluntary fire brigade then put out the fire. After another six months of inactivity, the same six members of the fire brigade set fire to another building. The two instigators, Korolski, a member of the brigade, and Dezenke, assistant to the chief, were condemned to death. Three others were sentenced to ten years in prison; another one of the defendants was sentenced to eight years.

Retrying the Case

**Dedicated to the Chief Justice of
the Superior Court: The Honorary
Doctor, Mr. Justice Bumke°**

First Day

Presiding Judge: Well and———?

Witness: And so—well, he just—

Presiding Judge: What?

Witness: (silence)

Presiding Judge: But go ahead—speak. No
one here is going to hurt you! Remember
you're under oath.

Witness: (very quietly) And so he just spent
the night with me—

A juror: That is, the night of the murder?
Between 16 and 17 November?

Witness: Yes . . .

Presiding Judge: But for heavens sake! Didn't
anyone question you at the last trial?

Witness: The gentleman was terribly stern
—and it all went so fast—

Presiding Judge: And so you let an innocent
—so you let a man be sentenced to death,
and then go to prison for life, without saying—no really, I can't understand that!

Witness: (weeps) My parents are so religious
. . . and the disgrace———

Second Day

Witness: But I said all that. The investigating
judge didn't want to hear about it.

Presiding Judge: Mr. Justice Pechat?

Witness: That's right. I kept pointing out
that the scream couldn't be heard very
clearly: it was a very rainy night and the
house was a long distance away . . .

Presiding Judge: In your testimony . . . but
there's nothing about that in the record.

Witness: The judge told me if I didn't sign,
he'd just keep me locked up.

District Attorney: But that's quite impossible! Judge Pechat—please?

Judge Pechat: I don't recall the incident.

Third Day

Expert Witness: The first thing any professional would do, would be to examine the second revolver. But that wasn't done at the time.

District Attorney: But why didn't you testify to that effect?

Expert Witness: Mr. District Attorney! I've been a specialist now for twenty-three years —but something like that trial—I wasn't allowed to say a thing. The District Attorney, Mr. Pochhammer, and the Presiding Judge, Mr. Brausewetter, just kept repeating that those were my personal opinions, and that they weren't at issue . . .

Presiding Judge: In your opinion, would it have been possible to aim at and hit the target with the first gun, at the distance assumed by the first decision?

Expert Witness: No. It's absolutely impossible.

Fourth Day

District Attorney: . . . although we cannot be absolutely certain, we can nevertheless assume with some degree of probability, that the accused was not the culprit. I don't say that he could not have been. Although his alibi has now been confirmed by the witness, Miss Koschitzki; although the testimony that a cry was heard has been shaken; although—I continue—the failure to examine the second army revolver leaves a missing link in the chain of evidence; we are still faced with the question, what became of August Jenuschkat? The murdered man's body has never been recovered. Therefore we cannot assert that a circumstance might have been wrongfully omitted during the first trial. That would be unjustified exaggeration. The circumstances, as I have just———

(Disturbance among the spectators)

Presiding Judge: I must request order. Bailiff, close the . . .

Bailiff: All right out . . . now this way . . . out . . .

Voice: Hey Frank—what're you doing in the dock?

The defendant: (stares wildly and faints)

Bailiff: Here now . . . here now!

Presiding Judge: Order! What's this? What do you want? Who are you?

A strange man: Me, I'm Jenuschkat!

Presiding Judge: If you wish to enter a claim in the case of your murdered relative . . .

Stranger: Aw no! It's me—August Jenuschkat himself!

Presiding Judge: Order! You're August Jenuschkat? Are there two men of that name in your family?

Stranger: Naw. I heard I got murdered—but I think it aint so!

Presiding Judge: Step forward please. Have you identification papers? Yes . . . well so you are . . . well then, you must be . . .

Stranger: Yooo—when I got home that morning, the police was all in front of the house. So I left—thought they'd come to get me. There was something with the taxes. So I took my horses over into Lithuania. Fell in love there and got married—forester's daughter. Nobody wrote—didn't have my address anyway. And this morning when I came over again, with the horses, well, I heard all this. Well, I tell you———!

Presiding Judge: Court adjourned.

Recent Promotions

District Court Justice Mr. Pechat, to Chief District Court Justice.

District Attorney Dr. Pochhammer, to Chief District Attorney.

Chief District Court Justice, Mr. Brausewetter, to Speaker of the Senate in Königsberg.

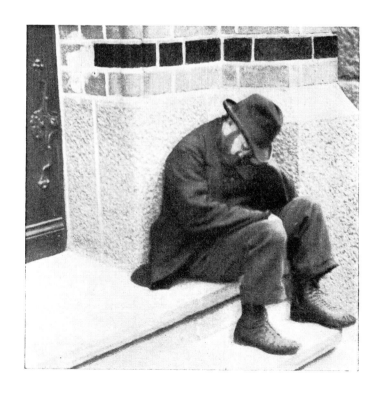

Mr. Wendriner Goes
Shopping

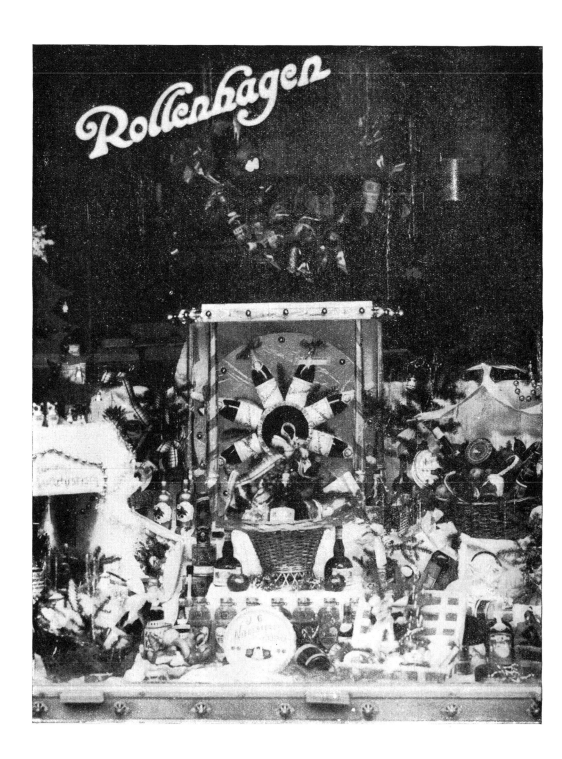

". . . How'd'ydo . . . nice crowd here . . . well, let's see . . . how about stepping back, Mister? . . . Of course I'm not pushing! . . . Ox! . . . You wouldn't believe it. It's our turn next. We were here first. Are you waiting too? A goldmine, this business, what do you think! They must make a bundle.

Well, I wrote them that I'll make the deal if they'll take the mortgage at fifteen. They're good people—but with the freeze the way it is—nobody has any money. You're telling me? I told them, either decide now or I'm out—Oh Miss, Miss! Yes, we were here first. Pardon me! . . . Well, let's have some

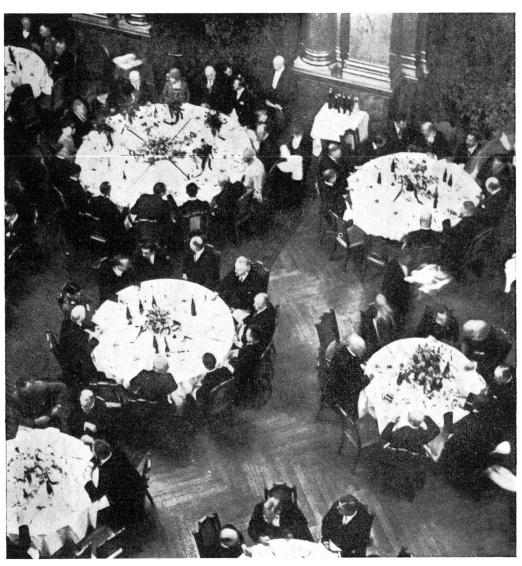

of these sardines—you're sure they're fresh? O.K., a half. Either you decide right now, or be responsible for the commission—Not such little ones, Miss. That's right—from underneath there! And then half a pound of the vegetable salad . . . You know, I always eat at home with my wife during the week— it's cheaper, and at least you know what you're getting. Tonight I've got a confer- ence, but I want to eat first. Stuffed tomatoes? No—but you could give me some of those cold cuts. Did you see HER? Reminds me a little of Fred's Clara. That's a fabulous woman all right. You know, if I were what I used to be—but you get so busy. But get a load of that little piece back there. That's something! The roast pork, Miss, but not too fat. Yes, Schüh's involved too. No, it's not finalized yet—you know, tax-wise, it's not so simple—but we've got a good agent. Jack still makes waves—always countering directives. My God, I took him on because I thought he'd at least keep the personnel in line. A bottle of English Sauce, Miss—the sharp kind! And you know Lach- mann don't you? That boy goes in to Jack this morning and asks for a raise! What do you think of that? Miss, I'll take some of the Kalvil apples! I gave that boy a piece of my mind! Now—in these times—what's in the kid's head anyway? Have you been to the new shows? That one's supposed to be a wonder! We're going Saturday. I'm going to see if I can't get complimentary tickets through Lachmann. Did you see the paper tonight, about the ghosts? I don't know— occultism . . . Say? Is that singing outside? Communists? I thought that was done with. Oh well, it's O.K.—just hikers. Listen, today the army marched by our shop and let

me tell you—fantastic! Like the old days. Really good. You have to hand it to Hinden- burg°—he does a good job. The trial in Leipzig? I haven't heard—Well, let's have the bill! I don't follow politics. No, you know, on principle. Nothing but headaches! Twenty-four eighty? How come? Oh, I see. Let's go—I see Number Nine coming. I don't know, my liver's bothering me again when I walk—I guess I'll have to see the specialist. No, we go to a good one, my wife's cousin. First-class man. He takes fifty Mark for a consultation. Well, naturally, for me he does it for less. The pains start up here, you know, and stop down there. Not at night—just during the day. And I'm always dieting even so. What's that you have? Neuralgia? You should take a hot bath. Well, my regards to your wife! So long.

That's human too! Makes you wonder. How does he get by?

Still a Joke

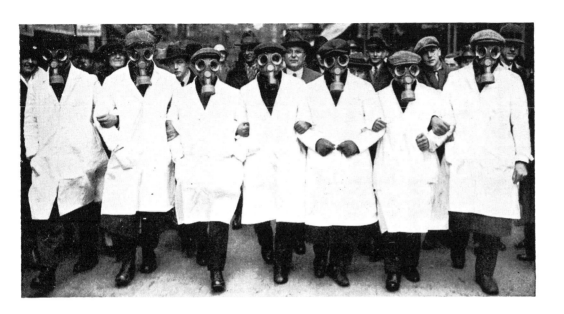

One day it will be serious. The snout-face will be ordinary reality. No one will think it's funny anymore. Many people will weep. But, of course, we can't prevent it: the hat manufacturer proclaims straw-hat week, the Canadian fruit-grower propagates peaches, and the defense industry needs war.

How Stupid They Were—!

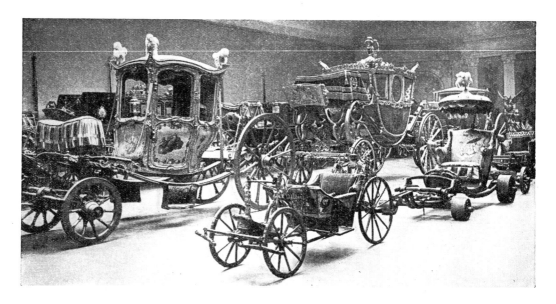

They really rode around in golden coaches, just as the fairy tales say. A glance would tell you who was king—you were supposed to be able to tell. It's different today.

The most powerful man rides hidden in the back of his big car. The car, an unusually elegant and expensive make, has only a small monogram on its dark door. The passenger, who may control half the world's oil supply, has no golden coach. The passenger, who can make war and—if it's good for business—peace, does not decorate his car with ostrich feathers. You can't see that he owns half your country: you aren't even aware of it. True power is anonymous. The passenger in the car only smiles when the people outside throw rocks and want to hang some little wrong-doer from the lamp-post. The passenger in the car knows better. Few people know him. If he's very smart, the newspapers never mention his name.

Revolutions used to be simpler. The symbols were so convenient. A ruler's palace . . . the Bastille . . . golden coaches—help yourself, please. And today . . . ?

Anywhere in Europe

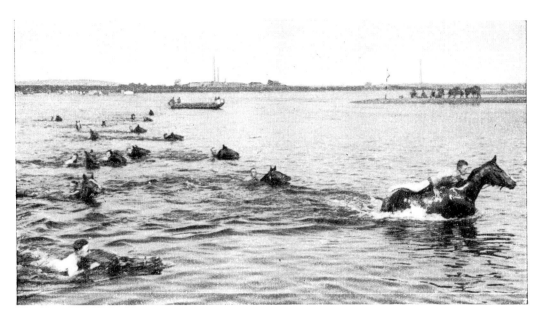

when healthy young people on horseback cross a river the chances are a hundred to one that it is not for sport, or pleasure, not because they feel a joyous relationship to animals, or a love of nature—such activity always goes on "in the interests of national defense." Here, for instance, the army is crossing the Elbe at Magdeburg.

Thousands of young men would enjoy this sport—but there is no money for it. No river. No horses. No time. Money, horses, rivers, and leisure hours belong to the state. The state uses them to build up defensive fronts against other states which do likewise.

> the steel industry
> the defense industries
> the coal-mining industry
> the banks

gain profits. The taxpayer loses

> money
> health
> happiness.

The river which separates the small taxpayer from the state is a broad one—a hundred times broader than the Elbe.

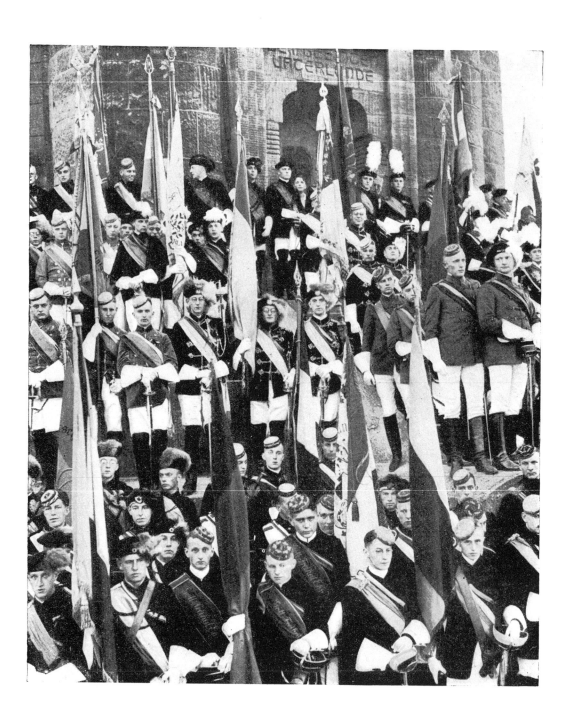

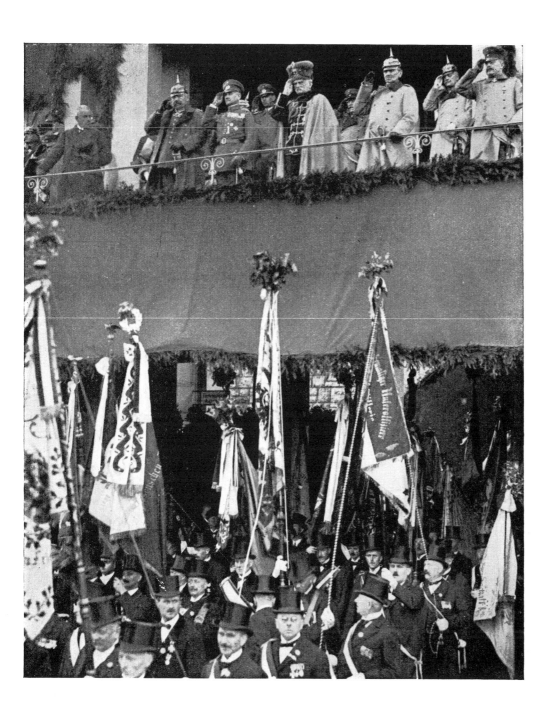

For Some Unknown Reason

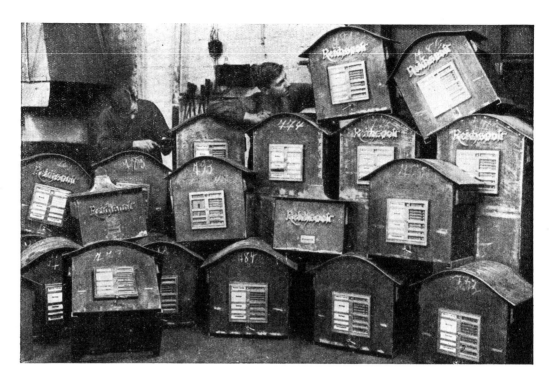

mailboxes have to be ugly. Why?

These mailboxes aren't quite as scary as their predecessors—those excrescences overgrown by ornamentitis. But you wouldn't call these German postal official's creations, with their silly little roofs and clumsy lettering, beautiful. These mailboxes were designed in complete ignorance of the principle that simple things can be beautiful if their proportions are related. Why?

Because the post office mentality is limited. Because the post office has a monopoly. Because bureaucracies, in their limitless self-importance, will take a single step forward only when technology is already miles ahead. Because, Honored Mailbox Users, there is no reason in the world why the state should employ people for life.

Because it is insane to breed apathy, and because the country needs interested workers, not an army of officials. Would you kill yourself at a job, if you knew you were unassailable? I'm an official for life—I'll get my salary no matter what. I'll always have a right to my pension. What would you do? What they all do: the minimum.

The state isn't nearly as sacrosanct as it thinks. The state takes actions, as if it were granting us unusual privileges. It graciously consents to modernize some department. Not much happens though—any well-run business moves faster. A multitude of bureaucrats is death to the taxpayer.

And that's why mailboxes are so ugly.

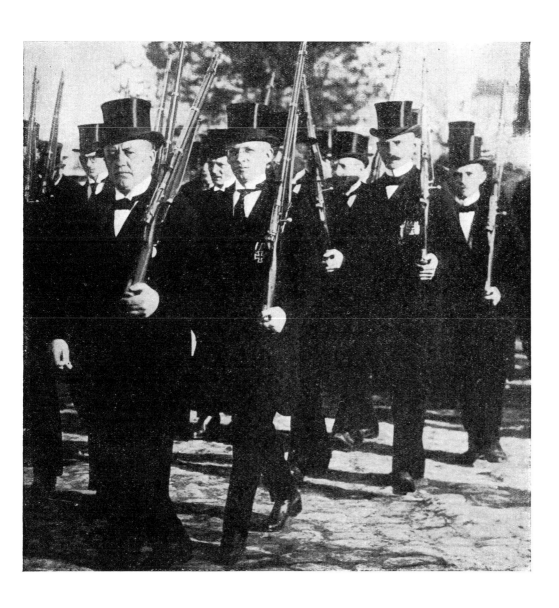

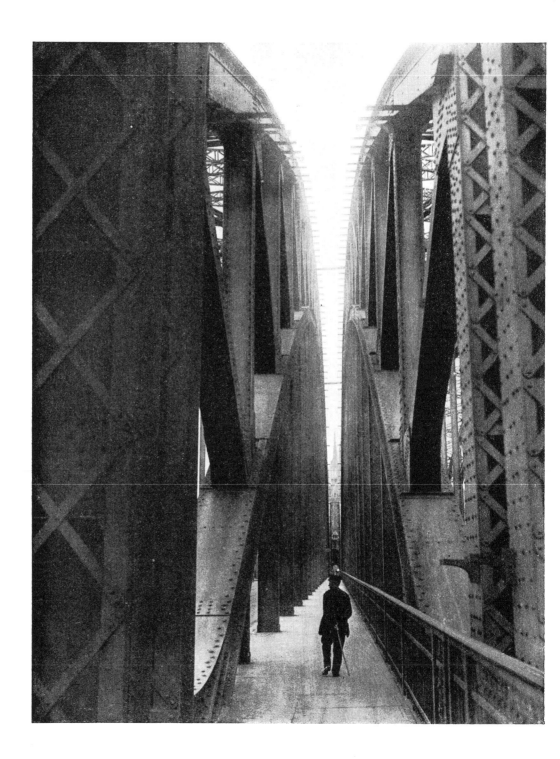

The Bridge over the Rhine at Cologne

Here is the big railroad bridge that crosses the Rhine at Cologne. On one end, our Dear Departed° rides forever in the same place on his monument; they have let him stay, riding, there—one has to be tolerant.

Cars and trains cross the bridge. This way leads to Paris. A man walks on the bridge. A lot has crossed the river here. A whole lot.

Many millions of paper Mark crossed the Rhine here; they were rushed into the Rhineland to keep it from becoming independent. At the time, it hung by a hair.

Today the historians open their mouths and shout about "traitors" and separatists and Mr. Matthes° and Mr. Dorten° (who, incidentally, don't belong in the same pot) and . . . and . . . but it hung by a hair.

If you bend over the railing, you can look down into the Rhine. If you stare long enough, you may see something down there, shining. It is the Rhinegold. A beautiful old story, in which a certain Hagen played a certain part . . .

But just ask where Mr. Hagen° and Mr. Adenauer° and all the rest were, when the question of the Rhineland's independence hung by a hair. The hair from which the province dangled was silver—or, should we say, paper? They held a giant auction. Paris bid, and the autonomists bid, and poverty-stricken Prussia, never excessively beloved by the Rhinelanders, placed a bid too. When the gavel fell, it was revealed that Prussia had once again bought the Rhineland. Old stuff.

Certainly, it's old stuff. But let's not pretend that the happy populace just drips with loyalty to the state. It never has. The Rhinelanders are too smart for that.

Well you see, the bridge is there.

Many people crossed it. Mr. Sollman°, who is so *Real*-political that he doesn't notice his party taking on the role of the old liberalism and being pulverized in the process, crossed the bridge. Fat priests crossed the bridge to survey their territory, while the territory itself has no idea who rules it. The people of the Rhineland have only two passions: beer and anti-Semitism. They keep staring at the handful of Jews, who are only a fly-speck compared to Rome. The cleverest Jews are in the Vatican.

And couriers crossed the bridge, taking thick briefcases full of instructions to the ambassador in Paris. That's a great game. The ambassador can't stand the French; the Foreign Office feeds him rumors; he sits on a hornet's nest with intrigues buzzing under his bottom; everybody contradicts everything and, finally, the French have the last laugh. But you mustn't tell anyone that.

And the pitiable "traitors" who, the courts believe, revealed the sad lie of Germany's disarmament on the other side— they rode and walked across the bridge. When truly, there is nothing that isn't already known over there. We have nothing more to betray.

The wind whistles on the bridge. On this end—not in the picture—they held *The Press*, that marvelous exposition of the world press. You could see everything there, except how newspapers really come into being—who makes them and who controls them. That, you couldn't see.

Yes, below this bridge flows old Father Rhine: surrounded by myth and crowned with *Kitsch*. Workers labor and gentlemen get drunk on its shores. It's a defenseless river and Rudolf Herzog lives on its shores, composing one novel after the other.

Is the man still on the bridge? Yes. A lot has crossed the river here. What a lot!

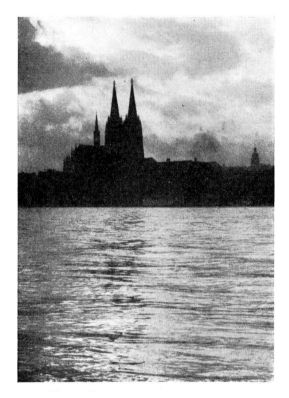

The Time Cries Out for Satire

for Walter Hasenclever°

I

By special messenger:
My Dear Sir:

If you are interested in working on the book for a major literary revue with satirical emphasis, would you telephone our General Director, Mr. Bonheim, today? We will be ready to receive your call between eleven and eleven-thirty A.M. Hoping to receive an affirmative answer at your earliest convenience, we remain,

respectfully yours,
German Literary Company, Inc.
Theater Division
for the managing director (signed)
Dr. Milbe

2

"Hello!"

"German Literary Company."

"Peter Panter,° here. You wrote that your General Director Bonheim wanted to talk to me. About a revue . . ."

"Just a minute . . . Yes?"

"You wrote me . . ."

"Who's speaking please?"

"This is Peter Panter. You wrote me. General Director Bonheim wanted . . ."

"I'll connect with the General Secretariat, General Director Bonheim."

"This is the General Secretariat, General Director Bonheim."

"This is Peter Panter. You wrote that your General Director Bonheim wanted to talk to me. About a revue . . ."

"Just a minute. Well, what's the problem?"

"This is Peter Panter. You wrote me.

Your Director Bonheim wanted to talk to me about a revue . . ."

"You mean *General* Director Bonheim! The General Director can't be reached. He's out of town. If he were here he'd be in an important conference."

"But the letter said it was urgent. A Dr. Milbe signed it."

"That's the Theater Division. I'll connect with Division, Theater."

(Heart Attack)

Finally, an appointment with Dr. Milbe.

3

"Well, here's my thinking on this. We produce a revue. You get me, a revue—that is, something completely new in Berlin! Something really sharp, understand me, witty and catchy—why it's common knowledge: the time cries out for satire! This is really big! So we naturally thought of you— have a cigarette?—no question of anyone else. We'll cast Pallenberg, Valetti, Paul Graetz, Ilka Grüning, Otto Wallburg°— Hello? Say, excuse me a minute—! (fifteen minute phone conversation) Well, yes, where were we? Oh, right. We'll cast Massary, Emil Jannings, Lucie Höflich°— But there's one catch: gotta have manuscript delivery in eight days. That's the way it is. Waiting's too expensive. Theater's rented —have to move: fish or cut bait. Well, that should be right up your alley! The director? Piscator,° naturally. He's accepted already. If he can't, then Jessner.° Or Haller.° Anyway, the best. Depend on us for that. And really go to town on the chansons! No, just a minute, chansons are out: better write songs.° Songs are in. Don't have them too literary, you know? We want to reach all the public—so keep it sort of average—we thought more or less on the order of *The Threepenny Opera*° with a shot of Lehar.° The music? Probably Meisel and Kollo, or else Hindemith and Nelson°—the thing's got to have some unity. Terms? Yes, we'll certainly need to discuss that. Our business manager's in Moabit today, as it happens. To give evidence. You know, I used to write myself—let me tell you, I really envy you. How I'd love . . . Hello?—No, don't leave yet. Have to tell you something else. (Forty-five minute phone conversation) All right, it's settled then. We're agreed. Right. You'll deliver the manuscript on the eighteenth, rehearsal starts the nineteenth. This way out—"

4

"But Dr. Milbe asked me to come at ten-thirty."

"I'm very sorry. Dr. Milbe is in an important conference."

"Then I'll wait. For goodness sake—what are you doing here, Mehring?° And who else? Old Kästner?"°

"What d'you know, Panter? Yes, we're here—met downstairs—don't know how ourselves. Mehring says he's working on a show. I'm working on a show too."

"So'm I. Some joke! The guy never told me he was getting other people. We could have been working together. What a—"

"Dr. Milbe will see you now, gentlemen."

(hissing sound) "Didn't I tell you, not all three together!"

"Ah—yes. Very happy to see you. I asked you gentlemen to come together—easier,

don't you think, right from the beginning? Just as we decided in conference. Sit down, won't you? Well, yes, hmmm—yes, we've looked through your scripts—looked through—hmmm, yes, and I'm really sorry I have to tell you right now. It won't go. Look at it this way—Hello? Just excuse me a minute—(half-hour telephone conversation) Now, where were we? Oh yes—as I just explained to you, gentlemen, that's why it won't work. Mr. Kästner, it's too high-brow—the public won't understand a word. No, we want a good revue, but you know, it shouldn't be too good! And Mr. Panter, it's impossible, impossible, you understand. Now here, you see, here this scene with the canoe, that's good—"

"That's meant as parody. That scene's not serious at all—"

"No problem—we'll do it serious. That's the kind of revue we want. But here, this bit—

Red Rover, Red Rover
Let the bread-man come over

If you think our audience uses "bread" to mean money, you're making a big mistake. *I* know what you mean all right, but listen, after all, this is the carriage trade! And here —about the army—that certainly won't work—and the business about Zörgiebel° has to go—but otherwise, it's pretty— Hello? For God's sake! I'm in an important conference! I don't want to be disturbed! No! Yes! How should I know? Now listen— (half-hour telephone conversation) Well where? Oh yes, Mr. Mehring—please, don't be offended, but I just couldn't understand this. I mean, I don't get it! O.K. So I'm not as literary as you are—but I earned my spurs in journalism too! Listen, I just don't have

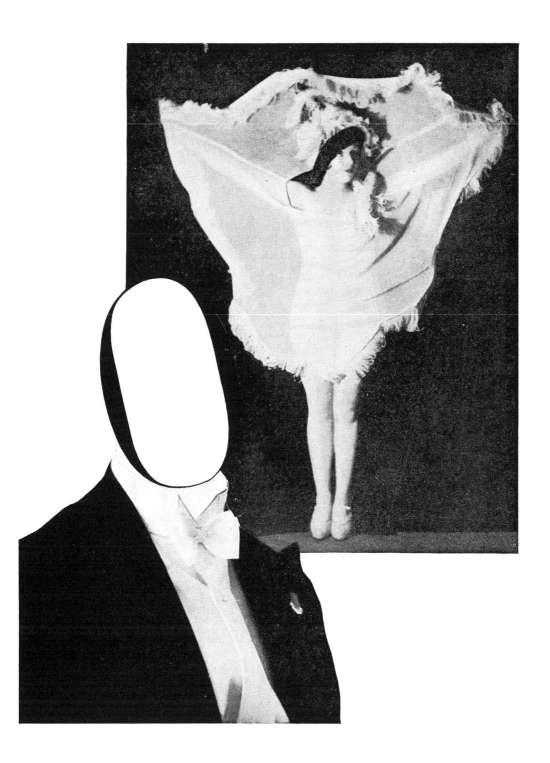

93

the nerve to show this to Mr. Bonheim. Why he'll laugh us out of the office! Look, here it says

The eskimo and broker don't communicate

That's why we can't relate. Oh no we can't relate—

Do *you* get it? How could they communicate —they don't even speak the same language! Well and this bit,

There's a corpse in the old Corps Canal

My little one, my fisher girl—°

Now in the first place, that's old fashioned— and besides, it's disgusting. People want to go eat after the show. No, gentlemen, it won't go. You'll just have to work on it. I mean, some wit, some raciness, some go— I'll be seeing Mr. Polgar and Mr. Roelling- hoff° and Mr. Marcellus Schiffer this afternoon—we've got to push through. Otherwise I may have to get Mr. Ammer° or Mr. Villon or—God forbid—Mr. Brecht. Hmmm. Well, gentlemen, four o'clock with the director. Good bye—!''

5

"I told him I wouldn't do the production under any circumstances. I have no idea why he asked you all to meet in my office. And if I did it, it'd have to be on my terms. Com- mitment! Commitment! Commitment! It has to mention the housing shortage! It has to include the repeal of Article 194 of the criminal code! The relevant problems! And besides, of course, there's the film."

"What film?"

"The film from Bronnen's play."

"What Bronnen play?"

"The play from the Remarque° novel.

That is, the film from the play from the novel—I'm making a sound-film—well, not really, but I do it a special way with a moving staircase,° and Jessner has—Oh, how do you do, Doctor; how do you do, Director Bon- heim. Nice of you to come—"

"Do you have a phone here?"

"Certainly, right over here—"

"Well, let's get going. Here it is, gentle- men. We begin tomorrow. Rehearsal starts —but there's a few things that still have to be changed. Right here—just give me a minute—this right here has to come out. We can't make fun of the law that way— that has to—just hand me the blue pencil— thanks—that has to go. And gentlemen, in case you don't know, we're associated with Bosenstein and Klappholz, and I. G. Farben's right behind them. So jokes like this about the stock market—no, excuse me, we mustn't be that tactless. Let's try to stay nicely within limits. Yes, and here—the part with the 'Internationale'—you could let them sing that if you really think it's necessary. People sort of like it before dinner. Well, now if you'll just make those changes for me—"

"General Director Bonheim is wanted on the phone."

"I am? Excuse me a minute."

(Pregnant pause. Whispering)

"Dr. Milbe thinks, Massary."

"But Panter, you could work that out for us? You always wanted to write for her. No thanks, I'm not smoking right now."

"Here I am again. Yes, I just heard, Emil Jannings sent a wire—he can't—and Otto Wallburg can't either. But it doesn't matter —we'll recast—I've got some really talented young people. (Milbe, I thought of—*whisper,*

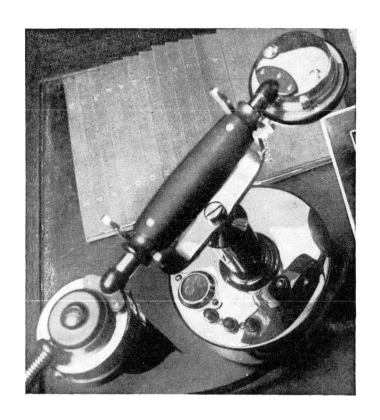

whisper, whisper—) Yes, all right, how far along are we now? With the excisions? Yes. Mr. Mehring, could you tell me what exactly you have against the Chancellor? Why'n't you leave the poor man alone? He's got a hard enough life—don't you agree? No, now look here—traffic in Berlin—now that's a *real* scandal! My car was stopped for five minutes by the clock just now on Wittenberg Square—now *that's* something to write about! Yes, hmm. And the title?

"Yes, the title?"

"Mr. Kästner, what do you call the thing?"

"Heart in the Mirror."

"And you, Mr. Panter?"

"Swedish Punch."

"And Mr. Mehring?"

"Witches' Sabbath."

"Good enough. So the show's *Berlin is Worth the Trip.*° Mr. Milbe will explain everything else, gentlemen. I have another important conference. Good-bye."

"Certainly, General Director. Good-bye, sir."

"Yes, gentlemen, as I said. The show's all set. Now get going on the revisions!"

6

"Stop!"

"Why?"

"How'd that alligator get on stage?"

"I asked for it. Mr. Klöpfer° wants it."

"But that's—that doesn't have a thing to do with the text! It's the marriage broker's song, for God's sake—"

"I'll throw the whole damn part over, if Mr. Panter keeps butting in! I can't rehearse like this! Take your rehearsal to the devil—not me! Here—"

"But Mr. Klöpfer, we're—"

"Shut-up! I'll choke you with my bare hands! If I don't do *something* with this trash, you won't get a single laugh. They'll die on you—they'll rot in their seats! They won't even come! All the nuances are mine, all mine—here the business with the tire and here, second refrain, my wrong exit—and here where I come with the gas mask; and if I can't hold the alligator here then you can—"

"Why not let him keep the alligator, Mr. Panter? It may even be sort of effective? (softly) I'll slip the monster some mineral oil tonight."

7

"I'm not singing that!"

"Well, friends, if you're not going to sing what's written—you really can't just make up your own words as you go along!"

"But why can't we? Of course we can. Or you could write better ones for us, darling."

"My dear lady, you really cannot. As far as I'm concerned, of course. Anyone here can sing whatever they please. But if my name's on the program—"

"Oh I can't do it! I can't stand it! My nerves won't stand it! You can have the whole damn business! Either *I'm* singing here, or else I'm not. And you—you old goat—why don't you get out? Disgusting—after Kate° all day—I'm surprised you don't bring your bedding along to the theater!"

"But my dear young lady—"

"This brothel's just a theater! I mean, this theater—oh, I'm leaving! Act your garbage by yourselves!"

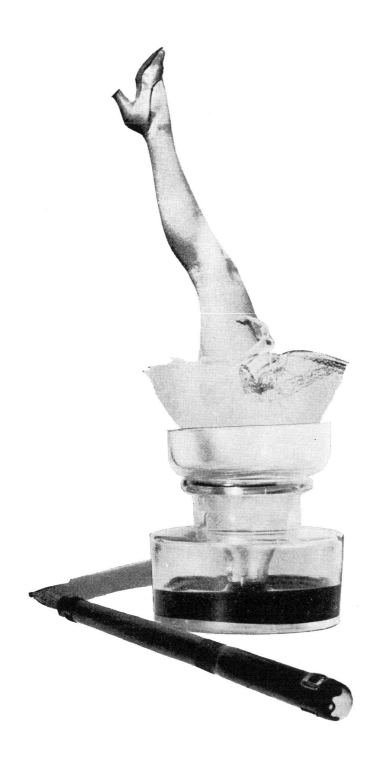

8

"Everybody on—No, stop! Don't start yet. What is it, sir?"

"Milbe, this has to be changed! Here, in the fourth scene. It's impossible! How could you let that get by? Stresemann° frequents the Theater Club—we can't treat diplomatic circles that way! Counselor Moosheimer already criticised me for being involved with this business—the whole thing's starting to turn sour on me—Yes, and the police in scene eight absolutely cannot wear those uniforms again! Put them in those French uniforms from the last show —get Pichorek to look for them right now. And that anti-Reichstag song comes out!"

"But it was really effective at the dress rehearsal, sir."

"What do I care? Who's boss here anyway—you or me? All this revolutionary stuff—I'm a loyal citizen! And that caricature of the Crown Prince in the courtroom scene goes too—get rid of it! It's easy to kick a dead lion—and anyway, why should my entire business connections—on your account—"

"Everybody on stage. Signals."

9

Deutsche Tageszeitung:—This red trash— *Vossische Zeitung:* Our friend, Peter Panter, probably had an off day. It can happen to anybody. But you shouldn't try to write, those days. After the Reichstag scene, which seemed strangely limp, the speaker exited and we stayed, unable to tell what it was all supposed to mean. Next, it seemed as if the actor playing the President still had something to say, but apparently the author's

invention didn't stay the course . . . what French policemen have to do with a German meeting will probably remain the author's secret forever . . . It was not one of his best days. Let someone throw this beast of prey a new side of beef and encourage him to jump through other hoops.

10

(Mrs. Wendriner on the telephone; 10:30 A.M.) ". . . she said she'll call me when she has a new girl for you. You can trust her absolutely—she always gets the cups for me—for the set—she's dependable. Yesterday? At the Majolica Theater, at the premiere of the new revue. No—oo—just fair. The Bois girl° is sort of good, but it's all so mixed up—we didn't even laugh. It was supposed to be something—but we were ready to leave at intermission. Oscar stayed because he still wanted to talk to Paul afterwards—on business. Really, what saved it was Graetz and Hesterberg,° otherwise it wasn't much. Margot called yesterday—why don't you call her—she's going to call back tomorrow—and you ought to call Lina and get her to get in touch with Trudi, about the varnish. Katie is quite satisf———"

11

"It's your fault!"

"Mine? That's fantastic! It's your fault!"

"Who said so from the beginning? Well, who said it from the beginning?"

"Not so much noise here in the office! We won't get our money back that way either! Instead of getting some decent writers! Presber!° Remarque! Ferdinand Bruckner!°

No, you have to get your charming friends . . ."

"You don't speak to me like that!"

"It's my business, Dr. Milbe—I speak the way I like! What are you all hanging around for anyway? Maybe you want money from me? You want money for that? What am I paying theater rent for then . . . just let me tell you something—"

"Aren't you taking a strange tone?"

"You're fired! And you too. I'll use an iron broom here . . ."

"And the same to you! What a shit theater—I'm going!"

"Get out! Personality like a toilet seat!"

"Come on, Panter, let's go!"

"You should . . ."

"I did . . ."

"Why you horse's ass—who said it from the very first day? But nobody listens to me, in my own business—but starting today— why, I'm an old theater-buff, and these idiot boys . . . I'll sell the business, see how you get along without me! I'll go into the film syndicate or back to the garment industry!"

"You're coming down? I'm going up to get my money."

"I wouldn't bother then. No money— just noise."

"For heaven's sake—what's going on up there? It sounds like bloody murder—who's screaming like that?"

"Who? Oh, that's the time. The time cries out for satire!"

German Sport

After debate and vote on the order of the day, the discussion in fact turned to the motion now put forward by the Board of Directors. This motion (as previously reported in brief) proposed that games with professional soccer teams might, after all, be approved by the German Soccer Association if they served instructional or exhibition purposes, or if they furthered the continuation of international relations. The Board of Director's action runs counter to every law of parliamentary procedure. (Subsequent to the denial of the more inclusive motion, it should have been impossible at this point to introduce a limited motion.)

Special and corporate members are not granted the right to display the German Automobile Club emblem on their automobiles—for regular members the "traditional" emblem (the shield of the Royal Automobile Club) which may be displayed along with the GAC emblem, is being revived. Although such members may not use the club rooms of the GAC, they can exert some influence on the leadership of the organization through the Executive Committee. This consists of a president and three vice-presidents, elected from the representatives of the regular membership, but includes by mutual agreement three further vice-presidents elected from the ranks of special and corporate members. These vice-presidents are required to become regular members of the GAC for the length of their term in office.

The German Bobsled Club has made its entry into the Fédération Internationale de Bobsleigh et Toboganning, with headquarters in Paris (F.I.B.T.), dependent on several conditions. Most important is representation on the Executive Board. The GBC felt entitled to set such conditions, because Germany is undeniably a nation in the lead among bob-sport practitioners. Although the F.I.B.T. would be pleased to grant Germany membership, it feels unhappy about accepting conditions set by the GBC. It is to be hoped, however, that the directorates of both clubs will come to a mutually agreeable arrangement when they meet in St. Moritz, and that internationalism will be established in bob-sledding, as it has been in other sports. Furthermore, the General Assembly saw no reasons why Germany should not participate in the Olympic contests, since these are sponsored by an International Olympic Committee rather than by the F.I.B.T.

It has come to our attention that it was the Bavarian Automobile Club, under pressure of strong competition from the AGAC in Munich, which moved to tighten its organizational agreements with other clubs, in an effort to strengthen its position against an inconvenient rival.

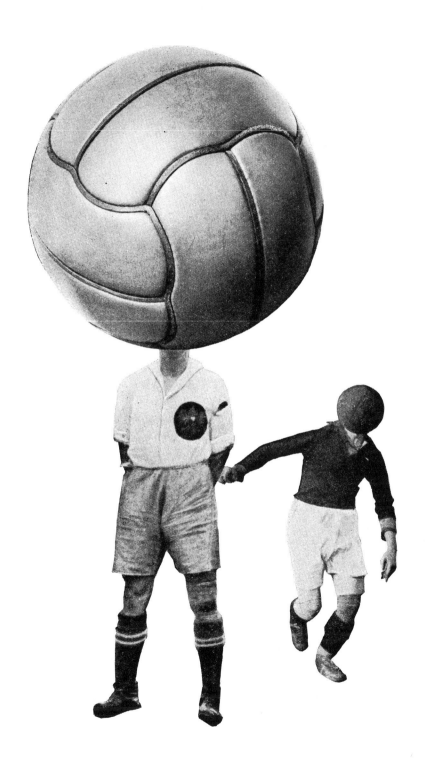

Here in Europe

You send us from the land of Fords
some pretty dreary human exports.
Your middling middle-class average
is flooding Greece and crowding Paris.
    Loud and boastful and unable
    (in spirit) to keep their feet off the table,
    their annoying omnipresence
    tells us every other sentence:
       "But in America we . . ."

You have good and bad. You have two kinds of law
(for rich and for poor) in America.
There's Lewis and Mencken. And then there are
the servants of the almighty dollar.
    Your America has republicans
    and stern and bloodstained Puritans.

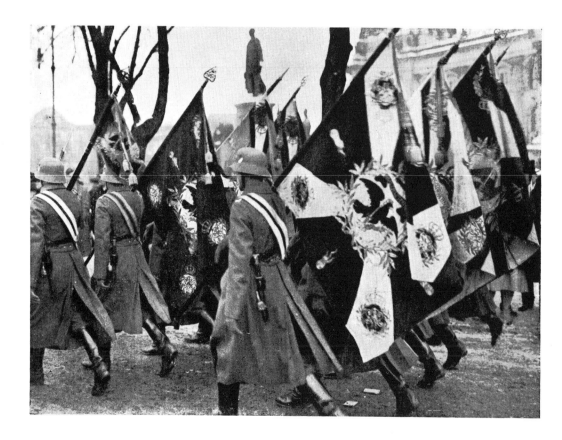

Your country's rich and young and strong
but that doesn't mean you can't be wrong
    sometimes, in America.

Here in Europe we have women,
not harem-ladies with no guts in them,
and we don't build special railway cars
for people with black skins to use.
    A man without money is forgiven
    and even allowed to go on living.
    In Europe people live quite well
    without ever going to Sunday-school,
    and almost no one stands up in church
    to make the kind of vapid noise
        that they do in America.

Of course there are plenty of you, who know—
but the rest hear what the trumpets blow:
they hear the flattering choruses
of their newspaper. Think they're first-class—
    Don't listen, worker. Let them be,
    the vanities of the bourgeoisie.
    Their passports, their flags, and their parades
    are only so many cement-façades
    —The boundary between worker and drone
    cuts straight down the middle of every nation
        in your America
            and in our Europe.

Where is the lion?

(a picture puzzle)

Hannover, 16/8/20

[Translation of handwritten note:]
His Majesty, the Emperor and King, did not desert the flag. I indignantly deny this slander. The Emperor left us because his people deserted him. It was impossible for him to die a hero's death at the head of his troops, because a truce was in effect at the time.

If His Majesty had remained with us, civil war and the resumption of hostilities with the enemy would have resulted. The unhappy ruler wished to spare the Fatherland both these consequences.

It is easy to kick a dead lion.

von Hindenburg
General Fieldmarshal

The lion has a monthly pension of approximately 50,000 Mark.

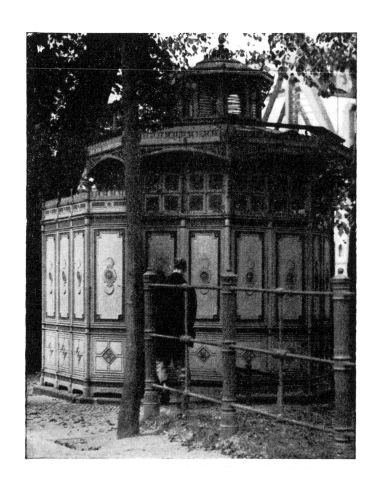

Excuse me—I'll Only be a Minute

The tin architecture of this little house reveals a whole world. The tin monster can tell us the story of decades. About citizens who felt that it was somehow indecent to have private needs in public places; about a society with absolutely no feeling for craftsmanship; about a society with no sense of beauty. Consider the miserable ornaments that spot the empty spaces like bird-droppings. Consider the meaningless angularity of the arrangement—ornamentation around a barrack's gate looks something like this. Although we admit, grudgingly, that something like a "sense of beauty" is said to exist, we basically reject it. The visual and olfactory image have been treated with absolute equality. But this little house is not the most grotesque example of architecture in Wilhelminian Berlin. Our cathedral is quite attractive too.

Things have gotten better since then. Although some of these little houses are still much too coy, and people in Berlin still think it's a good joke that there aren't enough of them. Paris ought to set us an example; on the other hand, there, these places tend to be of a really baroque ugliness. And dirty besides. But in Berlin and many other German cities you still have to "make a phone call" or order a cup of coffee, when you say, "Excuse me—I'll only be a minute."

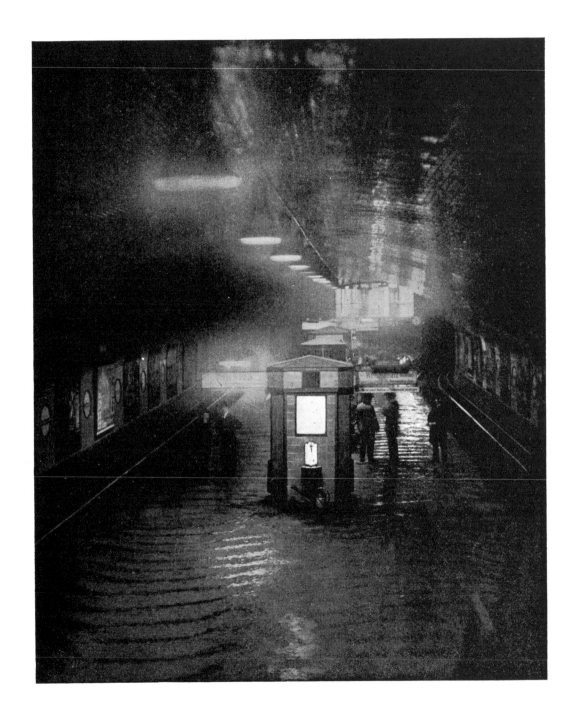

Subway

It doesn't look like this at all—only the
photographer ever sees it like this.

It does look like this. It doesn't.

You don't see the subway station if the
train has just pulled in, if you're in a hurry, if
you're riding with a pretty woman. You
only see it when you're bored and forced to
wait for the next train. Then the tired eye
stares, half-conscious, at the advertisements
—Chlorodol—the car in the social register
—scrub your feet with Abrador—you see
everything and nothing.

You see the subway, and perhaps the
whole huge city, the way the photographer
saw it, only once.

When you suddenly sense what it is you
live inside. A landscape. There can be a
special moment when you experience the
city like a forest, like mountains, like the sea.
You'll see the subway lights reflected in the
bright tiles and for a moment feel something
almost romantic—you can smell subway,
and feel the big city in your veins. Then the
black tunnel becomes a strange tube in-
habited by giants, and the stone walls and
the hundred rolling cars that you hear only
faintly, all seem to press down on you: you
know you're in a cellar. But the feeling
passes very quickly. And you're standing at
Kloster Street Station again, carefully feeling
for your ticket. You hope you haven't already lost it.

Start

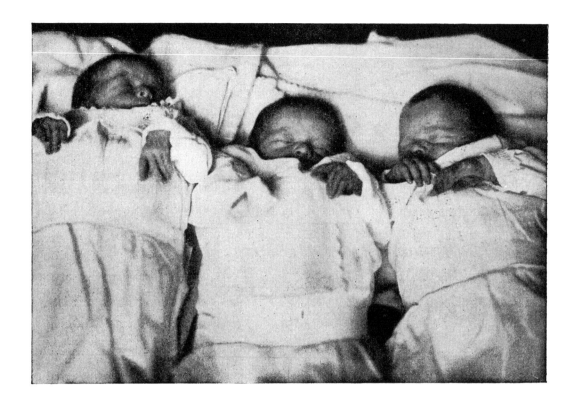

You'll be a government bureaucrat
    whaa—whaa—!
You'll have a belly big and fat,
stamp-collecting be your hobby,
you'll love authority and the army—
    hush little baby,
    hush, don't fret,
    there are dumplings in the oven
    but you can't see them yet!

You'll be a business boss-in-charge
    whaa—whaa—!
Your top is bald, your bottom large.
Your jaws rattle socialistic,
your heart beats German-nationalistic:
    hush little baby, don't fret.

District-Court-President, some day
    tickle—tickle!
You'll know what all the lawbooks say.
Your kisser duel-scarred and grim,
you'll doze through hearings in a dream.
    Tickle—tickle—tickle!

You're going to be a great, big whore.
    Nim—nim—nim!
You'll love the paying customer.
If you get caught, you'll know the score
and pay at the nearest abortion-store.
    Nim—nim—nim!

You'll be the leader of a union!
    Hush little baby, don't fret.
At first you'll be shy and unassuming,

but once you get to know the rich
you'll leave your comrades in the lurch.
　　There are dumplings in the oven
　　but you can't see them yet!

　　Hush-a-bye-boo—
　　Well, what about you?

And you, my boy, will grow up to become
a decent proletarian.
You'll keep your sympathy for your class,
　　and grow up human.
　　　　Hold fast, hold fast—!
When you're big you'll understand this
　　thought:
Each class determines its own lot!

Constricted Horizons

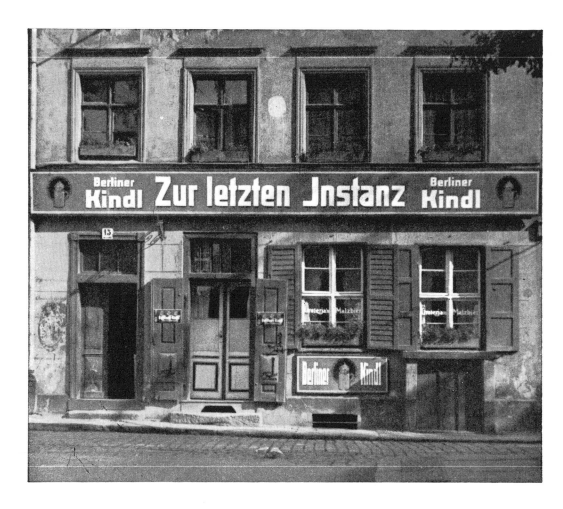

Little people, big noises. Listen at the door of this bar near the courthouse.

"And then he said, a midwife aint no corkscrew by a longshot!" "Whena judge jiggled his head I got the message, that was it!"— "If ya weren't so bullheaded stupid, ya'd given y're evidence like I told ya—but no, ya gotta do it your own way . . ."—"I'm wondering the whole time, like how come the other side, they never take up this point . . . well, now I got it: it's this way, because the judgment against . . ."—"And if I have to take it to the Supreme Court I want . . . (another beer, here) . . . I want my rights, or I'll know the reason why."—"But he can't! The guy can't do it! After the court order you gotta first get a expert's opinion, and then we'll see who in this neighborhood makes inferior quality boots!"—"Listen, even the counselor says . . ."—"Now just a minute. There's no decision on the books, regards of the value of the object in dispute

—here, whyn't you read it yourself—here's the law . . ."—"And then he said, a midwife still aint . . ."

The rest of the world has disappeared. The people have eyes and ears only for plaintiff and defendant. They are controlled by a spirit like that which animates the following announcement from a small, provincial newspaper:

I beg to deny the slanderous statements issued from the cellar.

Respectfully,
A. Grimkasch

The man forgot that there was more than one cellar in the city; he was aware of only one. His. *The* cellar. The people in the bar near the courthouse see only *the* cellar.

When the average German goes to court, he becomes a Roman after two sessions. And no wonder—given the way the legal process is carried on: pointlessly scholastic, wholly counter to simple human understanding, strictly according to an entirely non-German idea of justice. It's a far cry from the original boots or libel. The issue turns into destroying your opponent: flatten him! Root him out! Get him—with war cries! People tremble with the tension of it, and everybody's face is flushed: thousands of Kohlhaases° carry on around the courts. That right and justice may prevail! And how much self-righteousness is mixed with the right!

It's not just that the law is half-insane, inadequate to our economic conditions, and unable to protect the weak. People also expect too much from the law. First, they always expect a particular law to fit "their case" exactly; then, they always believe— oh charming German misconception—that they themselves are wholly and completely in the right, while their opponent must be wholly and completely wrong. "For heaven's sake—that's as clear as Grandma's dumpling-broth!" At the last judgment in heaven they'll still be appealing the verdict, because there's nothing the law-abiding little man puts more faith in than the court of last resort.°

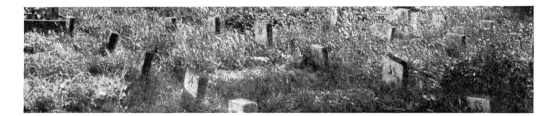

Dream on the Shores of
the Neckar

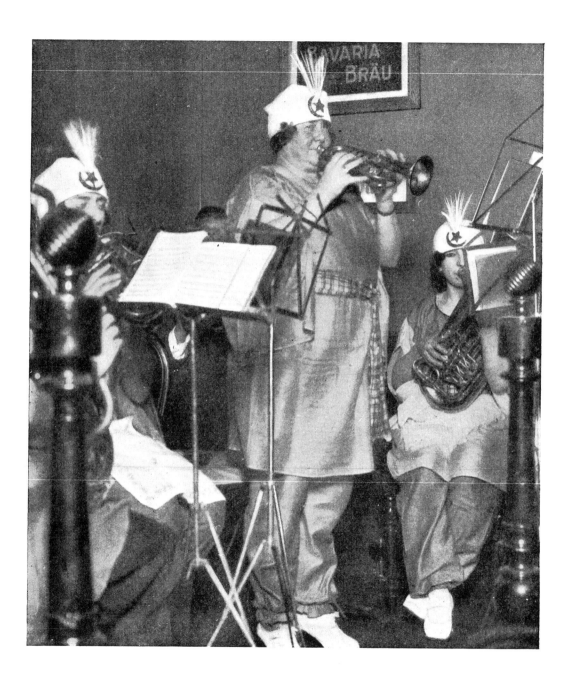

No other people has anything like this. This
gigantic woman, unassailable by water or
land, stands like a fortified island in an ocean
of beer. She represents many a German's
fondest dreams: strikeback ability, strength,
460 pounds of fleshly delight, and a conjunction of harem and drill-ground that ought
to fulfill every desire—hurrah!

Actually, there's another side.

These trumpeting women are surely not
sitting here for their own amusement. It's
no fun, working in a smoky beer hall until
two in the morning and making this kind of
music is harder than chopping wood.
But would working in a factory be
pleasanter, or better paid? The fat woman
with the trumpet probably has two children
and household worries. She plays for an
audience of sailors in Hamburg—sailors
who have had the last remnants of romanti-
cism knocked out of them by the big shipping
companies. Ahoy, ahoy—Bavaria-bräu!
We're not licensed for dancing, but the
waves of pleasure break, roaring, on Ger-
mania's breast, somewhere on the Reeperbahn at twelve-thirty in the morning.°

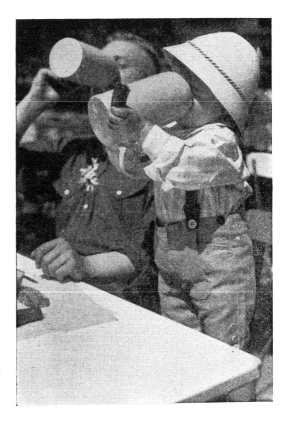

The Furnished Room

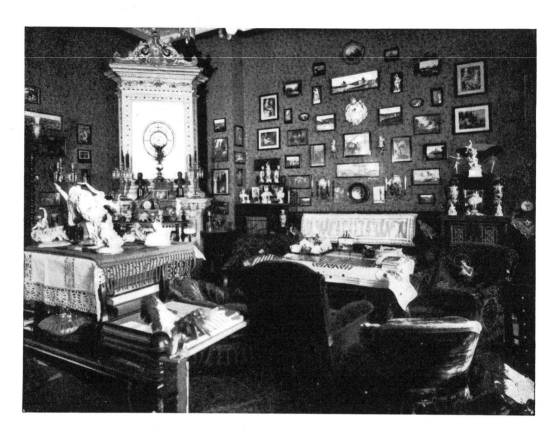

Spoken by the landlady:
Oh no, my tenants can't remove things—
I can't let them move pieces! It stays this
way—the room's decorated beautifully!
And every piece a memory! Here's the Isle
of the Dead by Bölkien° that my husband—
may he rest in peace—brought me from
Gollnow after our honeymoon—and this,
this is real china, also from my dear departed.
On Wings of Song, it's called. And this here
is Rome, including the Pope's palace, and
this was from Auntie Frieda, and here's the
Wartburg,° and this here was a bet. My son,
Max, won it at his bowling-club when they
bet who could hold a glass of beer on his
head the longest and he won, and they gave

him this. Constancy's Reward, it says. And
this here's Henny Porten° as Camelia lady,
and these are the candlesticks from my
wedding, and that's me as a young girl. Thank
God, I wasn't so bad! And that's Hindenburg, and that's Learn to Suffer Without
Complaining—the gentlemen should know
they're not renting from just anybody. And
no, that's the way it is, I can't let my tenants
remove the pieces!———

116

The Display Window

I

Sermon by Chaplain Untermoser, delivered in Upper Tupfingen, Lower Bavaria:

". . . but a pious Christian muuuuust recoil in horror from the city of Berlin, where the lusts of the flesh mount on high, and the devil throws his temptations in the straight path of Man. Therefore, I say unto you, beware the swinish Prussians who suckle at Sin's bosom and disport themselves licentiously, for aye and aye! But the Lord will not permit them entry into the gates of Paradise. Amen."

II

The Berlin hairdresser in front of his display window:

"I guess it'll do like this. Maybe move the middle one up a little, like so. Think they'll make a stink about it at the Station again? But go and find less cleavage! I order the most conservative ones he had—then the police act like it was God knows what! Well, all right, pull that lace up a little on the middle one maybe—let sleeping dogs lay. You know, that stuff about women's breasts —it's not such a big deal these days. But I'm not going to get worked-up about it, all right. If you want to see dirt, you can find it anywhere."

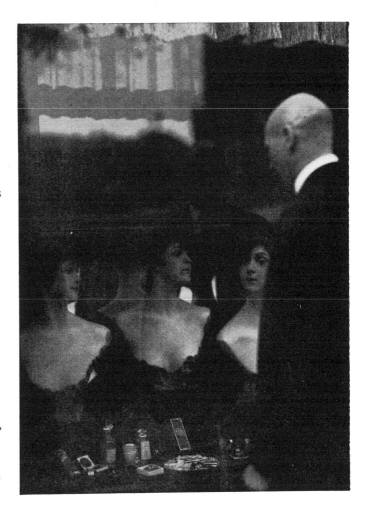

Never Alone

A rarely mentioned, tragic part of proletarian life in all countries is that the worker can never be alone. Here is his life: born either in a hospital ward, surrounded by other mothers in labor, or at home in the bedroom in which the family—and the roomer—crowd around him. That's how he grows up. The family, here, though, is better

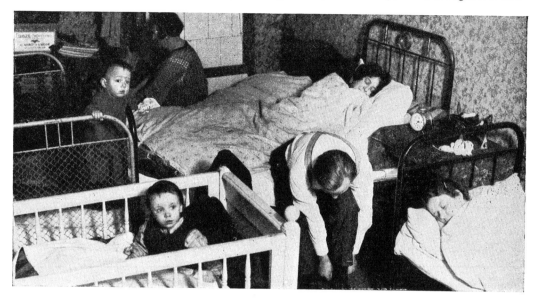

off than many, because each person has his own bed. People who live in such rooms live continually inside the lives of others. They are never alone. This is the worker's

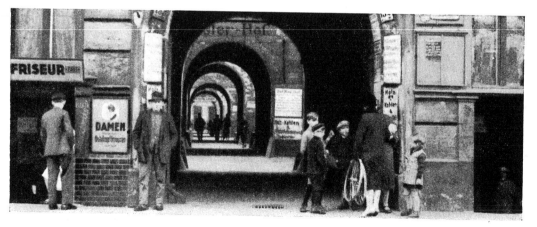

world. This house, for instance, has sixty courtyards; six hundred families live here; they go in and out, call each other and scream, cook and do the washing, and everyone hears everything. Each shares the other's lives in the most irritating way possible. That is, through the ear. A worker's ear gets to know silence only in prison, in solitary.

He works with others in the machine shop; he's with the others in the mineshaft and on the construction site. Never by

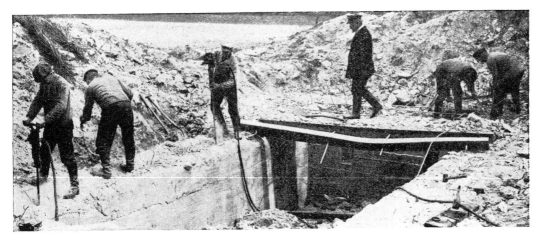

himself. Nor does he have privacy at home.

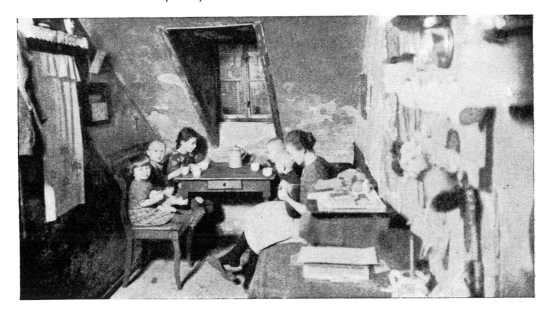

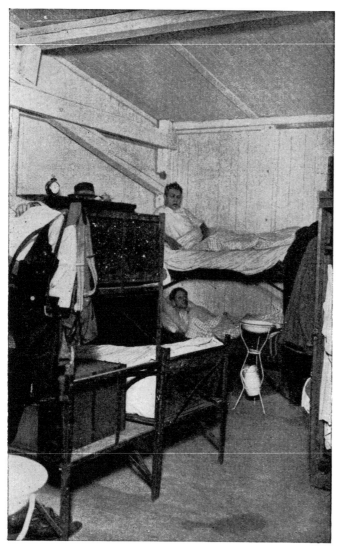

When he dies, he dies either in a greasy hole like this, or in the hospital. Still not alone. Let's not say "the people are used to it." That's like the waiter serving oysters. "Yes," he says, "oysters die as soon as you open the shell. But they're used to it." A life with never a moment to oneself is not a life to get used to. It is life lived to its end in continual deprivation.

The need for occasional privacy is not a false bourgeois ideal; it does not deny solidarity or the communal spirit. French peasants like high walls around their property; German small landowners have an immense preference for fences as symbols of ownership. But a new generation in Russia has brought a different spirit into the world and, it may be, that people there feel less enmity towards each other than has been usual. Of course comrades should feel solidarity, should live and work together. But is there a single human being, aspiring to be more than a labor-producing, re-producing, and digesting machine, who would not wish sometimes to be alone?

Not only bodies are pressed together here. Souls are sweated out. With so little room, the spirit pulls back—narrows, feels threatened, and shrinks.

People living under such low ceilings need enormous courage and energy if they are to go on hoping, working, and keeping alive the idea of class struggle. This room, as a

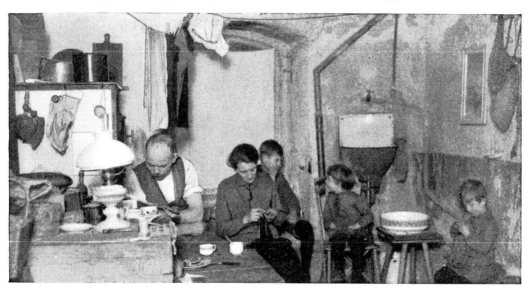

matter of fact, is not even a room, but an abandoned laundry. The man couldn't pay his former rent of 68 Mark and they threw him out. His wife and children are never alone either.

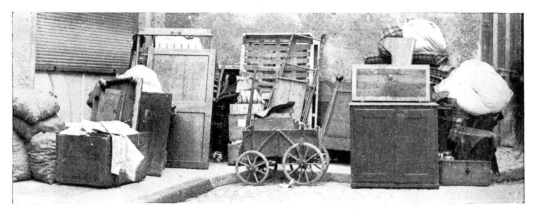

Human beings cannot be alone in 1929, as they used to be in castles and hermitages. Apartments are stuck together like cells in a honeycomb.

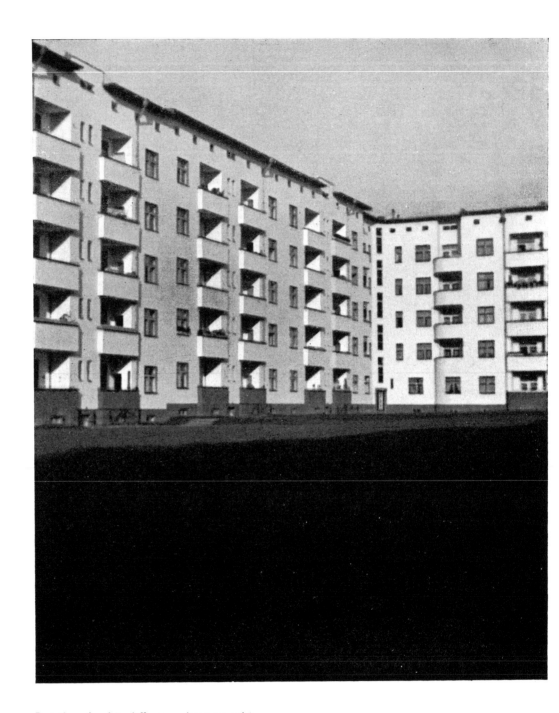

But there's a big difference between this

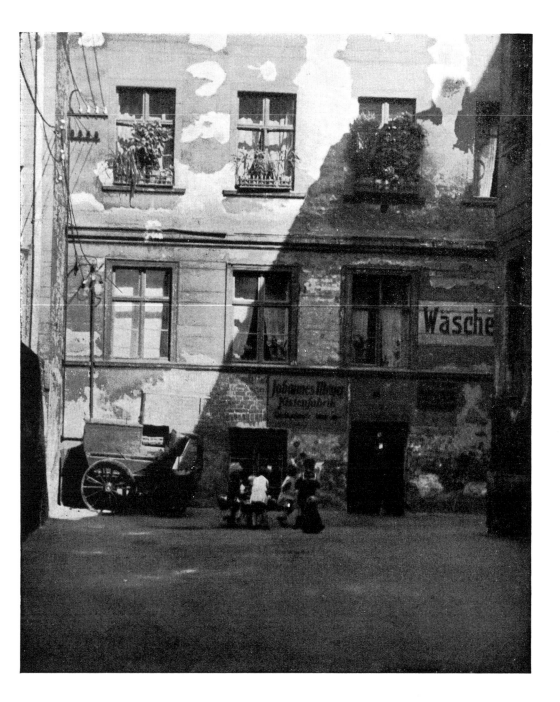

and this.

Unless the worker is very strong, his consciousness wholly permeated by the idea of fighting for his class, the world he in- habits is only this one, of the "third building across, to the right, second courtyard."

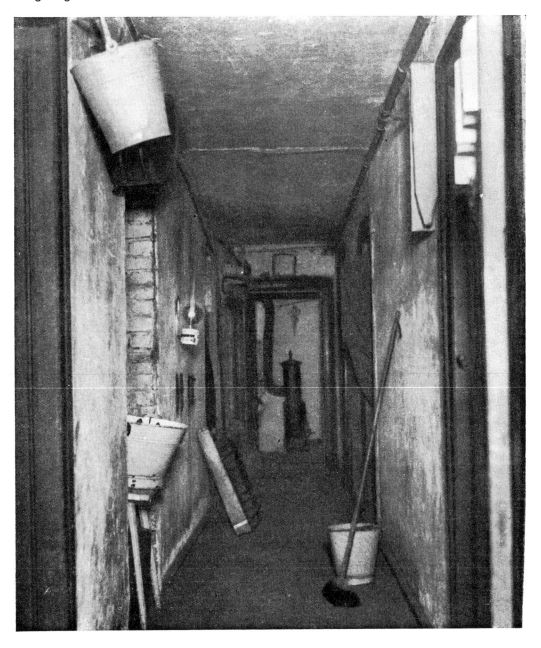

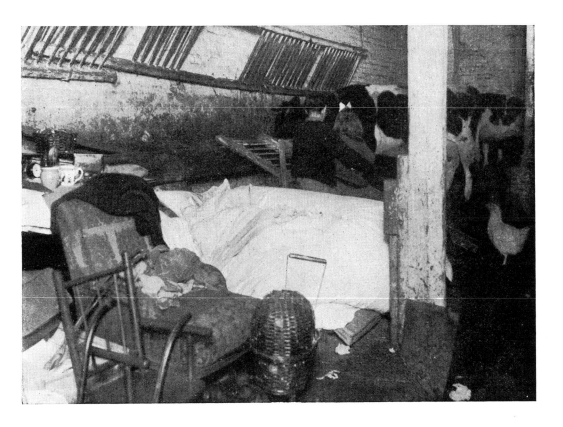

The passage is always dark and much more than pails clings to its walls. Mean gossip, small-mindedness that comes with need— the people growl at each other because they live too close together. Attempts to build something like a "home" in stables like this one are pitiful. Neighbor struggles against neighbor in constant fighting, in spiritual pain and bitterness. These people are never alone. And if other people will not take pity on them, perhaps the animals will. This room in the north of Berlin shelters a whole family. A horse rooms there, too, but it didn't get in the picture. It had gone to work.

Is this how German workers live?

Large numbers of them live like this, and do their work, and long for a different life. And wear themselves out, and suffer, and are never alone.

The People's Theater in
Berlin

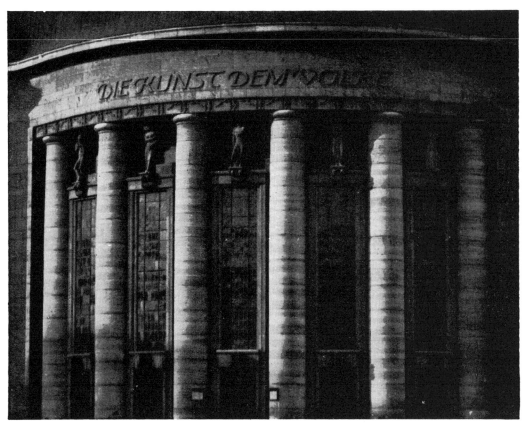

They gave us workers' pennies
to illuminate workers' lives.
    That was our job.
Our first programs said it:
"Proletarians! We'll stick together!"
    See inscription.°

A lot of water went down the Spree.
We did Hamlet for our comrades,
    often enough.
Farces were easy,
and comfortable plays that risked nothing.
    See inscription.

You mustn't laugh at the government.
Our plays are about peace: peace on earth,
    and organization is the secret of success.
Capitalism is about killing people.
But we're respectable,
    we admire purity and grace
      just like the censors.
    ART FOR THE PEOPLE?
    Whose art?

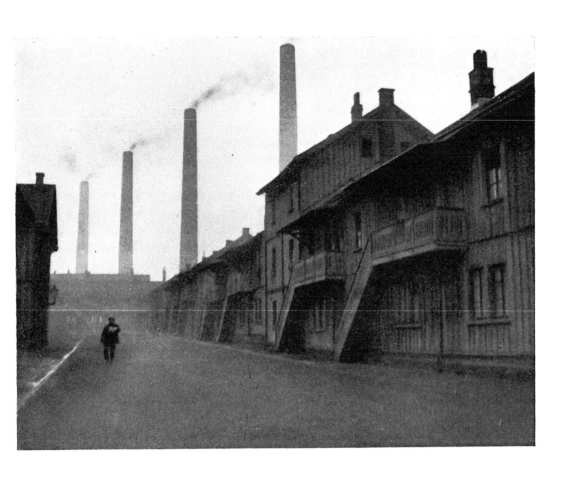

127

A Left-Handed Intellect

"He's a ghost from Munich."
—Alfred Polgar

It was a pleasant good-bye to Berlin: six weeks of Panke° and one evening of Karl Valentin.° The account balanced perfectly.

I got to the theater late. The hall was already warmed-up and full of laughter. The performance must have just begun, but the audience seemed animated and happy— the way they usually are after a good second act. A man who wore a pasted-on wig and looked like one's idea of a provincial comedian, sat—surrounded by the suburban kind of band—at the podium on the stage. I studied the scene closely but—with the best will in the world—found nothing to laugh at. But although the man hadn't said anything, the people laughed again. Suddenly my eye was drawn to the first row, down front. There was someone I hadn't seen before. He was the one.

A lattice-thin, tall fellow with spiky, stalky Don Quixote legs and angled, pointy knees. He had a little hole in the trousers of his shiny, threadbare suit. That hole—he rubs at it earnestly. "That's not going to get you anywhere!" the stern bandmaster tells him. And he, quietly as if to himself, "A little cleaning fluid would do it!" He speaks quietly—all his dramatic techniques are quiet. He is gentle and fragile and as irri-descent as a soap-bubble; if he suddenly burst, no one should be surprised.

The bandmaster knocks, "Ready! One, two, three—" but with just $\frac{1}{16}$ of a beat to go, the skinny trumpeter stops to point a serious finger. "Your tie's slipping out." The bandmaster angrily stuffs the thing back in place. "Ready! One, two, three—" the merest blinking of an eye separates the band from its crashing BAM—the tall one puts down his trumpet and looks around. The bandmaster signals a stop. What's the matter now? "I have to cough," says the tall one. Pause. The orchestra waits. But now he can't cough. One, two, three—taratara! It starts.

And here begins the oddest comedy we've seen in ages. It's a devilish dance of reason around both poles of insanity. He's a little man, this trumpeter, with a union button and a union scale, a neighborhood bar, and a gossippy local. He's worried about his con-tract, and also out for an advantage. "Play exactly what's there," the bandmaster says. "You don't catch me playing more," answers the union-member.

Up on stage, the curtain doesn't want to open. "Somebody go to the draper's," says the bandmaster. "But immediately. Tell him to stop by sometime when he has a moment." Done. The draper does have a moment: he comes by, bursting into the soprano's act. He climbs the stage with his ladder—"How I loved you in those days, oh my life" howls the soprano—and he unpacks his tools. He pounds, he hammers, he adjusts. But keep your eye on Valentin! You can't hold him! What's happening? What is it? He's in the grip of simple-minded curiosity. Fiddling away, because that's what he's paid for, he rears up and climbs on his chair and cranes his two necks—his own, and the violin's. He climbs down, walks through the orchestra, and climbs up on stage; there, he mounts the ladder right behind the workman; he fiddles and looks, works and watches the interesting things going on—I have to think back ages to re-member such laughter in a theater.

He's a left-handed thinker. Once, years ago, he preached in a Munich beer-cellar.

128

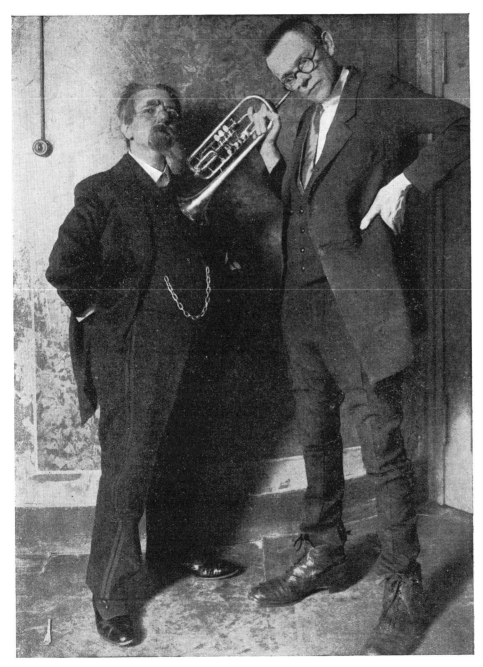

Lisl Karlstadt   Karl Valentin

"The day before yesterday I took Grandma to the opera. To see *Lohengrin*. Last night she dreamed the whole opera again. If I'd known that, we wouldn't have needed to go."

But this pen-pusher, who improves his daily bread with a little moonlighting, suddenly lights up, transparent, and other-worldly: he begins to glow. Do those long legs still touch earth?

A difficult problem arises: how to carry a bass drum from one end of the stage to the other. Valentin gets the job. "I'm actually a trumpeter," he says. Trumpeters don't transport drums. But—well—he ambles over. He can't do it alone. A colleague is supposed to help. And here it gets really moonstruck. "Get that drum over here!" the bandmaster calls impatiently. The colleague mumbles in his beard. "You mean right now?" The bandmaster, "Bring the drum!" Valentin, "Andy wants to ask you, when?" Right now. They circle the drum for a little while. Finally Andy says he has to stand over there—he's left-handed. Left-handed? Drum, bandmaster, and theater performance are all forgotten—left-handed! And now, almost Shakespearian, "Left-handed, are you? Completely left? Writing? And eating? Swallowing? Thinking?" And then triumphantly, "Andy says he's left." How much on our own side of experience we are. How distant the other is—how different. How separate we are—how far apart! Fellow-being? Parallel-being.

No doubt we're reading-in the philosophizing. Certainly Valentin had no theory worked out in his mind. But we'd like to see another comedian into whose work one could read such significances. You don't get ideas like this watching Mr. Westermeier.°

At the end of the performance there's a discussion of coincidence—a back and forth of little magical sparks, flashing from this oddly constructed intellect. He'd been walking along the main street, *Unter den Linden* in Berlin, with Nebenmann, and they'd been discussing a bicyclist—and just at that moment, one rode by. This to the theme, coincidence. The bandmaster rages. That's no coincidence. It's nonsense. Thousands of bicyclists pass there every day. "Well yes," Valentin says. "But that one came then." Imagine thinking, and writing and rehearsing, something like that!

The comedy of unreal potential statements—the monstrous analysis of the sentence, "I see that he isn't there." (What is touched on here, is beyond speech.) The simple foolishness of this irrational wit is unmarred by censoring human intelligence: he drinks beer from a mug at intervals, chews something he had saved in his pocket, reflects with his index finger, and takes his small private pleasure in the bandmaster's mistakes. Hans Reimann once circulated the question, "What would you wish for if a good fairy granted you three wishes?" Karl Valentin answered, "One, eternal good health. Two, a personal physician." A small soul.

And a great artist. Let's hope the Berlin producers don't get their hands on him. The secret of this primitive ensemble is its powerful naiveté. That's the way it is—if you don't like it, don't go. But God forbid training him to sing duets, or comic chansons. Not with the kind of evil-tempered, hag-ridden, nervous producers and directors at rehearsals, where no one listens, and the first response is always: No. Not with the whole unpleasant mess of Berlin types who insist that they know what the public wants —and for public, read their own not very pleasant circles. Not with these overworked and cheerless characters who can't laugh at anything simple, "Because it's been done." They themselves have certainly been done often enough. But Karl Valentin has been done only once, because he's a rare, sad, unwordly, incomparably funny comedian, whose mind works left-handed.

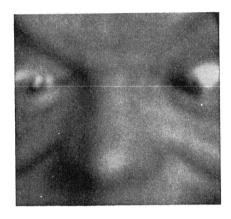

The Parliament

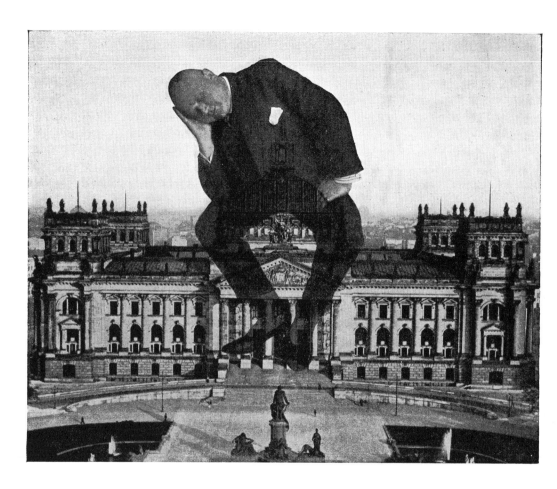

Were the Socialists elected—
　　forget it!
Has old Daddy Wirth° defected
to the left, or been ejected—
knuckled-under, as expected—
　　forget it!
Did Nationalists look cross-eyed at
and beat-up on a Democrat—
Who got his eyes blacked in debate—
　　forget it!
　　　forget it!
　　　　forget it!

Posters pasted up all over—
　　forget it!
Bilge for the city, bull for the farmer:
"A time for decision!"—"How long must
　　we suffer?"
　　forget it!
Do you know the fellows in the wings
behind the scenes, who pull the strings?
Joes in the beerhalls working up sweat,
making propaganda, haven't mattered yet.
　　forget it!
　　　forget it!
　　　　forget it!

132

So party-officers go to pot—
        forget it!
And pretty Rudi° gets his job
(it won't be cheap) in the cabinet—
        forget it!
Shipping, banks, and industry
decide the fate of Germany.
        The election's a cheap vaudeville act
no matter how worked up you get!
Go ahead, vote! What the people said
        forget it!
            forget it!
                forget it!

The Lighting-Crew

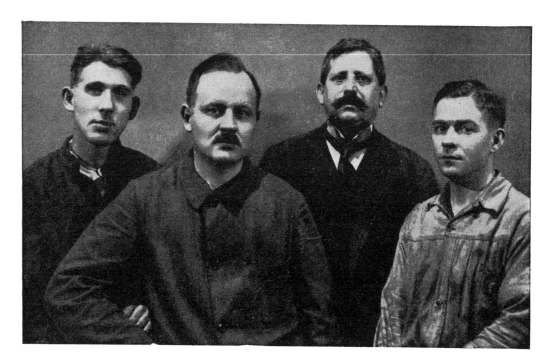

You can't get excited in theater. Where'd they be without us?

Not just anybody, see, can work lights—it's a skilled job. Takes training. We have to take the lamps apart and lay the wires, and like that—yeah, sure, they do that other places—but the theater, see, can really get to be a nut-house.

Actors are O.K.—but you know, they're crazy people. Man, even when they do make a rehearsal—always getting insulted. I ask myself, what's their trouble? It's always something. The part's too small, or then maybe it's too big—or say the director says, "At this point, you walk to the other side." He'll make a production out of it! He's not gonna walk! He's gonna stay right there, on this spot. He'll go complain to the producer! Well, I ask you—what's it matter to him? No—it's all showing-off.

We went on a real party the other day. Otto had a few—we went over to Beetz's first—and he stood some rounds, celebrating the old girl's birthday. O.K. good enough. Then I look at my watch and say, "Listen boys," I say, "Come on, or they'll start without us." So, we cross over, and I see Otto's walking kind of funny—sort of weaving—well, you'd hardly notice—but we got the idea. Anyway, we figure he's got experience—he's a pro—a few aren't going to hurt him. Good enough.

And so König comes on. Paul König, you must've heard of him. A famous man. The director thinks a lot of him too—and that night he's doing Hamlet. And we always have to be on the look-out for the place with the ghost. So we're all right there, at the switch in the wings, when I hear König call over to Otto. Sounds something like "lit—

lit—blooey—" And Otto points to his chest, like he means, who me? But he keeps on, "lit—lit—blooey—lit" and the others hear it too, and we all start laughing. But Otto's mad. "You mean me?" he yells real loud. Well by now the prompter's already shushing us, but Otto goes right on, "Who, me? What's the big idea?" And the fireman's looking by then, what's wrong, and König takes off and just walks right over to the wings. Shouting—we thought the audience heard him—"Get the blankety-blank blue spot lit, for Christ's sake!" Otto's so scared he switches on the red. Nobody noticed, anyway, and when it's all over, they made up. And after, König stood a few rounds at Beetz's too. And then when Otto went home, let me tell you, he was lit!

Well look, a theater without a lighting-crew—that's a shot without the beer to chase it.° Something missing."

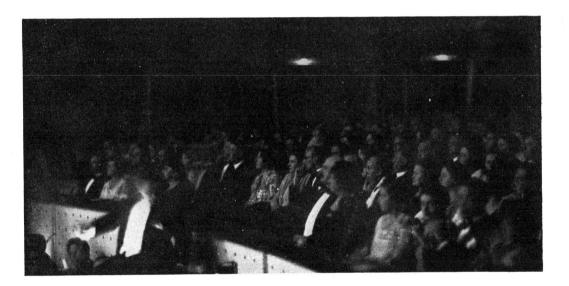

Hard of Hearing

Actually, I don't hear so good. Doctor says to get 'em rinsed—it'll come along. But it don't. Some days it's better, but if it's rainy and wet, it's like I don't hear at all. Yes. Those gadgets. That's no answer. You stick this black cookie on your ear, with a cord. People yell something at the bottom, and I'm supposed to listen on top. Naw—that's no way. What's that you say? Does it bother me? Well, there's times it does sometimes.

There's this thing with Kyritz on the Knatter, see. Poor land-owners, you know, that demonstrated? And it went to court, and the judgment was, everybody gets suspended sentences. You say that in plain German, nice people don't do time. What do you think? Take the workers, like in the Ruhr? Now if they do stuff like that—I hear about it—But I never hear nothing about no suspended sentences. I don't hear so good. It's a pain!

See, and then there's the Socialists, right? They got in the government, yelling in the elections before: Down with the battle-cruisers! Not a penny for this fleet! And like that. What d'y say? Yeah, and soon's they're in: Whammo! My Hermann's gonna O.K. the whole shebang. Well, that scream-ing at rallies! Man, did they sound off! But now . . . I keep listening; I prick up my ears. I can't hear nothing. It's my hearing . . . must be. A pain!

And then, you know, they just got through celebrating. Tenth anniversary, remember November ninth? Well, I remember pretty good—I was a noncom in them days. On the western front. When Erzberger° came through and they cheered him when they found out who he was. Yup—he did his job too. Funny—with tough jobs like that they always put in a civilian. Yeah, and they said the French really had it in for him, but Hindenburg, he said, you go. I'm sort of busy right now myself. And if you can't help it, accept. Just accept the terms, he says. Well and then, when they get after Erzberger afterwards, I sure thought, now he'll come out and say something—put in a word at least for the guy. After all. But listening and listening—I never heard no such thing. What he says is, I never shook this guy— Erzberger's—hand. You call that, a *demento mori*.° Yeah. But now I never heard no more about it. Must be because I don't hear so good. It's a pain.

How's that again? The ladies? Oh my old girl—she's a little deaf on one side too. Works out pretty good—if I don't hear everything she says, is just as well. But I want to tell you something: Too bad God didn't put lids on ears, like he did eyes. People'd feel better. Not that I need it—my damp days they can talk and talk—dedica-tions and in the Reichstag and sermons and for and against the annexation of Austria, and whatever they say, when they don't want to miss their connections—I don't hear nothing. And anyway, I could go in the army—be a officer, or get to be a judge. They don't hear so good either, when you want to tell them something. It all evens out. What's that you say? You want me to make up a sentence with "to hear" in it? Sure thing.

I think about those idiots in charge, and I've had it—up *to here*.° They never learn nothing. Well, yeah: Good Night.

136

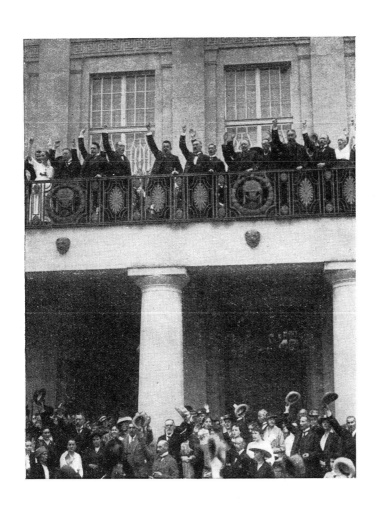

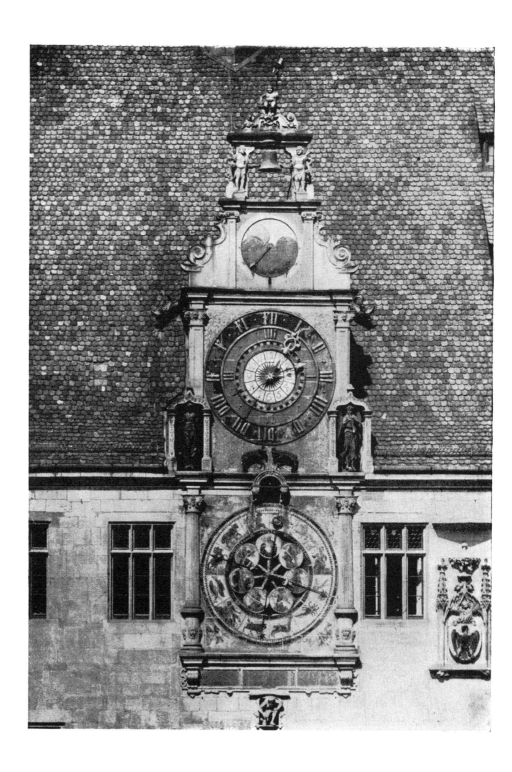

Little Exercise for Bells

The clock strikes 12—
God keep all good readers safe!

The clock strikes 1—
Hilferding° talks on. The Center bargains . . .
                              each to his own.

The clock strikes 2—
If England needs a roughneck, Germany never says, No.

The clock strikes 3—
Shouting "Long live the Republic!" is noncommittal, but noisy.

The clock strikes 4—
Once upon a time there was a republican *Reichswehr* officer.
                              (clock stops in terror)

The clock strikes 5—
We have too much good sense, here in Germany, to drive
ourselves crazy with nit-picking legalistics—
The clock strikes 6—
So why don't we just open the jails, and shove in—
The clock strikes 7—
those dirty Communists out on the street to demonstrate—
The clock strikes 8.

The clock strikes 9—
It must be broken?

Things have to move backward here—progress isn't German.
The clock strikes 10—

The clock strikes 11—
Martial law can be beautiful if the right condition's given.

The clock strikes 12—
May God still keep all readers safe!

Once upon a time a Socialist, really got the bosses hurting—
That made the clock strike 13!

The clock struck 14, 15, 16, 17, 18, 19, and 20—
We want to liberate our German brothers in Danzig, but Danzig isn't having any.

Thus day and night the clock strikes the hour,
according to its nature and its job up in the tower.
    A loudmouth in public,
    a beaten fink at the bone—
    That's the sound of the German carillon.

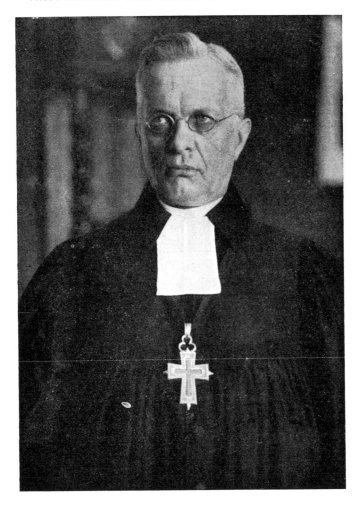

V.I.P.'s

We have decided, faced with a pressing need, to form a new organization: The German National Very Important Person Rental Agency (GNVIPRA).

Taking into account the fact that Germans occur only in groups, and that these groups tend to subdivide, until such time as the separate parts recombine in National Organization,

And furthermore, that the main function of such organizations is to hold meetings, congresses, yearly conventions, and organizational celebrations,

And that the presence of a Very Important Person is an indispensible part of such meetings;

The GNVIPRA undertakes to unify and coherently to organize the present confused and self-duplicating efforts in V.I.P. rental services. As follows:

The following basic equipment is available to borrowers:

V.I.P's	(town administration)	1.50	(hourly rate)	
,,	(county administration)	1.75	,,	,,
,,	(state administration)	3.00	,,	,,
,,	(national administration)	4.80	,,	,,
,,	(cabinet level)	5.10	,,	,,

With orders involving larger shipments, we will include two or three members of parliament for appropriate states at no extra cost. Bavarian officials 10% reduction.

One V.I.P. shipment will include all materials necessary for proper use:

Original frock-coat
Black trousers
Laced, square-toed boots
Furry top hat
Stand-up collar
Eye-glasses

Lessees are requested to take good care of borrowed material, and to return V.I.P.'s in the condition in which they would hope to receive them. Drunken merchandise is nonreturnable.

In general, our Agency deals only in V.I.P.'s equipped for speech-making. On special request, however, we can furnish a stoppered version at slight extra charge. Our V.I.P. is equipped to deliver an address, guaranteed to be absolutely inoffensive, at point of delivery; particular care is taken to avoid offense to Monarchists and the Republican Opposition. The speeches delivered by our V.I.P.'s are carefully pre-tested to guarantee lack of content.

All speeches contain short, universally comprehensible quotations from our esteemed classics—up to 1860.

The V.I.P.'s must be set up in a place of honor at all proceedings; they require police escort, or cordons, so that they may reach their places without interference. V.I.P.'s photograph well, and can be equipped with a white cross in the stomach region for efficiency in recognition.

We are confident we have rendered a valuable service to the German Nation and its organizational life with this summary of our agency manual.

Since the government has moved almost completely out of its offices and into the convention halls, we in no way hinder the administration. But the taxpayer learns that the administration sees it as its first duty to refrain, on festive occassions, from confronting those difficult situations for which it was originally created. We are happy to furnish references on request. Our most recent engagements include:

Appearances by the Secretary of Education during August:

6th: Weimar. Annual meeting of the Ladies Swimming Teams of decidedly Jewish Philatelists.

12th: Neu-Jannowitz. Annual meeting of the Association of Agricultural Proprietors, followed by dancing and tax-strike.

19th: Bitterfeld. Congress of Catholic Young Women's Associations to further Upper Bavarian Banana-Culture.

24th: Berlin. German Student's Convention.

25th: Berlin. Republican Student's Convention.

The Chairman of the National Committee for German Gymnastics, Permanent Secretary August Lewald, is engaged for the next two and a half years; in urgent cases, however, one of his frock coats may be borrowed.

We have discarded the principle of dispatching only specialists to the various conventions; rather, we encourage our V.I.P.'s to address themselves primarily to those subjects about which they know absolutely nothing. As follows:

Mr. Stresemann on music.

Mr. Hilferding on pharmaceutics.

Mr. Groener on lubricating oil.

Mr. Breitscheid on foreign policy.

All the above, on German culture.

We shall be most pleased to be recommended among your acquaintances and associates, and remain

Respectfully yours

German National Very Important Person Rental Agency

Borowsky   Heck°

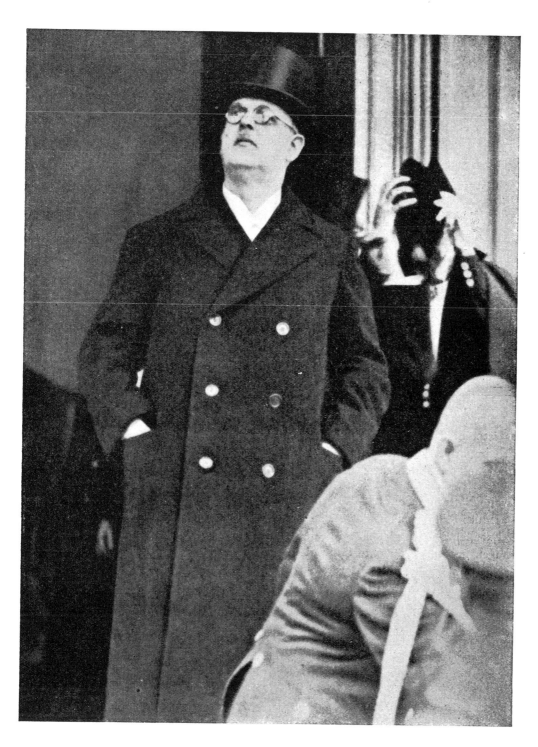

The Need

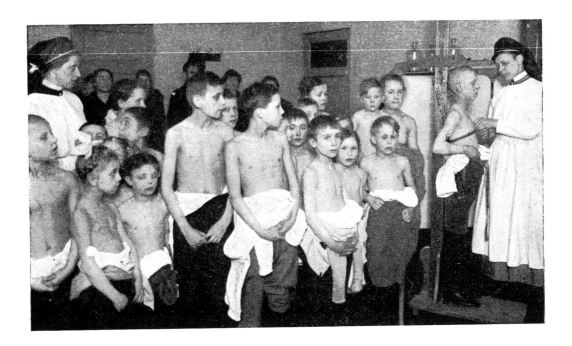

The children in this picture are taking physical examinations, given by a state insurance company. Oh, the poor children! Why, they're emaciated! What's the matter with them? They look so needy! Shall I tell you what these working-class children need?

"Second Battery: Fire!" Boom!

"The general staff moves into the castle. Make sure you requisition a piano for His Excellency, the first thing. There doesn't seem to be one in the castle—the others must have taken it out—damn piggishness! There's got to be one in the village somewhere—a concert grand, what do I know? But if it isn't here by three this afternoon, you're transferred!"

—In honor of the visit of his Royal Majesty, the Crown Prince of Bavaria:

MENU
Appetizers
Clear chicken broth
Pike in dill sauce
Very early green peas . . .

"I don't give a damn! In enemy territory I haven't heard of consideration! Cut down those fruit trees—all of them! All along the road. We have to hurt the enemy wherever we can! And don't forget to fill in the two wells at the village gate . . . !"

"Halt! A hundred eggs go to His Excellency! Put all that in a box—well, no—just wait here until the launch leaves for Kiel. We'll put in the two big crates of provisions too. For His Excellency's private kitchen . . ."

"Second Battery: Fire!"

"Well, so requisition it! What are you

waiting for? Just write:

> 28 place settings
> 2 carpets
> 100 panes of glass (40 × 80)
> 32 assorted pots and pans

"Third Battery: Fire!"

"Four tanks, of course. No, listen, we'd better make it eight. Eight tanks is safer. As long as we're ordering . . ."

"Fourth Battery: Fire!"

What the children need?

That's what they need.

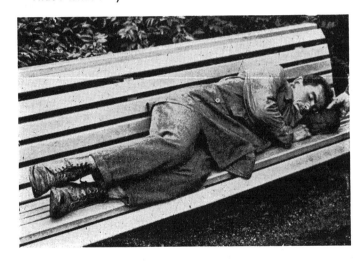

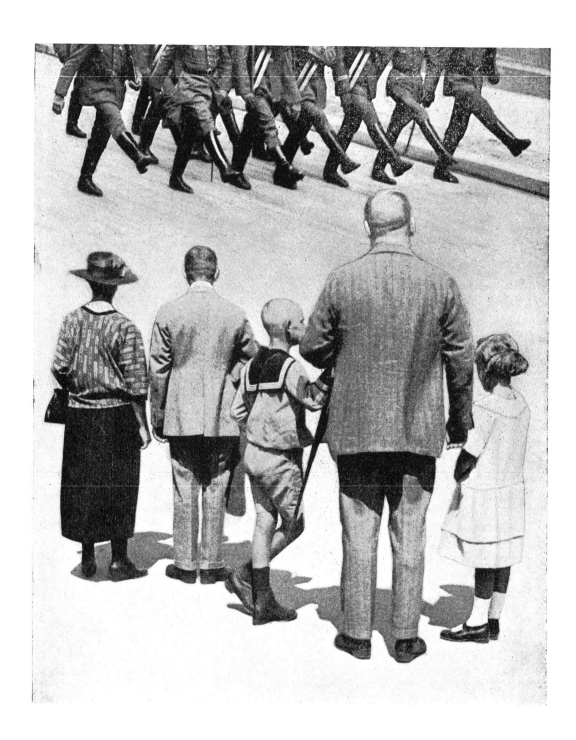

The Head in the Forest

A nineteen-year-old was condemned to
death and executed by the members of a
para-military, patriotic group. The body was
left in a shallow grave in the woods, but a
pack of hunting dogs has uncovered the
head.

The head speaks:

Just past Buckow, west of Old Lake
about thirty paces off the road
I lie buried.
My clothes have rotted into the ground—
it's swampy. Near here, I volunteered.
We were brothers-in-arms, we were patriots—
Oh our badges—our broad-brimmed colonial hats—

And somehow, it suddenly happened.

Yes, Lübecke attacked my honor
and started it all. Called me an informer.
He couldn't stand it, that I was pure—
he was always behind the barn with Völckner.
And he grabbed me one night, around half-past eight
to try it with me. But I'd been straight
and decent for the past two months—
one of our Order's few clean-living ones.
So I said, "I'll report it to the corporal—"
I felt so peculiar—
such a strange feeling—

Oh the ants! the ants! the ants keep circling!

Such a strange feeling: Lübecke knew about Bern
(that thing with Rathenau, with Fischer and Kern)°
and Lübecke was the real power in our *Bund*
and he always did exactly what he said.
So I missed next roll-call. And Lübecke
must have told more lies about me
just when Bröder was away, in Halle, on parade—
because he'd been an officer. That made it bad.
And they planned an action for the woods,
far enough away—a shot wouldn't be noticed.

There were four of them suddenly, without a sound—
not Lübecke though. They closed-in, and one said:
"You're no German! You traitor! We know you!"
Then I felt the blow.
One called, "You dog! This is the end!"
And I fell down. They trampled around
on me—and yes, their last words were
"Don't worry. No trouble. We're clear!"

I always went to church. Don't forget me, God.
Don't leave me unavenged. Let them find out!
Lübecke's to blame! And time is passing,
my mother's worrying about what happened—
They must be searching all over the world—

Dear God, now that it's too late
I can tell you—I know the secret.
It's France we have to fight! We'll be victorious!
The whole world's always been against us!
My swastika, God: it says everything I felt:
Deutschland, Deutschland über alles!
Über——— ——— ———

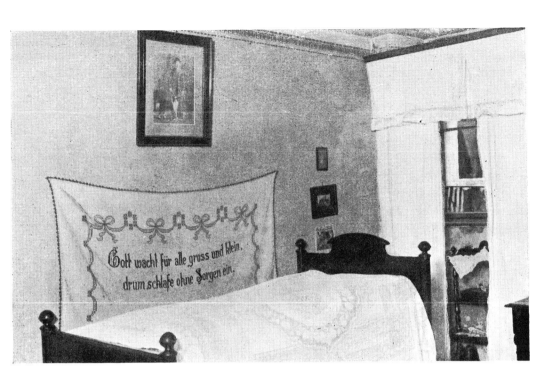

Gott wacht für alle gross und klein,
drum schlafe ohne Sorgen ein.

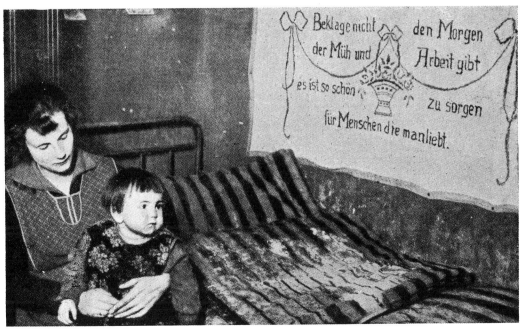

Beklage nicht den Morgen
der Müh und Arbeit gibt
es ist so schön zu sorgen
für Menschen die man liebt.

149°

German Judges

It's no longer accurate to say we face a crisis of confidence in the judicial system. A crisis is the uncertainty out of which decision comes: life or death—yes or no. The German workers have decided. No.

All trials, like everything else in this political world, are necessarily political. But we could ignore that, and still assert that we have no legal process that arrives at justice in specifically political cases.

No one in his right mind believes that an administrative decision—for example, the decision to deny someone a liquor license—is made for objectively valid reasons. The decision involves no more than the use—by an authority—of the power vested in it. The applicant who is denied a liquor license is not discredited by the denial; neither does the denial prove anything about the actual need for licensed liquor-dispensers. Such a decision is only an administrative measure, decided on grounds of expediency. No objective conclusions can be based on the decision—the actions of managing authorities tell us only about the nature of the authorities themselves.

We should look at the judgments which our courts have handed down in political cases during recent decades in exactly the same way.

The courts' decisions should be seen only as moments in the battle, as the clash of opposites in the class-struggle. The great majority of the politically enlightened German people has lost confidence in this political judicial process. And for good reason.

Neither a solemn edict pronounced by the smooth Herr Simons,° nor the amusing notion of appointing "Justice Department Press Representatives," could change the situation. We've had enough of official press conferences. We know the kind of lying that went on both during and after the war. It's an interesting old German superstition to hold that a thing is justified if you explain the technical processes involved in it. All that legal hocus-pocus carried on by bureaucrats with delusions of grandeur is irrelevant; when the Justice Department Press Representative asserts that one may not prejudice a case, he is irrelevant; when references are made to supposedly existing regulations, they are irrelevant. Especially since the recent Supreme Court decisions, since those pitiful attempts to use high-treason trials to cover expressed hatred of political dissidents, the people have rightly lost confidence in the judicial process.

Our political trials thus cannot be discussed seriously—nor do I believe that the rather lukewarm battle now being waged by that decent and well-meaning journal *Die Justiz*, edited by Mittermaier, Radbruch, Sinzheimer, and Kroner,° will serve any useful end. Their program isn't bad. They say that German judicature today overvalues legalism and undervalues humanity. It's a delicate enough statement, without excessive specificity. And even if one of the editors, Radbruch, had not failed in practice, and if another contributor, Wolfgang Heine,° were not a politician as evil as he is incompetent—it still won't work! Although I always except the one and only, Ernst Fuchs° of Karlsruhe. Let us honor his memory!

Reform of the German judicial process is unthinkable without the repeal by law of the recently established doctrine that a judge cannot be removed from office.

Let's see how a young, idealistic, future-oriented law-clerk enters the judiciary.

The new boy is always in the wrong. It's as true in the professions as in railway compartments. At first his position is weakened by technical inexperience and by youth, but most by the fact that the others have been there longer. During the "breaking-in process" the phrases, "We've always done it this way" and "I would strongly advise you to" play an important role. For the moment then he is powerless. And next, he is infected with the sneaking poison of routine. If he does reach an independent, leading position, it will usually be too late. We know from experience that if he rebels against the system, he will not long remain in the profession. He may possibly be allowed to stay, but then under such humiliating and difficult conditions of work that he will give up the unequal battle and resign.

The judiciary, as a matter of fact, utilizes a process of selection more pitiless and more dangerous than that used by its close spiritual relative, the Army. Each clearly perpetuates only itself: the group chooses only new members who fit into its definition of the group. New members always conform to the pattern, cannot be heterogenous. The process that begins before the examining board, goes on, through the fine sieve of the personnel-department chief. Our class of judges is the result.

The German judge views the world through distorting spectacles: his point of view is that of the middle and upper bourgeoisie. Life above or below this line of vision is not represented among the judges, and has little chance of being understood in

court. And further, the judge usually conforms to a particular type inside the middle bourgeois group—that is, the frozen, wooden, constricted type who is surrounded by hundreds of taboos, hemmed in by the boundaries which he has erected for his own protection, and nourished by a criminal psychology which old Villers° in his *Briefe eines Unbekannten* formulated rather well. "Every *Thou shalt*, means, *I can't*. Every *Thou shalt not*, means, *I am not permitted*."

Judgments of a group are always—and must be allowed to be—unjust. In social criticism we have the right to take the lowest type within a group, the one just barely tolerated on the edge of rejection, as the group's representative. Whoever is accepted is part of the group's definition. Thus the corrupt judge who can be bought is not typical of German judges. If one existed the profession would cast him out without mercy. We could not hold the profession responsible for him. But to place a laughable emphasis on something that ought to go without saying—that is, that a judge does not take bribes—diverts us from matters of real importance. A man is not virtuous simply because he does not abuse children.

We could say the following about the average German judge: very few intellectually sensitive persons could establish communication with him during a trial. Such a person will reject the judge's sentimentality, and his attempts at moral preachments; he will reject the judge's conceptions of decency and his idea of humor; he will reject the judge's response to pain, to pleasure, sorrow, and authority; he will reject the pictures the judge hangs on his walls, his wife, and his vacation plans

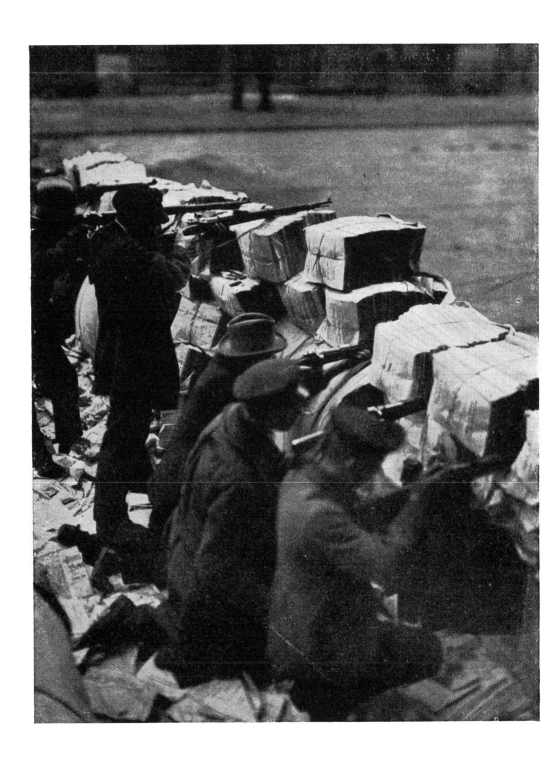

—the very air he breathes, the beer he drinks, and the children he rears. He rejects the judge's soul, rejects his caste, rejects his world.

The assistants with whom the judge surrounds himself are indicative. With the blind certainty of sleepwalkers, justice department officials select jurymen and lay assessors according to their preference for pinheaded, self-important members of the middle class: underlings who, as Polgar phrased it, delight in playing top-dog for a change. Like surrounds itself with like and a man like you or me, confronted with the likes of them, confronts a foreign world.

Why is no one brave enough to say that hundreds and thousands of self-employed and professional people, hundreds and thousands of enlightened workers, have nothing in common with our judges? Light-years separate them from us. Any one of us could more quickly establish some kind of relationship with any experienced lawyer, any progressive German nationalist, with any intelligent export salesman, in spite of vast political differences. The presiding judge of the district court is much farther away. We speak two different languages, follow entirely different lines of thought. Imagine, sending the victims of our courts on a trip to—for instance—Scandinavia, along with their judge: the trip would be an unbroken chain of false notes and dissonances from the first moonrise to the last porter's tip. They would always be incomprehensible to each other—speaking at cross-purposes.

If a person of our kind does enter the judiciary, he is so isolated that he is forced to assimilate very quickly. Schulz, the pro-gressive, can remain himself as a law-clerk; by the time he reaches the rank of district judge he has become unrecognizable. If we were to accept the principles of democratic thought, we would have to reject the spirit that animates our judges, and demand our full right to be represented there, where decisions are said to be handed down "in the name of the people." Although the people have nothing to do with the justice now among us.

But let's say our judging caste believes in dictatorship. Let's try to follow the reasoning of some judge who—having passed a few examinations and having the approval of the members of his caste—imagines himself all-powerful. We can demand something of him too. At least we should be ruled by the best among us. The best of us might—in the interest of the good—have the right to tyrannize over the majority. But what are our despots like?

Kindly look at our judges, and listen to them speak. Whole literatures have been written in vain; our trees do not bloom for them; both our laughter and our tears are strange to them. We are as far from them as we are from a distant planet. We have nothing in common. And we want nothing in common with them.

Our judicial reformers, often recruited from the ranks of lawyers, suggest reforms which are translations of their own thoughts into the judges' foreign tongue. They are only tactically clever attempts to propitiate the God with sacrifice, to quietly dent his sword a little, or to divert him from throwing one of his lightning bolts.

There can be no reform from the top. A progressive minister of justice shines like oil on the waters, but water and oil don't mix. And reform from the bottom is impossible by peaceful means. We should have to ignore the simplest relationships inside a social group, to believe that speedy, basic, internal change can ever take place without external pressure. Thus our judicial process, which a single class imposes on subjugated classes, will not be improved slowly with good advice, and cannot be corrected gently and piecemeal.

German judges are guided by a basic misconception about what they call penal law.

The state has no right to punish. Society has the right to protect itself against those who endanger its peace, but anything further is sadism, class warfare, a foolish arrogation of god-like powers on the part of men, the most abysmal injustice. Suppose that your nerves are steady enough to witness a German trial. The arrogant tone of the judge, the contemptuous treatment given the defense attorney, the prima-donna play of the district attorney, the rudeness of the marshals, will all combine to persuade you to answer the judge's moral sententiousness with "just the opposite!" The moral maxims uttered in the courtroom are on a level with the average confirmation-class instruction; they give off a musty odor of barracks, petty officials' homes, and small-town minister's married life. In this context the victim of a theft is partly to blame if he has "left his possessions carelessly lying-about." In this context sexual intercourse outside of marriage is immoral and an incriminating circumstance against the accused; in this context not being a German citizen leads to heavier sentence. All in all the motivations

that lie behind sentences conform to the lines of that popular drinking song in which it is asked, "Why drink?", and the answer comes back, "Every possible reason." Psychoanalysis, and research into every level of sexuality, have brought down the hollow pillars supporting the temple hundreds of times—it counts only outside of the courtroom.

You have to hear how the prosecutor would rather choke than say "Frau Grassman"—how it's always, "the woman, Grassmann." You have to hear how judges treat defendants if you want to discover from what source the muddied springs of justice flow. You have to see judges encouraging policemen to treat the public badly; you have to hear how "resistance" is punished—not as a criminal offense, but as sacrilege. You have to hear the subtle or silly questions used to influence witnesses in their testimony, and how answers are forced on witnesses, and how prosecutors intimidate independent witnesses, and how cavalierly the judge treats them. No one recognizes the first law of a hearing: to keep still and listen. And after all, there is very little real opposition. The judges are used to dealing with tricky lawyers who follow rigid tactical rules: a dead victim is always represented as a monster, but someone who survives an attempt on his life is always referred to with respect. The judge is habituated to discourse with people who accept the principle of his power and hope to circumvent it. Thus the judge never needs to reflect on the basis of his activities. Little functionaries twist life into accord with the penal code and—even in Berlin—one is often driven to wonder where in God's name such people spend their spare time. Can they really have so little idea of what life in the world is like, so little knowledge of what the customs of the country are? They're all watching the clock. Twelve-thirty. Finish-up, finish-up.

Let's add the judge's absurd belief that an acquittal signifies more than a defeat for the prosecuting attorney. And that the same judge who has participated in the schematic formulations of hundreds of "orders to proceed," can still believe that "there must be something to it—otherwise the fellow wouldn't be here," when he confronts the accused. The judge knows nothing about the controversial methods that police, the prosecutor's staff, and investigating judges use during pre-trial investigations; he is unaware of the bitter, silent, and mean-spirited campaign carried on in half-darkness against accused and defendant; he knows nothing about the defenselessness of ordinary people caught in the early stages of "legal proceedings"; he knows nothing about the preclusion of the defense, for whom access to the files is made as difficult as possible. None of this is within our judge's knowledge. Nor does he know anything about the effects of the sentences he passes. I deny that there are more than thirty criminal judges in Berlin who begin to understand the difference between a sentence of three, and one of four, years, although they pass them every day. What do those wearing the robes of office know about the execution of a sentence? What they were required to know for their examination. Absolutely nothing.

The German judge has constructed an ideal defendant with the help of his caste-soul and his group values. The well-behaved defendant. The first-grade-reader image thus constructed dominates the whole of the German judicial process, up to the highest court. We have, "the good son who supports his mother" and "the married man who travels to London with a female person not his wife." The lying images thus unrolled meet the standards of their creators. Small souls, small souls. The courts' most serious sexual morality is dictated by envy. They are ruled by the most superficial conceptions of human motives. A judge's favorable appraisal of moral character sounds like the Master recommending the stable-boy, whose loyalty, hard work, and humility he praises sternly from on high, as very useful traits. If it were known that a suspected murderer read during the night, slept by day, and was in love with two women at once, those facts would finish him off. Circumstances of that kind count for more than evidence. And—this seems to me worst of all—the accused has to defend himself against such allegations. As if he were being accused of crimes. The defense attorney does not—and cannot, for tactical reasons—suggest that the judge has no fundamental right to his moral excursions: he cannot destroy the moral foundation on which the whole tribunal rests. The defendant must be well-behaved: an underling, a first-grader, with that dog-like look in his eyes with which German soldiers used to regard their tormentors. Attention! You may steal.

It's horrible to watch an "academic education" confront a defendant who speaks German incorrectly and awkwardly has to search for words. Then the judge speaks "Teutonic," like a phony stepfather, in

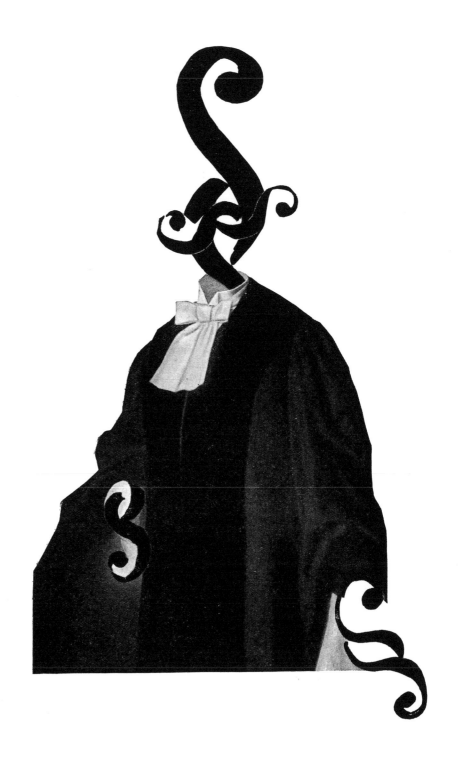

cheap silly phrases really meant for the ears of his fraternity or club-brothers. He may mock the defendant with supreme tasteless-ness, and deliver himself of the kind of irrelevant puerilities that themselves should be sufficient cause for removing him from office. And always underneath you sense the sound of, "Why am I wasting all this time on you? I made my decision long ago." The answer ought to be, why bother with the trial? Why not send the defendant a stamped, self-addressed postcard with his sentence? And again, why become a judge if you hate to listen to people? If it bores you for people to defend themselves? If having to deal with these people is so disgusting?

The judges are amazed that thieves and murderers exist! How false their exclama-tions of surprised horror ring! Such depravity! How could you? As if this were the first recorded case of breaking-and-entering, the first theft, rape, or fraud committed in a large city. Over and over a certain kind of judge registers his total amazement when he has to descend to the depraved lower levels of human existence. The defendant pays the price.

The German judge's attitude towards every authority clearly shows his class and group bias. Let's look at a thousand trial records. I'd take my oath on it—the German judge will have decided in favor of authority every time. He will decide not only for the state, but for anyone who exercises any kind of real or imagined authority. He will excuse the worst abuses and offenses if they have been committed by someone in some kind of "superior" position. Say a farmhand breaks his whiphandle on the stableboy's back. A German judge can do little or

nothing. What would happen to us if the "upper" no longer taught the "lower" that German society is stratified? Our examina-tion would show that—in the vast majority of cases—the "superior" always had the right.

Our judges' respect for authority results in outrageously light sentences in child-abuse cases. "Paternal authority . . ." The father, the inhuman couple, or the terma-gant mother, who misuse this certainly disputable authority, ought to spend in jail years equal to the tears shed by the abused child. But the more limited and narrow the point of view, the more uncompromisingly will it be represented. At these little trials, during which the judges are conscious of no outside pressures, their arrogant tone is really unbearable. "You should have!" and "You are completely . . ." But the judge is wrong. It is not his job to sit in moral judg-ment. Under present conditions he is neither qualified nor authorized to do so. No one has asked for his inexpert opinion.

But if we are to judge German judges, Berlin isn't even especially typical. The judge's manners, his general air and cultural level—no matter how ghastly—are bound to be a little bit more humane in the big city. Here a trial can occasionally appear to be fairly liberal in form, if not in real content. Further, the experiences of journalists and politicians cannot be considered typical court-room experience. They know how to appeal to the public. Thus the judges were seldom guilty of openly improper conduct in such cases, at least under the Kaiser. But in this Republic, and with this opposition party, the gentlemen have had to be less careful since 1918.

Our trials are miscarriages because they are conducted by one kind of judge, selected from only one group. There can be no change for the better without fundamental changes in the processes by which judges are chosen and educated. Though we might note that today's judge will look like pure gold, set beside those who will be judges in 1940.

The noisy petit-bourgeois gang-members at the Universities today have even less human kindness in their make-up than the dried-up old gentlemen we fight now. You can still meet with something like humor, find something to speak to—a shot of liberalism or bourdeaux joviality—in some of the old generation. The postwar *Freikorps* students have a cold, glazed, fishy look that forecasts a joyous future. When these boys don the judges' robes, it'll be an experience for our children! They have no sense of justice.

I'll summarize:

The caste out of which Germany recruits her judges, does not represent the line of Goethe, Beethoven, and Hauptmann.° Not for its sake do we love our country, like to speak its language, feel glad to be united in its spirit. The judges as they now are represent only one segment—one class—out of the whole. As such, they have no right to decide the right in the people's name. They should do it in their own name only. The opinions which their judgments embody must be fought, refuted, and denied— sentence by sentence, reason by reason, idea by idea. We may—in individual cases— grant them a personal good faith, but the effect of their activities is disastrous. Is there no defense against it? There is only one. An

all-inclusive, serious, and effective defense. That is, a scornfully antidemocratic and consciously unjust class-struggle for the idea of justice.

There are, further, some little nostrums, suggestions, pills, and mixtures, which may help against this incurable sickness.

Let's name some of the minor remedies.

An informed public would be some protection. It presents difficulties at the moment. The presiding judge "polices" his own court-room and tends to react to the slightest ripple among the spectators, while he lets pass all offenses committed by the marshals. It is therefore easy to eject inconvenient reporters. Appeals against this procedure will be handled by the judge's colleague—thus never without prejudice.

Nevertheless, and especially in the smaller cities, it would be useful for the press to keep watch on trials. Newspapers of all shades of opinion neglect this duty almost completely—they ought to assign a few dependable and knowledgable people to the courts. Of course, they would need reporters who know human nature and the law, and who can also write a readable German. As it is, even the biggest dailies use some kind of agency-report, often not even correct, and written from a point of view distasteful and dishonest in its pretended political neutrality. Such reports make a critique of the judge's public position impossible. In any case, a good many of the agency employees need—for business reasons—to keep the judge's good opinion.

As a minute down payment on reform, we should certainly demand that all criminal proceedings be carried on in public. The prisoner in investigative custody is delivered up—helpless—to the worst kind of arbitrary decisions. Ambitious investigators and investigating judges often remand or release for no discernible reason; they are ruled by the passionate hunter's devouring ambition —not to find the truth, but to bring down a quarry. They take a verdict of innocent as a personal affront; if the accused lies to protect himself—as he has the good right to do—they are insulted. It is always interesting to see the humbler employees of a large concern uphold group honor: how they insist—on pitiable salaries—that they have a right to be proud of their shop. Thus the slightest sign of disrespect counts against the accused. The judges know best what sins are committed during pre-trial investigations—but they choose not to know.

The German subject is purposely left in a profound state of uncertainty about his civil rights. Pre-trial investigations show this very clearly. Ask any of your acquaintances, whether—and when—you are required to obey a police summons to the station. No one will know the rights of even this ordinary situation. No one knows that —with minor exceptions—the police have no right to issue such summonses during preliminary investigations, or that no obligation to give evidence exists. Inquire whether the accused is obliged to give evidence in a preliminary hearing. Ninety of a hundred Germans will let themselves be intimidated by some little district judge eager to take a statement. None will suspect the snares and traps that can be hidden in the formulations of such a statement. This whole subject is unknown in primary and secondary school. The pitiful rights which our so-called "constitution" grants the German citizen are almost wholly unknown. We are even more ignorant of the few safeguards granted someone who is accused under the criminal code. The German code of criminal procedure, on the whole, reads like one of those delivery-contracts which have lately come into use: the customer agrees to assume full responsibility for everything, while the business takes absolutely none. An accused person gets the same treatment. From the moment of the first hearing he is pushed back and forth like a chesspiece with very little say in the process. But not one in a hundred Germans knows how he is cheated of his little bits of rights in a criminal case. The rulers like to leave the ruled ignorant, both about a criminal investigator's identifying marks, and a taxpayer's civil rights. They keep an exploiting organization veiled behind nationalist, metaphysical fog. We need enlightenment.

Since such enlightenment will not be granted voluntarily, it is up to proletarian organizations to find disaffected, sympathetic lawyers to serve the cause. They must begin to protect the worker with legal knowledge, and arm him for the battle against the bourgeois judge.

In the struggle against the dictatorship of the judicial establishment, we must remove the little bit of prestige which that establishment still enjoys in a few places.

We still attach too much value to the court's verdict, especially in political cases. This stock is still sometimes quoted above its true worth. In a political case we are dutybound to ignore all the findings on which the court bases its verdict. It's a basic mistake to draw conclusions from administrative measures. The verdicts don't count.

The court's verdicts are especially doubtful in defamation of character cases, and in cases in which a member of the ruling class is acquitted. Neither the SPD nor the powerful, so-called republican unions—sadly enough—have the courage to reject the wholly irrelevant notions of honor and patriotic duty which our judges still proclaim. What the judges call treason is nothing to us. The actions which they call high-treason do not dishonor us. What they label breach of the public peace, leaves us cold. The worker's movement ought to honor the victims of such judgments, if only to show that the men in robes wield a merely physical power—temporarily. The national newspapers that quote me will omit my next point, but it is understood that political fighters must keep to a high standard of personal integrity. That is, they must commit their crimes unreservedly in the interest of class-struggle.

Even in seemingly unpolitical cases, the judge's moral dictum is political. Maybe what a judge calls socially harmful, really is harmful. Usually it's good. Circumstances which the judge considers especially damaging are of no importance to us: they are usually extenuating. The German universities do not teach—nor do the German courts establish—moral justice, moral progress, or the people's ethical education. That the Superior Court is coldly rigid in moral questions, that it lacks totally any understanding for the demands of human life, that its pretended objectivity has never been a true one, are all facts which give us the right to deny that this caste of judges is in any way qualified to instruct the people in morality. Nor do the Supreme Court counselors simply implement the legal code: they do not feed data into the top of the Justice Machine and get results out at the bottom. Emotion, education and background, and class consciousness, all exert their influence at some point in every legal proceeding. And at that critical point the Supreme Court judge always lets the needle point due right. The judge may not be to blame personally, but we must declare guilty the caste which tenderly reared him, and put him in his place. That is why we deny these judges any spiritual legitimacy to grant any kind of justice. We despise their charges and their verdicts.

There has always been a minority of decent jurists that has fought against the enormities committed by their colleagues, against the obvious flaws in the system, and against a criminal code that has developed delusions of grandeur. But they fight like well-behaved children! I don't believe that the criminal code will evolve for the better. Progress within the institution is a slogan for the fearful. We can prove how useless the slogan is by pointing to a single year: 1918. The year when no one dared put out these same judges, these same officials, who "knew the regulations so beautifully."

There is only one way to clean up a bureaucracy. I will not write down the word here—it has lost its power to frighten the rulers. But it means, upheaval. Mopping-up operation, airing, and general clean-up.

Adults don't learn new lessons. If we wait for the law schools and the universities, for Hergt and Ebermayer,° to protect not just their own class but the whole society—if we wait for them to give up their presumptuous "right to punish"—we will pay dearly. We

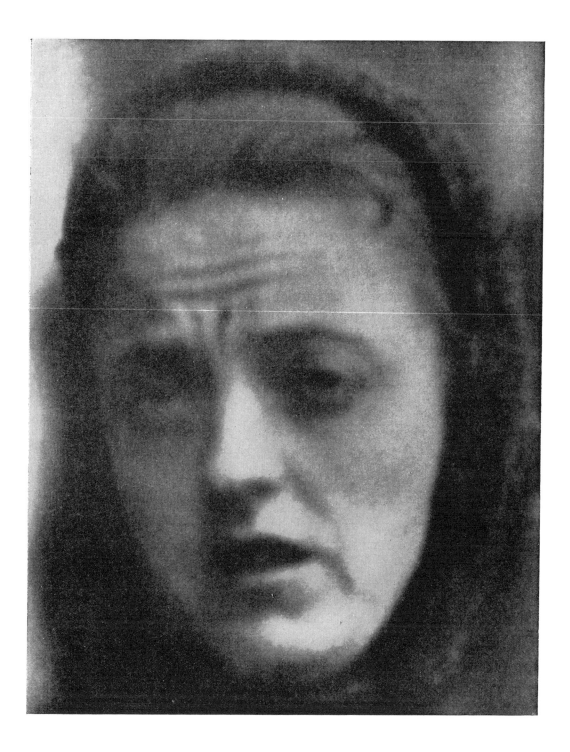

pay with the sufferings of the tens of thousands who are tormented and delivered up—harassed and defenseless—to the underpaid, abysmally low-grade, staffs of our prisons. Some of whose members are even drawn from the higher reaches of the military. A prison sentence is not an atonement. Very few people could deserve the moral torment which our prisoners are made to suffer. We know from experience that prison terms are no deterrent to crime. Neither do they rehabilitate the prisoners. Only a preacher who has never seen the inside of a jail could nourish that fantasy. Prison terms are made up of suffering on one side—of sadism, power-lust, laziness, and negligence, on the other.

And there is only one weapon, one way, and one goal, to set against the men who arrogantly take a power that none has granted them—against this bullheaded rabble whose qualifications consist solely in their own conviction of worth—against this group which is closed to all outsiders, these men who defend self-interest and an immoral economic system.

Bring down this shameful legal system; these shameful trials and sentencings: bring them down. Throw the statute-book at those who—with calculations and doubts and intellectual scruples—oppose the most important goal which could inspire a human being:

Justice for the oppressed!

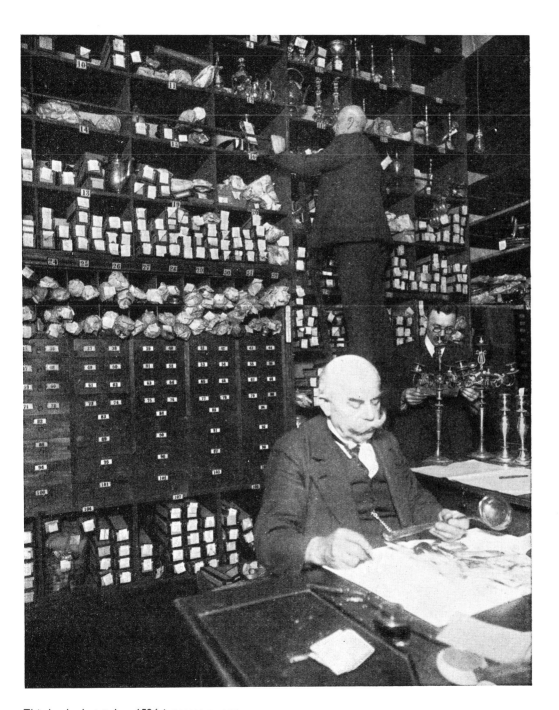

This hock-shop takes 45% interest a year.

163

Mother's Hands°

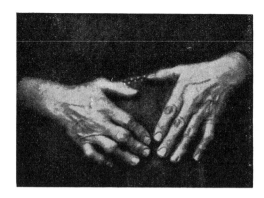

You cut the bread
and boiled the coffee,
    passed the dishes over
wiped and mended
fixed and patched . . .
    with your hands

Covering the milk
and bringing home candy,
    delivering newspapers—
you counted the shirts
and peeled potatoes
    with your hands

You slapped us plenty
bringing us up
    the eight of us—
six living
    with your hands

They felt hot sometimes
and cold
    Your hands look old—
You're almost finished.
And here we are
    to take your hands.

Theater in Berlin

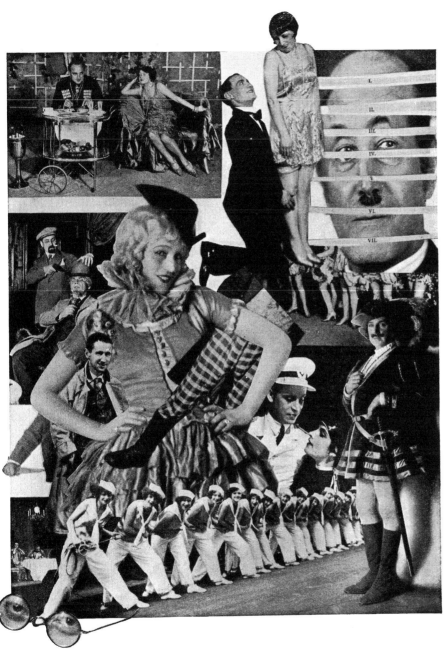

Berlin first-nighters want Goethe, plus Dante, plus Brecht, plus Bruckner, plus Claudel; at the fiftieth performance the audience wants the Follies with a shot of folk-lore.° So go and do a show in Berlin.

Hermione

People often ask for new books to read—well, I want to recommend one. It's so new it still smells of printer's ink. A highly entertaining novel. It's called *Hermione*, by Peter Guggenreit. (Poseidon Press, Chemnitz) You ought to read it. As far as I know, it's the first time an author has tried to get a particular aspect of modern life down on paper—what one might call the anonymous "functioning" of all things. Here's how it goes:

The hero, a young kid named Ludolf Gerold,° fresh out of school, is apprenticed to a large business concern. The book begins with his last school days. You find out at the start that Mr. Ludolf is no fighter, although he can be pretty aggressive behind people's backs. So he's apprenticed, and he learns the ropes, and fits in, very quickly. And now the book goes on to show exactly and beautifully how this modern machine—an office—really functions. How everyone works, but no one is responsible; how everybody steps on everyone else; how no one ever admits being stepped on. And especially how the machine itself dominates everything. Modern management, which reduces people to their functions, makes people resentful and vengeful. They revenge themselves on the system by throwing as many difficulties as possible in the way of the machine. That's how they demonstrate that they still exist. For instance, the messenger boy is supposed to take a letter to the post-office. Well, he does it of course—after all, he's only a messenger boy and not important. But he protests in the one way open to him: he devises infinite complications and problems about the letter. Thinks up so many formalities that—Oho!—he's no ordinary messenger boy—this is no simple matter—the job he does takes expertise! Ludolf, who's been asking everyone in the office, makes a surprising discovery. Everyone tells him the same two things. First, "The work I do here is more important than anyone else's!" And second, "My work's not easy. It takes practice, and some people could never learn how to do it!" The machinery moans and clatters—not the smallest action can be performed without some sacrifice to the worker's vanity. Otherwise, he won't do it. He won't. Ludolf learns. He learns a great deal very quickly.

Then he leaves business to become a civil servant in the Ministry of Finance. He gets to know a girl named Hermione. Hermione has just lost a law-suit—lost very badly in the courts. But she wants justice. It's a very complicated story and—because something like an assault may have happened at the police station—federal authorities may be involved. Anyway, she turns to young Gerold, who has meanwhile become quite influential, and he takes up her case with the various departments. He really wants to help her get justice. And he can't. He comes to a sudden realization. The people he deals with are—without exception—nice and polite. They even understand the troubles which he and the girl bring them. (He has to be very careful, of course. Occasionally people give him funny looks—as if he might have been at the station too.) But they all nod, and carefully straighten the heavy piles of documents on their desks. And then the big ball game starts—the game of channels. Nobody, but nobody, made the decision. And suddenly no one has the power to decide, and no one has any influence. Anyone who does admit that he might have influence, is suspicious and afraid of being used. A quarrel starts between offices—a palely gleaming competitive struggle of all against all in "the other departments." Hermione watches, unable to understand why her lot should be one of such bitter injustice. But once—and this is one of the best things in the book—she happens to be sitting in Ludolf's reception room, waiting for a document he's been holding for her. A young official comes out of Ludolf's office. Then Hermione goes in to him, calling, "Who was that?" After he tells her, she says, "You know, I really think he should show more respect for you. If he's only from the other department . . ." And Ludolf agrees. Then he sleeps with Hermione, and then he marries her, if only so that the case can finally end. And now, immersed in daily middle-class life, when the first floor fights the second, it's family against family, always and again department against department. It's masterful! For the first time in a novel, Hermione and Ludolf aren't really the main characters. The focus is on something else, usually unnoticed. The group.

There are still novels that explore the soul and give deeply reasoned analyses of men and women, and God knows what. But this other unknown, huge, mysterious, and dark and muddled power is one no novelist has yet dared to approach.

P.S. Unfortunately, there is no such novel.

Heads

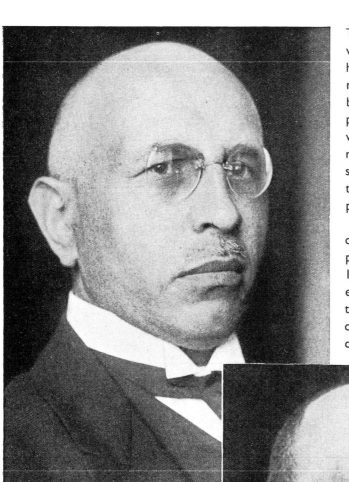

That people work hard in Germany is a well-established fact. But they work even harder at getting their work properly noticed and appreciated. Their vanity gives birth to a continual stream of business publications, memorial pamphlets, anniversary essays, all issued for "official business reasons." In general they make an immodest, somewhat embarrassing fuss about something that—one might have thought—could pass without special comment in Germany.

If you study such chronological sketches of businesses, you will usually find a series of portraits depicting the owners, say from 1684 to the present. And there's something extremely interesting about them. At least the last three generations are nicely and cleanly photographed, and unlike drawings, can be compared. Photographs are at least half-way dependable reports. Well, and what do these three generations look like? August Friedrich Wilhelm Schulze (1821–1889). An old, bearded, modest man with glasses and sparse white hair. A little bent with work and age, but a lot can be read in his eyes: the last glimmerings of a powerful will, sadness, a long life. He's a human being one could talk with. Rest in Peace. Then, Hans Erich Schulze (1854–1915). Bright eyes and the big skull that signifies an active man. There's a lot in his eyes too—inherited family features, cunning, certainly some human kindness. German humanism did something for him. He had some relationship to the best that Germany had to give. But he's already different from the old man, his father. *In pace.*

Dr. Ernst Emil Schulze (born 1885). God in Heaven!

A shaven pig-skull, little button eyes, a merciless collar, and toothbrush mustache. Around his wine-tasting underlip there's that strain of cold correctness that sums up all of the new Germany's heartlessness. *In pace? In bello.* "And the Hermundure whispers fearfully, My God, the place ain't what it used to be!"°

There never were any good old days. But bad new ones? You might say so. Just as the older generation of German judges was still bearable, because one could still find a tiny path to their hearts—most especially, because they still had hearts—while the brutality of the new generation is unprecedented, so the typical nineteenth-century German businessman, mostly silver plate though he was, looks like pure gold compared to the present nickel. You say it takes a good shine? That it gleams strong and hard? How horribly it will tarnish!

These are faces that belong inside trousers. But we show them to the world—with a challenging war cry out of *Götz*°—and then we wonder why everyone, everyone, is against us...

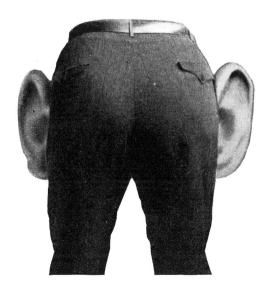

The Manly Pose

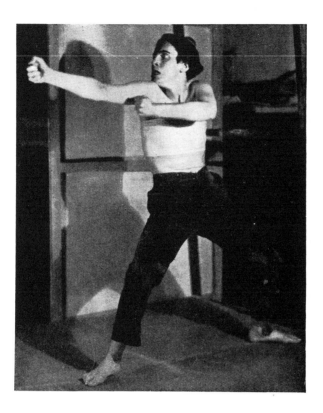

A somewhat effeminate generation of young people, which doesn't know beans about the manly art, depicts strength on our city stages. We have a whole literature of plays in which the Wild West, the machine, and—more recently—the proletariat, become the excuse for performances that are phony all the way down to their wobbly bones. Muscles are flexed defiantly—heads are thrown back! But the new age isn't like that. Not even on the surface. It's play-acting.

It's most horrifying when the weaklings, who worship strength, prop themselves up with nationalism, and passionately embrace its erect flags; this posture extends from our literary admirals down to some younger writers whose names I won't mention. But

one of them begins with the letter, B*ronnen*. You can find some moving scenes!

Now about the young man in the picture. I'm sure he's boxing in accord with the highest principles. I can almost hear the jagged, tightly-clenched, exaggerated verse accompaniment. It's not poetry, but it's bound to end with the *Internationale*. It's free, isn't it?

And there are those who fight just because they like blood. The characters in recent German literature seem to beat each other up a little too frequently. The monstrous success of trash like Löns' *Werewolf*° is founded on a latent sadism. I once read a story in the yellowing pages of a magazine called *The Dragon*. A member of the *Stahl-*

170

helm showed the hero a colored photograph of Schlageter's° execution. "You know," the hero says, "violence like that makes me———" He meant, it made him feel uncommonly good, but I wouldn't like to quote him more exactly. It's not nice. But what he said unequivocally reveals the underlying connection between sexuality and blood-lust. One man's Marilyn is the other's march into Munich.

In any case, none of it has anything to do with strength. It's just a pose. Wild sub-urbanites, who've never been to America, get high on cow-boys, the way their Pappas did on Karl May's° novels. Young gentlemen with barely the strength to work a type-writer love the Chinese revolution . . . Well, nothing in this life is simple. But we ought to laugh these affectations off the stage.

Go ahead and fight! But don't use fighters as sex-stimulants. Fight! But stop shouting, what great fighters you are. Just listening makes me hoarse. And it makes me laugh— the manly pose.

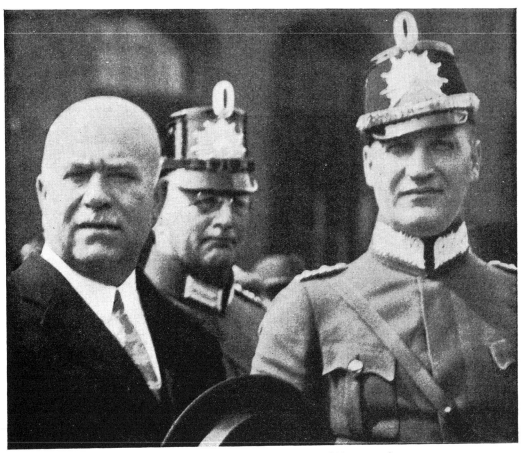

Police Commissioner Zörgiebel   Police Chief Heimannsberg

A Proletarian Faces the Judges

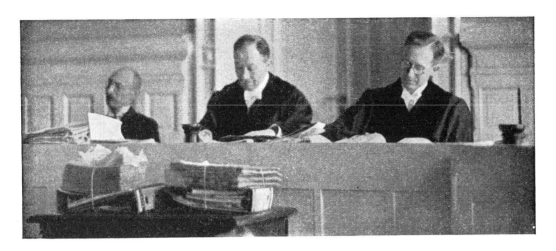

Have they got you in the dock
wanting to punish you now?
You look tired and pale and sick,
they—well-rested, energetic
and raring to go.
    The court is cozily agreed
    that justice will be done.
    Brother, keep your guard up!
        Three against one!

The egg-in-his-beer presiding judge
cuts you down to size:
Your character's bad! Don't dare answer
  back!
or—so the last question implies—
    With district attorney, with evidence
      barred,
    with the paid informer
                  with his police
                    guard—
  before they're done:
    Five against one!

The prosecutor has had his say.
Will you get home to say good-bye?
"Petition . . ." But Justice, Inc. detects
that lunch is on the schedule next.
    "Four years"—the pen—
    "Take him away—"
    Two women weeping quietly.
    See them again?
      No telling when—
      All against one!

They break your lives in cells, in prison
for something you have never known:
You paste brown-paper bags for freedom—
are freedom-fighters, everyone.
    Come up, you, from the mines and
      workshops!
    Build in the factories, stone on stone!
    The day of our revenge is coming
    and you will be the judges then—!

Treptow

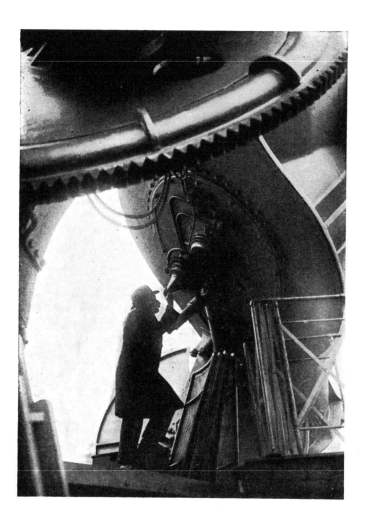

near Berlin, has an observatory and the observatory has a big telescope. The announcements say its the biggest in the world, but that won't make it any bigger.

There's a kind of mild, dusty summer evening, with military music blaring in the "Abbey," when the beer waiters sweat, the wine waiters perspire. And conversation. "Just a minute, there, that's my chair! What's the idea?" "Oh Gus, don't get so excited. Come on, sit over here." (Angry murmur) "The nerve—" Yes, well, on evenings like that we sometimes climbed up the little iron stairway. Sometimes it was very crowded; we would have to wait on the stairs to get our turn at Mars or Saturn. Well, we'd stand there. You had time to think a little, standing there, waiting for the Milky Way to become available.

The observatory in Treptow is a tiny arsenal of urban metaphysics. It's not very demanding metaphysics—but here, on the little iron staircase, the brain-radio rests a minute, and you sort of think, how high is heaven? I wonder how high the sky really is—Max, do you know how high? No, Max doesn't know either. If you stop to think, it's pretty far away—maybe they don't even know about us there. Funny—what a tiny being a man really is. Sophocles—Quickly death strikes down man.° Oh, baloney. But anyway, what was it the astronomer said before? Five million light years. That's— good God! Well, they're finished up in front now—let's see. I don't see anything—yes, now I do. There.

Ahh—!

Like a pea! Mars looks like a pea. You'd think—just wait a minute!—like a pea. Yes, and all yellow. Here, look—(still slightly submerged)—five hundred million light years—I guess we're really just a little pile of misery. What are they playing down there? Oh, the Merry Widow°—my goodness, what a life!

Once when we were standing there, immersed in our religious reflections, a little old grandmother tripped up and down, up and down, just in front of us. Something was bothering her. And finally she gathered up her courage and approached the astronomer, who supervises the planets up there on the flat, dark roof. She said:

"Haven't you heard about it too—that two giant suns are moving towards the earth at enormous speed? Yes, oh yes—" The astronomer hadn't heard. The woman turned to the rest of us, begging for support for her two suns. Two such good suns— "Have you heard about them?" Some people smiled scornfully, but others weren't so sure—they looked searchingly into the

black sky to see if they could see the suns coming. No, nothing. The double-sun lady left with her feelings deeply hurt.

But what if she's right?

Until the arrival of those suns, backsliding believers will work off the remnants of their religion on the roofs of the observatory. For a fifty-cent fee they understand the universe and arrive downstairs again, in full possession of their earthly dignity.

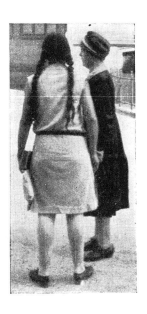

This Picture

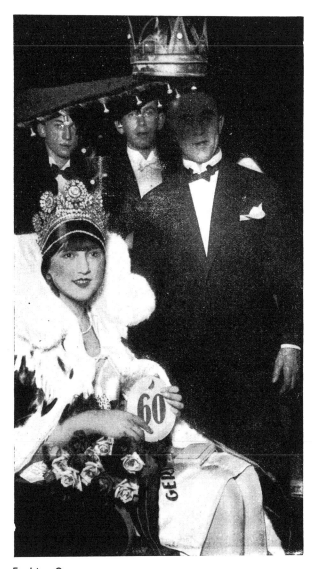

Fashion Queen

will look very strange in 1982. It shows a fashion queen—a creature most of us don't even experience as particularly attractive, or beautiful—just something to do with advertising. So far, so good.

But our grandchildren will look at this picture with the same mixture of anger and nostalgia with which we look at faded photographs from 1911 and 1913, those little years before the great war. And after our grandchildren have stopped talking about "those impossible fashions" they may go on to say:

"Yes, that was before the gas-wars. Look at those empty faces—they didn't know anything. Didn't you have anything else to think about? Couldn't you damn well have prevented them poisoning us? Didn't you have any idea that Europe was in terrible danger? How could you have done anything but hold meetings, tried to make sure that no one manufactured poison gas? Kept the insanity of nationalism from mounting higher and higher? Made clear to all the powerhungry bullies in all countries that there are powers stronger than they are, and stronger than the profit-hungry big industrialists, who collect Van Goghs and high culture in their houses? Didn't you know? Didn't you do anything for us? Didn't you see?"

We saw all right. We even worked against the gas, in our way. But you can't take pictures of that. And—human being of 1982, don't forget:

The world isn't purposeful. It isn't ruled by reason. The world wants to play. Fashion queens have always aroused more interest than future generations and their fate: they have to worry about themselves for themselves—and they'll be the same. Do you think those gentlemen in evening dress know anything about their real destiny? They're all caught up in dailiness—even more taken up by holidays—they don't know anything. Those who know something are gray and insignificant and not presentable enough for pictures. And don't forget, descendant, even during the French revolution women quarreled about the milk and clothes and their lovers—there has never been a time when an idea dominated the whole world.

Be grateful to those who cared about you. There aren't many of them. Take care of yourself. We had so much to do. We had to live.

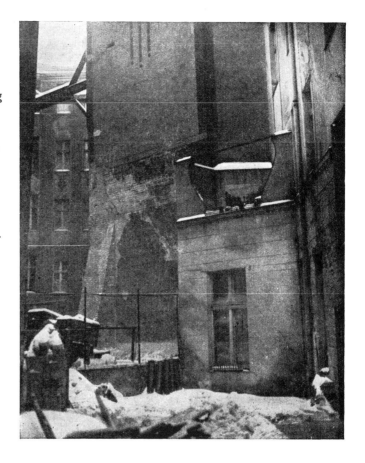

177

The Drummer

The small, almost triangular mouth opens a little.

> You
> only you
> make me blue

Bammbammbammbamm—the sticks rap on the dry wood that rings the drum. Many couples are dancing; others watch, looking ironic and superior because they're sitting down. The gents walk up and down the long room: casually, hands in pockets, faces bored, just a little afraid of the headwaiter.

> I want to belong
> to you alone

The drummer sings. He has deep-set eyes, a beaked horseman's nose, heavy lids, a round criminal skull. He sings idiocies. It's the same voice we once heard shouting in the yard in Lichtenberg: "Get over here, asshole! Stand there! Pig! Your wife'll see what we do to Commie-pigs! Damned dog!" Then a shot. Melodies rise above his beginning double chin.

> I'm waiting, Mamma,
> in Yokahama—

The ice-cold, slippery rhythm rattles on. The age of the whole band added together, isn't much more than that of the victim in the yard, then. That wasn't the only victim. It's fun watching that stuff.

The criminals, who joined the *Freikorps* to legitimatize achieving orgasm through blood, have not been punished. They're back among the people. They're all still around. They have jobs selling wine. Carrying suitcases at the railway station. And drumming.

Only occassionally, on nice days when they really feel alive, they remember a little. A confusion of voices sounds deep in the inner ear. "Mercy! I didn't do it! My wife! My children!" And the answer. "Shut up Bolshevik pig. Shut up. Against the wall, pig! Up against the wall!"

> In Nischni-Novgorod
> the kissing's free—

The drummer breaks off with a smothered sound. The melody breaks off too. He gets up gracefully—the fatal smell of strong disinfectant envelops him. He walks through the room with the funny bearing that people have when they are never quite sure whether they're masters or lackeys. He's clean-shaven and a triangular handkerchief hangs from his breast pocket. A gentleman. You'd think they'd give him a pension.

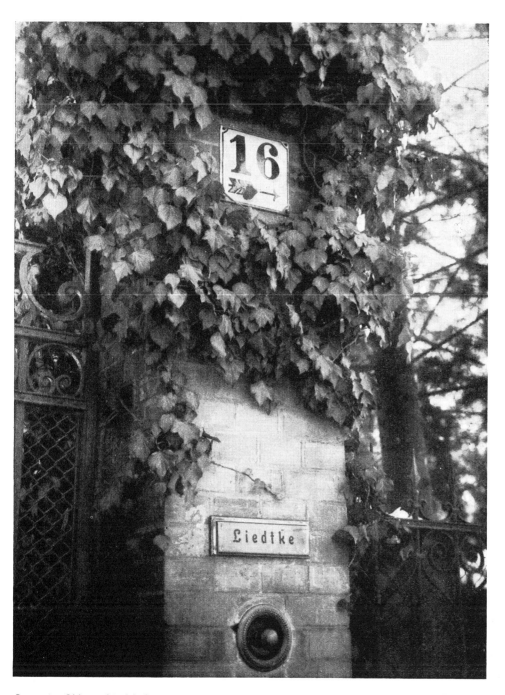

Portrait of Harry Liedtke°

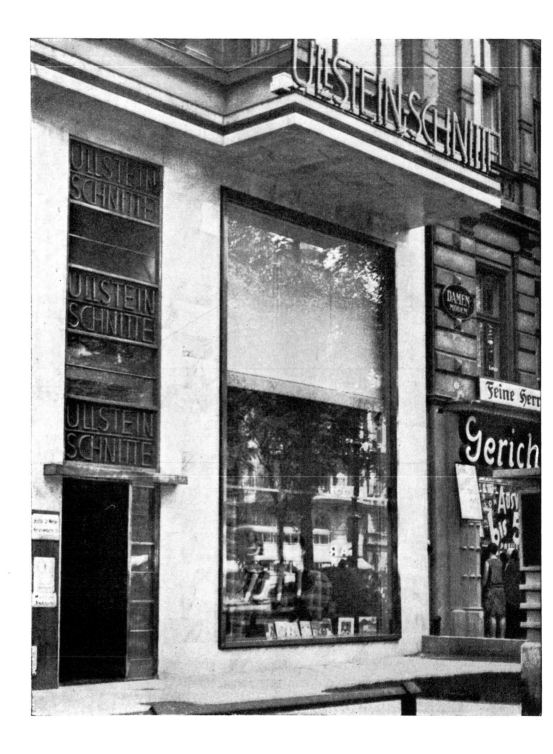

A House With Pants On

"They put pants on their houses." That's how a Frenchman once described this peculiar style of architecture. It consists of faking a façade around a shop and, in a sense, declaring independence on the ground-floor. The city dwellers' eye is so accustomed to this horror, that he hardly notices it. Above, and on the left and right sides, the house keeps its old, discolored, dirty-grey stucco. The proprietor of the ground-floor store, however, pastes new stucco—a few thin rectangles in "as-if" pretense—around his windows. Then he feels elegant. You could read it allegorically.

You could also say that urban architecture which does not start from the principle, that the only appropriate contemporary style is collective, creates a false image of the city. How does false individualism express itself? In a proliferation of "original" business signs and shop façades. In frivolities.

Worthwhile architecture in our century starts with a unified design for the whole; it plans whole city blocks and sections to include variation and interest within a coherent entity. What we have in the picture is a clear and exact image of what happens, when we allow falsely understood and badly utilized private property to tyrannize over us.

Monarchic Art

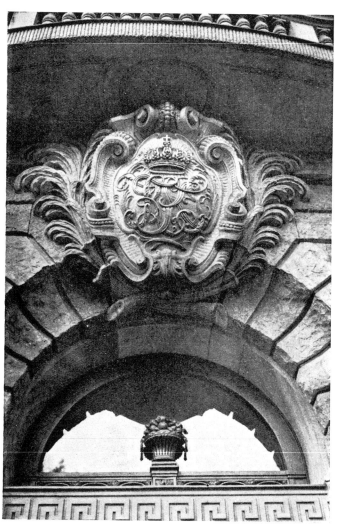

A new regime usually removes as much as it can of the public evidence of its predecessor's power. It's always been that way in the history of the world. The German Republic, however, has a guilty conscience . . .

Imagine if we had a dictatorship of the army—not a single historical stone that might awaken memories of the Republic would be left standing. But the Republic has a very guilty conscience . . .

If you should draw attention to the many emblems of old privilege that survive—not only in Bavaria—but in all our states, you're answered with a general concerned head-shaking. The life-long employees of the firm proclaim that, "According to the directives, only those emblems which have no artistic value may be removed." The wedding-cake ornament pictured here, has artistic value.

But it may be best, after all, for the ornament to stay in its place. At least we can see what HE was like—down to the last curlicue. Inflated, bombastic, derivative in form—a second rater in the Silesian poets' school,° but even less valuable. And by the way, our justice is meted out inside this little edifice. It's the High Court in Berlin.

Grock the Clown, and Conrad Veidt°

"We're both very famous. When I—Grock —shuffle out on stage, everybody laughs and claps; A lot of people know me, but they still laugh. I say, 'Woffor?' and 'Sans blague—' I can be funny in all languages. My legs never know what my feet are up to, and my long arms give me a lot of trouble too. I can play the piano and imitate a bass-fiddle and I put on thick white gloves to finger better, before I sound-off on the violin. I can jump up on the back of a chair without knocking it over —I hold it up with my legs. Once I'm up there, I sing a beautiful song. My laugh reaches from ear to ear. I wear a little grey cap. The cap covers all the comedy in the world. After I've worked forty-four minutes, the audience is weeping with laughter and they refuse to let me leave the stage. I'm very famous."

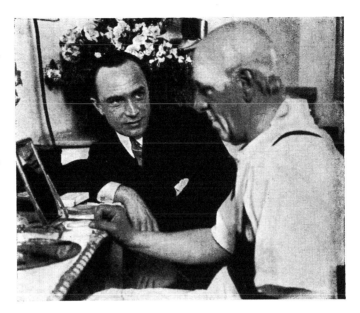

"We're both very famous. When I—that is, Conny—bending at the waist that special way, enter the scene, a hush falls on the audience. The ladies concentrate, the way they do at special sales; a thrill passes through all the rows. I don't move around very much; I know my trade and my medium, the film. You'd never guess that I speak a great Berlinese. People all over the world know my face. A lot of them write me con-fessional letters, and I never make fun of them. There must be something about me that moves women to open their hearts— I'm not Harry Liedtke. Sometimes my own face amazes me. I have a good sense of humor. I love Grock. We're both very famous."

"But nobody knows how much hard work and luck it took to become famous. How much cleverness, organization, intelligence, sophistication, luck, and hard work it takes for us to keep our fame. We work like slaves. We know all the agents' and business men's tricks—and the people we deal with aren't necessarily nobility. We're as tricky as horse-dealers. Our lives are a constant struggle to stay on top. It's true, we're not hungry these days, but we both remember what being out of work was like—what it felt like, not being able to buy a cup of coffee. We haven't forgotten. We've known innumerable people and we've experienced a lot—numerically, that is. No big tragedies, if you please, only little ones. Now everywhere we go, our names on posters precede us. Wherever we go, people stand aside for us. But there's plenty of competition to crowd us—the young people, the new ones coming up—and we have to keep working. We work and people love us. We're very famous.''

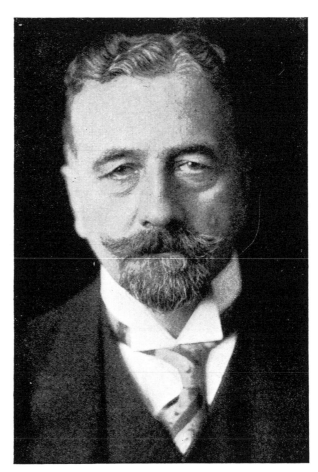

Külz°

184

From the Bottom

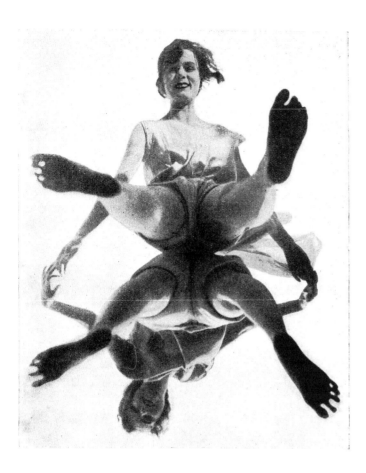

With all due ceremony, we dedicate this picture to the "Union of Militant German Women," particularly to those of its members interested in sniffing-out immorality.

It's how this special pornography section° sees the world. Many a pious parson° does, too. Blushing, and from the bottom.

We laugh and view our world from the top.

"... for once, let us admit here, what is so saddening in the development of German theater. That is, the great old names fade away and the new generation, able as some of its members individually may be, often cannot live up to the standards set by those others. Minor actors, who can show respectable achievements within their limited capabilities, are labeled "stars." Sadly enough, we must admit that the stage is often occupied by an artificially over-valued actor in a leading role. Such a prospect cannot please."

From *A History of the German Theater*

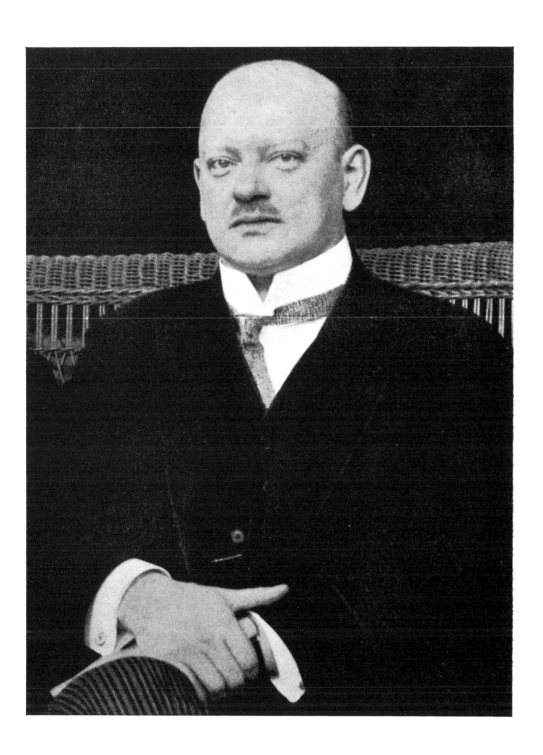

The Kitchen on Wilhelmstrasse°

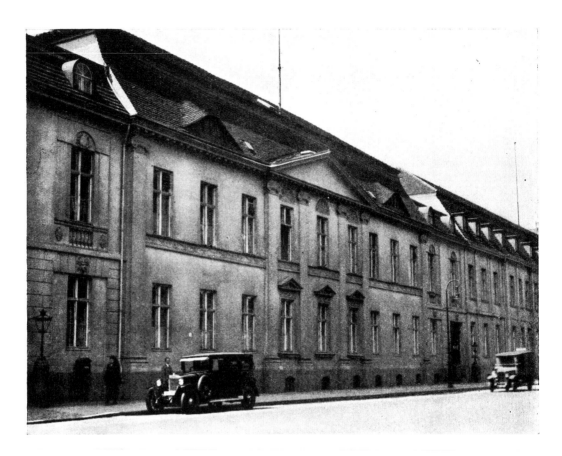

Your country's foreign policy is cooked-up inside these houses, dear taxpayer. Looking at the old façades so innocently lined-up, makes it hard to believe all the things that have emerged from these houses . . .

On the surface there isn't much to see. You can look at nicely furnished offices, long corridors, and messengers who differ from the higher officials only in that they take themselves with even greater seriousness. The whole department of state has an atmosphere of ceremoniousness that is almost Chinese. If you haven't heard the people here arrange to meet for lunch, you haven't heard anything. They have so much time and enjoy intrigue so much, that it's no exaggeration to say, three-quarters of their energies go into fighting the office next-door.

Their "affairs." Oh dear God—

You're their affair. You're the person who has to take what they dish out. And who are "they"?

Are they the nation? Don't make me laugh. These political kitchens look plain and clean and have an air of Prussian simplicity, but the cook uses rancid fat and he has innumerable helpers. All kinds of people spit in the soup. The nation that seems so powerful, is dependent on its defense industry, on the chemical manufacturing concerns, on the land-owners. It doesn't achieve a very satisfactory balance among all these conflicting interests, nor between workers and owners. Our state is a very one-sided business—it's a class-state. It's hounded by its creditors, up to its ears in debt to big industry. It's completely at the mercy of industry, which can put a disobedient state's workers on the street any time it pleases. "All right, then. Take care of them yourself!" So they cook up protective tariffs and tax remissions and subsidies. The state is dependent on an agriculture eighty years behind the times and unable to live or die (they arrange for the big land-owners to live, while babies in the city die without milk)—but if you listen to the farmers, they've been at the edge of the abyss, perishing, for the last hundred years. There's an inordinate amount of perishing going on in Germany generally. Well, there they are— the political kitchens.

The cooks assigned to the most sensitive spots are all fraternity brothers. You can't see the *Reichstag* from here. It's just a nuisance. Nor do the sometime "democratic" members of the cabinet have much to say here—they're just intruders who don't belong to the club. These few houses don't give a hoot for the people, about whom they know very little. They only need the people when somebody has to die in the trenches, while the cannons which Krupp and the other German factories sold the enemy, thunder overhead. Business is business.

Newspaper reporters say that "all the loose ends are tied up" in these houses. Don't you believe it.

It's like Penelope's garment. What others have woven together with painstaking care, the noble schemers unravel just as carefully. And the tangle of left-over, colored thread—that's German foreign policy.

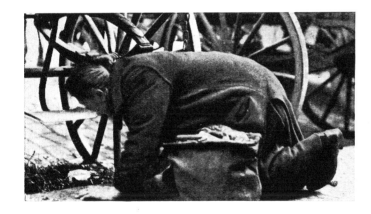

Small Official Journey

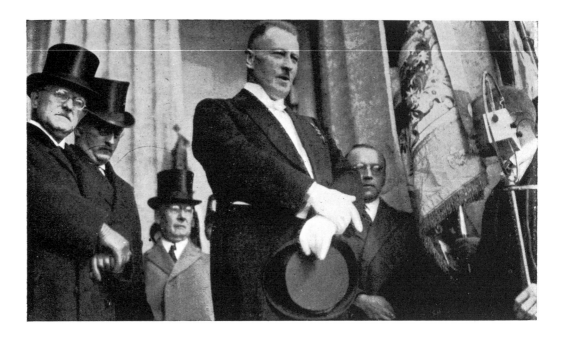

The people of Frankfurt planned a dedication
to open their new bridge across the *Main:*
with a great procession, with songs of celebration,
ringing of the church-bells and drinking apple-wine—
  Well, fine.

Our President-in-Office was formally and fitly
invited. But he didn't come. I think His Grace
couldn't forgive that—phew!—disgusting city
for being such a nasty, democratic place.
So he answered, *Nein.*
  Well, fine.

Frankfurt wiped its hurt nose
Frankfurt could dispense
without too much trouble
with Presidential presence.

But where—let us ask—where was the honored guest
who almost
fell into democratic, painful experience?

Was he in Berlin? *Nein.* In Cologne, *Nein.*

in Königsberg? *Nein.*
He went where good folk entertain ya—
to Stolp. (That's Farthest Pomerania.)
   Well, fine.
Oh there—!
It's family, it's pound-cake, the good old German pattern—
you can hunt out democrats, with your *Reichswehr* lantern;
the notables, at evening, sit solidly spread,
calling down damnation on the Jew Republic's head.
They've got discipline and order God's law and German respect
   down to a *tee*
   but no W.C.

It was Stolp, Pomerania, where our headman opened
a stadium. No bridge is so important—
though it bridge North and South in allegorical stone:
   Well—to each his own.

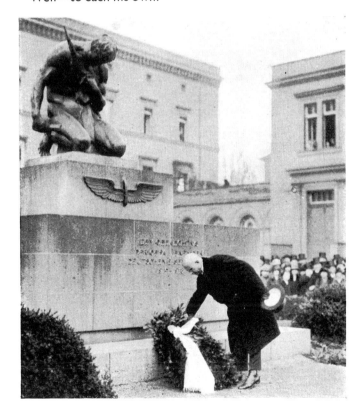

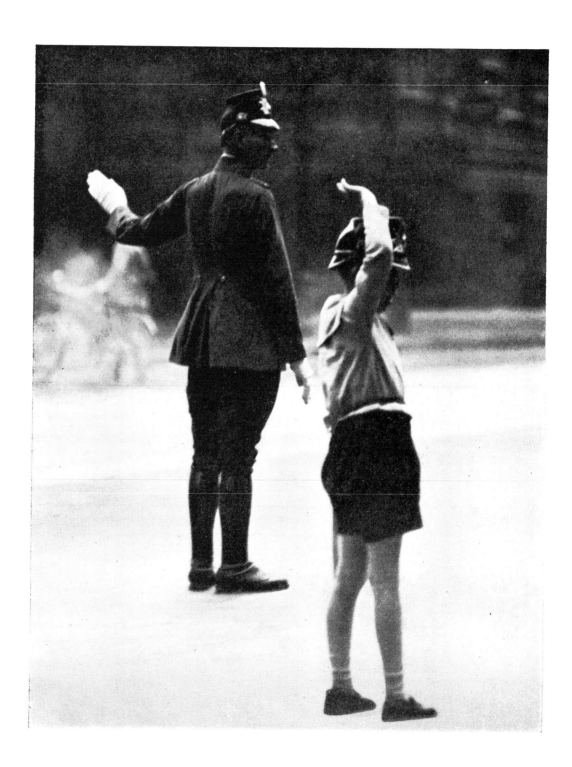

Traffic

Traffic has become a national obsession in Germany. In the first place, German cities are proud of their traffic. I've never been able to find out why. Noisy streets, dust, and a lot of cars, are symptomatic of city-design unable to cope with modern realities. Is that something to be proud of?

Probably, individuals have to feel important—and people's urge to ˙ount for something—stopped, braked, and denied in so many instances—finds its hissing outlet here. "Well, how do you like our traffic?" We answer that no German city has as great a traffic problem as—for instance—Paris. But that the Parisians are thoroughly miserable about their disfigured boulevards; that they mourn the beautiful old days when you could still go for walks. Today you are forced to listen to the din of a thousand beeping horns.

It would be much nicer if every large German city had an inner business district and—farther out—a healthy, green residential section. For the time being, we still have everything mixed together; people live in the narrow, interior streets of Cologne; and in Berlin the people spoil every pleasant residential district because they are too lazy to go "into the city" every morning. We have a dreary mixture of businesses and residences everywhere—neither one thing, nor the other. But the regulation of our still nonexistent traffic is even more ghastly.

The German citizen needed to find something to replace compulsory military service. For a while, our housing-offices seemed like a good bet, but they didn't quite fill the bill. The athletic-clubs were a good possibility. The army had become too small. So a few able public servants travelled to America and to London. They came, they saw, they took notes—the substitute was found. German traffic regulations now replace universal military service.

What gets organized here is no joke.

In their rage for organization, the administrators have lost all sense of purpose and proportion. The gesticulating, light-flashing, bell-ringing, and arm-waving that goes on, is terrifying: with so many directors, organizers, and regulators you hardly see the traffic.

First of all, we have far too much traffic regulation. In other countries a single policeman stands quietly on a corner and ocassionally gives a helpful signal. But we have a beadle. He's often not in the least concerned with helping either the driver or the pedestrian. As is usual in Germany, the letter of the law rules, and traffic policemen exist to enforce the rules for their own sake. It's the Authority of the State, operating at intersections.

The senselessly mechanical regulations prove it. Driving through Berlin, for example, you see cars stopped at a hundred different points, merely because the light in front of them is red. The light, by the way, is hung so that the first driver in line—if he has a closed car—can hardly see it. The light changes automatically—it's operated from that ideal of all organizers, a central control. They have a machine to shut-off fourteen streets—big and little, crowded and empty —it doesn't make any difference. Everything depends on the red light. The cars stop. They wait. They lose time.

Driving through Berlin is torture.

Of course, the results of all this regulating are catastrophic. A car too close to a corner becomes a "problem." Bicyclers dismount; people watch avidly, with that funny look in their eye—they're doing traffic-duty. No one can relax. The smallest difficulty, and strained tempers explode. They're all on duty.

What this nonsense involves is, people enjoying ordering other people about. Especially in the cities, the faces and actions of traffic policemen show that they consider themselves commanders. It never occurs to them that they're there to smooth the flow of traffic, not to enforce the rules. The citizens are so firmly drilled in this attitude, that they hardly notice it. You can sense the tune that accompanies the traffic policeman: "Before you do anything, Stop. Then maybe we'll see. But don't start-up, just like that, either. This is serious business. You'd better show some respect." And do they show respect! They're proud to obey with alacrity. It's the old military spirit, ineradicably in the blood. A sudden jolt—a quick stop— that's how they drive! That's how—with the least possible sense of comradeship. I don't even want to mention the martyrdom of ladies who aren't pretty and drive by themselves. And because of Germany's insane tax-politics with its systematic destruction of consumer power, the little man's envy accompanies every automobile. The people are not very friendly towards cars, even if they don't always throw knives at them as they do in Bavaria. But the drivers are even less friendly towards each other.

German drivers aren't like others. They drive to be in the right. Against the policeman, against the pedestrian (who, incidentally, has the same goal), but especially against each other. Should the driver be considerate? Let someone into his lane? Loosen up? Realize that consideration is practical? Why, you must be . . . !

In all seriousness, the major newspapers already run columns in which the single "right solution" for a traffic situation is theoretically arrived at—after the fact. The analyses are untranslatable. As if there were solutions! As if it didn't always depend on giving-in gracefully, on skill and presence of mind, and—except in a very few obvious cases—on the perception of a rounded, not a sharp-cornered, total pattern. But they don't see it. With blind obstinacy that seems directly imported from the barracks, cars ram other cars because they have the right of way. People shout at each other instead of trying to help—after all, they're in the right! Then the policeman comes and plays the Sergeant, and everybody else is wrong.

Elegant people in Berlin are proud, that their most popular traffic policemen get so many Christmas presents from drivers. More than would ever be available for poor children. What a lot of hypocritical humility, scared submissiveness, and knuckling-under to authority! They know you have to have order, and they can't imagine any other kind.

It's not order: it's organized boorishness.

Faced with driving in Paris, they're completely impotent. There, the drivers blend into a single stream without false individualism, with few rules but a great deal of tact, a lot of consideration for pedestrians, a lot of fluidity in the relationship between drivers —in short, in spite of all Mr. Chiappe's° police regulations, all kinds of things you can't put into rule-books. How come?

Germans imagine that any given thing can

be organized completely. But it can't be done. You can't codify everything, decide ahead of time, foresee once and for all every possible future occurrence and, discounting all objections, make a rule for it. That's an image of our so-called law, and it works out as you'd expect. On the streets we get the kind of grotesque distortion in which the pedestrian becomes the driver's enemy: he's jealous and ignores cars disdainfully—he'll show those guys. The driver, at the same time, is the pedestrian's enemy: I'll drive where I want! He'd rather die than brake carefully; he won't drive around—that guy could get out of the way! And the man who regulates the traffic, the policeman, is everybody's enemy.

Our ideal is to regulate traffic in every German city from a National Traffic Control Center at the Brandenburg Gate. Green light everywhere at once: 63,657 cars start up, unhesitatingly obedient. Pure joy . . .

Too bad it can't be done. But even so it's rather pretty—our German traffic. Better take a detour.

Week-End

Someone says it, first.

Then, there's quiet.
No one to buy it.

Next comes the pile-up of popularizers,
and organization-organizers—
civil-servants and newspaper-men,
other Jews—even Christians—want in—
a whole committee, hot-inspired,
including officers, retired.
Propaganda? Wow!
Let's go!

Posters and billboards
and founding of groups,
illustrating inserts,
incorporating clubs—
an honorary chairman?
(—he's still breathing, is he?—)
Germany's Oldest Veteran!
Busy, busy, busy—

No fit habitat for truth
is the house that takes the *News*.

And a gentle madness spreads,
addles all the people's heads:
"Week-end" bubbles embryo,
"Week-end" whispers Grandpopo.
Forgotten Chiang's spectacle,
the People's Theater debacle—
forgotten the whole of the *Stahlhelm* shit—
A call resounds!°
And this is it:
	Week-end!

Wik-end-cigars and wiek-ent-spats,°
wiegänd laces in wiekänt boots
and three-handled, special wieghennd pots—
wiehk-end diaper, wigent dummy
weegent bungalow
wiekennt tummy—

And we can so if London can go!

           Although
The minor employee's salary
seldom gets raised in Germany.
If you make 144
you haven't got much week-end-power.

    Our class-struggle
    shapes up clean:
    One side, country-house
    and imposing stream;
    the other gets the picture,
               and the week-
                end dream.

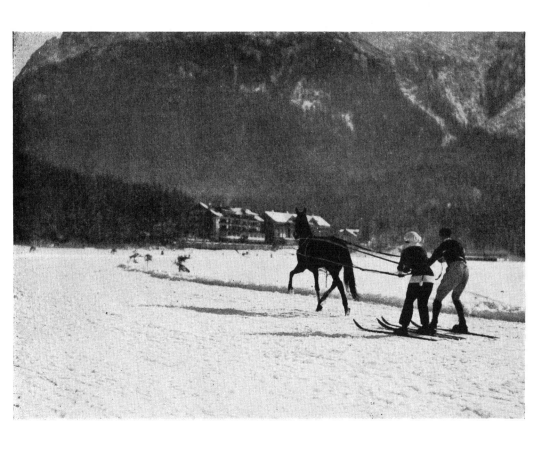

People's Interpellation

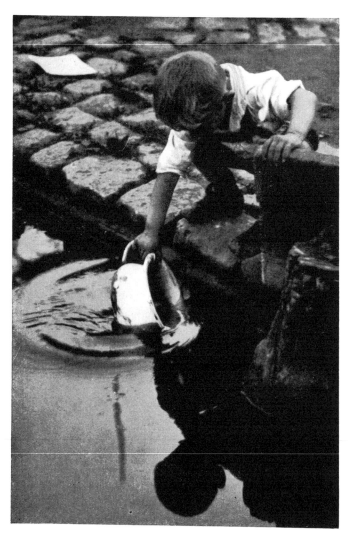

"Is it known to the government that the Minister of Public Worship has sexual relations with a certain Miss K. from Schöneberg? That it is his custom to meet her twice a week in a hotel on Frederick Street?

  "How does the government intend to combat this evil?"

United We Stand

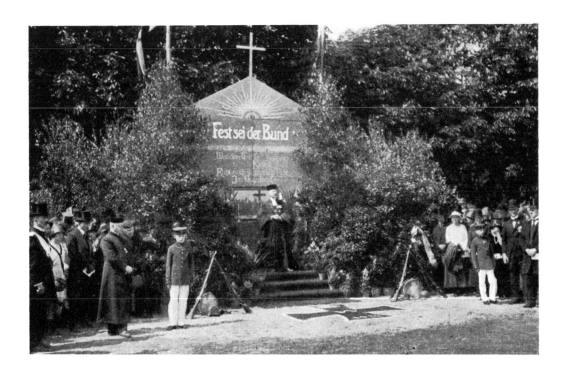

Guns to the right—guns to the left—Baby Jesus in the middle.° Can you imagine a more horrifying sight? There is none.

At this affair, something like, "Always follow your Lord, Jesus Christ" seems to be inscribed above the altar. And there is certainly no doubt, that Christ said, "Thou shalt not kill." A thousand passages in the Bible tell us whose side—the murderer's, or the victim's—Christ, who was one of the world's most courageous revolutionaries, would have chosen. Even if some rabble-rouser in disguise tries to tell me he also said, "Render unto Caesar . . ."

I have no way of knowing what—under Protestant skies—animates this congregation. I have no idea what is being dedicated on such a ceremonious, well-brushed, summer Sunday morning. It's unfathomable.

Chances are, the people have confused feelings, which include diluted metaphysics, the pleasure of wearing a top-hat, some after-breakfast digestive satisfactions, and an anticipation of noontime hunger-pangs. United we stand.

You bet we do!

The apparently congenital characteristics of the councilors who control the church, defeat all the rather touching attempts that young, sincere Christians make to combine the basic moral demands of their religion with the immoral demands made by the state. On August 1, 1914, all the church council was annointed with the same tincture of arrogance and faith. On the 26th of July they still had no idea what was going on; on the 27th they were still unaware of the crimes the government planned to commit behind its future frontline soldiers' backs; on the 28th they were unfamiliar with the documents; on the 29th and 30th, they read falsified telegrams; on the 31st they had the churchbells inspected—

And on August 1, God became a Prussian. The ministers prayed so hard they needed their bands and collars for slobber-bibs. They pronounced the cause they had not yet understood a holy and a just one. United we stand.

The whole business seems petty, trivial. Their crimes don't have the grandeur that the Catholic church's had under the Medici. These people are truly what they call themselves—church-officials. They think of death as something you enter in a register; the government is always right; holiness is granted by city-ordinance every Sunday morning between ten and twelve. And the country lets the day of rest be imposed on it—although it exists not to protect the workers, but to maintain the fiction that everybody goes to church. We have evidence that neither the most numerous, nor the best, part of the people do so. But no one wants to touch the problem: they become pious very quickly, if you mention how silly it is to sell cake at 9:30 and at 1:30, but not at 11:45. What a Prussian exactitude of belief! But bad conscience isn't quite the same as religious faith.

I predict that two church-councilors, and one upper-church-councilor, will now stop attending to their faith in order to hold a meeting. They have to determine whether this chapter needs to be brought to the Attorney General's attention. Paragraph 166 . . . blasphemy . . . defamation of the institutions of the established church . . . Well, friends, come ahead! United we stand.

A Journeyman with an Umbrella

This is a picture of—no, that's not the point now.

Well, it's a photograph from the nineties. It has a painted backdrop. It's a posed, studio portrait. The photographer put on an impressive show—"a dozen identification photos," with every comfort—to immobilize his subject. The man's not to blame, nor is he responsible for his rather comic, not very appropriate travel gear. People probably didn't know any better in those days . . . he may not have had any money either . . . Our criticisms exist on the same level as the jokes that used to be told about Frau Ebert.° Nor can the photograph tell us with certainty what kind of a man this youth will become. We know plenty of insignificant or comic photographs, taken of great men in their youth.

The wanderer here is the president of the Reichstag, Paul Löbe.° He started as a type-setter; went on to be an editor; he became important in the Silesian Social Democratic Party. What made him important?

He was a decent man. He certainly was. He worked hard. He was well-behaved. He was always on time on pay-day. Excellent. But there hasn't been much follow-up.

As Reichstag president, he does a well-organized, neat job. And after all, he doesn't have to deal with anything like the French parliament, that body in which real passions sometimes flare up, and in which the members react to the slightest nuances of language. He deals with decent, broad-bottomed regular fellows, just like himself.

And these are the workers' leaders. Successors to those men who made sacrifice upon sacrifice for the cause they considered holy—these are the men for whom a flame

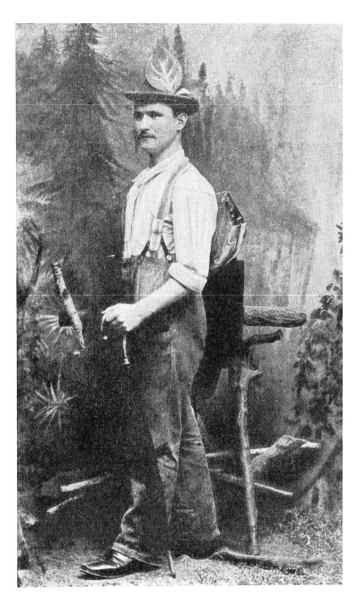

once blazed to the sky. Paul Löbe is one of the better people in his unspeakable party. His vest is clean, and he never betrays his principles. He doesn't have any. But he has a good heart. He always makes me think of a chorus-director. He lifts his little baton as the fellows—glowing with beer, in shirt-sleeves, their coats slung over their arms—gather round: "*one* and *two* and Oh Beautiful Forest———"° (Whereupon a policeman emerges from the beautiful woods and informs the quaking group in thundering tones, that "the singing of songs without a singing-permit is forbidden and punishable.") That's the kind of man.

He's touchingly ignorant in intellectual questions; he's dependably on board when some patriotic idiocy is in the works; he's the much-applauded bard of the annexation of Austria and of Viennese music festivals. Whose deal? Diamond, club, Jack of clubs—Paul, you've got another trump there. That's the kind of man.

There are worse kinds, of course. Breit-scheid's tail-coat, for instance. I have it on good authority that there's a politician inside it—but I don't believe it. Though I wonder whether it looks handsomer full-face, or in profile. And there's High-Secretary Hermann Müller°—oh, why name them all? You know them. This eternal journeyman isn't one of the worst. If only—at least—he were a real wanderer. But his background is painted cardboard, and the bumbershoot shows that he rejects the sublime, and let's have a beer, Paul, in the nearest bar. To the Party!

The End of Monarchy

In abject political disgrace,
he's still a most news-worthy face.
But never mind. He's humorous:
he's got the last laugh—and it's on us.
Because—get yours, while get you can!—
he's still Germany's richest man.

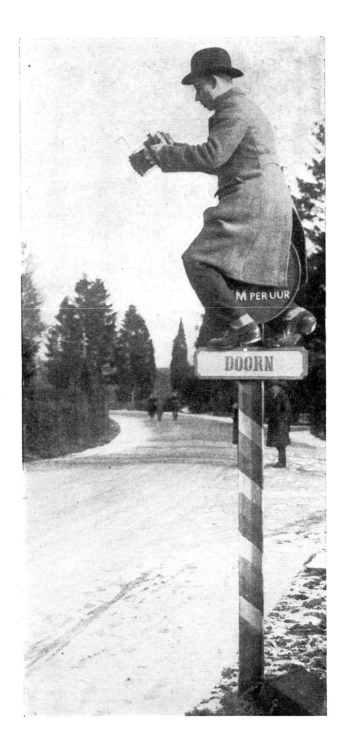

Faces

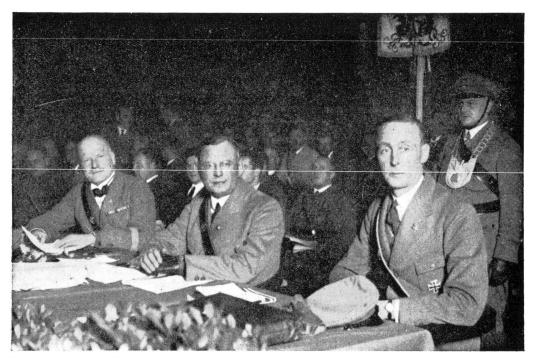

Leaders of the Stahlhelm *convention*

The man on the right has possibilities.

We should look carefully at all the other faces, one by one. Especially at those that begin to be lost in the background shadows. A few stand out clearly. Let's look at this scene, and ask a few questions.

Would we want to be judged by the likes of them?

Would we want to be dependent on these men's notions of right and justice?

Can we imagine that even one of these men has ever wondered about the nature of human existence?

Can we imagine one of these faces bent— for instance—above a dead horse to ask, "What's death all about?"

Could we imagine any of these eyes ever expressing anything that we could call "human kindness"?

Could we imagine any of these men lying in a meadow, and feeling in the humming of bees, what nature means?

We can't.

The uniform isn't even the final external expression of their lack of soul. The uniforms are too big: even a uniform has too much room inside it. Something exists that could be called the Escape into Uniform. The uniform works like a visor: it hides fear, gives protection, provides internal support. They're deserters from civilian life.

This is the nation's flower. The fruit looks it.

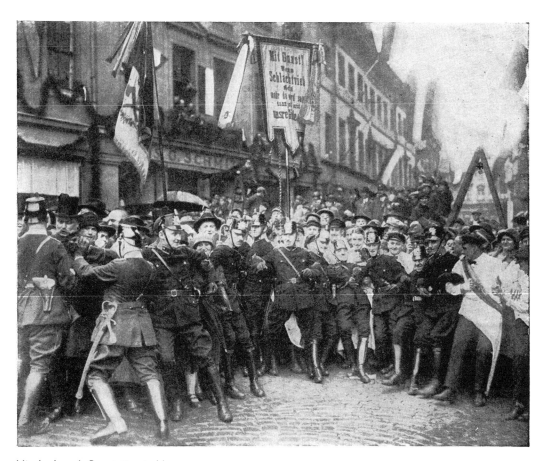

Hindenburgh-Reception in Hannover

  Banner inscription:
Permit this word: The while there's cattle left to slaughter
Will our guild survive and prosper

As the Twig is Bent

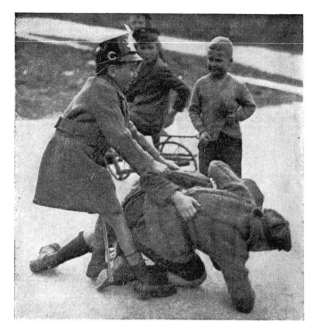

It's possible that this photograph may have been posed. In any case, the participants seem to know that the nice boy, in the policeman's helmet, is the good guy; the other boy, wearing the rowdy-cap, is bad.

When boys used to play "cops and robbers," they were almost always on the side of the noble, free, wild robbers. Today we have begun to see the "representatives of law and order" romantically, and, thus, all our supressed drives can suddenly find marvelous release. We may not like to admit it, but we all like to beat up other people. And here the beating has a higher— yes, even a moral—purpose, as any minister of the gospel would be glad to affirm. The aggressor gets double satisfaction: first, his sadistic drive, and then, his supposedly ethical impulse. A way of making hot air useful.

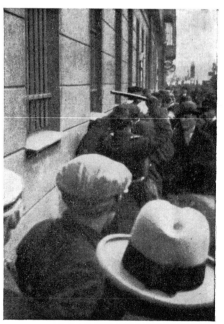

It is shocking to contemplate the brutalizing and corrupting effect of such things on women and children. By nature, they are always on the side of power. If you let power appear in a colorful costume, their enthusiasm will know no bounds—we all know how important a part in mass-delirium the uniform plays. Dress the military in sack-cloth and ashes, and the pleasure of war would diminish by half. But give the soldier a helmet—something out of the ordinary, a totem that separates the wearer from the mass, and sanctifies him— or a saber, and they will be unable to resist him. Sad that the equipment for which we all pay so dearly serves such disgusting purposes.

Song of the Piledrivers

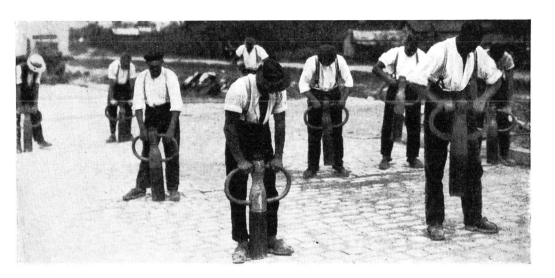

If every stone could be a judge
or general—we'd make them budge—
   Or high official dressed in black—
we'd ram so strong
it wouldn't take long—
    whack—
        rack-a-tack—
            whack-whack.

That every stone and every stone
should be as hard to hammer down
as the simple fact:
The working-man will not go on
slaving for another's gain—
    whack—
        rack-a-tack—
            whack-whack.

Who marches to music, who drives with a
  roar
over the pavement we labored for?
  Who'll answer for our wrong?
    Pick up the rammer,
    All together: hammer:
      Not long.
        Not long.
          Not long.

Memorabilia from the
Royal Yacht "Caesar's Eagle"

No. 1 : **Painting depicting His Majesty the Kaiser on
shipboard on the high seas.
Above the lower frame, dedication by His Majesty,
in the following words:**

Wednesday, 5 March 1890

In my travels I purposed not only to become acquainted with
foreign countries and their governments and to cultivate friendly
relations with the rulers of neighboring nations. My travels—
subject though they were to many misinterpretations—had the
high value for me of removing me from daily, partisan activities,
and allowing me to evaluate calmly and from a distance the
conditions at home. Whoever has communed with himself,
alone on the high seas and standing on a ship's bridge under
God's starry sky, will not deny the value of such a journey. I
would wish a number of my fellow citizens the experience of such
hours, in which a man can justify his ambitions and achievements
to himself.

Oh, that you had!

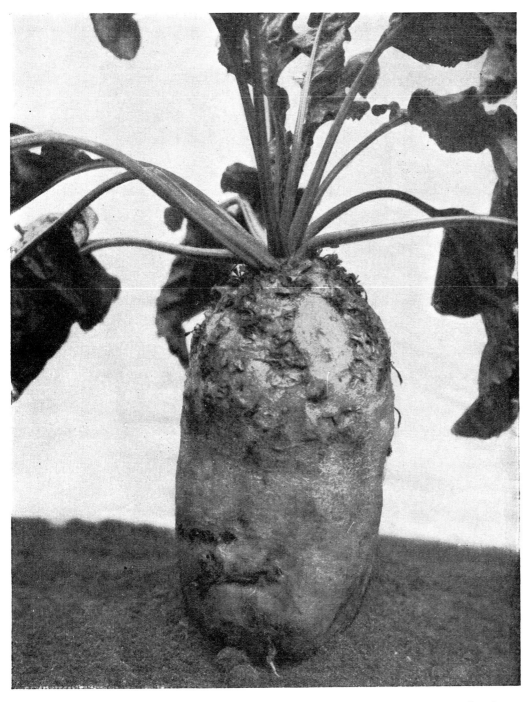

Rutabaga

At Last, the Truth about Remarque

The yellow press of Berlin has for months been howling advertisements for a disgusting production by Erich Maria Remarque. As a matter of fact, the very title of this work, *All Quiet on the Western Front*, was stolen from the High Command° (Mr. District Attorney?), and it describes war the way only a typical shirker could imagine it.

The next issue of the *South German Monthly* will finally reveal the truth about this traitor to his country; the data, checked by Professor Cossmann,° is almost reliable. Thanks to a special arrangement with the editors of the monthly we are able to give our readers special prepublication information today.

Erich Salomon Markus—that's this little Jew-boy's name°—had been a minor Synagogue caretaker (a so-called *salat schammes*)° in the Jewish Synagogue on Oranien Street in Berlin. This scion of Judah was born in Zinnentzitz in Silesia, where his father, Abraham Markus, had—a kosher butcher shop. (Notice anything?) The years during which Daddy Markus followed his noble calling there, are marked by the disappearance of an unusually large number of Christian children from the region; of course, they were always found very soon after their disappearance, but it has never been established [! the editors] whether they really were the same children!

Erich Salomon never had a mother; as is customary in Jewish families two mothers are recorded on his birth certificate: a certain Sarah Bienstock and an unmarried [!!] Rosalie Himmelstoss (we will have occasion to return to this name).

At nine years of age, the young Markus began his "service" in the aforementioned Synagogue. His duties were lighting the candles, dusting the Bible, and holding the Jewish boy-babies who were to be circumcised. (This last is most important for his later development.) It is said, that on one of these occassions the son of a well-known Berlin department store proprietor was accidentally circumcised twice. For this reason Markus was removed from office. Salomon Markus next became an unemployed drifter in Berlin; he tried to find employment in the theater and, it is said, that he played all the title roles in Brecht's *Criminals*° several times, under the direction of his race-fellow, Reinhardt.° Subsequently, the young Markus was active in Berlin as a candy-butcher, pimp, dog-barber, and editor. Markus is a free-mason, and a Jesuit.

The war came.

Markus went to the front. That is, he was assigned to the Mounted Supply Corps but —because of an illness which we will not specifically name here—he was unable to serve, and was employed behind the lines. Because of an incomprehensible carelessness on the part of the military authorities, Markus worked as a clerk in the Main Headquarters of his Majesty, the Crown Prince; thus he never saw the enemy, even from a distance.

After the war, he settled in Osnabrück as a ladies' dressmaker; he next became assistant-brakeman for the Jewish hearse in Breslau, and later moved to Hannover. Professor Cossman leaves open the question of whether Markus may not have known Haarmann,° or may even have been his accomplice . . .

This worthless swindler dares to write a report, with falsehood written on its very forehead, for Berlin's yellow press! In his

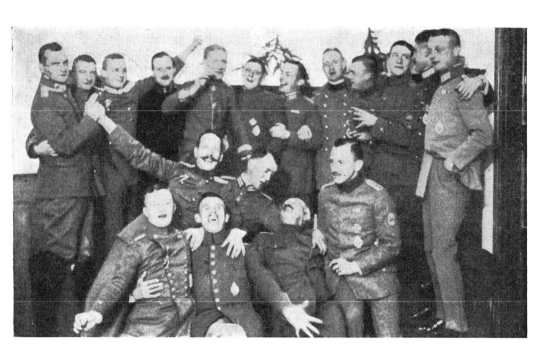

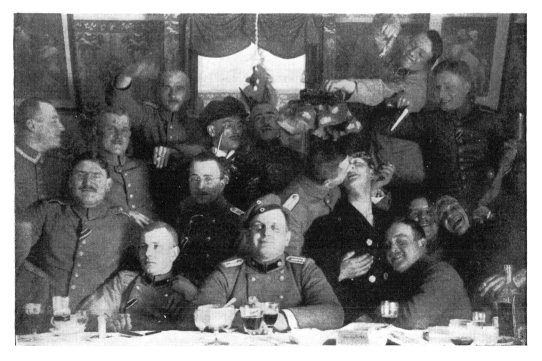

book he not only uses his own mother's name (Himmelstoss!) to denigrate one of his superiors (Mr. District Attorney?), but he also accuses German soldiers of cruelties of which they would never have been capable. Wasn't the German soldier famous for painless hand-to-hand combat, and humane drum-fire? Salomon Markus, of course, is unaware of this fact; while his comrades at the front marched to occupy Paris to the tune of "Deutschland, Deutschland, über alles"—but unhappily found it already occupied, the Jew Markus lived a riotous, gluttonous life behind the lines. When the German troops left, eighty-four illegitimate children were found in the environs of the Crown Prince's Headquarters alone—and who, if not Markus, could have fathered those children?

We must thank God that the book has not met with unreserved success.

The women of Germany, in particular, know what is proper. We must be grateful to them for knowing how to distinguish between heroic Germans and unheroic non-Germans; it is they who look up to Siegfried, Hagen & Co. and to the other heroes of our true German tradition. The German woman wants to look up to a hero. We have lately established this joyful and pleasurable fact at an evening get-together in Berlin.

As we noticed on that evening, her husband's life matters less to the German woman, than that he die a hero's death; she is ready to die with him, and will call out "I'm dying!" each and every time—even if she should have to marry ten times over! We know a man's character by the length of his sword, and the German woman demands that her husband be strong to defend his Fatherland—and if it be not attacked, why, we'll see to it, that it *be* attacked! [A true German sentiment! the Editors.] A noble German woman, wife of a high official, recently told us, "For me there is nothing more beautiful in our marriage, than the moment when I button hubby's uniform, or unbutton it. It's an indescribable feeling!"

Salomon Markus, however, has been judged. In the imperishable published pages of the "South German Monthly Review" his work is exposed for what it is: A black torch, bought and paid for by our enemies and the Marxists, which cannot hold its water beside the bright armour of German defensive strength—!

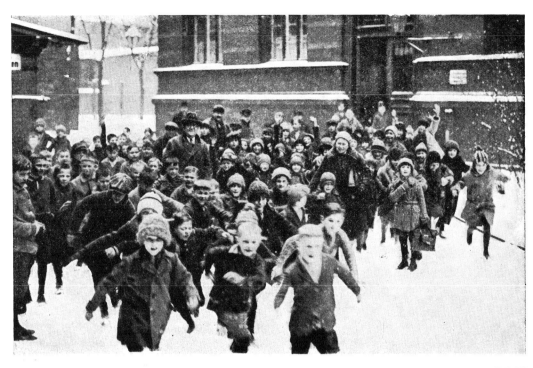

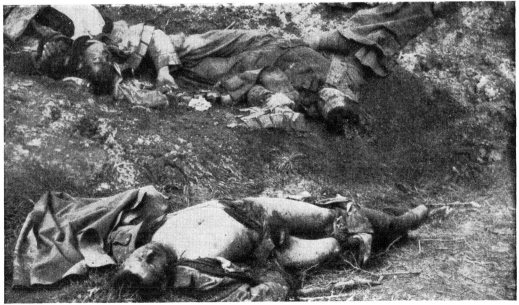

213

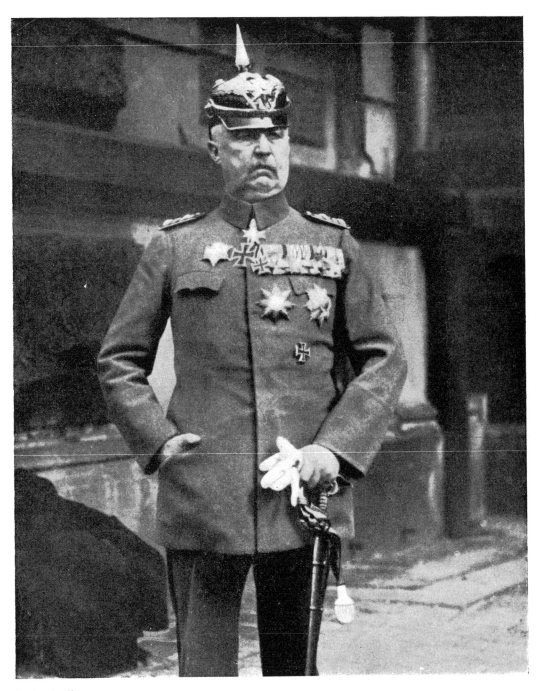

Ludendorff

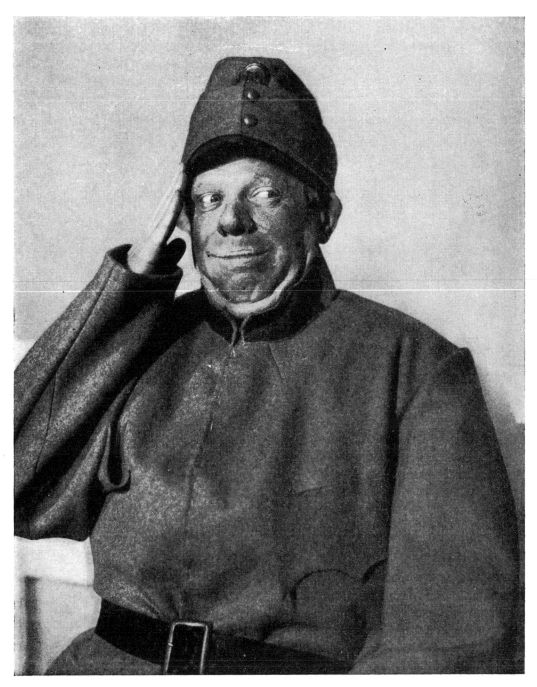

Schweik°

Only

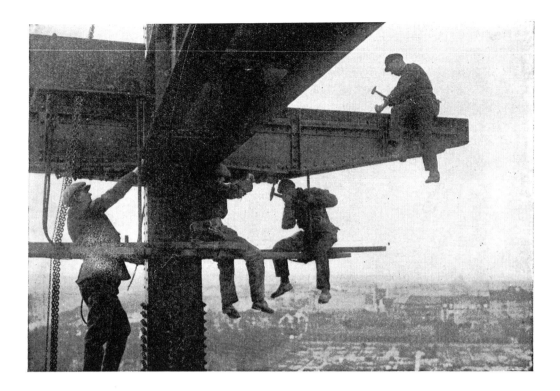

I recently learned something from a very elegant writer. "It is a mistake to think that the workers built the towers. They only put them up." Only—"only" is good.

That more towers don't collapse, more railroad bridges don't cave in, more wheels don't jump the tracks, seems continually amazing. What is it all founded on? It has a double foundation.

It rests on the intellect that conceived it— and on the infinite conscientiousness that carries out the plan. The intellectual worker, at least some of the time, gains more than his own inner satisfaction from his work; he shares in the profits and can buy stock; he gets fame and his name becomes known—at least sometimes. (Even though large concerns have learned how to suppress the engineer, the inventor, the intellectual jack-of-all-trades until he is forced into the dismal role of employee; the worker ought not to overvalue the white collar: it can be a delusion.) But what does the worker gain?

An inadequate wage. Little satisfaction. At the very most, a word of recognition from the foreman who knows his men. Who will know that Schulze IV is O.K. That whatever job you put him on gets done. But, that's all.

It's even more amazing, then, that all these labors get done with a great deal of devotion, attention to detail, and serious technical knowledge. Of course, the worker has to consider, first of all, that he'll be fired if he doesn't do a good job. And then what? But besides that, he often has the pride of his trade and takes pleasure in the job itself —in spite of everything and even though so many forces are busy trying to take it away from him. Occasionally, the worker can even forget for whom he's really working— the human being is made in such a way that his work can absorb him completely; he can tighten screws as if they belonged to him, as if he got paid for it. He doesn't get paid. He only gets his weekly wage.

So they hang on the sides of towers, lie on the bridges, pull themselves up and down the scaffoldings and wield paintbrushes, hanging in midair—I forgot to say, only. They're only putting things up. They're only seeing that the intellectual vision of the builder becomes a reality—after all, that's not much, is it? Anyone could do it. I doubt whether the elegant writer, who wrote that "only," could. Which is why I think:

The manual laborer is equal to the intellectual worker. The former cannot plan the tower on paper; doesn't know the heated nights in which the work—still only a concept—cries out for completion. The latter can't get up at five every morning and be at work in all weathers, work without dizzyness, offer up the strength of his body . . . Each does his own thing.

"Only?"—a petit-bourgeois philosopher is the most superfluous thing in the world.

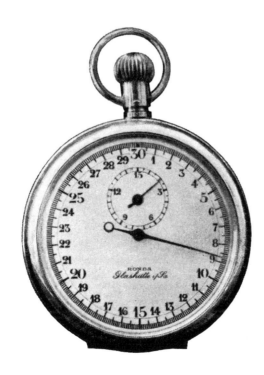

Charity

See the convalescent home
owned by the stock-holders' group:
Mornings, they dish-out gruel,
and evenings, barley-soup.
   And the workers are allowed in the park . . .
   Good. That's the penny.
     But where is the Mark?

They give you hand-outs now and then
with pious protestations;
pregnant women get medicine—
they need new generations.
   They'll send a charity-coffin 'round . . .
   And that's the penny.
     But where's the pound?

Thousands and thousands have flown away
filling strangers' hands;
after much argument, the board
agreed on the dividends.
   A few get marrow. Soup's for the many.
   They get the dollar. You have the penny.

Proletarians:
   Don't be taken in!
They owe you more than they're giving.
They owe you the lot! Factory and mine—
   the large estate and the shipping-line . . .
And the pleasures and powers of living.
   Take all you can get! Don't take the guff!
   Remember your class! Grow strong enough!
   The Mark and the penny are yours by right!
     Fight—!

German Movie

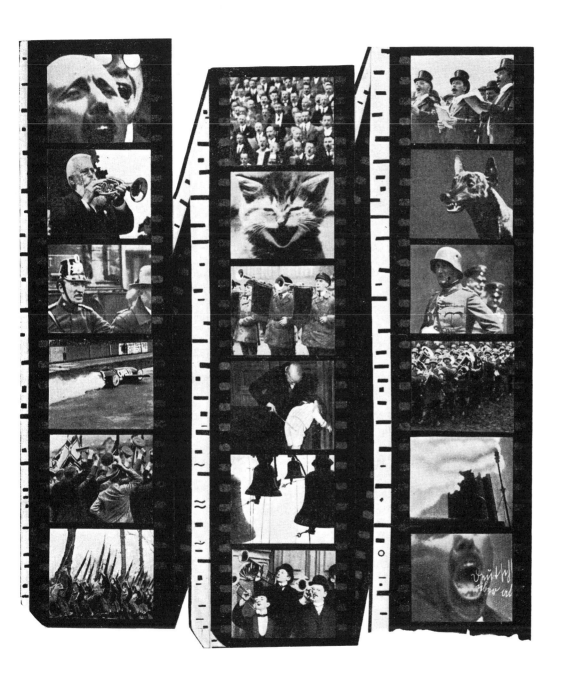

Home

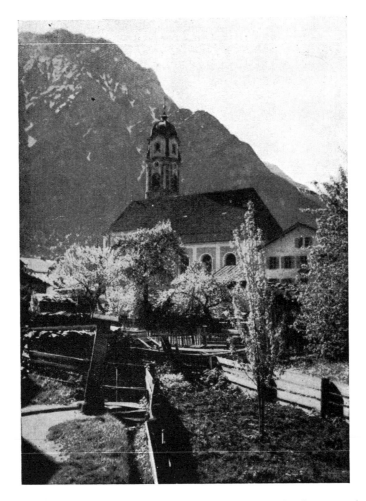

"But you always have one comfort, a refuge, an escape. There are trees even on the flat plains around you, shining pools of water look up at you, the horizons are far and even through the darkest fogs you can still breathe in the scent of the fields."
—Alfons Goldschmidt, *Deutschland heute* [*Germany Today*]

We have said *No* in 219 pages—*No* in pity and *No* in love, *No* in hate and *No* in passion. Now at last we want to say *Yes*. *Yes*, to the landscape and to the land, Germany.

The land in which we were born and whose language we speak.

Let the state get out of the way—we love our home. Why? Why this land when there are so many others? There are such beautiful countries.

Yes, but our heart doesn't speak in those other countries. Or if it does, it speaks a foreign language. We're unfamiliar with the earth: we admire and appreciate—but it's not the same.

There is no earthly reason to kneel down in front of every spot in Germany and to lie, "How beautiful!" But there is something common to all the regions—and it's different for each one of us. One person may be most intimately moved in the mountains, where field and meadow peer into the little streets. Or at the edge of mountain lakes where the air is full of the scent of water and wood and rock, and where one can be alone. If that's where one is at home, it will make one's heart pound faster. All this feeling has been cheapened in bad books, stupid verses and films, so that one is almost afraid to say, I love my homeland.

But if you can hear the music of the mountains and feel the rhythm of a landscape— No, it's enough, really, just to feel that you've come home—that this is your country, your mountain, your lake, even though you do not own a single foot of ground.

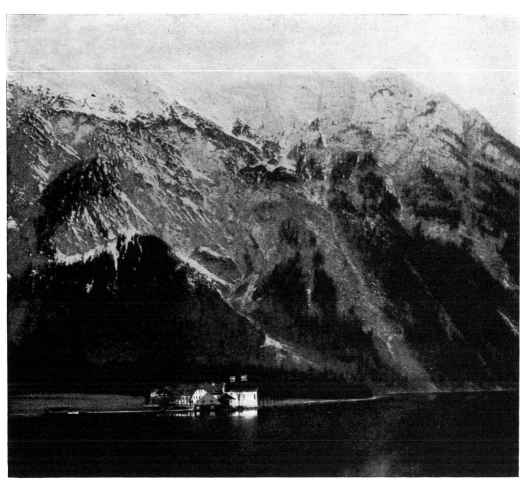

This is a feeling separate from all politics, and it is out of this feeling that we love this land.

We love it because the air flows through its little alleys, this way, and no other; because of the quality of the light that we recognize; for a thousand reasons that cannot be enumerated—that are not even conscious, but nevertheless deep in the blood.

We love it, in spite of the horrible false notes of anachronistic architecture around which one has to detour. We try to avoid looking at monstrosities like this one. We love this land, in spite of the pastry-cook's images of our rulers that threaten us in the woods and in many a public place.

Let them threaten, we say, and are on our way over the heath. Which is lovely, in spite of everything.

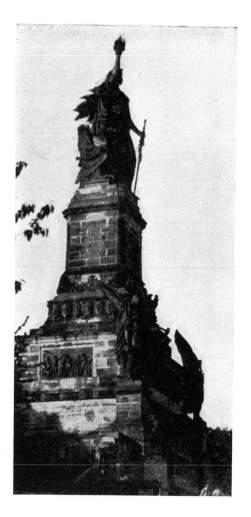

The loveliness can be aristocratic and no less German ; I don't forget that hundreds of peasants lived in poverty so that this might be built—but nevertheless, it is beautiful. Although we have no intention of turning our book into a picture album suitable for someone's birthday—there are so many of those, and they're always incomplete—there's always another spot in Germany, another corner, another landscape that the photographer forgot to take along. And besides, we all have our own private Germany. Mine lies to the north. It begins in middle Germany, where the air seems to rise so luminously above the roofs. As you get farther and farther north, your heart beats louder and louder, until you finally sense the sea. The sea—still miles away, every fence post and every thatched roof suddenly takes on a deeper significance. We are here, they say, only because the sea lies just behind us. We're here for the ocean. The vegetation moves in the wind. You feel the fine sand between your teeth.

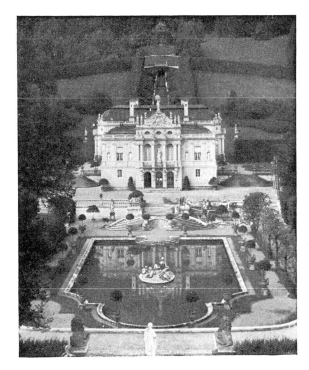

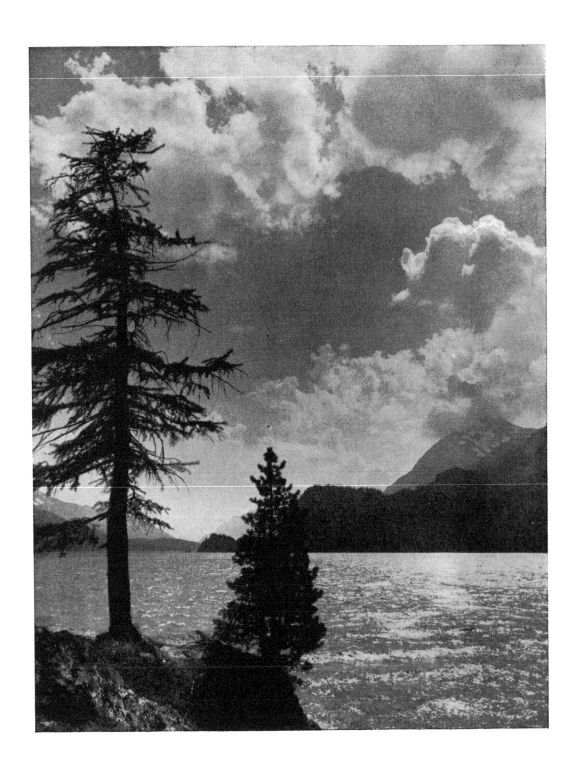

The sea. Childhood impressions are unforgettable; the hours you spent here can't
be erased. Every year you feel the same joy in
the first greeting, no matter how blue the
Mediterranean. The German sea. And the
beechwoods, and the moss that's so soft
under your feet, that your step cannot be
heard; and in the midst of the woods the
little pool on which the midges dance. You
can touch the trees and understand what the
wind in their branches says. We called this
book "Deutschland über alles" as a joke—
such a foolish line from a big-mouth poem.
No, Germany doesn't count above all and
isn't over all—never. But let our land be
with, including all. And let the confession,
with which this book ends, stand here:

Yes, we love this land.

And now I want to tell you something:

Those who call themselves nationalists
and are really only bourgeois-militarists,
don't have an exclusive lease on this land and
its language. That's not true. Neither the
member of the government in his morning
coat, nor the professor, nor the ladies and
gentlemen of the *Stahlhelm*, make up
Germany by themselves. We're here too.

They open their mouths wide and yell "In
Germany's name . . ." They yell, "We love
our country and we're the only ones who
love it." It isn't true.

We'll let anyone who wants outdo us in
patriotism. Our feelings are international.
But no one can outdo us in our love of home
—not even those who have registered the
country in their name. It is ours.

I am disgusted by the nationalists-in-
reverse, who find nothing good in our
country—not a single hair, no words, no sky,
no ocean wave. But I will certainly not fall

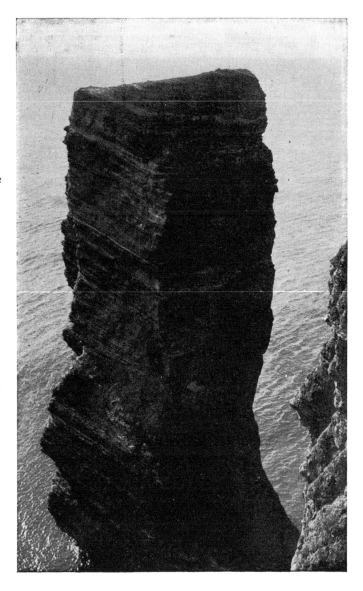

over into "fatherland-ish" excesses either. The flags are nothing to us—but we love the land. And we, who were born here, who write and speak better German than most of the nationalist asses, have the same right to our country as the nationalist organizations that drum up marchers along the roads. With the very same right, we take possession of stream and forest, beach and house, clearing and meadow: it is our land. Because we love Germany, we have the right to hate it. When others speak of Germany, they must take us into account: the communists, the young socialists, the pacifists, and the lovers of freedom of all degrees; they have to think of us, when they think, Germany. It's too simple to pretend that Germany is made up only of the nationalist organizations.

Germany is a divided country. We are one part of it.

And in the midst of all its contradictions—without flags, without barrel-organs, without sentimentality, and without drawn swords—we assert our firm and quiet love for our homeland.

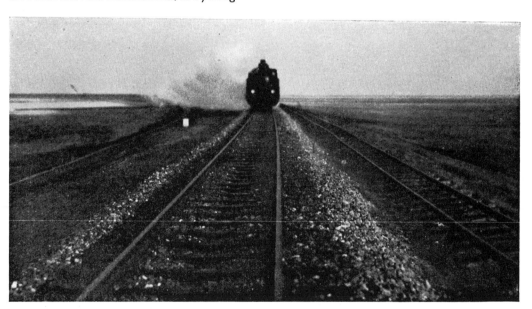

Notes

Annotated items are signaled in the text by the superior symbol °, and are arranged by page number and catchword below.

1. Hölderlin: From Friederich Hölderlin's novel *Hyperion* (1797–9).

6. "standing at attention": *"durch Anlegen der Hände an die zu diesem Zweck angebrachte Hosennaht."* Literally, "by putting their hands on the trouser seams which have been provided for this purpose."

7. Ludendorff: Erich Ludendorff (1865–1937), German general in the First World War, used the pseudonym Erich Lindström when he fled to Sweden toward the end of 1918.

7. Kitchen-help: An allusion to the lines *"Doch jeder Jüngling hat wohl mal/'N Hang fürs Küchenpersonal"* from Wilhelm Busch's *Die fromme Helene* (1872). In H. Arthur Klein's translation of *Hypocritical Helena*: "A young man often feels a hankering/For kitchen help and hanky-pankering."

15. Ignaz Wrobel: One of the four pseudonyms under which Tucholsky wrote (in addition to using his own name). He called this situation "gay schizophrenia." Tucholsky thought of Ignaz Wrobel, a name he regarded as particularly grating and distasteful, as an acid, bespectacled, closely shaven, slightly hunchbacked redhead. He used this name for his more aggressive and mordant political and social satires.

18. "black, red, and gold": Official state colors of Wilhelminian Germany. See note below on Fritz Ebert.

20. Democracy: Translations of signs in the picture are, top to bottom: "Side Entrance/for deliveries and service personnel/this way." "Entrance around corner."

"Stairway/Masters and mistresses only."

25. Philipp Sh.: *"Philipp, dessen Namen rechtens mit einem Sch. anfängt"*—"Philip, whose name properly begins with Sch." (for *Scheisse*, in English a scatological four-letter word). The reference is to the politician Philipp Scheidemann (1865–1939), who in 1918 served as state secretary in the Cabinet of Prince Max of Baden and on November 9 of that year proclaimed the German Republic. In the following year Scheidemann served as its first chancellor, but he resigned in opposition to the Treaty of Versailles.

25. Fritz Ebert: Friedrich (Fritz) Ebert (1871–1925), Social Democratic politician, German Chancellor in 1918 and Federal President from 1919 to 1925.

25. Groener: Wilhelm Groener (1867–1939), general and politician, Minister of the Army from 1928 to 1932, Minister of the Interior, 1931 to 1932.

27. Liebknecht, Luxemburg: The Social Democratic politician Karl Liebknecht (1871–1919) and the Communist leader Rosa Luxemburg (1870–1919) were co-founders of the revolutionary Spartacus League. Both were murdered.

27. [Posters]: Translations of headlines in posters are as follows: *Center*—"Socialization is here!/ . . . The Coal syndicate/ . . . Socialization of potash mining/ . . . German collective-economy/ . . . *And that is/Socialism!"* *Right*—"Socialization of Mining."

31. *Stahlhelm*: Der Stahlhelm (Steel Helmet) was a paramilitary organization of World-War-I veterans founded in 1918 by Franz Seldte and active in the nationalistic politics of the Weimar Republic.

32. Reimann: Hans Reimann (b. 1889), Leipzig-born author especially noted for his

satirical anecdotes (*Sächsische Miniaturen,* 1922 ff.) written in the Saxon dialect.

32. A Kaiser costs 50,000 Mark: In 1929 the exchange value Marks to Dollars was approximately four to one; hence this represents something like $12,500.

37. Prince Eitel Friedrich: Prince Eitel Friedrich of Prussia (1883–1942), the second son of Kaiser Wilhelm II, led a battalion of guardsmen in the First World War.

42. Mr. Tirpitz: Alfred von Tirpitz (1849–1930), grand admiral and architect of the German war fleet, resigned in 1916.

42. [Placards]: Translations of placards in the picture are, from left to right: "We are starving!" "We, veterans of labor, ask only our rightfully earned secure old age." "Employed Workers: We are sacrifices to the Capitalist Profit Economy. Help us and you help yourselves." "We, pensioned Krupp empl . . . at last demand . . . instead of empty election promis . . ." "Krupp, the city of Essen, and the government let us go on starving."

50. *I. G. Farben:* A combine of dye and chemical factories, the largest industrial organization in Germany between 1925 and its dissolution in 1952.

52. old Kahl: Wilhelm Kahl (1849–1932), professor of Protestant canon law, co-editor of the *Deutsche Juristenzeitung,* member of the *Reichstag* from 1920 on and chairman of its committee on criminal law and penal reform.

53. Dr. Georg Michaelis: Georg Michaelis (1857–1936), Prussian prime minister, Federal Chancellor in 1917.

53. Dr. Wilhelm Cuno: Wilhelm Cuno (1876–1933), ship-owner and politician, chancellor in 1922–1923. He formed a

"government of economy" and after the French occupation of the Ruhr region pursued a policy of passive resistance.

53. Gottlieb von Jagow: Gottlieb von Jagow (1863–1935), state secretary in the German Foreign Office 1913–16, member of the Prussian parliament.

53. Dr. Lewald: Theodor Lewald (1860–1947), state secretary in the Ministry of the Interior and promoter of sports in Germany, member of the Olympic Committee and commissioner of the Olympic Games in Berlin in 1936 (even though of Jewish descent).

54. Mr. Gustav Bauer: Gustav Bauer (1870–1944), Social Democratic politician, Chancellor 1919 to 1920.

54. Mr. Hermes (Mosel): Andreas Hermes (1878–1964), economist agronomist, Minister of Nutrition, 1920 to 1921, Minister of Finance, 1922 to 1923. "Mosel" refers to a series of articles in which it was charged that Hermes had given money and supplies to the Mosel, Saar, and Ruwer wine growers' associations in return for cheap wine.

54. Mr. Emminger: Erich Emminger (1880–1951), member of the *Reichstag* from 1920 to 1933. As Minister of Justice (1923–1924), he created a new jury system.

55. "Animals looking at you": *Tiere sehen dich an* was the title of a popular picture book (1928) by Paul Eipper (1891–1964), an artist and author of animal and travel books.

56. Hauser: Kaspar Hauser, one of Tucholsky's pseudonyms, derived from the name of the mysterious foundling (ca. 1812–1833).

56. Grumbach: Salomon Grumbach (1884–1952), Alsatian-born French Social Democratic politician and journalist.

56. Breitscheid: Rudolf Breitscheid (1874–

1944), economist and leader of the Social Democratic party, Prussian Minister of the Interior, 1918–19.

56. Brüninghaus: Franz Willi Brüninghaus (b. 1870), admiral in the First World War, leader of the *Deutsche Volkspartei* in the *Reichstag* since 1920, proponent of the "stab-in-the-back" legend concerning the war.

56. Killinger: Manfred von Killinger (1886–1944, suicide), leader of the Bavarian Free Corps, later in the SA.

57. Noske: Gustav Noske (1868–1946), Social Democratic politician, commanded the troops that ruthlessly crushed the Spartacus uprising in Berlin in 1919. He served as Minister of Defense from 1919 to 1920 and subsequently was president of the province of Hanover.

57. "With swastikas on our helmets": *"Hakenkreuz am Stehl . . . am Stahlhelm"*— play on words in the original, literally "on the steal . . . the steel helmet."

59. Rudolf Herzog: Rudolf Herzog (1869–1943), novelist, dramatist, and poet. *Die Wiskottens* (about the Ruhr district) appeared in 1922, *Kameraden* in 1922.

60. Mrs. Courts-Mahler: Hedwig Courts-Mahler (1867–1950), prolific writer of pot-boilers. Some 30 million copies of her more than 200 novels have been sold.

60. Clauren: Heinrich Clauren was the pen name of Carl Gottlieb Samuel Heun (1771–1854), a writer whose sentimental, pseudo-romantic stories and novels were once widely read.

60. Arnolt Bronnen: Arnolt Bronnen (originally Bronner) (1895–1959), Austrian-born expressionistic dramatist and novelist, a political activist who began as a leftist and moved to the extreme right.

60. Ewers: Hanns Heinz Ewers (1871–1943), author of bizarre, demonic novels like *Alraune* and *Vampir*.

60. Bonsels: Waldemar Bonsels (1881–1952), novelist, author of travel and animal books (*Die Biene Maja*, 1912).

62. Baron von Lersner: Kurt Freiherr von Lersner (b. 1883), imperial legation counselor, diplomat, chairman of the German Peace Commission at Versailles in 1919, member of the *Reichstag*, 1920 to 1924.

62. Baron von Grünau: The embassy counselor Kurt Freiherr von Grünau.

62. Colonel Heye: Col. Wilhelm Heye (1869–1946), army chief of staff in the First World War and from 1926 to 1930.

63. Freikorps: Literally, free corps, volunteer corps. Nationalistic home-guards formed in Germany after World War I. Cf. note on *Stahlhelm*.

64. Gustav Landauer: Gustav Landauer (1870–1919), German-Jewish scholar and Socialist activist, murdered while serving as a Minister of the Bavarian soviet republic.

65. Arthur Eloesser: Arthur Eloesser (1870–1938), German-Jewish literary historian and drama critic.

67. August the Strong: Augustus II of Poland, "the Strong" (1670–1733), Elector of Saxony and later King of Poland.

67. Herzog is the Duke: *Herzog* is the German word for "duke."

67. Walter Bloem: Walter Bloem (1868–1951), novelist and dramatist of nationalistic persuasion.

68. Mr. Höcker: Paul Oskar Höcker (1865–1944), editor of *Velhagen und Klasings Monatshefte* and author of novels, including *Die Stadt in Ketten: Ein Liller Roman* (The City in Chains: A Novel About Lille).

70. Fuad: Fuad I (1868–1936), Sultan and King of Egypt (from 1917 on).

71. Ludwig Thoma: Ludwig Thoma (1867–1921), Bavarian storyteller and dramatist.

75. Mr. Justice Bumke: Erwin Bumke (1874–1945, suicide), jurist, president of the Federal Court since 1929. As section head in the Ministry of Justice from 1919 on, Bumke attempted to make reforms in criminal justice.

80. Hindenburg: Paul von Beneckendorff und Hindenburg (1847–1934), German commander-in-chief in the First World War, *Reich* president from 1925 on.

89. "Dear Departed": *"Der Selige,"* Tucholsky's frequent reference to Kaiser Wilhelm II, who had departed for Doorn, Holland, after Germany's defeat in the war. See also illustration on page 203 above.

89. Mr. Matthes: The Social Democratic journalist Joseph Matthes was driven into exile in France in the early twenties because of his muck-raking opposition to Germany's Ruhr policies and his support of the separatist movement.

89. Mr. Dorten: The separatist Hans Adam Dorten (b. 1880).

89. Mr. Hagen: The banker and industrialist Louis Hagen (originally Levy) (1855–1932). The other Hagen was the villain, Siegfried's killer, in the *Nibelungenlied*, the German national epic.

89. Mr. Adenauer: As lord mayor of Cologne from 1917 to 1933 and as a member of the provincial diet of the Rhineland, Konrad Adenauer (1876–1967) fought for an autonomous Rhineland.

89. Mr. Sollmann: Wilhelm Sollmann (1881–1951), editor of the *Rheinische Zeitung* from 1913 on, Minister of the Interior in 1923 and a *Reichstag* member until 1933, opposed France's Rhine policies and separatism.

91. Walter Hasenclever: In 1932 the dramatist Walter Hasenclever (1890–1940, suicide) collaborated with Tucholsky in the latter's only dramatic work, the comedy *Christoph Columbus*.

91. Peter Panter: Peter Panter ("round and agile") was yet another of Tucholsky's pseudonyms. Names like Panter and Theobald Tiger were not originally meant to suggest the ferocity of wild animals, although that may have been their effect later on. One of Tucholsky's teachers in law school used to coin such alliterative animal names in discussions of law suits as equivalents of our "John Doe."

91. Pallenberg, Valetti, Paul Graetz, Ilka Grüning, Otto Wallburg: Max Pallenberg (1877–1934), Viennese-born actor in both dramatic and comedy roles; Rosa Valetti (originally Vallentin) (1878–1937), Berlin-born actress of stage and screen, cabaret singer and film star *(The Blue Angel)*; Paul Graetz (1890–1937), stage and film actor, cabaret star; Ilka Grüning (1878–1964), Vienna-born actress; Otto Wallburg (originally Wasserzieher), stage and film actor, cabaret performer, especially noted for his comic roles, who perished in Auschwitz in 1944.

91. Massary, Emil Jannings, Lucie Höflich: Fritzi Massary (originally Friederike Masarek) (1882–1969), Viennese-born actress and singer, star of operettas and revues; Emil Jannings (1884–1950), Swiss-born actor and film star *(The Blue Angel)*; Lucie Höflich (1883–1956), comic stage and film actress.

91. Piscator: The theatrical producer and director Erwin Piscator (1893–1966).

91. Jessner: Leopold Jessner (1878–1945), theatrical director, head of the Prussian State Theaters until 1933.

91. Haller: Hermann Haller (1871–1943), author and director of revues in Berlin.

91. "songs": Tucholsky wrote "Sonx"—to indicate the German pronunciation of the word which denoted cabaret songs or chansons.

92. *Threepenny Opera*: The *Dreigroschenoper,* the most famous collaborative effort between Bert Brecht (1898–1956) and Kurt Weill (1900–1950).

92. Lehar: Franz Lehar (1870–1948), Hungarian-born Austrian operetta composer.

92. Meisel, Kollo, Hindemith, Nelson: Will Meisel (b. 1897), composer of film scores, chansons, and operettas; Walter Kollo (1878–1940), Berlin operetta composer; Rudolf Nelson (originally Lewysohn) (1878–1960), director of cabarets and composer of chansons. The inclusion of the serious composer Paul Hindemith (1895–1963) in this list is not as far-fetched as it may seem, for 1929 witnessed the premiere of Hindemith's topical comic opera *Neues vom Tage* (News of the Day), with a libretto by Marcellus Schiffer (1892–1932), a writer of revues and composer of chansons.

92. Mehring: Walter Mehring (b. 1896), social satirist, poet, and writer for the cabaret.

92. Kästner: Erich Kästner (b. 1899), social satirist, poet and storyteller, author of children's books.

92. Zorgiebel: Karl Frierich Zörgiebel (1878–1961), commissioner of police in Berlin from 1922 to 1933.

94. "There's a corpse . . . fisher girl": *"Es liegt eine Leiche im Landwehrkanal/Fischerin du Kleine"*—lines from Walter Mehring's sardonic *Wiegenlied* (Cradle Song); the second line alludes to a hit song then popular in Berlin.

94. Mr. Polgar, Mr. Roellinghoff: The essayist, storyteller, dramatist and theater critic Alfred Polgar (1873–1955); the cabaret writer and performer Charlie (Karl Gottlieb Josef) Roellinghoff.

94. Mr. Ammer: In 1908 the Austrian Karl Klammer (1879–1959) published translations from François Villon under the pen name of K. L. Ammer. Bert Brecht later was accused of using some of these translations almost verbatim in his *Dreigroschenoper.*

94. Remarque: The novelist Erich Maria Remarque (1898–1971). (See also p. 210 ff., above.)

94. "moving staircase": Presumably a reference to the so-called "Jessnertreppe." Leopold Jessner had a special feeling for the various planes of the stage and was noted for his effective use of steps and shifting levels to achieve spectacular tridimensional effects. Jessner also made a film, *Die Hintertreppe* (The Back Stairs), in 1921.

96. "Berlin is Worth the Trip.": A 1970's tourist slogan, to correspond to the original, *"Jeder einmal in Berlin,"* from the twenties.

96. Mr. Klöpfer: Eugen Klöpfer (1886–1950), stage and film actor, became director of the Berlin Volksbühne in 1936.

96. Kate: Presumably a reference to the cabaret singer Kate Kühl (originally Elfriede Katarina Nehrhaupt), who, like most of the above-mentioned cabaret performers, sang many of Tucholsky's own chansons.

98. Stresemann: Gustav Stresemann,

1878–1929, Chancellor and Foreign Minister from 1923 on.

98. the Bois girl: Ilse Bois, actress and cabaret performer especially noted for her parodistic impressions of other performers, member of the *Kabarett der Komiker* in Berlin from 1926 on.

98. Hesterberg: Trude Hesterberg (1892–1967), actress, star of the Berlin cabaret.

98. Presber: Rudolf Presber (1868–1935), storyteller, dramatist, poet, essayist, and editor.

98. Ferdinand Bruckner: The dramatist Ferdinand Bruckner (pen name of Theodor Tagger, 1891–1958).

113. "last resort": The establishment in the photograph is called The Last Resort, *Zur letzten Instanz.*

113. Kohlhaases: A reference to *Michael Kohlhaas,* a novella by Heinrich von Kleist (1810) in which a wronged sixteenth-century horsedealer fanatically takes justice into his own hands.

115. "on the Reeperbahn at twelve-thirty . . .": *Auf der Reeperbahn nachts um halb eins,* the title of a hit song about the honky-tonk and brothel district on Hamburg's waterfront.

116. Bölkien: Arnold Böcklin is the correct name of the Swiss artist (1827–1901).

116. Wartburg: A castle in Thuringia, the site of a legendary poetic contest in the Middle Ages and of student festivals in more recent times. Luther translated the New Testament there.

116. Henny Porten: Henny Porten (1890–1960), popular stage and film actress.

126. Inscription: Art for the People.

128. Panke: The Panke is a brook in Berlin which has given the district of Pankow its name. Here it serves to indicate Tucholsky's aversion to living in his native Berlin.

128. Karl Valentin: Karl Valentin (originally Valentin Ludwig Fey) (1882–1948), popular Munich comedian. From 1911 on he usually appeared together with Lisl Karlstadt (originally Elisabeth Wellano) (1892–1960).

130. Mr. Westermeier: The actor and operetta and cabaret performer Paul Westermeier (b. 1892).

132. Old Daddy Wirth: Joseph Wirth (1879–1956), Center Party politician, Chancellor from 1921 to 1922, later Minister of the Interior. After the assassination of Walther Rathenau he was instrumental in bringing about a law for the protection of the Republic.

133. pretty Rudi: The reference is to Rudolf Breitscheid.

135. "without the beer . . .": *"wiene Weisse ohne Schuss"*—a reference to a Berlin specialty, light beer with (in this case, *without*) a dash of raspberry syrup.

136. Erzberger: Matthias Erzberger (1875–1921), leader of the Center Party, signed the armistice at Compiègne in 1918, served as Finance Minister in 1919–20, and was assassinated in 1921.

136. *demento mori*: An obvious corruption of *memento mori* (remember that you must die).

136. "up *to here*": The German pun is *Jeheer* and *Je hehr* (*Gehör,* "hearing," and *Je höher,* "the higher," in the Berlin dialect).

139. Hilferding: Rudolf Hilferding (1877–1941), Socialist politician, Minister of Finance 1923 and 1928-9.

142. *Borowsky, Heck*: Tucholsky borrowed the names of the men signing the announce-

ment of the *Deutscher Reichs-Behörden-Verleih* from Christian Morgenstern's witty poem "Die Behörde," which is included in his *Galgenlieder (Gallows Songs)*.

147. Fischer, Kern: Hermann Fischer and Erwin Kern were the men who murdered Germany's Jewish Foreign Minister Walther Rathenau in June of 1922. Surrounded in Saaleck Castle, their hiding place, three weeks later, Kern was shot and Fischer killed himself.

149. [Wallhangings]: Translations of the wallhangings in the picture are, top to bottom: "God watches over big and small/ so go to sleep free of care." "Do not bewail the morning/that brings you pain and toil/ it's beautiful to be caring/for people that one loves."

150. Herr Simons: Walter Simons (1861–1937), head of the Federal Court, 1922–29, sometime Foreign Minister and deputy to the Federal President.

150. Mittermaier, Radbruch, Sinzheimer, Kroner: Wolfgang Mittermaier (1867–1956), jurist and professor of criminal law; Gustav Radbruch (1878–1949), Social Democratic politician, Minister of Justice from 1923; Hugo Sinzheimer (1875–1945), jurist, professor of labor law at the University of Frankfurt, 1920–1933; Richard Kroner (b. 1884), neo-Hegelian and religious philosopher, professor at German, British, and American universities.

150. Wolfgang Heine: Wolfgang Heine (1861–1944), member of the Reichstag and Prussian Minister of the Interior.

150. Ernst Fuchs: Ernst Fuchs (1859–1929), jurist at the Karlsruhe Superior Court, author of works on sociological jurisprudence.

151. Villers: Alexander von Villers (1812–1880), diplomat in the service of Saxony (at Frankfurt, Paris, Berlin, Vienna, etc.). *Briefe eines Unbekannten* appeared in 1881.

158. Hauptmann: The playwright Gerhart Hauptmann (1862–1946).

160. Hergt, Ebermayer: Oskar Hergt (1869–1967), leader of the National People's Party, Minister of Justice and Vice-Chancellor, 1927–28; Ludwig Ebermayer (1858–1933), attorney-general.

164. "Mother's Hands": This poem, written in the Berlin dialect, is probably Tucholsky's most popular creation.

165. "the Follies with a shot of folk-lore": *Das Dreimäderlhaus*—Heinrich Berté's romantic operetta based on the life of Franz Schubert (1916).

166. Ludolf Gerold: Gerold was the maiden name of Tucholsky's second wife Mary, and Ludolf was their fanciful name for the child they never had.

169. "And the Hermundure . . . used to be": *"Und der Hermundure flüstert [stottert] beklommen:/'Gott, ist die Gegend runtergekommen'"*—the concluding lines of Theodor Fontane's poem *Veränderungen in der Mark*, about changes noticed around Berlin by men of A.D. 390 who returned from Valhalla in 1890. The Hermunduren or Ermunduren were members of an old Germanic tribe that lived along the Elbe and Saale rivers.

169. "a challenging war cry out of *Götz*": An unmistakable and widely quoted scatological invitation ("Tell him he can . . .") from Goethe's Storm-and-Stress play *Götz von Berlichingen*. The photomontage illustrates a German vulgarism: *"Ein Arsch mit Ohren"* (an ass with ears).

170. *Werewolf*: *Der Werwolf* by the story-teller Herman Löns (1866–1914) appeared in 1910.

171. Schlageter: Albert Leo Schlageter (1894–1923), German officer executed by the French for sabotaging their occupation of the Ruhr. The Nazis glorified him as a martyr, and he was the subject of a play by Hanns Johst (1933).

171. Karl May: Karl May (1842–1912), author of popular novels of adventure set among American Indians, in the Near East, and in other exotic locales, most of which the author had never seen.

175. "Quickly death strikes down man": *"Rasch tritt der Tod den Menschen [an]"*—from Friedrich Schiller's play *Wilhelm Tell*.

175. *The Merry Widow*: the popular operetta, of course, by Franz Lehar (1905).

179. Harry Liedtke: Harry Liedtke (1888–1945), popular German film star.

182. "Silesian poet's school": *Zweite schlesische Dichterschule*—a reference to the bombastic style of late Baroque literature in Germany in the latter part of the seventeenth century (writers like Lohenstein and Hofmannswaldau).

183. Grock, the Clown; Conrad Veidt: The real name of the Swiss musical clown Grock (1880–1959) was Charles Adrian Wettach. Conrad Veidt (1893–1943), was a Berlin-born stage and film actor.

184. Külz: Wilhelm Külz (1875–1948), German Minister of the Interior, 1926–7, author of the controversial *"Schmutz und Schund"* (antipornography) law.

185. "special pornography section": *Schmutzsonderklasse*, the concluding section of a "black list" put out by a federation of women's organizations. Tucholsky explained that the two young women stood on a glass table and were photographed from below.

185. "parson": *Pfaffe*, a word denoting a hidebound, narrow-minded clergyman.

188. Wilhelmstrasse: The seat of the German government in Berlin.

194. Mr. Chiappe: Jean Chiappe, the Paris chief of police.

196. "A call resounds!": *"Es braust ein Ruf wie Donnerhall"*—a quotation from Max Schneckenburger's patriotic poem *Die Wacht am Rhein* (The Watch on the Rhine, 1840).

196. "Wik-end-cigars and wiek-ent-spats": The word "weekend" has long been part of the German language. Tucholsky here plays with some popular misspellings and mis-pronunciations of it.

199. "Guns to the right—guns to the left—Baby Jesus in the middle.": *"Gewehre rechts—Gewehre links—das Christkind in der Mitten."* An allusion to Goethe's autobiographical *"Prophete rechts, Prophete links, das Weltkind in der Mitten."*

201. Frau Ebert: Presumably a reference to the lowly antecedents of Friedrich Ebert and his wife. People did not let Ebert forget that he had once been a journeyman harness-maker.

201. Paul Löbe: Paul Löbe (1875–1967), president of the Reichstag from 1920 to 1924 and 1925 to 1932.

202. "Oh beautiful Forest": *"Wer hat dich, du schöner Wald"*—the beginning of a folk-song based upon Joseph von Eichendorff's poem *Der Jäger Abschied* (The Hunters' Farewell).

202. Hermann Müller: Hermann Müller (1876–1931), Social Democratic politician, Federal Chancellor in 1920 and from 1928 to 1930.

210. "stolen from the High Command": The original title of Remarque's book, *Im Westen nichts Neues*, was a standard phrase in German war communiqués.

210. Professor Cossmann: Paul Nikolaus Cossmann (1869–1941), editor of the *Süddeutsche Monatshefte*.

210. "the little Jew-boy's name": Despite numerous canards and much propagandistic misinformation to the contrary, Remarque was born in Osnabrück, Westphalia, as Erich Paul Remark, the son of a non-Jewish bookbinder.

210. salat schammes: More properly, "*shelatenshammes,*" a Yiddish expression for a factotum or performer of menial tasks.

210. *Criminals*: The play *Die Verbrecher* (1928) is by Ferdinand Bruckner, not by Bertolt Brecht—an indication of these circles' knowledge of, and respect for, facts.

210. Reinhardt: The Jewish theatrical director Max Reinhardt (originally Max Goldmann, 1873–1943).

210. Haarman: The name of a convicted and executed mass murderer.

215. Schweik: "The Good Soldier Schweik", the protagonist of Jaroslav Hašek's satirical novel by that name (1920–3) about an ingenious World World War I "sad sack" who outwits an entire military bureaucracy, is here portrayed by Max Pallenberg.

Afterword

If the old Chinese adage according to which one picture is worth ten thousand words has any validity, this afterword to a powerful book based on pictures may well be deemed superfluous and anticlimactic, especially since Kurt Tucholsky has already supplied thousands of words to go with the pictures. It would be too bad if these additional words as well as the notes that precede them lent respectability to Ernst Pawel's preposterous statement that Tucholsky's work as a whole is "the record of a dead world in a dead language, increasingly difficult to decipher,"[1] a statement that is most effectively refuted by the fact that as of May 1970 a total of four million copies of Tucholsky's books had been sold in numerous editions and in many countries. (This compares with 306,500 copies sold until 1933, when Tucholsky's books were burned in Nazi Germany.) It may be belaboring the obvious to say that to Americans of the late sixties and early seventies the problems of the Weimar Republic have become painfully relevant, to use a much abused word that is currently in vogue. As Carl Schorske has suggested, American interest in Weimar is due to a certain sense of kinship. "Caught in a crisis ourselves, we turn to Weimar, because its tragic experience of dissolution—political, social, and cultural—seems to promote understanding of our own situation."[2] Miss Halley's idiomatic, lively, and frequently ingenious translation of *Deutschland Deutschland über alles* can only aid this process of understanding by making as plain as

American English can what Tucholsky was trying to do. In this book a master satirist graphically catches Germany (and holds her in suspended animation, as it were) at a time of political and economic instability and social disintegration, a few years before the philistinism, indifference, stupidity, perversion, and brutality rampant in public life produced the tragedy of Nazism. Yet this particular book and Tucholsky's purposes and methods in compiling it have often been misinterpreted. The following remarks, then, are intended to set the record straight and present Tucholsky's own feelings about it as well as some of the reactions to it.

Habent sua fata libelli. . . . Books not only have fates of their own but are also capable of influencing the fates of others. In his autobiography and workshop book *From Cover to Cover*, Stefan Salter, who left his native Germany to become one of America's leading book designers, gives *Deutschland, Deutschland über alles* credit for changing his life.

I have seen many picture books in my life, beautiful ones, interesting ones, and even amusing ones. But never before or since, such an impressive one as Deutschland, Deutschland über alles. *This was the book which made it abundantly clear to me, a young man who knew nothing about politics or economics, that there was trouble brewing. Naturally, I did not know exactly what was about to happen, but the author of the book, Kurt Tucholsky, and the illustrator, John Heartfield, knew. . . . What impressed me at once about the book were the photographs, the photomontages, and the way the text ran with the illustrations. Dramatic statements were made not only by the text or illustra-*

1. "A Voice Before the Silence," *Commentary*, December 1968, p. 106.
2. "Weimar and the Intellectuals," *New York Review of Books*, May 7, 1970.

tions but by the way they were laid out. It was a great textbook of our time, teaching important lessons which few people were willing to learn. It was like the handwriting on the wall, and it sent me away forever and in ample time.[3]

Salter's is an uncommonly honest and refreshingly positive voice in the chorus of critical condemnation which greeted this controversial book upon its publication and which has started up again in recent years. Tucholsky has been cast in the role of a journalistic *enfant terrible* and a political simpleton, a man who committed numerous transgressions against tact and taste and with his satirical sniping stunted the fragile growth of the Weimar Republic. *"Deutschland, Deutschland über alles,* a vicious attack on German militarism," writes Pawel, "was so far ahead of its time in avant-garde vulgarity that even many of [Tucholsky's] friends felt constrained to disavow the book, if not its author."[4] Josef Nadler, the nationalistic Austrian literary historian, said that "no people on earth has ever been so vilified in its own language as the German people has been vilified by Tucholsky." Writing in 1939, Thomas Mann's children, Erika and Klaus, thought that the picture book lacked taste (a frequent and partly justified criticism) and that it was part of Tucholsky's "unremitting, truculent, and contemptuous warfare with the nature of the German people."[5] (It should be noted that when they wrote this, Erika and Klaus Mann were filled with a youthful and vibrant belief in the existence of "the other Germany." Tuchol-

sky, on the other hand, by his own admission had since 1913 "been among those who think that the German spirit is poisoned almost beyond recovery, who do not believe in any improvement, who regard German democracy as a façade and a lie.") A contemporary German critic, Paul Sethe, says that while the leaders of the Weimar democracy "exhausted their energies in hard combat with Hugenberg and Hitler, Tucholsky stood aside and jeered at them. They could have used help. All they got was scorn and laughter."[6] Even a sympathetic critic like Gordon Craig, who refers to Tucholsky as "this greatest of German satirists since Heine, this master of prose style, this nonpareil of comic invention, this indefatigable fighter against the forces that were eroding the basis of the German republic" feels that whenever Tucholsky turned to politics, his work was "flawed by a lack of moderation, a failure of perspective, and a violence of tone that weakened its effect and served the cause of people he detested."[7] "No one with any historical sense who rereads *Deutschland, Deutschland über alles,*" writes Craig, "can escape the feeling that this atrabilious collection of essays did more to weaken the cause of democracy in Germany than to help it. . . . Tucholsky's great weakness was that he was indiscriminate in his selection of targets and immoderate in his expenditure of ammunition."[8] Even though Craig speaks of Tucholsky's "staggering naiveté," "incomprehension of the realities," and

3. Englewood Cliffs: Prentice-Hall, 1969, pp. 25–6.
4. Op. cit., p. 104.
5. *Escape to Life* (Boston: Houghton Mifflin, 1939), p. 179.
6. "Tucholskys tragische Irrtümer," *Die Zeit,* April 10, 1964, p. 7. Alfred Hugenberg (1865–1951) was a nationalistic politician and industrialist.
7. "Engagement and Neutrality in Weimar Germany," *Journal of Contemporary History,* April 1967, p. 57.
8. Ibid., p. 59.

"rather cheap delight in exposing . . .
personal and intellectual inadequacies,"[9]
he does realize that Tucholsky was too
much of an artist to be capable of seeing
life in anything but absolute terms.

Some years ago only those on the political
right spoke of the corrosiveness or destruc-
tiveness of Tucholsky and men like him,
using phrases like "fouling their own nest."
Now it is the leftists who counsel moderation and tact in an effort to avoid the personal tragedy of Tucholsky and the fate of his
country. One of these critics, Walter
Laqueur, who regards this picture book as
"a caricature of Weimar Germany, some of
it quite true, much of it distorted—all in
questionable taste,"[10] sees a "Tucholsky
Syndrome" spreading in some American
circles: "A radical force has come into being
even more emphatic in its rejection of
America, its way of life and the aspirations of
most of its citizens than the opposition of the
writers of the *Weltbühne*[11] to the Weimar
Republic. . . . There are countless publications which take up with a vengeance the
theme of *Deutschland, Deutschland über alles,*
opposing not just American policy at home
and abroad but deriding patriotism, the
national symbols, traditional values, valuable
traditions."[12] Laqueur expresses concern
over the fact that many leaders and followers
in this group are, like Tucholsky, Jews.

Tucholsky and men like him "had no real
roots themselves and, therefore, they lacked
the sensorium for the patriotic feeling of
their fellow citizens."[13] Apart from this
regrettable talk about rootlessness, which
one has come to associate with Jew-
baiting writers, Laqueur apparently believes
that any radical criticism is bound to lead to
reactionary repression and that radical
criticism by a Jew necessarily gives rise to
anti-Semitism. Missing Tucholsky's point
completely, Laqueur asks this question
about the photomontage entitled "Animals
Looking at You": "Did Tucholsky mean to
imply that the German army and police
needed better-looking officers? If so, they
certainly got them a few years later; Hey-
drich, for instance, was a man of striking
appearance."[14] Laqueur points out that
Tucholsky's time was one of unprecedented
political freedom in Germany. "Tucholsky
and his friends thought that the German
judge of their day was the most evil person
imaginable and that the German prisons
were the most inhumane; later they got
Freisler[15] and Auschwitz. They imagined
that Stresemann and the Social Democrats
were the most reactionary politicians in the
world; soon after they had to face Hitler,
Goebbels, and Goering. They sincerely believed that Fascism was already ruling Germany, until the horrors of the Third Reich
overtook them."[16]

Laqueur has raised the issue of Tucholsky's
Jewishness. (Like Heinrich Heine, Tucholsky

9. Ibid.
10. "The Tucholsky Complaint," *Encounter*, October
1969, p. 78.
11. The left-wing weekly in which most of Tucholsky's
writings first appeared. Cf. Istvan Deak, *Weimar
Germany's Left-Wing Intellectuals: A Political History of
the* Weltbühne *and Its Circle* (Berkeley: University of
California Press, 1968).
12. Op. cit., pp. 79–80.

13. Ibid., p. 79.
14. Ibid., p. 78.
15. Roland Freisler, the Nazi head of the "People's
Court" who sat in judgment on the conspirators of
July 20, 1944.
16. Op. cit., p. 78.

239

converted to Protestantism in his youth.) A further target of criticism has been Herr Wendriner, one of Tucholsky's most felicitous and most memorable characterizations, who is represented in the present book with a relatively innocuous monologue, one of fifteen written by Tucholsky. Wendriner is the personification of a Berlin businessman of Jewish origin, a lightweight in mind and morality, a spiritually empty, assimilated Jew whom Tucholsky exposed in all his unctuous, propitiatory servility. Ernst Pawel feels that the Wendriner monologues were "brilliantly apt and perceptive in their time, but not in ours. Both Herr Wendriner and his author have paid too dearly for their very human failings."[17] The German-born Israeli scholar Gershom Scholem has said about Tucholsky that "it remained for one of the most gifted, most convinced, and most offensive Jewish anti-Semites to achieve on a high level what the anti-Semites themselves were unable to do."[18] A corrective to such curiously emotional statements is supplied by Kurt Grossmann, who, in an article on German Jews on the political left, points out that "the Wendriner type existed and despite the Jewish tragedy is still among us."[19]

During his lifetime Tucholsky attempted to come to terms with some of the criticism levelled at his satire in general and his picture book in particular. Writing about the latter in the *Börsencourier*, Herbert Ihering deplored the blunting of intellectual weapons and the decline of polemics and satire in his time and said it was a polemic without risk if Tucholsky kept lashing out at the same old subjects. A gifted person like Tucholsky, he wrote, ought to be in Germany, in the thick of the battle, and not view things from the comfortable but distorting distance of Paris or Sweden. (Having left Germany in 1924, Tucholsky had chosen Sweden as his permanent domicile by the time his picture book appeared.) Replying to Ihering in October of 1929, Tucholsky admitted that his book was a bit of an anachronism, a final balance-sheet, as it were, and said that it was hard to find photographic documentation for emotions or psychic states. "Perhaps it is boring to take Salvarsan year after year," he wrote. "Camomile tea might offer greater variety, yet one has to take the real cure. The spirochetes, too, always remain the same. . . . I'd rather be reproached with being artistically unsatisfactory or of having missed the mark out of indignation than be indolent." Elsewhere Tucholsky wrote: "I am slowly becoming a megalomaniac as I read how I have ruined Germany. But for twenty years I have been bothered by one thing: that I have not succeeded in getting a single policeman dismissed from his post." And a letter to Franz Hammer dated May 5, 1931, contains these revealing remarks: "What sometimes worries me so is the effectiveness of my work. Does it have any? (I don't mean success; that leaves me cold.) But it sometimes seems to me so terribly ineffective. I write and work—and what practical effect does it have on the way the country is run? Do I get a single one of those foul, perverted, tormented and tormenting female wardens

17. Op. cit., p. 106.
18. "Juden und Deutsche," *Judaica II* (Frankfurt: Suhrkamp, 1970), p. 37.
19. *Gegenwart im Rückblick*, ed. by H. A. Strauss and K. R. Grossmann (Heidelberg: Stiehm, 1970), p. 97.

fired? Do the sadists leave? Are the bureau-crats dismissed? . . . This is what depresses me at times."

Those who take umbrage at Tucholsky's satiric method and expect of a practitioner of "total satire" tact, taste, and unerring political right-mindedness might do well to consider Tucholsky's own conception of political satire as enunciated as early as 1919:

Because the fight against the living is rocked by passions, because one's eyesight is dimmed at close quarters, and because for the fighter it is not a matter of detachment but of fight-ing: that is why the satirist is unjust. He cannot ponder—he must pound. And he generalizes and writes questions on the wall and blames a whole group for the sins of individuals because they are characteristic, and he exaggerates and minimizes. . . . And, if he has the stuff, he does in the final analysis hit the nail on the head. . . . If the author rushed into his time with open arms, he did not see the things as historians will see them in a hundred years, nor did he want to. He was so close to things that they cut him and he was able to hit them. And they tore his hands open, and he bled. . . .

In a piece also written in 1919 and entitled "What May Satire Do?" (the answer to that question is "Everything"), Tucholsky wrote: "Satire must exaggerate, and it is in its innermost nature to be unjust. It inflates truth to make it more distinct, and it cannot help but operate in accordance with the biblical saying that the just suffer along with the unjust. . . ." It would be easy to compile a catalogue of institutions and individuals to whom Tucholsky may be said to have been "unjust" in this picture book. One of them

was the long-lived Löbe, a man whom an outstanding historian of the Weimar Re-public, Erich Eyck, has described as "one of the best presidents the German Reichstag ever had: objective and just, calm, self-assured and polite."[20] (Yet this same Paul Löbe in 1926-7 declined Tucholsky's request that two visitor's passes to the sessions of the Reichstag be made available to the Welt-bühne.) By indirection, Tucholsky was unjust also to the Breslau Germanist August Hein-rich Hoffmann, known in literary history as Hoffmann von Fallersleben, whose "foolish line from a big-mouth poem . . . a really bad poem which a really demented Republic chose for its national anthem" supplied the mordant title of this picture book. When the patriotic professor wrote his poem "Lied der Deutschen" (Song of the Germans) in 1841 while living in exile on the island of Heligoland, at that time a possession of the British crown, he did not intend to produce a paean of praise to aggressive expansionism or to advocate the creation of a saber-rattling, nationalistic empire. Rather, he was appalled at the reactionary police-state methods and the demagogy of princelings in the petty principalities of a fragmented Germany and naively dreamed of the exten-sion of German culture beyond its political boundaries. Hoping for the metamorphosis of servile subjects into citizens, he urged his fellow countrymen to place the idea of a Germany united in brotherhood above factional strife. It was hardly his fault that the key line of his poem was given the kind of interpretation that led Nietzsche to remark,

20. A History of the Weimar Republic (Cambridge: Harvard University Press, 1963), vol. 2, p. 291.

in his *Twilight of the Idols*: "Deutschland, Deutschland über alles—I fear that was the end of German philosophy."

Deutschland, Deutschland über alles may not be Tucholsky's best book, but it certainly is his most aggressive and possibly his most characteristic one. Fifty thousand copies of it were sold within a year of its publication in 1929 by the Neuer Deutscher Verlag, a publishing house owned by the Communist Willi Münzenberg. (The facsimile editions issued in 1964 by the satirist's longtime publisher Rowohlt and in 1967 by the East German publisher Volk und Welt have not diminished the value of first-edition copies as cherished collector's items.) The book follows the familiar pattern of the numerous Tucholsky anthologies that appeared in his lifetime and after World War II, containing satiric vignettes, political essays, muck-raking editorials, literary satires, poems, and cabaret-type chansons. The main targets of Tucholsky's satire are there: abstract concepts like patriotism and nationalism as well as concrete facts like war or a state organized along national lines; classes or castes like officers and judges; organized religion; injustices of the great moloch State which cows the individual and impairs the quality of his life; deep-rooted flaws in the German national character; entrenched privilege; hero worship; intellectual fads and prejudices of all kinds; the German brand of Babbitry; and human stupidity, cupidity, and indifference in their myriad guises. The uniqueness of the book lies in the pictorial material and its interaction with the text.

The work had a long gestation period. As early as 1912 Tucholsky had called, in a brief article entitled *"Mehr Fotografien!,"* for more muck-raking photos "with contrasts and juxtapositions" and little text. "It must be shown systematically: this is how you are being whipped, this is how you are being educated, this is how you are being treated, this is how you are being punished." In an article published in 1925, *"Die Tendenzphotographie,"* Tucholsky called for a fighting periodical that would be illustrated along these lines. Tendentious photos and pictorial juxtaposition would be "irrefutable" and "unbeatable," and their effectiveness could not be surpassed by any editorial in the world. "Ludendorff in civilian clothes; a banker's automobile and the apartment of his doorman; the faces of Prussian judges and those of their victims; students at a drinking party . . . subjects that cannot be treated in words as strikingly as unretouched, truthful, and unobjectionable photographs can do it, photos that are made tendentious only by their arrangement and their captions . . . an immensely dangerous weapon." In Berlin-born John Heartfield, whom Bertolt Brecht once called "one of Europe's outstanding artists," Tucholsky found the perfect collaborator. The communist artist's real name was Helmut Herzfeld; he "translated" his name into English as a symbolic protest against *"Gott strafe England,"* "Perfidious Albion," and other evidences and excrescences of chauvinistic hatred during the First World War. In the 1920's Heartfield created book jackets, many of them involving photomontages, for the Malik Verlag, the Berlin left-wing publishing house headed by his brother Wieland Herzfelde. "If I weren't Peter Panter," wrote Tucholsky in 1932, "I'd like to be a dust jacket in the Malik Verlag.

This John Heartfield really is a little wonder of the world."[21] Raoul Hausmann, one of the outstanding representatives of Dadaism, has explained that "photomontage was an explosion of views from different angles and mixed-up levels, far more extreme in its complexity than futuristic painting. . . . We called this process 'photomontage' because it underlined our aversion to playing the artist. We regarded ourselves as engineers and pretended to assemble our 'work' like fitters." For this reason Heartfield was known in the movement as the "Monteur-dada."

"We have no intention of turning our book into a picture album suitable for someone's birthday," Tucholsky wrote. "We want . . . to extract the typical from snapshots, posed photographs, all kinds of pictures. And all the pictures together will add up to Germany—a cross-section of Germany." Official cross-sections, he pointed out, always cut the cheese without the maggots feeling hit; "we wanted to do it differently. Whatever you see moving as you cut is a maggot. And part of Germany." As Tucholsky wrote to his estranged wife Mary on August 30, 1930, all the photos used had originally been intended for publication by various correspondents and editors, and none of them violated the private life of anyone depicted. Among the readers and critics who have disagreed is Walter Laqueur, who recently wrote: "Some of the pictures . . . are embarrassing or, in a perspective of forty years, simply inexplic-

able."[22] While most of the original readers of this book must have been able to identify many of those depicted, this is not true of readers of 1964 or 1972. But even if all the pictorial subjects could still be identified, this would not necessarily enhance the subtle typology, so effective in the aggregate, that Tucholsky and Heartfield wished to create or clarify what Marcel Belvianes has described as a "sociology of the photograph." Does it, for example, add greatly to one's appreciation and understanding of Tucholsky's satire on show business to know that the man depicted in the upper-right-hand corner of the picture on page 165 is the theater critic Alfred Kerr and that his face is chopped up by the section numbers into which he customarily divided his critiques? An explanatory note for pages 186 and 187 seems more indicated, for by juxtaposing that particular text and that particular picture Tucholsky meant to indicate that he regarded Gustav Stresemann as a mediocre, vastly overrated politician. About the montage on page 55, probably the most famous or notorious in the book, Tucholsky wrote to the writer Jakob Wassermann on March 1, 1931, that it had been inserted by John Heartfield at the last minute and that he was not too happy with it, for "insulting animals is not to my taste." In their totality, the pictures constitute the photographic equivalent of the graphic art of George Grosz and Käthe Kollwitz. (Tucholsky's prose vignette *"Gesicht."*[23] written in 1924, is dedicated "to George Grosz, who taught us

21. It is interesting to note that both Tucholsky (1890–1935) and Heartfield (1891–1968) appear on postage stamps issued in recent years by the German Democratic Republic.

22. Op. cit., p. 78.
23. Included as "Face of a German" in *What If—?* *Satirical Writings of Kurt Tucholsky*, ed. by H. Zohn and K. F. Ross (New York: Funk & Wagnalls, 1968).

to see such faces.") The various things to be seen on the cover of the original edition—the color scheme black, red, and gold with a black, white, and red jack, a helmet and a top hat, a rubber truncheon and an officer's saber, the line "Brothers sticking together" from Hoffmann von Fallersleben's poem, etc.—are trenchant prototypes symbolizing the transition from the Hohenzollern monarchy to Fascism via the weak-kneed democracy of the Weimar Republic, and they express Tucholsky's view that this Republic was but a continuation of the imperial social order in republican guise. Harold Poor puts this in somewhat extreme terms when he writes: "For all of its shock effect, the dominant quality of the book seemed to be a lack of timeliness. Ostensibly the critique was of Weimar culture, yet the book appeared to be far more a catalogue of Tucholsky's dislikes of the old imperial regime."[24]

As for the text, with the exception of those pieces and captions that were inspired by the pictorial material, most of the selections had appeared earlier in the *Weltbühne* and other periodicals and newspapers to which Tucholsky was a contributor. The piece on Rudolf Herzog, for example, had first appeared in 1924, the year in which Herr Wendriner went shopping and Tucholsky went to see Karl Valentin, and the long essay on German judges first appeared in the *Weltbühne* in 1927 as a series of three articles. Lacking any consistent ideological thrust, the nondoctrinaire Tucholsky liberally and unsystematically mixed the tragic with the trivial to produce a great slice of life

which constitutes a strange mixture of involvement and alienation, of a reformer's zeal and complete withdrawal. Tucholsky concisely expressed his dissatisfaction with his book in a letter to his friend and sometime collaborator Walter Hasenclever, dated July 25, 1933: "As an artistic accomplishment the book is crude [*klobig*]. And weak. And much too mild."

This book, which came out just a few years before Tucholsky's final period of silence, represents one of the last, pathetic attempts by the sophisticated satirist to be the mouthpiece of the little people, to lash out at the killers of the dream, the republicans who had betrayed the revolution, to point to the bankruptcy of those institutions of the Weimar Republic that were not worthy of support, to show that the nationalists and the militarists, the politicians, the academicians, and the judges "don't have an exclusive lease on this land and its language." Harboring a *Hassliebe* for his native land in the manner of Heinrich Heine, he said that "because we love Germany, we have the right to hate it." For three more years Tucholsky frantically "poked about the roots of the German oak tree," as he once put it. In October of 1934, about a year before the man who despaired of a society without democratic traditions sought "the truest of all democracies, the democracy of death" by poisoning himself in Sweden a few weeks before his forty-sixth birthday, he wrote to Hasenclever: "What is taking place there [in Germany] partly reflects the deepest instincts of the German people." *Deutschland, Deutschland über alles* is a document of despair. We read it and view it today with the grim wisdom of hindsight and the

24. *Kurt Tucholsky and the Ordeal of Germany, 1914–1935* (New York: Scribner's, 1968).

chill realization that it contains most of the
ingredients of the witch's brew of Nazism.
Beyond what this book has to teach us about
Germany and the Germans, it presents a
poignant picture of Kurt Tucholsky, one of
the great exemplary figures of his time
and of ours. One is reminded of the words of
Walt Whitman: "This is no book; who
touches this touches a man."

Brandeis University   Harry Zohn
August 1971

**A note on the design and production
of this edition**

The original edition of *Deutschland,
Deutschland über alles* was issued by Neuer
Deutscher Verlag in 1929. In 1964 a facsimile edition was published by Rowohlt
Verlag. The University of Massachusetts
Press edition has been designed to convey
as much as possible the spirit of the original
layout. Because many of the original photographs no longer exist, the illustrations for
this edition have been made from the repro-
ductions as they appeared in the 1929 and
1964 editions. They are necessarily reproduced in the same size as in the first edition.
The type style and size, although different
from the original, were chosen in an attempt
to be true to the feeling of the original
design and the era. Variation in type style
and type size and placement of text and
photographs have also followed the first
edition wherever possible.

   The assistance of Mrs. A. Becker-Berke of
Rowohlt Verlag and Nicholas Burridge and
Martin Pegler of Oliver Burridge Filmsetting
Ltd. is gratefully acknowledged. — RH